BMA

Practical Manual of Minimally Invasive Gynecologic and Robotic Surgery

A Clinical Cook Book

Third Edition

Practical Manual of Minimally Invasive Gynecologic and Robotic Surgery

A Clinical Cook Book

Third Edition

Edited by

Resad Paya Pasic MD, PhD

Professor of Obstetrics and Gynecology
Director of the Fellowship in Minimally Invasive Gynecologic Surgery
University of Louisville, Kentucky

Andrew I. Brill MD

Director of Minimally Invasive Gynecology
California Pacific Medical Center, San Francisco, California

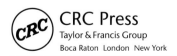

CRC Press
Taylor & Francis Group
Boca Raton London New York

CRC Press is an imprint of the
Taylor & Francis Group, an **informa** business

CRC Press
Taylor & Francis Group
6000 Broken Sound Parkway NW, Suite 300
Boca Raton, FL 33487-2742

© 2018 by Taylor & Francis Group, LLC
CRC Press is an imprint of Taylor & Francis Group, an Informa business

No claim to original U.S. Government works

Printed and bound in India by Replika Press Pvt. Ltd.

Printed on acid-free paper

International Standard Book Number-13: 978-1-4822-1632-5 (Pack- Hardback and eBook)

Library of Congress Cataloging-in-Publication Data

Names: Pasic, Resad, editor. | Brill, Andrew I., editor.
Title: Practical manual of minimally invasive gynecologic and robotic surgery : a clinical cook book / edited by Resad Paya Pasic and Andrew I. Brill.
Other titles: Preceded by (work): Practical manual of laparoscopy and minimally invasive gynecology.
Description: Third edition. | Boca Raton, FL : CRC Press, Taylor & Francis Group, [2018] | Preceded by A practical manual of laparoscopy and minimally invasive gynecology / [edited by] Resad P. Pasic, Ronald L. Levine. 2nd ed. c2007. |
Includes bibliographical references and index.
Identifiers: LCCN 2017028014| ISBN 9781482216325 (pack (hardback and ebook) : alk. paper) | ISBN 9781482216332 (ebook) |
ISBN 9781498715874 (ebook)
Subjects: | MESH: Gynecologic Surgical Procedures--methods | Minimally Invasive Surgical Procedures--methods |
Robotic Surgical Procedures--methods
Classification: LCC RG104 | NLM WP 660 | DDC 618.1/059--dc23 LC record available at https://lccn.loc.gov/2017028014

Visit the Taylor & Francis Web site at
http://www.taylorandfrancis.com

and the CRC Press Web site at
http://www.crcpress.com

CONTENTS

PREFACE

In keeping with the philosophical underpinnings and design of the original book, this third edition has been extensively updated to provide the gynecologic surgeon with a state-of-the-art and practical resource that can be used to review or learn about commonly performed surgical procedures in minimally invasive gynecology. To meet the needs of both novice and experienced surgeons, the text is engineered to cover the clinical decision-making, key instrumentation and technical cascade for each surgical procedure. Wherever possible, discussion is focused on methods to optimize outcome and reduce risk. The content in this latest edition has been substantially bolstered by the addition of chapters covering vaginal hysterectomy, tissue retrieval in laparoscopic surgery, single port laparoscopy, robotic hysterectomy, robotic myomectomy, robotic sacralcolpopexy, radical robotic hysterectomy, and hemostatic agents for laparoscopic surgery.

We are very honored that contributors in this edition continue to be established surgeons from the United States and abroad. We are deeply grateful for the generous guidance from our mentors and for the courageous pioneers throughout the world whose collective endeavors served to legitimize minimally invasive gynecologic surgery. We have no doubt that with the advent of robotic surgery and the growing numbers of gynecologic surgeons now trained in minimally invasive operative techniques, surgical paradigms will continue to evolve as innovation and truly disruptive technology continue to emerge.

We would like to thank the many members of industry whose support has made our work possible: Cooper Surgical, Ethicon Endosurgery, Halt Medical, Karl Storz, and Medtronic.

We are also indebted to the talents of our illustrator and graphic designer, Branko Modrakovic, for his creativity and guidance.

Most importantly, we dedicate this latest edition to the tireless permission and support from our wives.

Resad Paya Pasic
Andrew I. Brill

CONTRIBUTORS

JASON ABBOTT
Department of Gynaecological Surgery
School of Women's and Children's Health University
    of New South Wales
Randwick, Australia

BARUCH S. ABITTAN
Hofstra-Northwell School of Medicine
Hempstead, New York

MAURICIO SIMÕES ABRÃO
Obstetrics and Gynecology Department
Hospital das Clínicas
São Paulo University
São Paulo, Brazil

LEILA V. ADAMYAN
Federal Research Center for Obstetrics, Gynecology,
    and Perinatology
Moscow, Russia

ALI AKDEMIR
Department of Obstetrics and Gynecology
Ege University School of Medicine
İzmir, Turkey

JEFF W. ALLEN
Norton Surgical Specialists
Director Bariatric Program
Health and Weight Management
Louisville, Kentucky

MASAAKI ANDOU
Kurashiki Medical Center
Okayama-ken, Japan

ALI AZADI
Female Pelvic Medicine and Reconstructive Surgery
Norton Urogynecology
St. Matthews, Kentucky

ELIZABETH BABIN
Department of Obstetrics and Gynecology
Division of Female Pelvic Medicine and
    Reconstructive Surgery
Athena Women's Institute for Pelvic Health
Blackwood, New Jersey

SHAN BISCETTE
Department of Obstetrics, Gynecology & Women's
    Health
University of Louisville School of Medicine
Louisville, Kentucky

ANDREW I. BRILL
Department of Obstetrics and Gynecology
Center for Advanced Surgical Options in Gynecology
California Pacific Medical Center
San Francisco, California

MELCHOR CARBONELL-SOCIAS
Department of Obstetrics and Gynecology
Hospital Materno-Infantil Vall d'Hebron
Barcelona, Spain

LAURA CLARK
Department of Anesthesiology and Perioperative
    Medicine
University of Louisville School of Medicine
Louisville, Kentucky

MARK DASSEL
Department of Obstetrics and Gynecology
Cleveland Clinic
Cleveland, Ohio

NICOLE M. DONNELLAN
Department of Obstetrics, Gynecology and
    Reproductive Sciences
University of Pittsburgh Medical Center
Pittsburgh, Philadelphia

ADAM R. DUKE
Department of Obstetrics and Gynecology
University of Tennessee College of Medicine
Chattanooga, Tennessee

ERICA C. DUN
Department of Obstetrics, Gynecology, and
    Reproductive Sciences
Yale School of Medicine
New Haven, Connecticut

KEIKO EBISAWA
Kurashiki Medical Center
Okayama-ken, Japan

LUIZ FLÁVIO CORDEIRO FERNANDES
Obstetrics and Gynecology Department
Hospital das Clínicas
São Paulo University
São Paulo, Brazil

SEAN L. FRANCIS
Department of Obstetrics, Gynecology & Women's Health
University of Louisville School of Medicine
Louisville, Kentucky

DOBIE GILES
Departments of Obstetrics and Gynecology and Urology
University of Wisconsin
Madison, Wisconsin

ANTONIO GIL-MORENO
Department of Obstetrics and Gynecology
Hospital Materno-Infantil Vall d'Hebron
Barcelona, Spain

TOMONORI HADA
Kurashiki Medical Center
Okayama-ken, Japan

PATTAYA HENGRASMEE
Gynecological Endosurgery Unit
Department of Obstetrics and Gynecology
Bangkok, Thailand

S. PAIGE HERTWECK
Departments of Obstetrics, Gynecology & Women's
    Health and Pediatrics
University of Louisville School of Medicine
Norton Children's Gynecology
Louisville, Kentucky

SAM H. HESSAMI
Mount Sinai School of Medicine
Urogynecology and Reconstructive Pelvic Surgery
New York City, New York

BRIGID HOLLORAN-SCHWARTZ
Department of Obstetrics, Gynecology & Women's
    Health
Saint Louis University
St. Louis, Missouri

JOSEPH L. HUDGENS
Department of Obstetrics and Gynecology
Eastern Virginia Medical School
Norfolk, Virginia

TRACI ITO
Department of Obstetrics, Gynecology & Women's
    Health
University of Louisville School of Medicine
Louisville, Kentucky

GRACE M. JANIK
Medical College of Wisconsin
Obstetrics and Gynecology Residency
Milwaukee, Wisconsin

SUSAN KHALIL
Department of Obstetrics and Gynecology
Jamaica Hospital Medical Center
Jamaica, New York

ROSANNE KHO
OB/Gyn and Women's Health Institute
Cleveland, Ohio

ALAN LAM
Centre for Advanced Endoscopic Surgery
Royal North Shore Hospital
St. Leonards, Australia

THOMAS G. LANG
Charles E. Schmidt School of Medicine
Florida Atlantic University
Boca Raton, Florida

and

Minimally Invasive Gyn Surgery
Bethesda Hospitalist East
Boynton Beach, Florida

TED LEE
Department of Obstetrics, Gynecology and
    Reproductive Sciences
University of Pittsburgh Medical Center
Pittsburgh, Philadelphia

DAVID J. LEVINE
Minimally Invasive Gynecologic Surgery
Mercy Hospital St. Louis
St. Louis, Missouri

RONALD L. LEVINE
Department of Obstetrics, Gynecology & Women's
    Health
University of Louisville School of Medicine
Louisville, Kentucky

C.Y. LIU
Department of OB/GYN
University of Tennessee College of Medicine
Chattanooga, Tennessee

JAVIER F. MAGRINA
Department of Gynecology
Mayo Clinic Arizona
Scottsdale, Arizona

PAUL MAGTIBAY III
Department of Gynecology
Mayo Clinic Arizona
Scottsdale, Arizona

PAUL M. MAGTIBAY
Department of Gynecology
Mayo Clinic Arizona
Scottsdale, Arizona

TIMOTHY B. MCKINNEY
Department of Obstetrics and Gynecology
Athena Women's Institute for Pelvic Health
Blackwood, New Jersey

SUKRANT MEHTA
Department of Obstetrics and Gynecology
Kaiser Permanente Woodland Hills
Woodland Hills, California

CHARLES E. MILLER
The Advanced Gynecologic Surgery Institute
Naperville, Illinois

SUKHPREET SINGH MULTANI
Department of Ob/Gyn
St. Vincent's Medical Center
Indianapolis, Indiana

LIDIA HYUN JOO MYUNG
Endometriosis Division
Obstetrics and Gynecology Department
Hospital das Clínicas
São Paulo University
São Paulo, Brazil

CEANA H. NEZHAT
Nezhat Medical Center
Emory University
President Society of Reproductive Surgeons
Atlanta, Georgia

FARR NEZHAT
Nezhat Surgery for Gynecology/Oncology, PLLC
Weill Cornell Medical College of Cornell University
Stony Brook University School of Medicine
Mineola, New York

YOSHIAKI OTA
Kurashiki Medical Center
Okayama-ken, Japan

RESAD PAYA PASIC
Department of Obstetrics, Gynecology & Women's
    Health
University of Louisville School of Medicine
Louisville, Kentucky

HARRY REICH (RETIRED)
Dallas, Philadelphia

J. STEPHEN RICH
Department of Obstetrics and Gynecology
The University of Tennessee College of Medicine
Chattanooga, Tennessee

ROBERT ROGERS
Surgical Gynecologist, The Health Center
Kalispell, Montana

KIRSTEN SASAKI
The Advanced Gynecologic Surgery Institute
Naperville, Illinois

TAMER SECKIN
Department of Obstetrics and Gynecology
Endometriosis Foundation of America
New York City, New York

FATIH ŞENDAĞ
Department of Obstetrics and Gynecology
Ege University School of Medicine
Lenox Hill
Hostra University
İzmir, Turkey

LINDA SHIBER
Division Minimally Invasive Gynecologic
    Surgery
Metrohealth Medical Center
Cleveland, Ohio

DAVID SHIN
Department of Urology
Rutgers University
New Brunswick, New Jersey

JONATHON SOLNIK
Head of Gynaecology
University of Toronto
Toronto, Ontario, Canada

ASSIA A. STEPANIAN
Academia of Women's Health and Endoscopic
    Surgery
Atlanta, Georgia

J. RYAN STEWART
Department of Obstetrics, Gynecology & Women's
    Health
University of Louisville School of Medicine
Louisville, Kentucky

BENJAMIN D. TANNER
Norton Surgical Specialists
Health and Weight Management
Louisville, Kentucky

CLAIRE TEMPLEMAN
Department of Obstetrics and Gynecology
KECK School of Medicine
Los Angeles, California

JOHAN VAN DER WAT
Vaginal Hysterectomy Special Interest Group
    AAGL (American Association of Gynecologic
    Laparoscopists)
and
University Witwatersrand
Netcare Parklane Hospital
Johannesburg, South Africa

KATERINE L. YAROTSKAYA
Federal Research Center for Obstetrics, Gynecology,
    and Perinatology
Moscow, Russia

PATRICK YEUNG Jr.
Department of Obstetrics, Gynecology & Women's
    Health
Saint Louis University
St. Louis, Missouri

JOHNNY YI
Department of Medical and Surgical Gynecology
Mayo Clinic Arizona
Phoenix, Arizona

CHAPTER 1

PATIENT PREPARATION

Shan Biscette and Andrew I. Brill

Although laparoscopic surgery is by its very nature minimally invasive, it must always be considered to be major surgery. Therefore, it is important to carefully prepare the patient for surgery both psychologically as well as physically. The surgeon must also possess adequate training and experience in the operative techniques that are necessary to complete the proposed surgical procedure in a safe and efficient manner. The decision to perform any surgical procedure in a minimally invasive fashion must be consistent with the best interests of the patient. When indicated by either the patient's condition or surgeon experience, the decision to perform a laparotomic alternative can also serve the patient. *Primum non nocere!*

PATIENT EVALUATION FOR MINIMALLY INVASIVE SURGERY

Initial patient evaluation should consider the indications and contraindications for laparoscopic surgery. Given the variations of surgeon experience as well as surgical pathology, there are no hard and fast rules; even the term *absolute contraindication* must be considered as a guideline, rather than an admonition.

TRADITIONALLY ESTABLISHED ABSOLUTE CONTRAINDICATIONS

There are few absolute contraindications for laparoscopic surgery. With the availability of advanced anesthesia techniques, even some of these may be considered relative.

- Patients with severe cardiac disease (class IV) may not tolerate the deep Trendelenburg positions necessary for operative laparoscopy or the variable amounts of pneumoperitoneum that are frequently required for satisfactory vision and instrument movement (see Chapter 4).
- A hemodynamically unstable patient with the need for control of active bleeding is best approached by laparotomy. However, many surgeons believe that they can rapidly enter an abdomen safely by laparoscopy, such as in the midst of a ruptured ectopic pregnancy.
- Intestinal obstruction with distended bowel is best approached by laparotomy. However, by adopting open laparoscopy techniques for peritoneal entry, it may be possible to employ laparoscopy in this circumstance.

TRADITIONALLY ESTABLISHED RELATIVE CONTRAINDICATIONS

- Multiple previous abdominal surgeries must be considered a possible contraindication, depending on both the chosen technique for peritoneal access and the experience of the operating surgeon. However, utilization of left upper quadrant insufflation techniques or open laparoscopy may afford safe entry even in the event of multiple previous surgeries (see Chapter 5).
- Morbid obesity may be daunting for the inexperienced laparoscopist. However, with the use of operative techniques described in Chapter 5, patients with body mass index (BMI) as high as 60+ *often* may in fact be candidates for laparoscopy.
- Pregnancy beyond 5 months' gestation must be approached with a great deal of caution as the pelvis is almost completely filled with the gravid uterus. Whereas some surgeons have advocated gasless laparoscopy techniques for more advanced pregnancies, some studies have demonstrated that pneumoperitoneal CO_2 gas and hypercarbia do not adversely affect the fetus.
- Severe, chronically ill patients may present problems for general endotracheal anesthesia. Nevertheless, given the judgment of the anesthesiologist, it may be possible to cautiously move forward with a laparoscopic surgery.
- If malignancy is a possibility, the outcome should not be compromised by the use of laparoscopic surgery. If a mass is known to be malignant and the surgeon does not have the necessary skills to laparoscopically remove it without rupture or dissemination, then laparotomy should be the method of choice.

INFORMED CONSENT

Appropriately conducted informed consent should fulfill more than the established legal doctrine to address risk and benefit. It needs to also be humanistic by addressing the significant emotional and social needs of the situation. A full understanding of the surgical procedure develops personal ownership of the proposed surgery and can help alleviate anxiety before the operation. The utilization of exemplary video, still images, plastic models, and artwork can be very useful for explaining in layman's terms both the underlying pathology as well as the proposed surgery. The patient should be given ample time to integrate new information and ask any questions. It is always best, if possible, to have a member of the family or a close friend present during these discussions. Because of nervousness and apprehension, patients frequently forget the information that has been explained to them, and the support person can then help fill in the blanks. The patient should be honestly informed of the alternative surgical and nonsurgical methods including watchful waiting. She should be told that general anesthesia is typically employed, which necessitates the use of a tube being placed into her throat which may cause soreness. She should be seen preoperatively by the anesthesiologist to explain the procedure and risks of the selected anesthesia regimen. It can be useful to develop an informed consent sheet specific to laparoscopic surgery that is written in layman's language. The anticipated position during surgery and the method used to create a pneumoperitoneum should be explained. The placement and locales of trocars need to be identified, including the possibility of injury to underlying bowel, blood vessels, or the urinary tract. The general risks of surgery must be explained, including transfusion and death. It is important to never promise that surgery will be accomplished by laparoscopy. Rather, it is better to explain that if surgery can be performed by laparoscopy, there will be certain comparative advantages including quicker recovery, less pain, less infection, and less scarring. She also should be informed about the anticipated postoperative course, including the degree and nature of any pain that may or may not be expected. Importantly, the patient should be encouraged to call the office at any hour for nausea, vomiting, fever, vexing constipation, or any abdominal or pelvic pain that is progressive despite the proper use of prescribed analgesics. Any of these symptoms may be indicative of a visceral injury.

PREOPERATIVE LABS AND PREPARATION

The patient should be seen within 1–2 weeks of the surgery at which time a review of the history and a physical exam should be conducted that at least cover the following:

1. Weight
2. Blood pressure and pulse
3. Auscultation of the lungs and heart
4. Palpation of the abdomen for organomegaly and hernias
5. Complete bimanual pelvic examination including Papanicolaou smear if indicated

Many hospitals require laboratory tests within 1 or 2 weeks of the surgical procedure. Most laparoscopy requires a minimum of laboratory tests usually consisting of only hemoglobin with hematocrit and urinalysis. A coagulation profile may be needed for any patient with a history of bleeding problems. Patients who have other medical problems may also need further evaluation by their general medical doctor who may require other laboratory testing, such as a multipanel test.

Patients who are over 40 years old may benefit from a chest x-ray if one has not been obtained within the last 2 years. It is important to review her medicines and to inquire about the use of aspirin. Many patients do not consider aspirin a drug and neglect to inform the doctor of its chronic use. If the patient has been taking aspirin, it should be discontinued for 7–10 days prior to surgery.

It is recommended to eat lightly for 24 hours and be nil by mouth for at least 12 hours prior to surgery. Recent studies have shown that bowel preparation for routine gynecologic procedures is not necessary and may have little to no benefit in improving visualization or decreasing complications. In cases where pelvic adhesive disease is suspected and possible bowel resection is anticipated, consideration should be placed on the practice preferences of potential consulting specialists when deciding on bowel preparation.

DAY OF SURGERY

Patient preparation extends beyond the preoperative period and well into the day of surgery. Since most laparoscopic surgery is performed on an outpatient basis, it is recommended that surgery be started in the morning, if possible. The patient is instructed to arrive at least 1.5 hours prior to surgery to allow adequate time for the anesthesiologist to see the patient, and for all laboratory results to be checked. Before the patient receives any medication for anesthesia, it is important to review the anticipated surgery with her and again allow any questions.

Successful and efficient laparoscopy requires attention to detail and patient safety. The operating table should ideally be placed centrally to allow access to the patient by both the surgeons and anesthesiologists; access to monitors; and access to surgical equipment and support staff (Figure 1.1). The operating table should be appropriate for the patient's size and height to ensure proper support of the patient in both the supine and lithotomy positions. Although most operating room tables are equipped to support a patient weighing ≤500 lbs, it is important to also be mindful of the girth and BMI of the patient and when indicated give consideration to specialized bariatric operating room tables that make allowances for the morbidly obese patient.

It is imperative that the patient be correctly positioned on the operating table at the start of the case to allow for access to the abdomen and perineum, but most importantly to ensure the safety of the patient and operating staff. The lithotomy position allows access to the pelvic structures and is the preferred position for the majority of laparoscopic gynecologic surgeries. Boot stirrups provide physiologic support to the lower

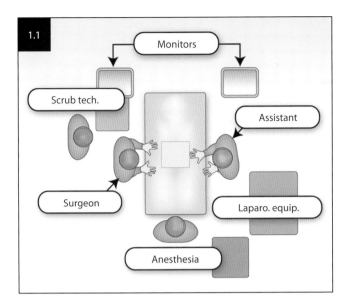

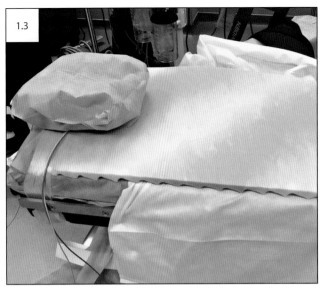

extremities; however, care must be taken to avoid prolonged instances of hyperflexion of the hip, which can lead to varying degrees of femoral nerve injury (Figure 1.2). Compression of the lateral aspect of the leg can lead to peroneal nerve injury, although this is seen more often with candy cane stirrups as compared to boot stirrups. Gynecologic laparoscopic procedures have been implicated in compartment syndrome due to patients being in the lithotomy position for prolonged periods of time; care should be given to proper positioning and padding of the lower extremities.

In addition to the lithotomy position, most laparoscopic gynecologic procedures require the patient to be in a head-down tilt (Trendelenburg position) to allow visualization of the pelvic structures. This places the patient at risk for slipping in the cephalad direction and is of great concern in cases utilizing steep Trendelenburg. Cephalad displacement of the patient in this position increases the risk of undue compression and stretch on the brachial plexus as well as the nerves of the lower extremities and

can result in injury. The use of antiskid devices such as gel pads, egg crate foam, and bean bag positioners can potentially decrease the risk of slippage and subsequent nerve injury. The egg crate foam and gel pad can be placed directly against the patient's skin to decrease slippage, with a surgical sheet placed beneath these devices to tuck the patient's arms (Figure 1.3). The bean bag conforms to the patient's body when it is inflated; therefore, it is not always necessary to use extra devices to secure the arms in the average size patient (Figure 1.4).

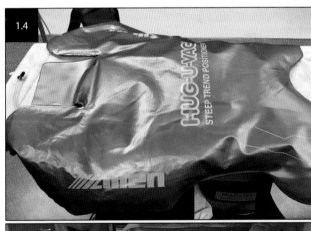

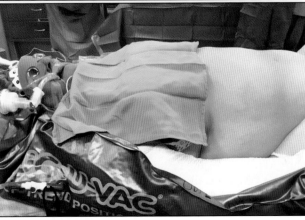

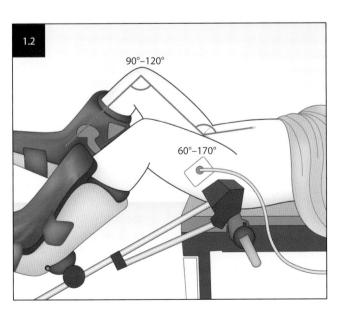

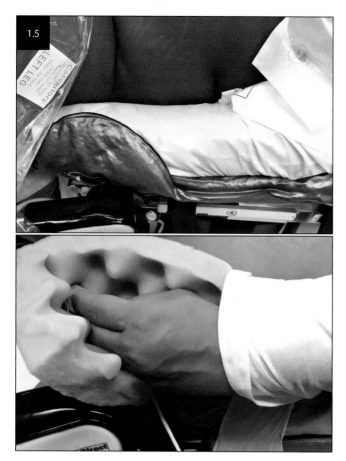

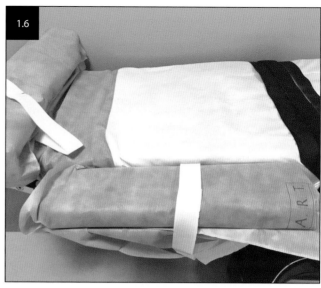

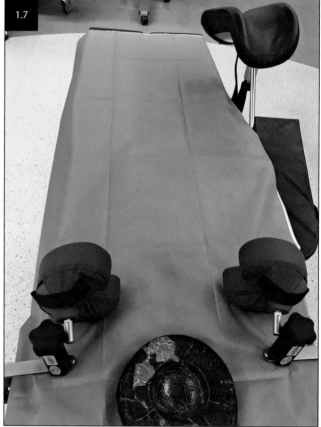

It is important that these devices be securely fastened to the bed before tilting the patient. Once the patient is properly positioned, the arms should be placed in the supine "military" position, padded at all pressure points, and securely tucked at the patient's side. This allows the surgeon access to the patient and decreases the risk of nerve injury that may occur if the arms are left outstretched. Padded arm sleds can be utilized in the obese patient to further protect and stabilize the arms if needed (Figure 1.5). In obese patients, surgical table expanders can be used to make sure that the patient's arms are properly supported (Figure 1.6).

Shoulder braces, body straps, and body restraints should be avoided as they may increase the risk of neurovascular injury and are implicated in brachial plexus injuries. If the shoulder braces are used, they need to be positioned against acromion and not close to the patient's head to avoid brachial plexus injury (Figure 1.7).

An orogastric tube is recommended for decompression of the stomach in cases of difficult intubation, which may lead to gastrointestinal distension; in cases of trocar insertions above the umbilicus as is seen in the left upper quadrant (Palmer point) entry; and in cases of incomplete gastric emptying in instances of emergency surgeries. This helps to minimize the risk of stomach injury during the initial, blind entry into the abdomen with the Veress needle or primary trocar.

The bladder should be drained prior to starting any gynecologic laparoscopic procedure. For shorter cases, the patient may be asked to void prior to entering the operating suite or an intermittent catheter may be used to empty the bladder after the vagina and urethra have been sterilely prepared. A Foley catheter should be considered for cases anticipated to last more than 30 minutes to allow for continuous emptying of the bladder. This step is important to avoid inadvertent bladder injury during port placement (especially during placement of a suprapubic trocar) and also to allow for adequate visualization of the operative field.

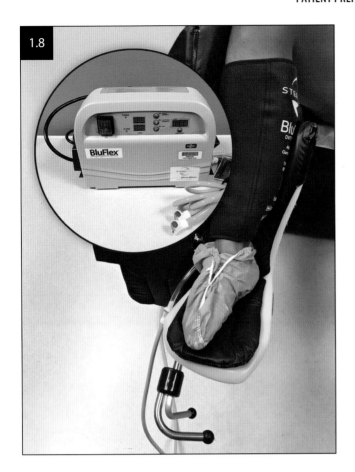

Venous thromboembolic events occur in 15%–40% of patients undergoing major gynecologic surgery in the absence of thromboprophylaxis—with the most serious sequelae being death in some cases involving pulmonary embolism.

It is important that proper risk stratification is undertaken in the perioperative period and that appropriate measures are utilized to minimize the risks of thromboembolic events. The procedure type, duration of surgery, age of the patient, and presence of other risk factors should all be addressed when stratifying risk. No specific prophylaxis is needed in patients at low risk for venous thromboembolism undergoing procedures anticipated to last ≤30 minutes. Mechanical compression devices and/or medical prophylaxis are suggested for patients at moderate to high risk of thromboembolism, in accordance with current institutional and medical guidelines (Figure 1.8).

Prevention of surgical site infection is an important consideration in the preoperative period. Although there is no surrogate for proper surgical technique, other measures have been shown to augment the efforts of the meticulous surgeon in decreasing perioperative infection. Antibiotic prophylaxis is recommended before gynecologic procedures, when entry into the reproductive tract is planned or contamination of the peritoneal cavity by vaginal contents is anticipated. Antibiotic prophylaxis is not recommended for diagnostic laparoscopy, tubal occlusion, adnexal surgery, and adhesiolysis. Aseptic preparation of the abdomen and vagina are also important measures in decreasing surgical site infection. Povidone-iodine is typically used in aseptic preparation; however, emerging data suggest that chlorhexidine products reduce the bacterial load and have longer residual activity compared to povidone-iodine. Additionally, alternative solutions may be needed in patients with an iodine allergy. Chlorhexidine gluconate–alcohol preparations with a lower alcohol content (4%), or sterile saline can be used for vaginal preparation in patients with a known iodine allergy. Vaginal preparation with chlorhexidine gluconate is considered off label in the United States, and restrictions on use for this application may be in place at certain institutions.

When the surgery is completed and the patient is sufficiently conscious, she is given written instructions regarding follow-up visits and how to take care of herself. The instructions should cover when she can bathe (anytime), begin to drive (after 24 hours), perform household duties, resume intercourse, restart exercise, and return to work. Instructions should be carefully worded to explain expected postoperative discomfort and how to differentiate it from types of pain that require contact with either the surgeon or a designated contact person using a telephone number that is answered 24 hours a day.

Ideally, on discharge, the appropriate instructions are in hand and any postoperative analgesics prescribed at a designated pharmacy.

SUGGESTED READING

Ballantyne GH, Leahy PF, Modlin IM, eds. *Laparoscopic Surgery.* Philadelphia: W.B. Saunders; 1994.

Fanning J, Valea FA. Perioperative bowel management for gynecologic surgery. *Am J Obstet Gynecol.* 2011;205:309.

Levine RL, Pasic R. Surgical setup for minimally invasive surgery. In: Bieber E, Sanfilippo J, Horowitz I, eds. *Clinical Gynecology.* New York, NY: Elsevier Science; 2006;543–548.

Pasic R, Levine R, Wolfe W. Laparoscopy in morbidly obese patients. *J AAGL* 1999;6:307–312.

CHAPTER 2

THE ART OF THE COMPETENT SURGEON: ANATOMY AND SURGICAL DISSECTION

Robert Rogers

THE ART OF SURGICAL DISSECTION

The purpose of surgical dissection is to expose vital anatomic structures while safeguarding their normal structural and physiologic functions. In doing so, the competent surgeon also minimizes any bleeding and discoloration of the tissues in the dissection field. The actual progression of dissection is a purposeful and efficient "millimeter by millimeter." No surgeon can expect his or her surgical outcomes to be any better than his or her skills of surgical dissection. Therefore, by mastering the hands-on skills of surgical dissection, the competent surgeon minimizes blood loss and surgical complications in his or her patients.

The purpose of these maneuvers is simply to thin, stretch, and open the visceral connective tissues and any scarring so that the vital structures can be clearly identified by sight and/or palpation (Figure 2.1). The surgeon must not cut, ligate, or coagulate any tissue that he or she cannot see or understand. Therefore, any surgical dissection, sharp and blunt, must proceed millimeter by millimeter. The ultimate goal of dissection is to reveal the anatomy and not obscure the dissection field or confuse anatomic appearances. This is only accomplished by the bloodless thinning of the connective tissues in which are embedded the anatomic structures—therefore, it is necessary to master dissection techniques (Table 2.1).

By progressing millimeter by millimeter in his or her dissections, the operator achieves four goals. First, the surgeon maintains correct orientation and direction of dissection. Second, the surgeon has step-by-step control of instruments and techniques employed. He or she has time to evaluate and change instrumentation, techniques, or direction. This is part of the art of the master surgeon. Third, the surgeon safely exposes the anatomic structures and dissects around them. Fourth, the surgeon minimizes blood loss and any injury to a viscus or structure by only 1–2 mm. Therefore, significant bleeding from a blood vessel or large visceral injury to a ureter, the bladder, or bowel should be minimized. Such small injuries are easily and quickly repaired in most cases, saving much surgical time when compared to repairing much larger, more extensive injuries.

The surprising result is that millimeter-by-millimeter dissection techniques actually save surgical time and increase surgical efficiency since the surgical dissection fields are more clearly seen and defined with little blood loss. This saves much time in having to look for and control bleeding from more aggressive tissue handling by the surgeon or from having to take the time to repair a large viscus injury.

Laparoscopic technique enables the surgeon to achieve better dissection than in open surgery. In laparoscopy, we are working with a laparoscopic camera and robust illumination that enable us magnification of anatomy and better recognition of tissue planes. Another important factor is that CO_2 under pressure in a closed laparoscopic environment dissects planes and enables us to follow the right planes during laparoscopic dissection.

The techniques of expert surgical dissection are "grasp and tent," "mm" incisions under direct visual control, "push-spread," "traction-countertraction" (Figure 2.2), "gentle wiping/teasing" of tissues, and hydrodissection.

Hydrodissection is the pressurized delivery of sterile fluid into the surgical field in order to tent and thin out the underlying connective tissue fibers (Figure 2.3). By grasping and tenting the peritoneum or tissue to be incised, the operator elevates the tissue away from the vital structures lying underneath—ureter, artery, vein, bowel, bladder, and somatic nerve. Grasping and tenting of the tissues also thins out and stretches the grasped tissue so that the edge of the bowel or a large blood vessel can be better seen. A mm incision can be safely made without concern for injury to underlying structures. With the gentle push-spread ("poke and open") technique, the operator further thins out the embedding connective tissues and fibrosis to further reveal what structures lie therein. This step is further aided by gentle traction and countertraction, and tenting before further cutting or gentle wiping proceeds. These maneuvers are repeated millimeter by millimeter and over and over until the tissues are completely thinned, revealing the vital anatomic structures in that anatomic region. Always stay parallel to vital structures when performing blunt traction and countertraction for tissue exposure.

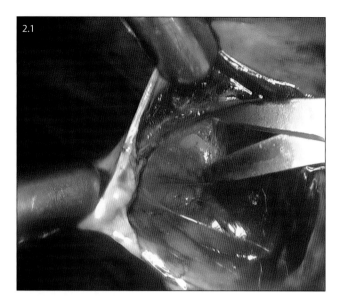

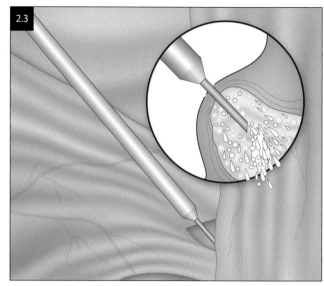

TABLE 2.1

DISSECTION TECHNIQUES

"Grasp and tent"

"Millimeter by millimeter"

Small tissue incisions under direct visual control

"Push-spread"

"Poke and open" technique

"Traction-countertraction"

Gentle wiping/teasing of tissues

Always stay parallel to vital structures

Always dissect from the known to the unknown

Dissection should proceed millimeter by millimeter from easy-to-dissect and known areas of anatomy to denser, more difficult areas of dissection. Always dissect from the known to the unknown. With experience, the

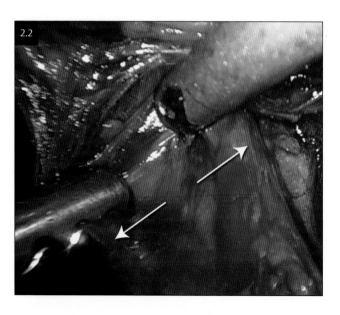

operator will become conditioned to the sight and feel of these safe dissection techniques—they can be effectively used in each region of the pelvis. Wiping must proceed gently and millimeter by millimeter to further thin the tissues surrounding the structures. Broad blunt and quick strokes of wiping may result in uncontrolled entry into a viscus or blood vessel. The technique of hydrodissection can facilitate dissections in the pelvic sidewall and potential spaces, such as the retropubic space, vesicovaginal space, paravaginal and pararectal spaces, and rectovaginal space. Hydrodissection is especially useful in vaginal surgery when performing vaginal dissections in the spaces surrounding the vagina in preparation for the various reparative vaginal procedures.

HOW TO LEARN DISSECTION TECHNIQUES

In order to learn these dissection techniques and the anatomy of specific surgical dissection fields, the student of surgery must observe the competent surgeon live in the operating room or via a video. When observing, the student must ask two important questions: "Where in the pelvis is the surgeon operating?" and "Which dissection techniques is the surgeon using?" The first question makes the learner think of the anatomy contained in the field of dissection (next section). The second question makes the student concentrate and focus on learning the true skills of the competent surgeon. In using this pattern of asking himself or herself questions, the less-experienced surgeon can prepare his or her eyes to observe and his or her mind to concentrate for relevant learning—learning that can and will immediately improve the surgeon's skills of tissue dissection used in his or her next surgical procedure. The student can only learn what his or her mind has been prepared to learn, and what his or her eyes have been prepared to see and observe and transfer to his or her mind.

The next level in mastering dissection techniques involves the student having hands-on experience with animals or human cadavers. These dissection techniques must be practiced in repetitive and precise exercises under the teaching of experienced surgical mentors. The student must have his or her mind and eyes actively engaged in the precise millimeter-by-millimeter hands-on practice of each dissection technique alone and in sequence. This active practice of expert dissection techniques is immediately transferred to his or her improved surgical skills in his or her next live surgical case.

The student of surgical technique must own his or her training and have confidence in improvement. The goal is to "do no harm to the patient," and to become a safer, more efficient surgeon.

SURGICAL ANATOMY OF THE FEMALE PELVIS

For laparoscopists, surgical female pelvic anatomy is the anatomy of surfaces and underlying abdominal and retroperitoneal structures. Surface landmarks on the anterior abdominal wall locate safe areas in which to pass laparoscopic trocars to establish ports through which laparoscopic instruments can be passed into the pelvic cavity to perform the planned surgery. Superficial peritoneal landmarks within the pelvis alert the operator to key anatomic structures in the retroperitoneal spaces. A sure knowledge of surgical and laparoscopic anatomy is a requisite for performing laparoscopic dissections that are safe for the patient and which achieve the desired goal of the surgery. The three-dimensional field of pelvic anatomy as seen through the two-dimensional plane of the laparoscope is a difficult challenge to master. The diligent laparoscopic gynecologist must always study and then observe carefully in order to gain this working knowledge. Just as technical skills can be consistently improved through frequent and proper practice, so can one's working knowledge of gynecologic surgical pelvic anatomy.

The following are discussed in this chapter: the anterior abdominal wall, the presacral space, the area of the pelvic brim, the sidewall of the pelvis, the area at the base of the broad ligament (cervicouterine junction), the various spaces within the pelvis, and the anatomy of the retropubic space (space of Retzius).

THE ANTERIOR ABDOMINAL WALL

The various ports needed to perform laparoscopic surgery must traverse the anterior abdominal wall. Thus, knowledge of this anatomy is important to avoid a primary complication of injury to the arteries and veins contained therein. Landmarks of interest are the umbilicus, the anterior superior iliac spines, and the pubic symphysis. In addition, landmarks on the anterior abdominal wall assist the laparoscopist in safely placing trocars in order to avoid injuring deeper vascular structures such as the aorta, common iliac vessels, and external iliac vessels.

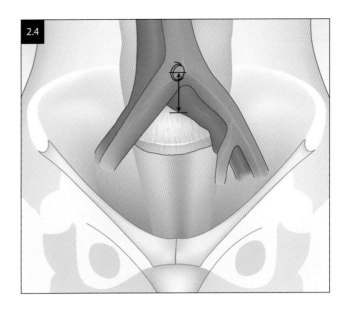

Depending on the habitus and weight of the patient, the umbilicus may lie slightly above, at, or below the bifurcation of the aorta. In obese patients, the umbilicus may be shifted several centimeters below the bifurcation of the aorta and commonly lies on top of the right common iliac artery. In all patients, the left common iliac vein covers at least part of the sacral promontory as it crosses the midline approximately 3–6 cm inferior to the bifurcation of the aorta and is inferior to the level of the umbilicus (Figure 2.4). In the thinner patient especially, the surface of the anterior abdominal wall is significantly closer to these great vessels.

In placement of lower lateral abdominal trocars, the surgeon must avoid lacerating the inferior and/or superficial epigastric arteries and veins and their branches. The inferior epigastric artery and vein travel on the posterior surface of the rectus abdominis muscle on its lateral third, particularly in the lower quadrants of the abdomen (Figure 2.5). The superficial epigastric arteries and veins travel

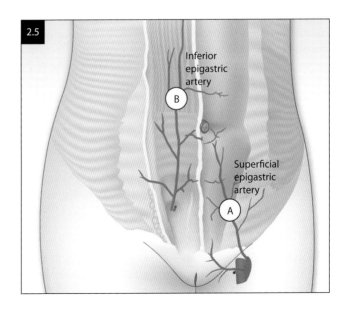

Inferior epigastric artery

Superficial epigastric artery

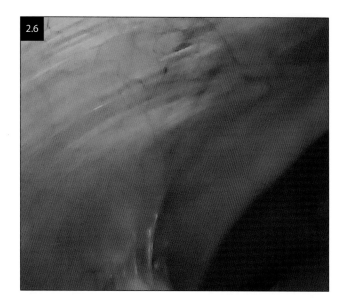

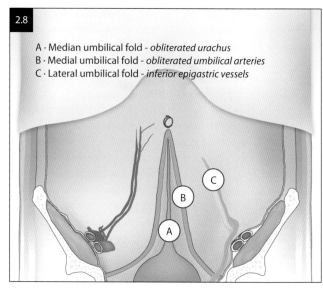

A · Median umbilical fold - *obliterated urachus*
B · Medial umbilical fold - *obliterated umbilical arteries*
C · Lateral umbilical fold - *inferior epigastric vessels*

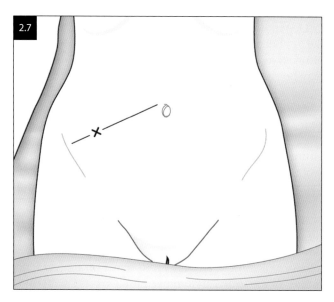

within the subcutaneous tissue of the anterior abdominal wall in variable locations lateral to the umbilicus. The superficial vessels can usually be seen by transillumination of the anterior abdominal wall, while the inferior epigastric vessels cannot be seen due to shadowing from the rectus abdominis muscles. These latter vessels must be identified directly through the laparoscope (Figure 2.6).

Most injuries to these vessels within the abdominal wall can be avoided by placing the lateral ports approximately 8 cm from the midline and 8 cm superior to the pubic symphysis. This area also happens to be known as McBurney point, which is anatomically located at one-third of the distance from the anterior superior iliac spine along the line from that spine to the umbilicus (Figure 2.7).

SUPERFICIAL PERITONEAL ANATOMY

All laparoscopic procedures must begin with a systematic inspection of the surface areas of both the pelvis and upper abdomen. Such examinations should not only

visually document the condition of the pelvic viscera and the surfaces within the pelvis, but also include inspection of the appendix, ascending colon, falciform ligament, liver and gallbladder, omentum, transverse colon, stomach, right and left hemidiaphragms, and descending colon. The operating laparoscopist must visually search for evidence of adhesions, inflammation, endometriosis, cul-de-sac fluid, peritoneal studding, tumors, or distortion of any pelvic or abdominal anatomy and structures.

Only through the laparoscope can the operating surgeon appreciate the structures on the undersurface of the anterior abdominal wall. Running from the dome of the bladder underneath a peritoneal fold is the obliterated urachus, known as the median umbilical fold. Just lateral to the median umbilical fold are the medial umbilical folds (Figure 2.8). These are formed by the peritoneum covering the obliterated umbilical arteries. Each obliterated umbilical artery, when followed back underneath the round ligament into the broad ligament, will lead the surgeon to the superior vesical artery, and then back to the terminus of the internal iliac artery (Figure 2.9). Lateral to the medial umbilical fold is the lateral umbilical fold, which is formed by the tenting of the peritoneum over the inferior epigastric artery and vein. These latter vessels exit the external iliac artery and vein just medial to the exit of the round ligament from the body through the internal inguinal ring. Direct identification through the umbilical laparoscope will allow the laparoscopist to place lateral trocars through the anterior abdominal wall well lateral to these epigastric vessels.

Anterior traction on the uterus will place the uterosacral ligaments on tension and lead the surgeon to visualization of the ureters in the pelvic sidewall (Figure 2.10). The dome of the bladder is a semilunar outline overlying the pubic symphysis.

PRESACRAL SPACE

The presacral space is important to laparoscopic surgeons performing "presacral neurectomy" for the hopeful

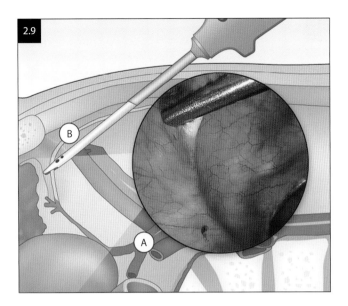

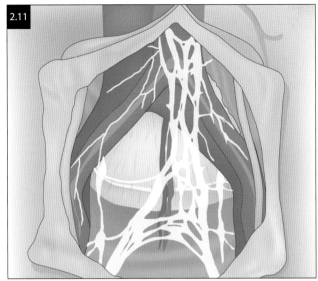

alleviation of central and chronic pelvic pain. At this time, presacral neurectomy is considered a controversial procedure (see "Suggested Reading"). The space is bounded anteriorly by the parietal peritoneum. Posteriorly it is bounded by the periosteum and anterior longitudinal ligament over the lower two lumbar vertebrae and the promontory of the sacrum. The middle sacral artery and a plexus of veins are attached to the posterior boundary of the space. The superior extension of the visceral endopelvic fascia in this area embeds fatty areolar tissue, presacral lymph nodes and tissue, and visceral nerves (Figure 2.11). There is not one presacral nerve but a multitude of finer visceral nerves that have great variability in their course and distribution within this space. These "presacral nerves" are simply the multiple afferent and efferent visceral nerve fibers of the superior hypogastric plexus. The right lateral boundary of this space is the right common iliac artery and ureter. The left lateral border is the left common iliac vein and left ureter, as well as the inferior mesenteric artery and vein traversing the

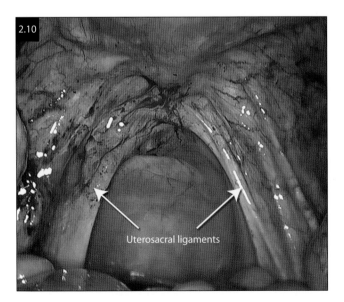

Uterosacral ligaments

mesentery of the sigmoid colon. Great care must be taken by even experienced laparoscopic surgeons in order to dissect safely within this space. Damage to the ureter and the possibility of massive hemorrhage exist here.

PELVIC BRIM

The pelvic brim region at the location over the sacroiliac joint is the important location for the entry of multiple structures into the pelvic cavity. These structures course over the pelvic brim in a vertical manner and then rotate in a 90° fashion to form the structures of the pelvic sidewall. From the peritoneal surface working posteriorly to the sacroiliac joint, the following structures are found coursing one over the other: the peritoneum; the ovarian vessels in the infundibulopelvic ligament; the ureter traversing over the bifurcation of the common iliac artery; the common iliac vein; the medial edge of the psoas muscle; and in the same plane, the obturator nerve overlying the parietal fascia just over the capsule of the sacroiliac joint (Figure 2.12). In the same plane as the obturator nerve, but more medial, the lumbosacral trunk is found coursing from the lumbar plexus of nerves to the sacral plexus of nerves that are found overlying the piriformis muscle in the pelvis (Figure 2.13). When ligating the ovarian vessels in the infundibulopelvic ligament, the surgeon must lift the infundibulopelvic ligament well away from the course of the ureter in order to avoid injuring it (Figure 2.14).

THE PELVIC SIDEWALL REGION

Based on avascular planes, the pelvic sidewall consists of three surgical layers. Medially, the *first layer* is the parietal peritoneum with the attached ureter in its own visceral fascial capsule. When this peritoneum is incised and retracted medially, the ureter comes with it (Figure 2.15).

The *second surgical layer* consists of the internal iliac artery and vein and their visceral anterior branches, all

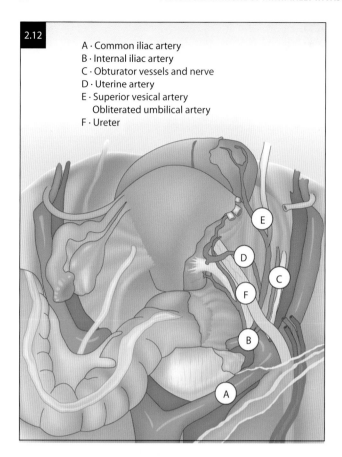

2.12

A · Common iliac artery
B · Internal iliac artery
C · Obturator vessels and nerve
D · Uterine artery
E · Superior vesical artery
   Obliterated umbilical artery
F · Ureter

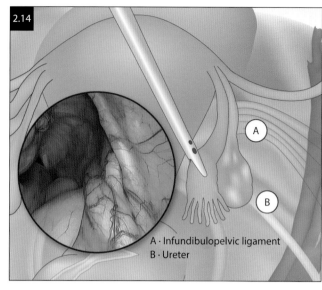

2.14

A · Infundibulopelvic ligament
B · Ureter

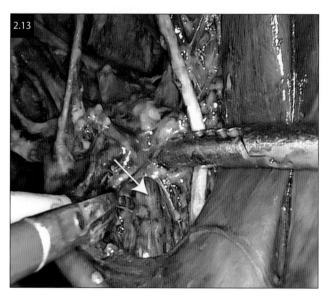

2.13

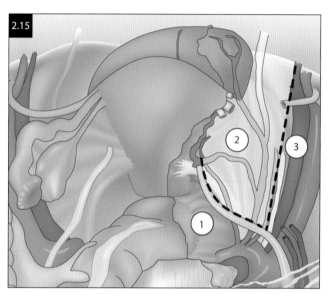

2.15

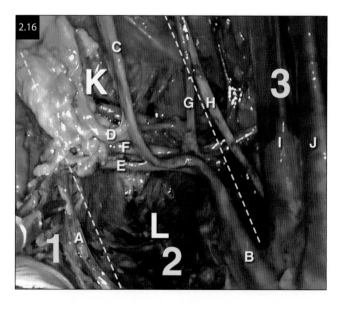

2.16

enveloped within the surrounding visceral connective tissue containing the lymph tissue and the visceral hypogastric nerves. Figure 2.16 shows three layers of the pelvic sidewall 1, 2, 3 on the patient's right side; A, ureter; B, internal iliac artery; C, obliterated umbilical artery; D, uterine artery; E, vaginal artery; F, uterine vein; G, obturator artery; H, obturator nerve; I, external iliac vein; J, external iliac artery; K, paravesical space; and L, pararectal space.

The *third surgical layer* consists of the parietal fascia over the obturator internus muscle with the obturator artery, nerve, and vein allowed to remain on this muscle. However, during obturator space dissections, the nerve can be retracted safely medially. In addition, the third layer consists of the external iliac artery and vein on the medial aspect of the psoas muscle, on top of the bony arcuate line of the ilium (linea terminalis).

Blunt dissection by the laparoscopic surgeon easily separates the first surgical layer from the second surgical layer and the second surgical layer from the third surgical layer—all in an avascular manner. The second surgical layer of the pelvic sidewall can also easily be found by tracing the course of the obliterated umbilical artery back to the superior vesical artery within the broad ligament, and then back to the terminal root of the internal iliac artery. The medial offshoot at this junction is the uterine artery.

THE BASE OF THE BROAD LIGAMENT

The base of the broad ligament is that anatomic region where the cardinal ligament inserts into the pericervical ring of endopelvic fascia for upper vaginal suspension. It contains the ureter traveling underneath the uterine artery in an oblique fashion, approximately 1.5 cm lateral to the side of the cervix (Figure 2.17). This region is an important anatomic area where the ureter makes a "knee-bend" in order to turn anteriorly and medially across the anterolateral fornix of the vagina to enter the bladder. This area of the knee-bend is approximately 2 cm medial and anterior from the ischial spine. This area is also called the *parametrium* (anatomically next to the cervicouterine junction). The area located lateral to the vagina is called the *upper paracolpium*.

PARARECTAL SPACE

Posterior to the base of the broad ligament is the pararectal space, which is easily developed by dissecting the ureter medially toward the rectum, away from the

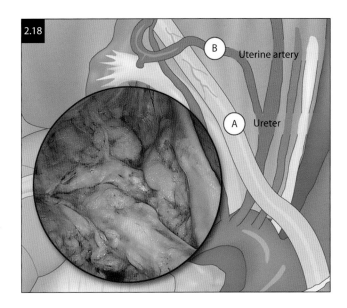

internal iliac artery and vein, and posterior to the origin of the uterine artery. The anterior border of this space is the base of the broad ligament. The lateral and medial borders are the internal iliac artery and the ureter, respectively. This space also contains the uterosacral ligament laterally as it passes posteriorly toward the sacrum (Figure 2.18).

PARAVESICAL SPACE

The paravesical space is found anterior to the base of the broad ligament and is bounded medially by the bladder and laterally by the obturator internus muscle fascia. The paravesical space simply leads into the lateral space of Retzius (Figure 2.19). The space within the paravesical space lateral to the obturator nerve is known as the obturator space. Figure 2.20 shows the obturator space on the patient's right side; A, ureter; B, obliterated umbilical artery; C, obturator artery; D, obturator nerve; and E, external iliac vein. From this region above the level of the obturator nerve, the operating laparoscopic gynecologist will harvest the obturator lymph nodes.

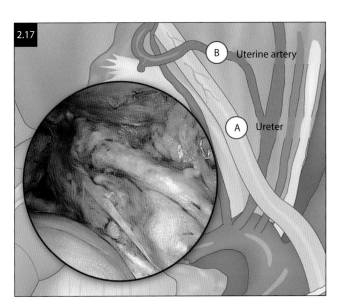

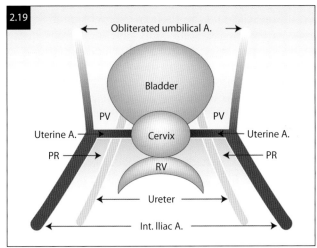

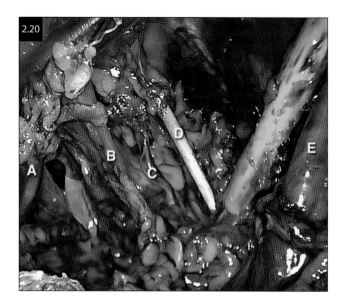

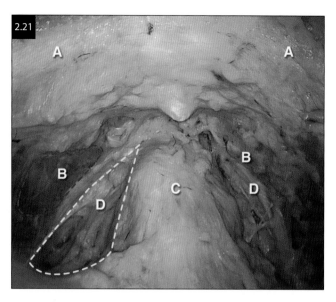

SPACE OF RETZIUS

The space of Retzius or retropubic space is a potential space containing much areolar tissue between the back of the pubic bone and the anterior portion of the bladder. Surrounding the bladder is a visceral bladder capsule that contains the rich network of perivesical venous sinuses that are very fragile and bleed easily when surgery is performed in this space. Centrally over the urethra is the deep dorsal vein of the clitoris that feeds into these venous channels. The lateral border of the space of Retzius is the obturator internus muscle and its parietal fascia, with the obturator nerve, artery, and vein just beneath the bony ridge of the ilium on its anterior border. The posterior border (toward the sacrum) is a visceral fascial sheath surrounding the internal iliac artery and vein and their anterior branches. Remember in the standing female patient, the internal iliac artery starts at the bifurcation at the pelvic brim over the sacroiliac joint and travels in a vertical direction along the anterior border of the greater sciatic foramen down toward the ischial spine.

The floor of the space of Retzius is simply the pubocervical fascia inserting into the lateral fascial white line. The fascial white line (arcus tendineus fasciae pelvis) is a thickening of the parietal fascia overlying the levator ani muscles and travels from the pubic arch straight back to the ischial spine. Just anterior to this fascial white line is a more variable and thinner thickening of the parietal fascia overlying the obturator internus muscle called the *muscle white line* (arcus tendineus levator ani). The muscle white line is the origin of the levator ani muscles from the lateral and posterior aspects of the pubic bone in a curvilinear fashion back toward the ischial spine that meets with the fascial white line. Figure 2.21 shows a dissected space of Retzius: A, pubic bone and Cooper's ligament; B, internal obturator muscle; C, bladder; D, pubocervical fascia.

When working in this space and performing a paravaginal defect repair or a Burch retropubic colposuspension through the laparoscope, the surgeon must clear the areolar tissue off the white glistening pubocervical fascia before placing sutures directly into its thickness, which is attached to the underlying vaginal epithelium.

THE VESICOVAGINAL SPACE

The vesicovaginal space is found between the anterior surface of the vagina and the posterior aspect of the bladder down to the trigone. This space is bordered laterally by the bladder "pillars" that allow for the passage of the inferior vesical arteries, veins, and ureter to the bladder (Figure 2.22). This space is important to the

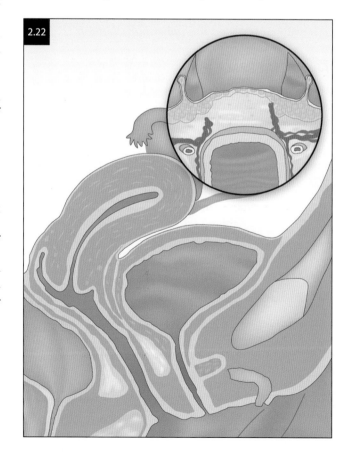

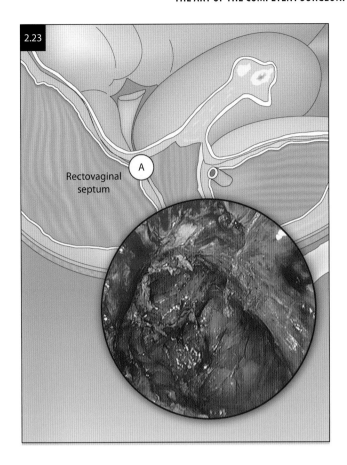

Rectovaginal septum

A

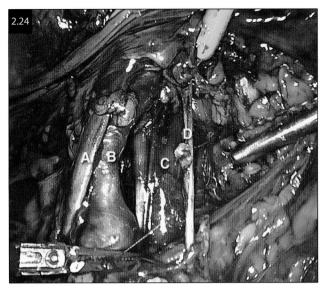

surgeon performing a hysterectomy since he or she must incise through the vesicouterine peritoneal fold in order to mobilize the bladder off the lower uterine segment and upper third of the vagina. This potential space is created by dissecting between the visceral fascial coat around the bladder and the pubocervical fascia, found on top of the cervix and anterior vaginal wall, down to the level of the trigone. Care must be taken not to dissect too vigorously and laterally to avoid injury to the ureter and vasculature found within the bladder pillars.

RECTOVAGINAL SPACE

The rectovaginal space is bounded superiorly by the cul-de-sac peritoneum and the uterosacral ligaments, laterally by the iliococcygeus muscles of the levator ani, posteriorly by the visceral fascial capsule surrounding the anterior surface of the rectum, and anteriorly by the visceral fascial capsule surrounding the posterior aspect of the vagina. The rectovaginal septum is found just behind the vagina, somewhat adherent to it and yet dissectable away from it (Figure 2.23). The rectovaginal fascia is more and more commonly being used for repair of rectoceles.

DISSECTION OVER THE PSOAS MUSCLE TO HARVEST LYMPH NODES

The anatomy of the pelvic brim has already been discussed. The pelvic brim is also important for the surgical oncologist for harvesting pelvic lymph nodes from around

the external iliac artery and vein. This area is entered by tenting up and opening the peritoneum between the round ligament and the infundibulopelvic ligament, and then, extending the incision superiorly in a millimeter-by-millimeter progression. The external iliac artery and vein can be visualized on the medial aspect of the psoas muscle and are surrounded by the lymphatic chain of nodes enveloped in the yellow, fatty areolar connective tissue. The external iliac artery and vein most commonly do not have any branches in this area. This fact is important to know when performing a pelvic lymphadenectomy procedure. The first branch is the deep circumflex iliac vein, which represents the lower border (near the inguinal ligament) of the external iliac node dissection. Parallel and lateral to the external iliac artery and vein on the surface of the psoas muscle is the genitofemoral nerve. Care should be taken not to injure this sensory nerve when removing nodes in the area. Figure 2.24 shows the patient's right side (A, external iliac vein; B, external iliac artery; C, psoas muscle; D, genitofemoral nerve).

AFTERTHOUGHT ON YOUR TRAINING AS A SURGEON

Own your training. Teach yourself how to learn from your surgical mentors and from surgical videos. Ask yourself the important questions concerning the anatomy in the field of dissection and in identifying the individual techniques of tissue handling and dissection. Answer those questions to yourself. Appreciate the directed flow of purposeful anatomic dissections. Always remember that the only purpose of surgical dissection is to thin and open visceral connective tissues and scar fibrosis. This process reveals the anatomic structures embedded within in a safe manner. Tissue dissections by the competent surgeon are clean and elegant. The anatomy is clearly demonstrated in a bloodless field. The expert surgical operator is known for his or her millimeter-by-millimeter dissection techniques and low rates of surgical complications. Learn, practice, and master these essential components of safe and efficient surgery. Your surgical successes are directly proportional to your working knowledge of surgical anatomy and your hands-on expertise in tissue dissections. Be disciplined, be caring, and evolve into an expert surgeon. This chapter gives you that essential guidance and learning.

SUGGESTED READING

Hurd WW, Bude RO, DeLancey JOL, Newman JS. The location of abdominal wall blood vessels in relationship to abdominal landmarks apparent at laparoscopy. *Am J Obstet Gynecol.* 1994;171:642–646.

Netter FH, ed. *Atlas of Human Anatomy.* West Caldwell, NJ: CIBA-GEIGY Medical Education; 1989.

Rogers RM. Pelvic denervation surgery. *Clin Obstet Gynecol* 2003; 46(4):767–772.

Rogers RM, Pasic R. Pelvic retroperitoneal dissection: A hands-on primer. *J Minim Invasive Gynecol* 2017;24:546–551.

Rogers RM, Taylor RH. Surgical dissection and anatomy of the female pelvis for the gynecologic surgeon. In: Gomel V, Brill AI. eds. *Reconstructive and Reproductive Surgery in Gynecology*, New York and London: Informa Healthcare; 2010; 38–45.

Rogers RM, Taylor RH. The core of a competent surgeon: A working knowledge of surgical anatomy and safe dissection techniques. *Obstet Gynecol Clinic of N Am* 2011;38(4):777–788.

CHAPTER 3

INSTRUMENTATION AND EQUIPMENT

Resad Paya Pasic and Andrew I. Brill

GENERAL ROOM SETUP

The setup should be designed to optimize efficiency using the team concept. The team usually consists of the surgeon, a first assistant, a scrub nurse, and a circulating nurse. The most recent addition to the traditional team is the biomedical technician. He or she may not be required for the entire case, but it is helpful if the technician is in attendance at the start, as well as intermittently, and at the end of the case. The technician should be trained and skilled in the use of all electronic equipment, the video camera, laser equipment, and other electronic supplies, and be able to possess on-site troubleshooting skills. Since operative endoscopy is completely dependent on high-tech equipment, all should be thoroughly checked prior to the start of each case.

The circulating nurse is the main coordinator of the team, and he or she will be responsible during the procedure for running the video, checking suction and irrigation equipment, and generally providing support and maintaining the steady rhythm of the operating team.

The operating room setup requires an operating table that can be placed in deep Trendelenburg position. It must have rails that will accommodate the stirrups, shoulder braces, and other possible equipment. Most gynecologic surgeons perform laparoscopy from the left side; however, this is an individual idiosyncrasy that started when laparoscopy was performed without a camera and therefore required holding the laparoscope with one hand while leaving the right to manipulate instruments. Generally, if the surgeon is right handed, then he or she should stand on the patient's left side in order to introduce the Veress needle and trocars with the dominant and more ergonomic hand. In the ideal operating room (OR), to decrease the floor clutter and to allow more room for lasers, fluid monitors, and other large equipment, monitors and most electronic equipment may be suspended from the ceiling using overhead mechanical booms along with all gas lines and electric outlets. To increase efficiency, many of the commands in the modern ORs can be voice operated and controlled by the surgeon's voice with the help of the Hermes system (Stryker Endoscopy, Santa Clara, California) or OR1 (Karl Storz Endoscopy, Tuttlingen, Germany) (Figure 3.1). This technology uses electronic control systems to integrate devices and environmental components of the OR, including overhead mounting systems, lighting, operating room tables, endoscopic equipment, cameras, image capture systems, and information networks. It brings all of these technologies under the direct control of the surgical team.

Ideally, two monitors would be available with one to each side of the legs; however, if only one monitor is available, it should be between the legs.

The back table should hold all of the handheld instruments that may be needed during the case. They should be grouped in an orderly manner just as the back table is arranged during open surgery. A Mayo stand can either be placed between the legs or adjacent to a leg with the equipment that will be frequently exchanged during the procedure (i.e., suction irrigator, scissors, and several different types of graspers).

VIDEO IMAGING AND CAPTURING

Modern video cameras are based on the solid-state microprocessor chip. Historically, there were one- or three-chip cameras with a head that attaches to the eyepiece of the laparoscope and connects to the camera controller by a cable. The signal is then fed into the monitor to display the image. The quality of the video display advances along with technology. It is important to understand that the composite image on the video monitor is related to both the resolution of the camera and the monitor. If one has a resolution capability of 750 lines and the other 500 lines, it is only possible to visualize at the lower level. High-definition endoscopic video cameras have now become conventional in most ORs. The HDTV camera and widescreen monitor have more than twice the number of scanning lines (180p) than the frame of conventional videos, making the images clearer and of higher resolution. Most of the currently marketed cameras utilize HD technology with 180p resolution. High-definition systems may prove quite useful in diagnosing endometriosis and early metastatic spread.

The Spies camera system (Karl Storz) features a new three-chip camera head technology providing unique and brilliant imaging with excellent color rendition and details in full HD. An optical zoom guarantees magnification of the viewed image without a loss in quality. The Spies Clara automatically identifies and brightens dark areas in video images for enhanced illumination, and the Spies

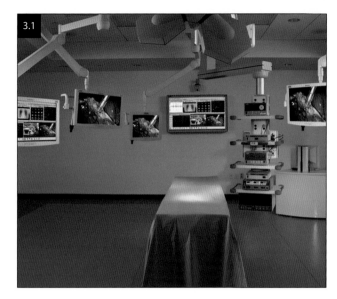

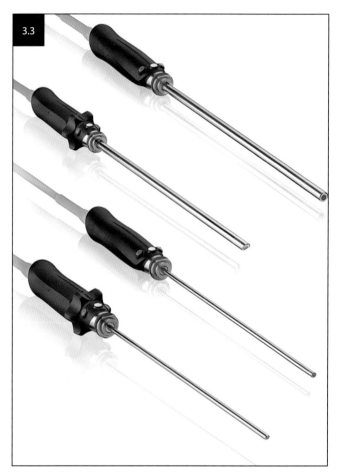

Chroma intensifies color contrast of the video so that differentiation of tissue is enhanced. The Spies Spectra makes it easier to differentiate between tissue types and allows recognition of the finest tissue structures by filtering out the bright red portions of the visible spectrum and expanding the remaining color portions (Figure 3.2).

Another type of video camera system consists of a combination telescope and camera, which are fully integrated with a camera chip mounted at the distal end of the laparoscope (EndoEye video laparoscope, Olympus Surgical America, Orangeburg, New York) (Figure 3.3). This configuration eliminates the use of optical lenses by directly transmitting a digital image from the chip at the distal tip.

The 4K is the latest standard for digital cinema and computer graphics resolution. Comparative advantages include higher image definition quality, a more detailed picture, better fast-action, and larger projection surface visibility. The 4K format was named because it has approximately 4000 pixels of horizontal resolution.

Standard 1080p and 720p resolutions were named to describe vertical resolutions. The new standard renders more than four times higher image definition than 1080p resolutions, for example (Figure 3.4).

No perusal of instrumentation would be complete without looking even further into the future. It is recognized that there are some limitations to using the two-dimensional view of the surgical field. Depth perception potentially helps surgeons to develop their hand-eye coordination and to more efficiently perform advanced laparoscopic tasks such as laparoscopic suturing. The Olympus 3D Imaging System Videoscope (Olympus Surgical America, Orangeburg, New York) produces a bright, natural three-dimensional (3D) image that provides up to 100° of articulation in all directions, enabling observation of the entire peritoneal cavity. The articulating, chip-on-tip design and dual optical channels enable anatomical views in 2D and 3D that are simply not possible with traditional laparoscopes (Figure 3.5).

Video capturing has also become an important part of supplying documentation for record keeping. A high-definition capture system such as the AIDA (Karl Storz Endoscopy) (Figure 3.6) is designed to capture and route the high-definition images without loss of quality. This equipment allows the surgeon to document his or her cases on several types of media, such as CD or DVD, as well as route pictures directly to a printer or to the electronic medical record.

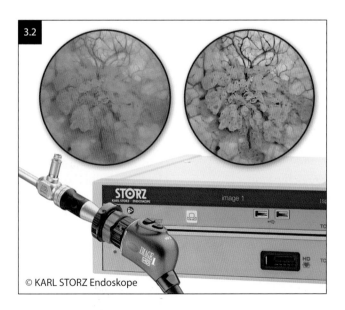

© KARL STORZ Endoskope

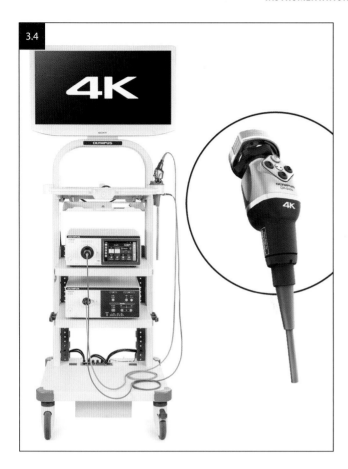

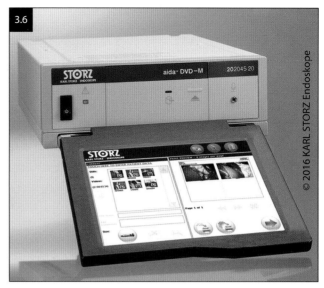

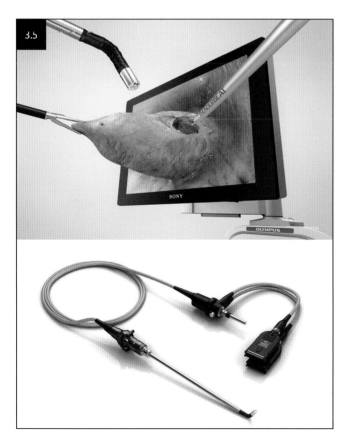

UTERINE MOBILIZATION

Most laparoscopic surgery is expedited by the use of a good uterine manipulator. It may be the most important ancillary tool for the laparoscopic surgeon. This device should ideally be able to rotate, antevert, and retrovert the uterus depending on the anatomical needs of the procedure. If a standard uterine manipulator is not available, one may insert a uterine sound or dilator high into the fundus and then attach it with surgical tape or sterile rubber bands to a tenaculum previously placed on the anterior lip of the cervix. There are many types of commercial manipulators that are reusable, such as the Hulka Uterine Elevator (Richard Wolf Medical Instruments, Vernon Hills, Vermont), Pelosi (Apple Medical Corp., Bolton, Massachusetts), and the Valtchev Uterine Mobilizer (Konkin Surgical Instruments, Toronto, Canada). Partially disposable manipulators, such as the Rumi (Cooper Surgical, Shelton, Connecticut), have disposable tips that are available in different lengths from 6 cm to 12 cm along with a sized disposable cup used to delineate the vaginal fornices and an inflatable balloon to occlude the vagina after culdotomy (Figure 3.7). Completely disposable manipulators, such as the Vcare (ConMed Corp., Utica, New York) or Cooper Surgical Delineator, can also be adjusted for the length of the tip and has opposing in-line plastic cups to mechanically occlude the vagina for culdotomy. These manipulators also typically have the ability to chromopertubate. The tips of these devices are usually held in place by a small distal balloon that may be inflated with sterile fluid after being properly positioned in the uterine cavity.

INSUFFLATION INSTRUMENTS

The various techniques of insufflation are addressed in Chapter 5. Most techniques utilize a Veress needle. These spring-loaded needles are available as reusable,

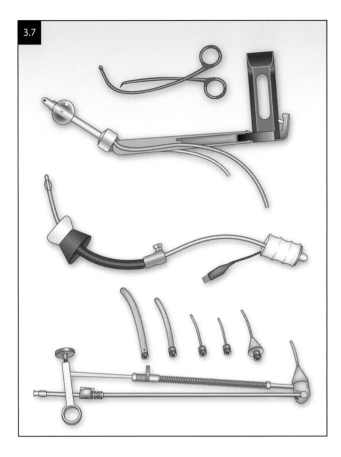

3.7

partially disposable, or completely disposable instruments. It is a delicate instrument that has a sharp outer sleeve and contains an inner sleeve with a dull tip on a spring mechanism that retracts back when a resistance is encountered. Without resistance, the dull tip springs forward to protect intraabdominal structures from the sharp tip (Figure 3.8). If the reusable needle is sharpened frequently, it is as functional as, and certainly less expensive than, the disposable type. The disposable Veress needle has an advantage in always being sharp, which enhances its use. The spring mechanism should be checked prior to insertion, even with the disposable instruments.

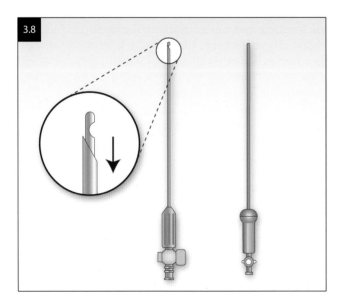

3.8

INSUFFLATORS

There are multiple insufflators on the market. The ideal insufflator can deliver rapid, accurate flow rates of CO_2 gas up to 15 L/min. However, it is obvious that the gas flow supplied at the outlet of the machine is not what is delivered intraabdominally owing to the diameter and the distance of the connecting tube. In actual measurements, the true amount delivered at the end of the tube may be only 60%–70% of the capable flow rate of the insufflator. Gas flow through a 5 mm trocar may be severely restricted whenever a laparoscopic instrument is placed through this port. Some insufflators such as the Thermoflator (Karl Storz Endoscopy, Tuttlingen, Germany) (Figure 3.9) have heating capability to warm the gas, thus decreasing the intraabdominal hypothermic effect of cold CO_2 gas and decreasing fogging of the distal lens of the laparoscope. The Insuflow device (Lexion Medical, St. Paul, Minnesota) is relatively inexpensive equipment that can be attached to the insufflator that will both hydrate and warm the gas.

The UHI-4 Insufflator (Olympus) provides a near smoke-free environment during laparoscopic surgery. When paired with a dedicated device, the insufflator automatically initiates suction while simultaneously delivering compensatory CO_2 whenever the Thunderbeat (Olympus) or Gyrus (Olympus) device is activated (see these devices described in Chapter 6; see also Figure 3.9).

AirSeal (Surgiquest) is a novel and integrated access system for laparoscopic and robotic surgery that stabilizes the pneumoperitoneum while providing continuous smoke evacuation and valve-free access to the abdominal

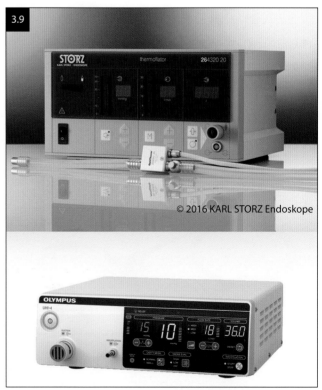

3.9

© 2016 KARL STORZ Endoskope

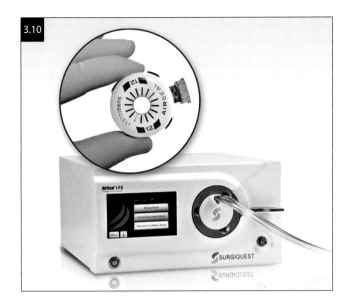

cavity. This is made possible by the high-flow, pressure-sensing capabilities of the Tri-Lumen Filtered Tube Set and the Access Port, which are the key elements of this system and come in 5, 8, and 12 mm sizes. Moreover, the Access Port does not contain any valves like conventional trocars, which prevents smudging of the lens and allows improved tissue removal from the abdominal cavity (Figure 3.10).

The basic information that should be supplied by the readout of the insufflator is

1. Insufflation pressure
2. Intraabdominal pressure
3. Insufflation volume per minute
4. Total amount of gas used (the least important)

ABDOMINAL ACCESS INSTRUMENTS

An entire chapter could be used to address this highly debated issue. There are several categories in which all of the instruments may be grouped:

1. Disposable or reusable
2. Open or closed technique
3. Mini entry techniques or direct view

DISPOSABLE OR REUSABLE

The argument of disposable versus reusable equipment may be focused on trocars and sheaths. The traditional disposable trocars have become popular mainly because the tips are always sharp, thus requiring a much smaller force to achieve penetration than the reusable instruments. The shield that springs out over the tip after entry into the abdominal cavity plays little, if any, role in safety. Providing significantly improved abdominal wall retention while ensuring minimum penetration into the operative field, the Kii Fios Advanced Fixation trocar manufactured by Applied Medical comes in 5 and 12 mm

diameters. The trocar sheet is equipped with the balloon that can be inflated with 10 mL of saline to secure it in place and prevent sliding of the trocar out of the abdominal wall. A retention disk slides down to maintain the sleeve position in the abdomen, securing the trocar in place and virtually eliminating unintentional displacement or forward migration while providing pressure on the incision site, which potentially reduces port-site bleeding (Figure 3.11).

There has been a continuing area of contention regarding the style of the trocar tip in reusable instruments. Some surgeons favor the pyramidal tip, while others extol the virtues of the conical tip. Most trocars today use the pyramidal-style tip. There are advantages to each, but sharpness is of most importance in the closed technique. Reusable trocars and sheaths have a distinct economic advantage; however, the necessity of frequent sharpening and cleaning may offset the savings.

Trocars are available in many sizes, from 3 mm up to 12 mm and greater. Most standard laparoscopy is performed using a 10 or 12 mm umbilical port for the laparoscope and 5 mm lower abdominal ports for the secondary instruments. There are even smaller trocars that may be used for 3 mm instruments.

OPEN OR CLOSED TECHNIQUE

Most closed-technique instruments have sharp tips, which may potentially injure bowel or large blood vessels. One alternative is to use a Hasson cannula while performing

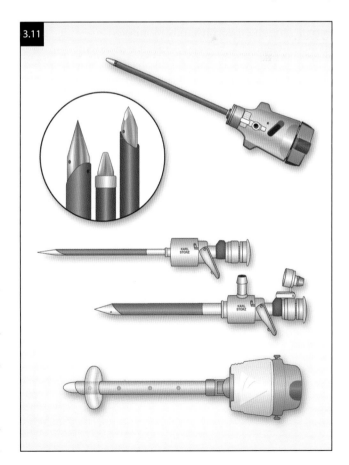

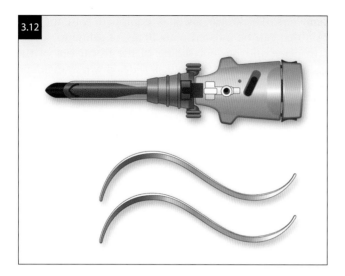

3.12

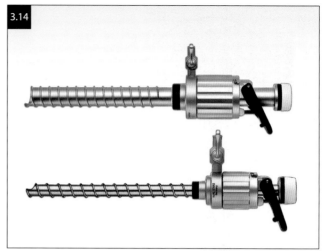

3.14

the open technique invented by Dr. Harrith Hasson (see Chapter 5). This instrument requires opening into the peritoneal cavity prior to the insertion of the sheath and does not develop a pneumoperitoneum prior to its use (Figure 3.12). The use of vision-directed trocars such as the Endopath bladeless trocar, a disposable instrument (Ethicon Endosurgery, Cincinnati, Ohio) (Figure 3.13), is a hybrid that combines a bit of each technique. Another innovation using visual access is the ENDOTIP device, which is a reusable threaded port that dilates the tissue as it is threaded in (Karl Storz Endoscopy, Culver City, California) (Figure 3.14). With each of these methods, a 10 mm 0° laparoscope is inserted into the trocar, and as the trocar is advanced through the abdominal wall layers, the passage into the abdomen is constantly monitored, and thus, damage to bowel or blood vessels may be avoided.

More recently, a larger and disposable single-port cannula to be used transumbilically was introduced to the gynecologic armamentarium providing improved cosmesis and potentially accelerated healing by removing the need for lower abdominal ports. The GelPOINT access platform (Applied Medical, Rancho Santa Margarita,

California) is exemplary and provides a flexible, airtight fulcrum to facilitate triangulation of standard laparoscopic instrumentation (Figure 3.15).

LIGHT SOURCE

An adequate light source is absolutely essential for performing laparoscopic surgery, as it is important to have good illumination in order to obtain image clarity and true colors. A 250 W halogen or xenon light source provides excellent light intensity. The temperature of 6000°K obtained from xenon provides true white light that enhances visualization to permit recognition of pathologic changes (Figure 3.16). A fluid light cable that connects the light source with the laparoscope may provide optimal light transmission. The fiberoptic light cord should be handled with care, since the fibers within the housing may be broken if the cord is kinked or dropped. If there is a decreased light transmission, one end of the light cord can be held up to a room light, and by looking at the other end, it is possible to assess whether a significant number of fibers are broken. Due to the

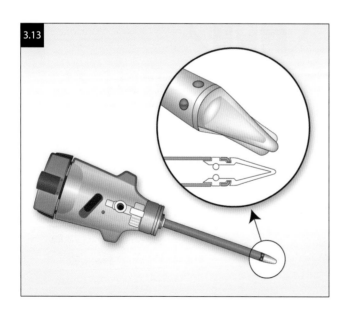

3.13

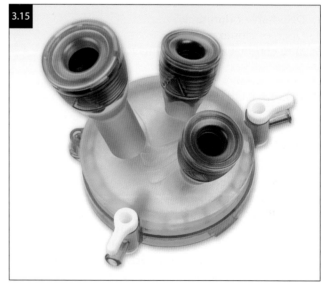

3.15

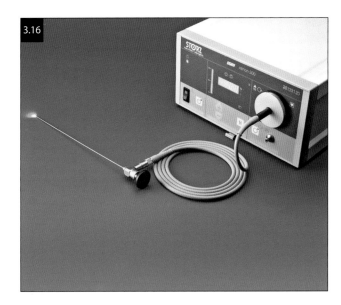

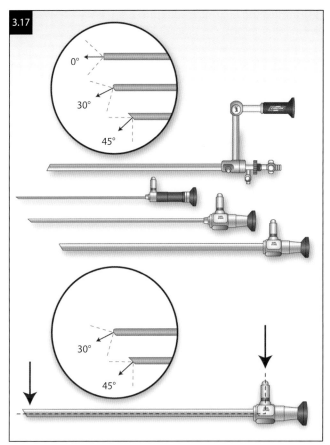

concentrated light intensity at the end of the light cable, a significant amount of heat is produced. Therefore, the end of the light cable should not be placed on drapes or allowed contact with the skin of the patient in order to prevent possible burns.

OPTICS (LAPAROSCOPES)

It is important to obtain as panoramic a view as possible, allowing the operator to coordinate proper placement of the instruments. Often the surgeons do not realize the magnification afforded by laparoscopy. Indeed, the magnification is one of the many advantages of this technique. The lenses in the scope enable magnification up to six times depending on the distance between the end of the scope and the object. At 3 cm from the tip to the object, the magnification is ×4 and at 4 cm it is ×6.

Angle of view: Whereas laparoscopy is still commonly conducted with a 0° view (i.e., looking straight ahead), it may be advantageous to have an angle of vision typically at 30° to facilitate visual access and to provide a more panoramic view of the pelvis. This may be particularly helpful during removal of large uterine fibroids and sacrocolpopexy. For laparoscopes with an angled view, the direction of vision is always pointing opposite the light post. There are also operative laparoscopes available with an operating channel for the insertion of instruments or laser beam (Figure 3.17).

ELECTROSURGICAL GENERATORS

Electrosurgical generators are designed to produce a high-frequency electric energy in either a monopolar or bipolar output (see Chapter 6). Generators have the ability to deliver the energy in either a coagulation/blend (modulated/interrupted) or cutting (nonmodulated/continuous) waveform. Some generators have an ammeter to permit either visually or by sound the monitoring of the current flow. This is important because it informs the

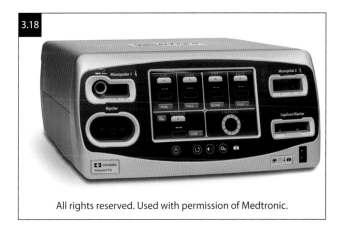

surgeon when complete desiccation of the tissue when sealing a Fallopian tube during sterilization has occurred (see Chapters 6 and 8). Some instruments have built-in circuitry to detect insulation failure or capacitive coupling. The generator may be connected to various instruments including scissors, graspers, needles, and bipolar forceps (Figure 3.18).

OPERATIVE INSTRUMENTS

The instruments used during operative laparoscopy may be divided into the following groups:

1. Graspers—traumatic or atraumatic
2. Cutting instruments

3. Hemostatic ligating and cutting devices
4. Staplers, bipolar graspers, ultrasonic energy instruments, bipolar vessel sealing instruments, ligation and suturing equipment
5. Morcellating and tissue retrieval instruments
6. Irrigation-suction instruments
7. Lasers
8. Specialty instruments (sterilization and mini-instruments)

A complete book would be needed to describe all of the various instruments produced by a myriad number of companies. Therefore, only examples of instruments will be described.

All graspers, whether atraumatic or traumatic, may be found in a variety of diameters and lengths. They usually range from 3 to 11 mm; however, the most commonly used graspers are 5 mm in diameter and 33 cm long. Longer instruments (44 cm) are designed to pass down the channel of operating scopes. Handles are generally of two basic types—those that will lock (box lock type) and handles that are not locked (Figure 3.19). The non-locking handles are best used on dissecting-type instruments. The tips vary in design depending on their use. Some have very rounded tips that are extremely dull, and the inside of the jaws are also blunt with rounded ridges. This style of instrument is best used for mobilization of the bowel and the fallopian tubes (Figure 3.20) and may be referred to as atraumatic. The authors prefer using the atraumatic grasper with locking handle and long jaws by Aesculap (Tuttlingen, Germany) (Figure 3.21). The best way to determine whether an instrument is atraumatic is to grasp the web space between the thumb and forefinger to register undue discomfort. If absolutely pain free, it may be considered atraumatic (Figure 3.22). The more pronounced and sharp the ridges in the jaw, the more traumatic the instrument. This type of instrument should only be used on tissue that will be removed or on tissue

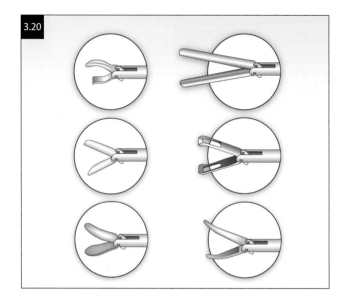

3.20

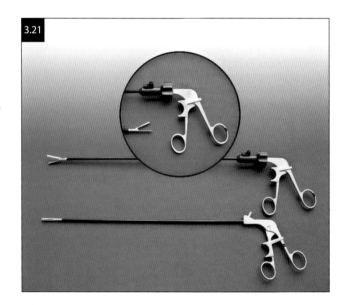

3.21

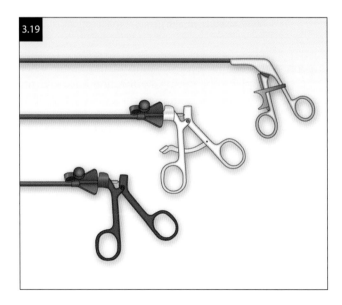

3.19

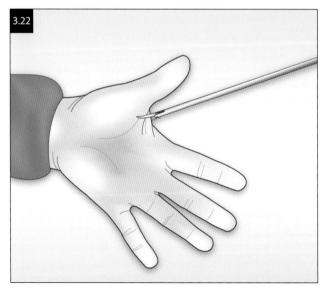

3.22

not expected to bleed (Figure 3.23). It does afford a stronger hold on tissue than the atraumatic type.

Cutting instruments are usually scissors. Laparoscopic scissors may be found in a multitude of forms: straight or curved or hooked and may be reusable or disposable. Some are designed with semidisposable tips that may be replaced after a number of uses or if they become dull. No matter which scissor is used, the most important aspect is having a sharp instrument (Figure 3.24).

Providing improved cosmetics without technical compromise, 3.5 mm mini-laparoscopy instruments by Karl Storz that include both reusable 3.5 mm trocars and a recently introduced 3.5 mm bipolar forceps, can be safely utilized during appropriately chosen cases (Figure 3.25). Pediatric laparoscopy has also necessitated a need for smaller instruments. Small trocar sheaths for 3 mm instruments may be used, but there are even smaller instruments such as the mini-retractor set and grasping instruments. The need for small instruments

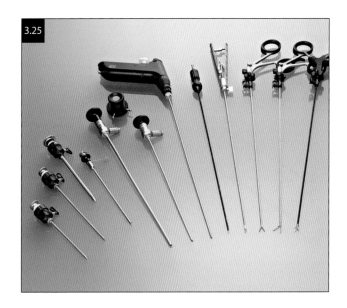

has also been fueled by the desire to produce improved cosmetics and less postoperative incisional pain.

Comprehensively reviewed along with all other currently employed energy-based surgical modalities in Chapter 6, monopolar electrical energy may be delivered to tissue using a laparoscopic scissors for simultaneous coagulation and tissue cutting. Ultrasonic energy may be used either in the form of a cutting blade alone, or as a combination ligating-cutting device that not only incises the tissue, but also coagulates for reliable hemostasis. The use of bipolar electrosurgery is a safe, inexpensive, and reliable modality to control either potential or active bleeding (Figure 3.26). The ROBI reusable laparoscopic bipolar grasper by Karl Storz is available with flat or Haeney-type jaws and provides exceptional desiccation without significant tissue sticking (Figure 3.27). The introduction of advanced bipolar devices provides simultaneous coagulation and cutting of vessels up to 7 mm with demonstrably less lateral thermal damage. The major types of lasers that are currently used for gynecologic

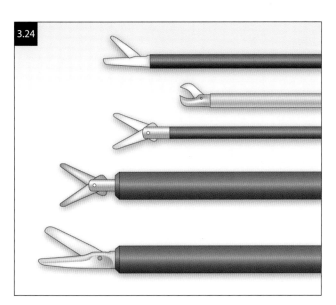

© 2016 KARL STORZ Endoskope

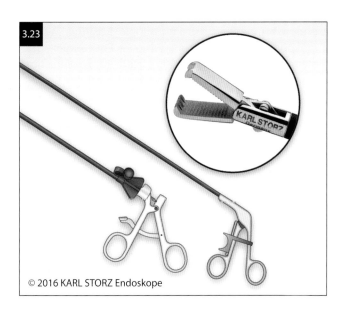

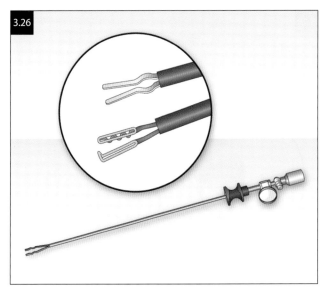

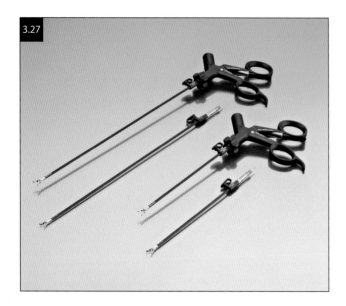

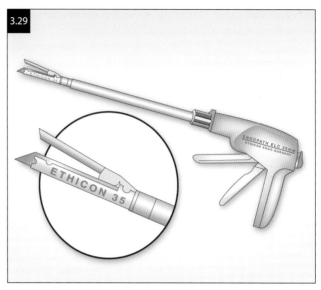

surgery are the CO_2, argon, KTP-532, and the Nd-YAG (neodymium-yttrium, aluminum, garnet). Each of these has various indications that are not within the purview of this chapter. The basic instruments that supply these different energy sources are fairly large, expensive, and require specific training in their use (Figure 3.28).

The initial popularity of linear stapler/cutter instruments to secure and cut vascular pedicles has waned with the introduction of bipolar ligating devices. These stapling devices may now be found in a variety of styles and are useful for rapid cutting of tissue while simultaneously firing a double row of titanium staples for the control of bleeding. The stapler fits through a 12 mm trocar sleeve. The staplers are disposable and use disposable cartridges that have either 48 or 54 titanium staples depending on which company manufactured the stapler. The staple line is approximately 37 mm with a cut line of 33 mm (Ethicon Endosurgery) (Figure 3.29). Another stapler is the Endo GIA Universal Multifire (Tyco Healthcare Inc., Princeton, New Jersey). which is also a

single-use stapler that rotates 360° and can be reloaded and fired multiple times. For bleeding control, another useful instrument is the Endoscopic Rotating Multiple Clip Applier Ligaclip Allport (Ethicon, Endosurgery Inc., Cincinnati, Ohio) that is loaded with 20 medium/large titanium ligating clips (Figure 3.30).

The traditional surgical use of suturing and ligation requires some special materials and equipment. Simple ligation is possible through the use of loop ligation as introduced by Dr. Kurt Semm. This requires an Endoloop (Ethicon Endosurgery Inc., Cincinnati, Ohio) that is a preformed, looped slipknot available in a variety of suture materials and suture sizes (Chapter 7). Endoscopic suturing can be accomplished using a variety of needles and suture materials. The techniques will not be addressed in this chapter; however, some of the instruments that may be required are needle drivers and knot pushers. The revolutionary introduction of barbed sutures such as V-Loc (Covidien), a unidirectional suture system with shallow barbs that are circumferentially distributed, and

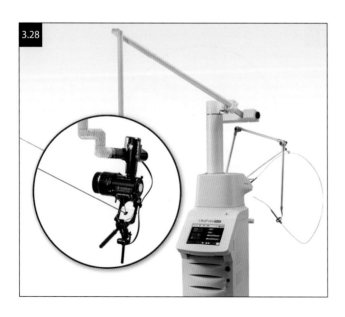

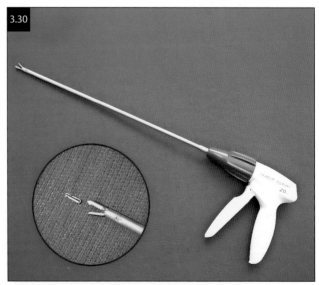

Stratafix (Ethicon), a double-wedged bidirectional system with spiral anchoring. Both systems facilitate wound closure by distributing the forces more evenly along the suture line, eliminating dead space by preventing slippage, and obviating the need to secure with a surgical knot (Figure 3.31).

There are many different types and sizes of needle drivers. Basically, differences are either in the type of handle or tips. A large number of laparoscopic surgeons prefer the pistol grip type of handles. Choosing a laparoscopic needle driver should ultimately depend on its personal handedness and perceived level of ergonomic advantage (Figure 3.32).

For many years, the "Holy Grail" of laparoscopy was the most effective method for removing mass tissue from the peritoneal cavity. Presently the two methods of tissue removal are either through tissue morcellation or by use of a sac, or some combination of both. The ideal method has to be safe and efficient and prevent spillage within the abdomen. A retrieval system plays a vital role in laparoscopic surgery. To supply this system, it may be necessary to use some type of extraction sack. The specimen bag must be used in the removal of ovarian tissue that has a possibility of neoplasia in order to obviate the dissemination of possible malignant cells and prevent spillage during removal of a benign teratoma. It is necessary that a removal bag be very strong so that it may resist breakage in the face of a large force in pulling it through a small opening. The sack also should be easily deployed within the abdomen and be capable of holding

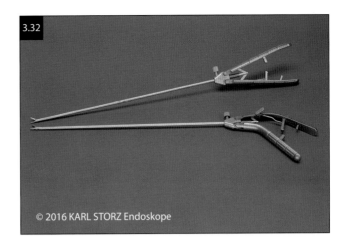

3.32

a mass larger than 10 cm. Newer bags are equipped with self-opening and self-closing mechanisms that facilitate easy removal of tissue. There are several bags on the market, such as the Inzii retrieval systems (Applied Medical, Rancho Santa Margarita, California). The Cook LapSac (Cook Urological, Spencer, Indiana) is a very strong bag made of nylon with a polyurethane coating; however, it is more difficult to place specimens inside of it (Figure 3.33). In response to concerns about the accidental dissemination of a uterine sarcoma, several manufacturers have produced larger and more resilient bags for tissue containment morcellation under directed laparoscopic view.

There are several motorized morcellators that efficiently remove mass tissue from the peritoneal cavity. The Rotocut Morcellator (Karl Storz Endoscopy, Tuttlingen, Germany) (Figure 3.34) does not require the trocar sheath and comes in 12 and 15 mm diameter. LINA Xcise (Lina Medical Formervangen 5, DK-2600 Glostrup, Denmark) is a cordless laparoscopic morcellator that is fully disposable, easy to handle, and effectively and safely morcellates all tissue (Figure 3.35).

Irrigation and aspiration are necessary for operative laparoscopy, because without a clear surgical field, the

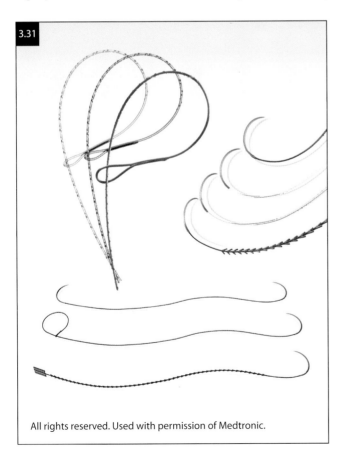

3.31

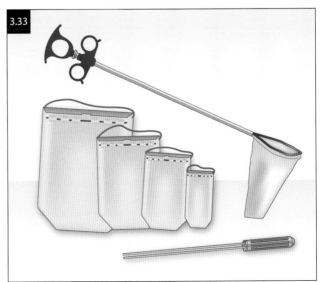

3.33

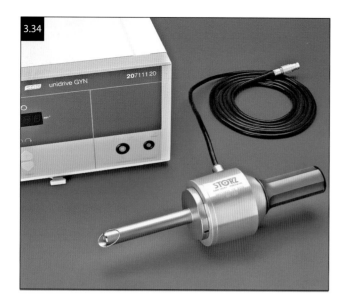

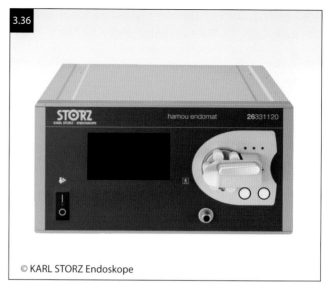

© KARL STORZ Endoskope

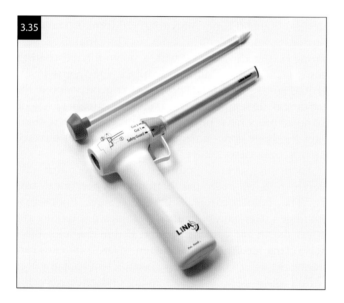

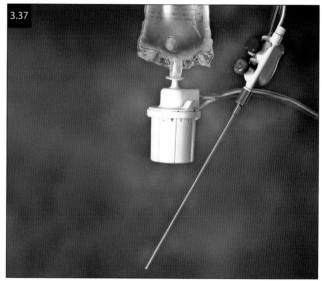

surgeon is blind. Irrigation is used to clear away debris, blood, blood clots, and char that may be produced by electrosurgery or laser treatment. The ideal irrigator must produce enough hydraulic pressure to disrupt clots and assist in hydrodissection. The hand-controlled valve should easily operate both the suction and irrigation. It is important that it be usable with a large enough channel so that large clots may be removed rapidly without clogging the instrument. If the probe tip is to be used for suctioning near the bowel, small holes near the tip are useful to avoid pulling the bowel into the probe. There are several different types of instruments with varied pumps to deliver the fluid for irrigation, such as Endomat (Karl Storz Endoscopy, Tuttlingen, Germany) (Figure 3.36). The disposable suction/irrigator made by Striker Endoscopy is gaining in popularity. It uses a battery-operated disposable pump that is attached to the irrigation fluid bag, and provides excellent fluid pressure (Figure 3.37).

Single-port laparoscopic instruments are described in Chapter 28.

Instruments that are unique to sterilization may be used either through secondary trocars or through the 8 mm channel of an operating laparoscope. The three most commonly used instruments are the Hulka Clip Applicator (Richard Wolf Medical Instruments, Vernon Hills, Illinois), the Filshie Clip Applicator (Avalon Medical Corp., Williston, Vermont), or the Fallope Ring Applicator (Circon Corp., Santa Barbara, California). Their use will be described in Chapter 8.

Although not part of a basic equipment list, robotics are the look of the future. Presently the use of robotics is limited in general gynecology, although there is increasing interest especially in gynecologic oncology (see Chapters 32–36). The most used device is the DaVinci Surgical System (Intuitive Surgery, Mountain View, California). This equipment consists of three parts: a surgeon's console, a video electronics tower, and the robotics' tower that supports three robotic arms. The surgeon sits at the computer console viewing a virtual operative field through a 3D imaging system. His or her hands are inserted into a

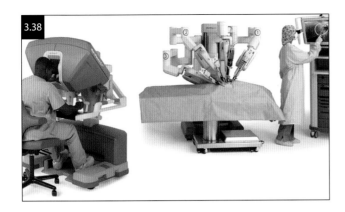

"master" that translates the motions of the surgeon's hands into motions of the robotic arms, which hold two surgical instruments and a video telescope. The hand-like surgical instruments move with 7° of freedom and 2° of axial rotation. The surgeon's feet activate several pedals that control various aspects of the robot's movements (Figure 3.38).

Despite the fact that new instruments are being invented and introduced at a steady pace, the surgeon must be aware of all basic instrumentation currently available and be familiar not only with their function, but how to assemble and troubleshoot their use. The onus for equipment choice and function are solely that of the operating surgeon.

SUGGESTED READING

Hulka JF, Reich H, eds. *Textbook of Laparoscopy*, 2nd ed. Philadelphia, PA: W.B. Saunders; 1994.

Mencaglia L, Wattiez A. *Manual of Gynecological Laparoscopic Surgery*. Germany: Endo-Press Tuttlingen; 2000.

Pasic R. All you need to know about laparoscopic suturing. In: Pasic R and Levine RL, eds. *A Practical Manual of Laparoscopy: A Clinical Cookbook*. 2nd ed. Taylor & Francis Publishing; 2007, Chapter 7, pp. 97–108.

CHAPTER 4

ANESTHESIA IN LAPAROSCOPY

Laura Clark

Many surgical procedures dictate the management of anesthesia. The procedure of laparoscopy creates its own subset of factors unique to the procedure itself. The impact of laparoscopy on the human body went relatively unnoticed in its infancy because the majority of cases initially were laparoscopic tubal sterilizations performed in a relatively short time on young, healthy individuals.

Barring complications, these individuals could adjust quite well to the changes that occur during laparoscopy. Only when the technique expanded, both in use and type of operations, was the full impact apparent. Presently, laparoscopic operations are frequently longer, and the population may have other disease processes and may even be elderly. This subset of patients has not been able to compensate as well as young, healthy patients, and the true impact of these physiologic changes is being delineated. This expansion has been a useful and productive development, but as shown later in this chapter, the choice of laparoscopy versus an open procedure is made by the physiologic impact of the laparoscopy on the individual patient during the operative procedure and not only on the physical factor of surgery without a major incision.

LAPAROSCOPY CAN BE BENEFICIAL

- LESS PAIN
- EARLY MOBILIZATION
- SHORT TO NO HOSPITALIZATION

VERY SICK PATIENTS MAY NOT BE CANDIDATES

- CANNOT COMPENSATE FOR CHANGES THAT OCCUR DURING LAPAROSCOPY

Anesthesia must accomplish amnesia, analgesia, and maintenance physiologic processes to maintain homeostasis during the surgery. Laparoscopic procedures may produce physiologic changes secondary to the procedures required to accomplish visualization of the anatomy in order to complete the surgery without opening the abdomen.

The creation and maintenance of a pneumoperitoneum in the Trendelenburg position are unique requirements of gynecologic laparoscopic surgery and produce responses that have specific impact on the physiology of the patient. How the patient responds depends on the initial health of the individual and what compensatory mechanisms the patient can maintain. The impact on the patient can be minor to severe. Complications can occur inherent to the milieu that must be created to successfully operate.

The major task of the anesthesiologist and surgeon is to recognize that anesthetic issues related to laparoscopic surgery exist and must be recognized. Awareness of these issues allows good outcomes, even in high-risk patients, comparable to those of low-risk patients. The anesthesiologist and surgeon working in concert with good communication will avoid or promptly recognize potential complications that can occur.

PHYSIOLOGIC CHANGES

The patient responses resulting during laparoscopy can be divided into mechanical and physiologic. Mechanical changes are a result of the physical pressure of superinflating the abdominal cavity and the challenges to the system from being placed in steep Trendelenburg position. Physiologic changes are a result of the absorption of CO_2 and the neurohormonal response to the procedure.

CHANGES

1. MECHANICAL
2. PHYSIOLOGICAL

CARDIOVASCULAR AND RESPIRATORY SYSTEMS ARE THE MOST INVOLVED.

The respiratory and cardiovascular systems are the primary systems involved. However, hepatic, gastrointestinal, renal, and cerebral changes have been described. These changes can range in severity from unnoticed to severe depending on the initial condition of the patient. A detailed preoperative assessment is imperative in the compromised patient when laparoscopic surgery is an option. For this reason, some severely ill patients are not candidates for laparoscopy even though the operation is possible by this method.

MECHANICAL EFFECTS

CARDIOVASCULAR

Pneumoperitoneum

Just as one might expect, there is a mechanical pressure effect on the large vessels from the pneumoperitoneum. Aortic compression will increase systemic vascular resistance (SVR) coupled with inferior vena cava and intraabdominal vessel compression, causing an initial brief increase in preload. This is short lived but results in a decrease in preload and, thus, in a decrease in cardiac output. The greater the intraabdominal pressure, the more pronounced these effects become on the patient. The compression of intraabdominal vessels is minimally decreased with insufflation pressures between 7 and 12 mm Hg if the patient is adequately hydrated. There is a direct correlation between intraabdominal pressure and perfusion. Any incremental increase in pressure must be justified as cardiac output, and impact to perfusion of internal organs may suffer. Pressure near 25 mm Hg should be avoided for any length of time due to a significant decrease in perfusion at this level. However, elevated pressures for a short period of time during placement of the initial port are usually well tolerated. Effects at any pressure will be pronounced in the patient with hypovolemia. It is important to maintain adequate intravenous fluids during the operation to augment perfusion pressure and venous return during pneumoperitoneum.

> IVC AND AORTIC COMPRESSION
> INCREASED SVR
> INCREASED PRELOAD FOLLOWED BY
>
> • DECREASED PRELOAD
> • DECREASED CO₂
> • INCREASED OR NO CHANGE HEART RATE

If deterioration is seen, it is prudent to communicate with the anesthesiologist and decrease the insufflation. Improvement is often achieved with a small decrease in pressure without affecting operating conditions. The act of inflating the abdomen and the ensuing distension may stimulate the vagus nerve resulting in marked bradycardia requiring vagolytic drugs.

PATIENT POSITION

Most gynecologic operations are accomplished in the Trendelenburg position. Elevation of the lower body and the head-down position will cause an initial increase in venous return by an increase in the preload as the lower limbs are elevated. This has minimal detrimental impact on the healthy patient.

For the compromised patient, this can present as an overload to the heart and precipitate or worsen existing congestive heart failure. Interpretation of pressures from a Swan-Ganz or central venous catheter should be interpreted with caution and may not be reliable in this position.

> A SMALL DECREASE IN INTRAABDOMINAL PRESSURE MAY BE ALL THAT IS NEEDED TO IMPROVE HEMODYNAMICS.

> TRY TO AVOID UNNECESSARY TRENDELENBURG.

PULMONARY

The effects of laparoscopy in the supine position are limited to a decrease in compliance and a possible increase in peak airway pressure. These are usually not a problem except in the obese patient. The effects of Trendelenburg on the respiratory system can be severe in all patients, but the possibility of serious compromise is magnified in the obese or those with asthma or other pulmonary disease. These effects may be so critical that the patient cannot be adequately ventilated in this position.

The compression of the viscera in the Trendelenburg position can cause the diaphragm to move cephalad (Figure 4.1). This may increase the work of ventilation resulting in increased airway pressure, decreased compliance, decreased vital capacity (VC), and decreased

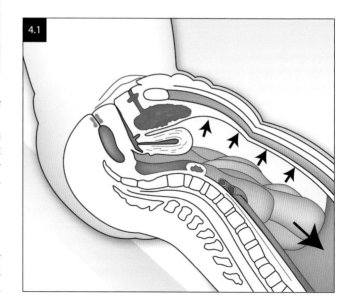

4.1

functional residual capacity (FRC). Even in healthy patients, these can be changed by as much as 50%.

PULMONARY EFFECTS INCLUDE THE FOLLOWING:

↓ COMPLIANCE
↑ AIRWAY PRESSURE
↓ FRC
↓ VC

The endotracheal tube may become endobronchial with the Trendelenburg position. The endotracheal tube does not actually move, but the movement of the abdominal contents forward may cause the tube to favor one bronchus or actually enter the bronchus creating a one-lung ventilation scenario. This also causes an increase in the peak airway pressure and a picture similar to Trendelenburg itself. One should not assume the position is responsible, but should listen to both lungs once the position is assumed and at any time during the operation that a drop in oxygen saturation occurs. Once two-lung ventilation is assured, and barring other physiologic effects, a decrease in intraabdominal pressure and a decrease in severity of Trendelenburg may result in improvement.

BE ALERT FOR ENDOBRONCHIAL INTUBATION WHEN PATIENT IS PLACED IN TRENDLEBURG

PHYSIOLOGIC CHANGES

PULMONARY

Carbon dioxide is absorbed into the bloodstream in a variable manner. Hypercapnea may increase moderately or profoundly and is thought to be due primarily to the absorption of CO_2 rather than decreased mechanical ventilation. The increase may occur early and become fairly steady state in most patients with an increase in minute ventilation of 30%. If compensatory mechanisms are not available to the patient because of other organ system disease, a significant acidosis can develop.

This trend can be observed to some degree from end-tidal CO_2 monitoring but is not reliable. There can be a significant difference in the end-tidal and arterial values. Arterial trends may be monitored with frequent arterial samples from an arterial line in very long cases or in medically compromised patients. The ability to eliminate CO_2 varies widely and may persist for several hours. It is not uncommon to see elevated hemidiaphragm in a postoperative x-ray. The absorption is greater if the insufflation has occurred in the subcutaneous or extraperitoneal tissue; thus, a larger increase in CO_2 in the arterial system should be expected.

NEED TO INCREASE MINUTE VENTILATION BY 30% OR MORE.
ARTERIAL LINE MAY BE NECESSARY TO MONITOR pH IN PATIENTS WHO WOULD NOT NEED ONE IN AN OPEN PROCEDURE.
↓ pH COULD BE SEVERE.
TWO IVs ARE RECOMMENDED

The anesthesiologist will increase the minute ventilation to help compensate for this change, but such increases may not be successful in ill patients. The patient could be placed in a severely acidotic state. Since this is temporary, bicarbonate use would outlast the operation and usually is not considered an option. This possibility must be considered, as the condition of some patients may not tolerate this situation even on a temporary basis. Respiratory status should also be considered. One study suggests that a forced expiratory volume of less than 70% or a diffusion defect less than 80% would identify patients at risk.

IF FEV IS <70% OR DIFFUSION CAPACITY IS <80%, THE PATIENT MAY NOT BE A CANDIDATE FOR LAPAROSCOPY.

CARDIOVASCULAR

Physiologic effects on the cardiovascular system are primarily related to the establishment of a pneumoperitoneum and the intravascular absorption of carbon dioxide. Cardiovascular effects may or may not be apparent initially on monitoring systems and vary according to the patient's inherent condition. Initial changes depend on preexisting conditions and on the ability of the patient to compensate.

CARDIOVASCULAR

↑ SVR
↑ SHUNT
↓ OR ↑ MEAN ARTERIAL BP
↓ OR NO CHANGE IN HR
↓ CO_2

Absorption of carbon dioxide occurs immediately and can affect the pH and lead to significant changes in the arterial blood gas after a variable amount of time depending on the condition of the patient. After 60–120 minutes, the storage mechanism for carbon dioxide can be impacted. The body can store up to 120 L of CO_2. Baseline adult CO_2 production is then augmented by absorption of carbon dioxide from the abdomen. This can lead to a pH of 7.1 or lower in longer cases or compromised patients.

Hypercapnea, $PaCO_2$ of 45–50 mm Hg is "normal" during this operation and may result in sympathetic stimulation. The initial effect is an increase in blood pressure, heart rate, and cardiac output. One study comparing nitrogen to CO_2 insufflation found a decrease in stroke volume and tachycardia that did not occur with nitrogen. These direct effects on the cardiovascular system are felt to be directly due to acid-base pH changes due to absorption of carbon dioxide.

While under anesthesia, the normal mechanism of increasing minute ventilation is accomplished by the anesthesiologist through the manipulation of ventilator settings. Changing minute ventilation can only accommodate minor absorption of carbon dioxide. The body's compensatory mechanisms of maintaining acid-base are primary. A $PaCO_2$ of 60 may be unavoidable and can cause severe acidosis, arrhythmias, and severe myocardial depression. Although time dependent, this can occur at variable times in compromised patients. Preexisting conditions must be considered when selecting candidates for laparoscopy. Certainly, this class of patients has a significant propensity to develop cardiac compromise requiring diligent monitoring by the anesthesiologist and a low tolerance by the surgeon to convert to an open procedure. Frequent blood gases should be obtained to monitor the patient's status, because end tidal CO_2 often does not correlate with arterial levels.

> Swan-Ganz is not reliable in Trendelenburg. May need transesophageal echocardiography (TEE) to monitor a compromised patient.

Acid-base changes resolve over time after release of the carbon dioxide at the end of the operation. Every effort should be made to minimize residual carbon dioxide in the abdomen, because hemodynamic effects will persist in the recovery room until normal acid-base balance returns.

OTHER SYSTEMS

Arrhythmias are very common, occur early, and therefore are not thought to be due to the presence of increased CO_2. Other than arrhythmias secondary to intubation, bradycardia most often occurs during insufflation due to distension of the peritoneum, vagal stimulation, or traction on viscera. They can manifest in patients without a history of cardiac disease. Although all types of arrhythmias have been reported and can occur, life-threatening

arrhythmias are rare. While ectopy is common, asystole is very rare and most often associated with severe complications such as gas embolism, and severe hypoventilation, hypertension, and acidosis.

OTHER SYSTEMS

- ↓ Glomerular filtration rate
- ↑ Gastric pH
- ↓ Splanchnic flow

---

*Pre-op visit: goal—to optimize the medical condition:

- Perform history and physical
- Order lab tests
- Modify treatment regimens
- Identify cardiovascular disease
- Optimize congestive heart failure
- Order pulmonary function tests, if indicated

* Recommend holding ACE inhibitors the day of surgery—continue other medications.

Although usually transient, arrhythmias should be treated if the underlying cause is known. Most often an anticholinergic drug such as Robinul or atropine, and slowing or stopping insufflation, will restore sinus rhythm.

PREOPERATIVE ASSESSMENT

The preoperative assessment of the patient is imperative for the successful outcome of any surgical procedure. In laparoscopy this is twofold. Obviously, any patient will have a better outcome if his or her medical condition is optimized. The surgeon and the anesthesiologist should assess the patient's condition as soon as the operation is planned, so that adjustments may be made to improve her condition and optimize her medical status prior to surgery. This is more important in the aging and elderly patient but should not be overlooked in the younger patient as well. Asthma or uncontrolled hypertension may have ramifications that can be magnified by laparoscopy and should, therefore, be well controlled. Many more elderly patients are now being placed on angiotensin-converting enzyme (ACE) inhibitors to optimize their cardiac status. These drugs should be stopped the day before surgery to minimize hypertension at the time of anesthesia induction. All other cardiac medication, other than diuretics, which can be administered at the discretion of the anesthesiologist during the procedure, should be maintained. All these issues can be addressed with a timely preoperative visit to the anesthesiologist.

ANESTHETIC CHOICES

1. MONITORED ANESTHESIA
2. REGIONAL
3. GENERAL

The preoperative visit is vital to the success of a tubal sterilization in which the patient and her physicians have elected to accomplish with monitored anesthesia, a sedated and conscious patient without general anesthesia. This is not a widely accepted method, and the surgeon and the anesthesiologist need to communicate with each other concerning the acceptability of each patient for this method. Several conditions must be met for the procedure to be successful. If steep Trendelenburg is required the patient should be informed of the likelihood of facial edema so that they are not alarmed. While optimum fluid management can decrease the edema it rarely can be totally eliminated.

MONITORED ANESTHESIA CARE

Although not as widely accepted as a common clinical practice, short procedures such as tubal sterilizations can be performed with a sedated but arousable patient with proper precautions.

Some anesthesiologists will not perform monitored anesthesia care (MAC) for this procedure, citing concern for the airway, patient comfort, and the ability to ensure adequate respiration in the Trendelenburg position. This also holds true for a regional technique, although spinal, epidural, and monitored anesthesia care has been used in this procedure. Many general surgeons also have reservations in performing this procedure without general anesthesia.

The surgeon must be efficient and adept at handling tissue gently, and adequately anesthetize the tissue with local anesthesia. The anesthesiologist must be able to sedate the patient adequately without losing the patient's protective reflexes. An informed, motivated patient is the best choice for this technique.

We have performed large numbers of these procedures in this manner with highly successful outcomes and pleased and satisfied patients. To be successful, this method requires more work and preplanning on the part of the surgeons and anesthesiologists. The main factor that would exclude the patient as a candidate for this procedure is morbid obesity because of the technical difficulties involved in each aspect of the operation. In the preoperative clinic visit, each patient is shown a video detailing all aspects of the procedure, which uses such phrases as "when the gas enters your abdomen you will feel as if you are pregnant" and "when your head is lowered it feels like you are standing on your head."

> SURGEON MUST BE REASONABLY EFFICIENT WITH SHORT DURATION OF OPERATIVE TIMES FOR MAC TO BE SUCCESSFUL.

Trendelenburg positioning may be duplicated on the stretcher prior to surgery to make sure the patient is comfortable with that position (Figure 4.2). Some surgeons require more Trendelenburg angle than others, which may exclude this method for certain patients for whom the excessive tilt is uncomfortable. The ability to accept this position is usually the most common limiting factor for the patient.

> • A VIDEO OF THE PROCEDURE IS VERY IMPORTANT TO INFORM THE PATIENT OF WHAT TO EXPECT.

The video of the procedure is extremely important because the patient becomes a participant in the procedure, and her understanding of every aspect is vital to the successful outcome. The patient is instructed that she will receive sedation by the anesthesiologist as she wishes, but it should be emphasized that there are aspects she may be aware of but that should not be painful. The pressure of the gas in her abdomen and insertion of the trocar are the main stimulating events. If the sensation is disturbing, a small release in pressure usually makes the patient more comfortable without compromising the visualization of the surgical field. During insertion of the Veress needle or trocar, the surgeon can time the insertion by observing the movement of the abdomen with respiration. No attempt is made to coerce the patient or give her unrealistic expectations, but if she is told of the likelihood of these sensations ahead of time, the patient can make an informed decision during surgery.

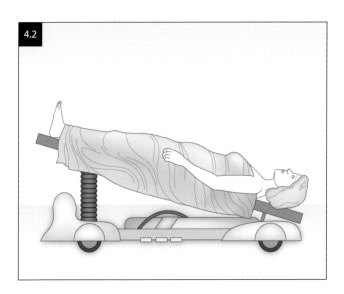

4.2

An important adjunct to the clinic visit is the clinic nurse. She helps to explain the procedure in her own words and past experiences are shared. Her adeptness at quickly establishing a rapport with the patient is vital as an additional source of information. She will also accompany the physician to the operating room, which greatly enhances continuity of care and an atmosphere of patient trust.

BIS INDEX RANGE

100   AWAKE
      • RESPONDS TO NORMAL VOICE
80   LIGHT/MODERATE SEDATION
      • MAY RESPOND TO LOUD COMMANDS OR MILD PRODDING/SHAKING
60   GENERAL ANESTHESIA
      • LOW PROBABILITY OF EXPLICIT RECALL
      • UNRESPONSIVE TO VERBAL STIMULUS
40   DEEP HYPNOTIC STATE
20   • BURST SUPPRESSION

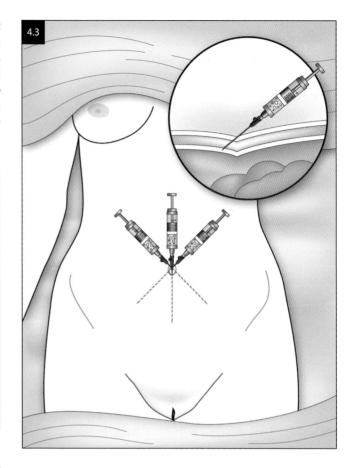

Given a motivated, knowledgeable patient, a safe and successful operation will depend on the skills of the surgeon and anesthesiologist. Enough volume and proper deposition of local anesthetic must be utilized. A paracervical block facilitates the tenaculum placement on the cervix. A uterine manipulator that can be used to perform transuterine hydrotubation is placed into the cervix.

The skin of the abdomen in the umbilical region is infiltrated with 1% lidocaine, usually with a small gauge needle initially (Figure 4.3). A 22-gauge spinal needle may follow, as its length is needed in a four-quadrant pattern to anesthetize the skin and subcutaneous tissue. It takes at least 15–20 cc of lidocaine to be adequate. The 22-gauge spinal needle is then inserted into the fascia, and approximately 10 cc of local anesthetic is deposited directly into the fascia. This should permit insertion of the Veress needle and trocar. At this stage, 20 cc of 0.5% xylocaine is infused through the uterine manipulator (Figure 4.4). After ensuring entry into the abdomen, lidocaine is dripped into each tube under direct visualization (Figure 4.5). This usually takes 10 cc per tube.

The anesthesiologist will provide sedation according to the patient's needs. Occasionally, some patients will watch the procedure on the monitors, although this is uncommon. Preoperative anxiolytics titrated with midazolam is usually adequate. Speech may begin to slur or a slight disinhibition may be observed. Occasionally, 50 μg of fentanyl is needed to augment the sedation. While the monitors are being attached, a propofol drip is started at 25 μg/kg/min. This allows a blood level to be

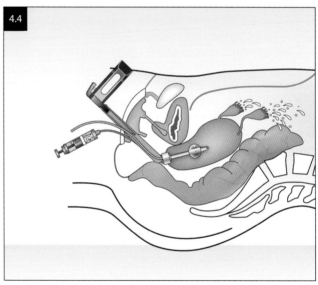

achieved gradually over time so that a bolus is not necessary prior to the beginning of surgery. It is important to maintain a level of sedation where patients are arousable but sedated. This is usually accomplished with a combination of midazolam, fentanyl, and propofol. Usually a propofol drip is the primary sedating agent with fentanyl given only as necessary. One method is a combination of 50 mg (1 cc) of ketamine to 50 cc (500 mg) of propofol for the maintenance infusion. If this method is chosen, very little fentanyl is necessary. The amount of ketamine is so small that dysphoria is not encountered. The ketamine,

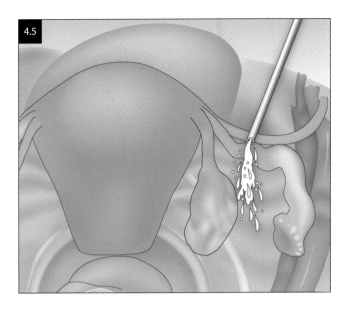

process. All of the routine monitors should be employed for this procedure.

In elderly patients, or during a prolonged procedure, an arterial line pressure monitor may sometimes be helpful to determine acid-base status. Other invasive monitors are used as the patient condition warrants.

General anesthesia for laparoscopy should always be accompanied by endotracheal intubation to ensure protection of the airway secondary to increased intraabdominal pressure and the Trendelenburg position.

After the airway has been secured and the endotracheal tube position is confirmed, an orogastric tube should be inserted for decompression of the stomach prior to instrumentation of the abdomen. This minimizes the risk of puncturing the stomach in addition to emptying it to help minimize nausea and vomiting during recovery.

however, provides some augmentation of analgesia and sedation with no respiratory depression. In addition to the usual monitors for general anesthesia, end-tidal CO_2 monitors as well as a BIS monitor are useful. This information will help monitor sedation levels and respiratory pattern without disturbing a sedated patient. It must be stressed that verbal communication should always be possible to assure the presence of adequate airway reflexes. The BIS levels for this type of anesthesia are somewhat patient variable, but are usually in the 75–85 range.

NITROUS OXIDE CAN BE USED FOR SHORTER PROCEDURES.

A HIGH CONCENTRATION OF OXYGEN HAS BEEN SHOWN TO DECREASE THE INCIDENCE OF NAUSEA AND VOMITING.

PROPOFOL HAS ALSO BEEN SHOWN TO DECREASE NAUSEA AND VOMITING.

SUSPECT SUBCUTANEOUS INFILTRATIONS WITH LARGE INCREASES IN END-TIDAL CO_2.

POSTOPERATIVE VENTILATION MAY BE REQUIRED IN SEVERE CASES.

- ELECTROCARDIOGRAM (ECG), 3–5 LEAD DEPENDING ON THE PATIENT'S CONDITION
- BLOOD PRESSURE
- OXYGEN SATURATION
- END-TIDAL CO_2
- INSPIRATORY AND END-TIDAL ANESTHETIC AGENT CONCENTRATIONS
- BIS MONITOR
- ESOPHAGEAL STETHOSCOPE
- MUSCLE TWITCH MONITOR

The anesthesiologist must be prepared at any time to intubate the patient and proceed with general anesthesia. This could be for surgical or anesthetic reasons such as complications or discomfort. The continuing communication between the surgeon and the anesthesiologist will allow the optimum conditions to be achieved for all parties.

GENERAL ANESTHESIA

General anesthesia is by far the most common method of anesthesia for laparoscopy. In an adequately prepared patient, laparoscopy has greatly accelerated the recovery

General anesthesia can be accomplished by the intravenous or inhalation method. The use of N_2O varies by anesthesiologist. Its effects on nausea and possible increased bowel distension are controversial. It has been reported that if the procedure lasts longer than 30 minutes, there is enough N_2O to support combustion.

If the patient gives a positive history of nausea, elimination of N_2O, as well as the use of antiemetics may be of some benefit. The use of 80% oxygen may also reduce nausea and vomiting and decrease the incidence of wound infections. Routine use of antiemetics is not indicated. A muscle relaxant that does not require reversal may also improve the chances of eliminating nausea during recovery. The use of propofol for induction and as the primary anesthetic, or as an adjunct to decrease the amount of inhalation agent, will also help to prevent nausea and vomiting and provide a quick recovery. However, in high-risk patients, treatment with an antiemetic, dexamethasone 4–8 mg, and Reglan or droperidol may be beneficial.

Different antiemetics used postoperatively in the recovery period may also be considered if nausea becomes a problem during that time.

Ventilation can be challenging in the steep Trendelenburg position. As previously mentioned, some hypercarbia can be expected and usually can be managed with an increased respiratory rate. If hypoxia despite PEEP and alteration of ventilator settings or very high pressures are necessary for ventilation, the patient may benefit from less Trendelenburg or less insufflation pressure. Good communication between surgeon and anesthesiologist is essential in this situation.

With the advent of suggamadex recent articles have introduced the possibility of less insufflation pressure (7–8 mm) with maintenance of a deep neuromuscular blockade till the end of the case rather than letting the neuromuscular blockade be moderate as the procedure progresses. Bruintjes found that deep neuromuscular blockade improved surgical space conditions during laparoscopic surgery and reduced postoperative pain scores in the postanesthesia care unit (Bruintjes et al. 2011).

Other articles have related lower insufflation to decreased referred pain. While not all studies have been positive and whether maintenance of deep blockade leads to fewer intraoperative complications, improved operating conditions or lower opioid requirements and a better quality of recovery, will be further delineated in future studies.

COMPLICATIONS

PULMONARY EMBOLISM

Pulmonary embolism, although rare, is possibly due to the venous stasis that may occur from the obstruction of flow secondary to the pneumoperitoneum. Even minimal insufflation values of 12 mm Hg can result in venous stasis that is not affected by external compression devices. Pulmonary embolism should always be considered in the differential diagnosis of cardiac compromise.

PNEUMOTHORAX, PNEUMOMEDIASTINUM, AND PNEUMOPERICARDIUM

Intraperitoneal gas may find its way through openings in the diaphragm and esophageal hiatus that are congenital or surgically created inadvertently. Any interruption in the falciform ligament may also allow access for movement of gas and unwanted accumulation in the mediastinum. Opening of pleural peritoneal ducts, as in ascites, may also lead to the accumulation of gas in the mediastinum or to pneumothorax. Pneumothorax is the most common of the three and can also occur from positive pressure ventilation. Pleural tears may also occur iatrogenically. End-tidal CO_2 will increase unless the pneumothorax is from a spontaneous cause. Tension pneumothorax is a possibility if the pneumothorax goes unrecognized. Whatever their origin, this must be recognized as quickly as possible. Risk factors include end-tidal CO_2 greater than 50 mm Hg and duration of operation greater than 200 minutes.

> GAS FOLLOWS OPENINGS IN THE DIAPHRAGM AND ESOPHAGEAL HIATUS OR PNEUMOTHORAX.
>
> AN INCREASE IN AIRWAY PRESSURE WITH DECREASE IN CARDIOVASCULAR STATUS IS SEEN.
>
> THIS RESOLVES WITH RELEASE OF INTRAABDOMINAL GAS.
>
> LIMIT PRESSURE TO LOWEST POSSIBLE LEVELS.

Recognition of increasing airway pressure is the earliest sign. Blood pressure may not decrease until some time has passed. End-tidal CO_2 and $PaCO_2$ will increase much sooner than blood pressure changes. Oxygenation itself may or may not be affected. Auscultation will reveal decreased breath sounds. The surgeon may be asked to look at the diaphragm for uncoordinated motion on one side. Tension pneumothorax should always be considered as a possibility. Other common causes such as migration of the endotracheal tube into one bronchus may be possible. Treatment consists of identifying the cause and supporting the patient by increasing the pressure in the alveoli to decrease the tendency for compression. Utilizing positive end-expiratory pressure, increasing the minute ventilation, and oxygen concentration will usually result in an improvement. If the patient tolerates this and improves, chest tube placement is not required, and spontaneous resolution usually occurs within 60 minutes of release of abdominal gas.

If N_2O is used, it should be stopped, and ventilator settings should be adjusted. Communication with the surgeon to reduce intraabdominal pressure as much as possible, and careful observation of the patient should correct the situation without thoracentesis. Limiting the intraabdominal pressure to the lowest possible levels will decrease the incidence. The most helpful monitor in this situation is transesophageal echocardiography.

PNEUMOMEDIASTINUM

Accumulation in these areas is rare in gynecologic procedures and occurs most often with retroperitoneal laparoscopy. These usually resolve spontaneously within 3–4 days. Pneumopericardium can be life threatening if large but should not be an isolated event.

Limiting the intraabdominal pressure to the lowest possible levels will decrease the incidence. The most helpful diagnostic tool is transesophageal echocardiography.

SUBCUTANEOUS EMPHYSEMA

Subcutaneous emphysema occurs as CO_2 dissects through peritoneal defects into the subcutaneous tissue. SQ emphysema can be seen on CT and ultrasound frequently. It can be subclinical or can range to moderate or severe with compromise of the physical airway or physiologically effect the carbon dioxide concentration. Any increase in end-tidal CO_2 that does not respond to increased minute ventilation should lead to suspicion of subcutaneous emphysema. A correlation exists with more than six ports and prolonged operative time. The patient should be physically observed and examined and preferably not totally covered with drapes. If crepitus and swelling of the tissue are seen, the case should be converted to open or aborted. The patient should be monitored after the procedure because absorption of carbon dioxide may cause hypoventilation due to a decreased respiratory drive and may even require mechanical ventilation. Depending on the level of arterial CO_2, the patient will often need mechanical ventilation until the CO_2 levels return to normal. This usually resolves within 24 hours or less depending on the severity.

GAS EMBOLISM

Gas embolism may occur from direct insufflation into a vessel or organ from direct needle or trocar placement. There appears to be an increased incidence during hysteroscopy more than laparoscopy. The volume of gas necessary to produce symptoms is 25 mL/kg of CO_2 as opposed to 5 mL/kg of air. It usually occurs at the beginning of surgery, so insufflation techniques that assure the surgeon of proper placement of the Veress needle are important. The Veress needle allows no more than approximately 2–3 L/min to be infused due to the diameter of the needle. If proper technique is used, then it is not necessary to limit the flow to 1 L/min. However, the patient is always watched carefully during initial insufflation. Signs of embolism include tachycardia, arrhythmias, hypotension, millwheel murmur, and ECG signs of right heart strain. End-tidal CO_2 may be decreased due to the decrease in cardiac output. Aspiration of gas, foamy blood from a central venous line, or air bubbles demonstrated on TEE will provide definitive diagnosis. To help reverse the symptoms, deflate the abdomen with the patient placed in the head down and left lateral position trying to keep as much CO_2 as possible in the right atrium, administer 100% oxygen, and aspirate as much gas as possible. Although gas embolism may be fatal, rapid diagnosis and treatment are highly successful as long as blood pressure is supported.

AIR (GAS) EMBOLISM

INCREASED INCIDENCE WITH HYSTEROSCOPY BUT CAN OCCUR WITH LAPAROSCOPY.
SIGNS: INCREASED HEART RATE, DECREASED BLOOD PRESSURE, ARRHYTHMIAS, MILLWHEEL MURMUR, ECG SIGNS OF RIGHT HEART STRAIN

TREATMENT: MUST ACT QUICKLY TO AVOID SEVERE COMPLICATIONS OR DEATH: HEAD DOWN, LEFT LATERAL POSITION, 100% OXYGEN, ASPIRATE GAS FROM CENTRAL LINE, SUPPORT BLOOD PRESSURE WITH ISOTOPES

NAUSEA AND VOMITING

PROPHYLACTIC TREATMENT NOT INDICATED UNLESS POSITIVE RISK FACTORS OR HISTORY
MULTI-MODAL ANALGESIA TO MINIMIZE OPIOID USE

- METOCLOPRAMIDE
- ANTIEMETIC OF CHOICE
- PROMPT TREATMENT IF IT OCCURS
- SMALL AMOUNTS OF STEROIDS AND BENADRYL MAY HELP
- ALLOW ENOUGH TIME TO EXPEL AS MUCH GAS AS POSSIBLE

POSTOPERATIVE RECOVERY AND THE TREATMENT OF POSTOPERATIVE PAIN

A significant advance in the treatment of postoperative pain has occurred with the implementation of multimodal analgesia. Multimodal therapy is based on the concept that multiple receptors transmit pain, and there is no one drug that acts at all receptors. In addition, with an insult such as surgery, numerous humoral factors are released in the blood. A local anesthetic block will not address those factors although a block may decrease the level of their release. More and more evidence substantiates that the overuse of one modality such as opioids will only increase the incidence of side effects and not the amount of pain relief. The World Health Organization and many other organizations promote a step-wise approach to pain therapy. The initial pharmacology should consist of nonsteroidal anti-inflammatory drugs (NSAIDs), if not contraindicated, and acetaminophen. Intravenous formulations of both have recently been U.S. Food and Drug Administration (FDA) approved. Since a significant component of the pain from surgery results from the incision or incisions in the abdominal wall, local anesthetic solutions have been utilized as a component of multimodal therapy. They should be the first line of therapy followed by adjunct opioids such as short-acting agents for moderate pain. For severe pain, the addition of long-acting opioids is warranted. Local anesthetic infiltration is applicable at any level. Ketorolac and COX-2 inhibitors are helpful adjuncts for the treatment of pain and will decrease the amount of opioids needed. Transdermal scopolamine and Benadryl may also be of benefit. At the time of skin closure, 60–80 mg of Toradol may avoid postoperative cramping.

Other adjuncts to consider are gabapentin or pregabalin, ketamine in small doses intraoperatively, magnesium, or alpha-agonists. A transition from intravenous to oral occurs when the patient's condition warrants. As uterine pain has a significant prostaglandin component, antiprostaglandins are quite effective in this population and should be a component whenever possible.

Postoperative nausea and vomiting can be significant problems. A positive history should be treated with preventive measures. Metoclopramide will help to empty the stomach preoperatively. Careful suctioning of the orogastric tube prior to emergence will relieve the stomach distension that may have occurred intraoperatively. For patients with a positive history, an antiemetic and 4 mg dexamethasone prior to emergence is indicated as well as a propofol-based anesthetic. Prompt treatment in the recovery room with antiemetics and a steroid will usually prevent a continuing problem. A multimodal treatment of pain will prevent total dependence on opioids and thus lessen the propensity for nausea and vomiting. Allowing enough time for as much gas as possible to escape the abdomen is an important and often neglected step in providing patient comfort.

A lidocaine-ropivacaine drip on the fallopian tubes will greatly decrease the pain of tubal ligation. Preemptive analgesia by local infiltration of the skin prior to instrumentation is a useful adjunct if done with a long-acting anesthetic in combination with lidocaine. Many maneuvers have attempted to decrease shoulder pain. Instillation of a long-acting anesthetic may help this condition in some patients. Some studies show that if the insufflation gas is heated and hydrated, the incidence of shoulder pain decreases.

Recently there has been an increasing application of local injection in the plane that is created between the transversus abdominis and the internal oblique muscle. The transversus abdominis plane (TAP) block has the advantage of no catheter site in contrast to the currently used multiport catheter and elastomeric pump. This technique can be used for any surgery involving the abdominal wall, including bowel surgery, cesarean section, appendectomy, hernia repair, umbilical surgery, and gynecological surgery.

Innervation of the anterolateral abdominal wall arises from the anterior rami of spinal nerves T7-L1. Branches from the anterior rami include the intercostal nerves (T7-T11), the subcostal nerve (T12), and the iliohypogastric and ilioinguinal nerves (L1). These give rise to lateral cutaneous and anterior cutaneous branches as they become more superficial. The intercostal nerves T7-T11 exit the intercostal spaces and run in the neurovascular plane between the internal oblique and the transversus abdominis muscles. The subcostal nerve (T12) and the ilioinguinal and iliohypogastric nerves (L1) also travel in the plane between the transversus abdominis and internal oblique, innervating both of these muscles. The branches of T7-T12 continue anteriorly from the transversus plane to pierce the rectus sheath and end as anterior cutaneous nerves (Figure 4.6). A combination of a TAP and rectus sheath injection or a subcostal TAP injection will provide coverage for above and below the umbilicus. It must be noted that this is a somatic block only and will not provide visceral coverage. Thus, this is an additional indication for a multimodal regimen.

A TAP block can be performed by the surgeon under laparoscopic guidance or by the anesthesiologist under ultrasound. El-Dawlatly demonstrated in laparoscopic cholecystectomy patients that the ultrasound method allowed for exact placement, and the perioperative opioid consumption was substantially reduced (Figure 4.7).

Petersen did a retrospective review of seven randomized controlled trials encompassing surgical procedures that included large bowel resection with a midline abdominal incision, cesarean delivery via the Pfannenstiel incision, abdominal hysterectomy via a transverse lower abdominal wall incision, open appendectomy, and laparoscopic cholecystectomy. These studies demonstrated clinically significant reductions of postoperative opioid requirements and pain, as well as some effects on opioid-related side effects (sedation and postoperative nausea and vomiting).

In 2012, Johns' systematic review of nine studies found that TAP block reduces opiate requirements within

---

TREATMENT OF PAIN

TAP block /infiltration of ports
Multimodal analgesia—IV/PO acetaminophen, NSAID, pre-gabalin, ketamine intraop infiltration of mesosalpinx

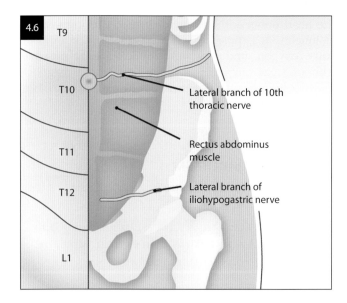

4.6

T9
T10 — Lateral branch of 10th thoracic nerve
T11 — Rectus abdominus muscle
T12 — Lateral branch of iliohypogastric nerve
L1

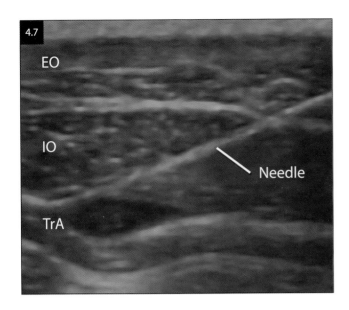

the first 24 and 48 hours postoperatively. This was the first meta-analysis to show a decrease in the incidence of postoperative nausea and vomiting with using TAP blocks. The TAP block continues to develop as far as applications, and at this time the best approach and dose have not been determined.

Pather looked at their experience in 61 successive cases of total laparoscopic hysterectomies. Women with a TAP block had a significantly shorter length of stay (1.45 versus 2.20 days, $P = .014$), lower total perioperative and postoperative opioid use (12 versus 19 mg in morphine equivalents, $P = .014$; 11 versus 21 mg, $P = .05$) when compared with those without a TAP block. Total opioid use significantly correlated only with a TAP block ($P = .005$).

Although complications have been reported, they are rare and consist of puncture of the abdomen, bowel, pneumothorax, and much more rare puncture of the liver. Hematoma can also occur. Most complications were associated with the older landmark approach rather than the more commonly used ultrasound approach in today's practice. There were no complications related to a TAP block in their study.

Sleep apnea and obesity goals of decreasing total opioids for improved management postoperatively are often challenging. Matthes reports an opioid-free single-injection laparoscopic cholecystectomy in a case reporting bilateral TAP blocks given after induction of anesthesia and multimodal analgesia.

However, the duration is governed by the local anesthetic, which is typically 10–12 hours with analgesia occasionally demonstrated to be a few hours longer. The usual current dosage is 30 cc of 0.25% bupivacaine bilaterally. An additional amount may be necessary for the subcostal or the rectus sheath. The aforementioned studies were using a long-acting local anesthetic such as bupivacaine.

A long-acting bupivacaine liposome incorporated into a DepoFoam agent, Exparel (Pacira Pharmaceuticals),

was FDA approved for infiltration in 2012. Trials and use of this agent in TAP blocks are increasing due to the duration of action to exceed 48–72 hours. The obvious advantages of an extended duration and no need for catheters presents a more mobile patient and perhaps a decrease in morbidity. Trials are currently underway and more needs to be done before the approximate dose and efficacy are known. The initial results are promising. Cohen looked at the economic impact in open colectomy patients and demonstrated less opioid consumption and a decrease in the median length of hospital stay from 4.9 to 2.0 days in a liposomal bupivacaine-based multimodal analgesic regimen versus standard opioid-based regimen.

The transversus abdominis plane has an excellent safety profile with a wide application. The TAP is applicable to open and laparoscopic gynecologic procedures. As more studies are being completed and with the development of longer-acting local anesthetics, the TAP block will be increasingly applied for its outstanding clinical utility and its advantageous for optimal pain treatment in the postoperative gynecological patient.

SUMMARY

Laparoscopy has shown obvious benefits to the patient and will continue to develop as better instruments, greater experience, and more knowledge about the effects on the body are further elucidated. As this occurs, our ability to apply this technique with greater expertise will improve patient morbidity and provide anesthetic challenges to supply a physiologic milieu in the presence of a myriad of physiologic variations caused by this procedure.

SUGGESTED READING

Bäcklund M, Kellokumpu I, Scheinin T, et al. Effect of temperature of insufflated CO2 during and after prolonged laparoscopic surgery. *Surg Endosc.* 1998;12(9):1126–1130.

Bardoczky GI, Engleman E, Levarlet M, et al. Ventilatory effects of pneumoperitoneum monitored with continuous spirometry. *Anesthesia.* 1993;8:309.

Bruintjes MH, van Helden EV, Braat AE, Dahan A, Scheffer GJ, van Laarhoven CJ, Warlé MC. Deep neuromuscular block to optimize surgical space conditions during laparoscopic surgery: A systematic review and meta-analysis. *Br J Anaesth.* 2017;118(6):834–884.

Cohen S. Extended pain relief trial utilizing infiltration of Exparel®, a long-acting multivesicular liposome formulation of bupivacaine: A Phase IV health economic trial in adult patients undergoing open colectomy. *J Pain Res.* 2012;5:567–572.

El-Dawlatly AA, Turkistani A, Kettner SC, et al. Ultrasound-guided transversus abdominis plane block: Description of a new technique and comparison with conventional systemic analgesia during laparoscopic cholecystectomy. *Br J Anaesth.* 2009;102(6):763–767.

Finnerty O, McDonnell JG. Transversus abdominis plane block. *Curr Opin Anaesthesiol.* 2012;25(5):610–614.

Goll V, Akca O, Greif R, et al. Ondansetron is no more effective than supplemental intraoperative oxygen for prevention of postoperative nausea and vomiting. *Anes Analg.* 2001;92:112–117.

Greif R, Laciny S, Rapf B, Hickle RS, Sessler DI. Supplemental oxygen reduces the incidence of postoperative nausea and vomiting. *Anesthesiology.* 1999;91(5):1246–1252.

Ho HS, Saunders CJ, Gunther RI, et al. Effectors of hemodynamics during laparoscopy: CO_2 absorption or intra-abdominal pressure? *J Surg Res.* 1995;59:497.

Howie MB, Kim MH. Gynecologic surgery. In: White PF, ed. *Ambulatory Anesthesia and Surgery.* Philadelphia, PA: W.B. Saunders; 1997:282–284.

Johns N, O'Neill S, Ventham NT, Barron F, Brady RR, Daniel T. Clinical effectiveness of transversus abdominis plane (TAP) block in abdominal surgery: A systematic review and meta-analysis. *Colorectal Dis.* 2012;14:e635–e642.

Joris JL. Anesthesia for laparoscopic surgery. In: Miller RD, ed., *Anesthesia*, 5th ed. Philadelphia, PA: Churchill Livingstone; 2000:2003–2023.

Matthes K, Gromski MA, Schneider BE, Spiegel JE et al. Opioid-free single-incision laparoscopic (SIL) cholecystectomy using bilateral TAP blocks. *J Clin Anesth.* 2012;24(1):65–67.

Mortero R, Clark L, Tolan MM, et al. The effects of small-dose ketamine on propofol sedation: Respiration, postoperative mood, perception, cognition, and pain. *Anesth Analg.* 2001;92:1–5.

Panther S et al. The role of transversus abdominis plane blocks in women undergoing total laparoscopic hysterectomy: A retrospective review. *Aust. N. Zeal. J. Obstet. Gynaecol.* September 16, 2011. DOI: 10.1111/j.1479-828X.2011.01369.x.

Petersen PL, Mathiesen O, Torup H, Dahl JB. The transversus abdominis plane block: A valuable option for postoperative analgesia? A topical review. *Acta Anaesthesiol Scand.* 2010;54(5):529–535.

Weingram J. Laparoscopic surgery. In: Yao F-S, ed. *Yao & Artusio's Anesthesiology: Problem-Oriented Patient Management,* 4th ed. Philadelphia, PA: Lippincott-Raven; 1998:732–759.

Wittgen CM, Ngunhein KS, Andrus CH, et al. Preoperative pulmonary function evaluation for laparoscopic cholecystectomy. *Arch Surg.* 1993;128:880–886.

CHAPTER 5

CREATION OF PNEUMOPERITONEUM AND TROCAR INSERTION TECHNIQUES

Thomas G. Lang and Resad Paya Pasic

The patient is placed in a dorsolithotomy position with the buttocks extended up to the end of the table. The thighs should be flexed (120°) to allow good laparoscopic instrument manipulation (Figure 5.1). Attention should be given to proper positioning of the patient's legs and feet to avoid peroneal nerve injury during lengthy procedures. Shoulder braces may be used to make the steep Trendelenburg position possible during surgery. If shoulder braces are used, they should be securely placed over the acromion to avoid possible nerve injury. A bean bag can also be used to effectively maintain the patient's position during steep Trendelenburg position. It is advisable that both arms be tucked along the patient's body in an adducted fashion to provide more space for the surgeons and to prevent brachial plexus injury. This is very helpful, especially if the monitor is positioned between the patient's legs, to permit the surgeon more backward mobility and to assume a comfortable and ergonomic posture during surgery. If monopolar electrosurgery is to be used, a dispersive electrode must be properly placed over the patient's thigh, in full surface contact. The bladder should be emptied to minimize potential injury during ancillary trocar placement; straight bladder catheterization may be performed for short procedures, whereas a Foley catheter is necessary for longer procedures.

After placement of a cervical tenaculum within the anterior cervical lip, a uterine manipulator is inserted transcervically into the uterine cavity to manipulate the uterus during the procedure (Figure 5.2). Manipulators with a capability for tubal lavage and that permit the instillation of dilute indigo carmine dye for chromopertubation may be used. If the patient does not have a uterus, or is pregnant, a moistened sponge stick, EA sizer, or Lucite rod can be substituted by placing into the vagina to push the vaginal vault and cul-de-sac upward. A rectal probe, moistened sponge stick, or open ring forceps can be used to manipulate the rectum to help identify the anterior rectal wall and rectovaginal septum during extensive laparoscopic dissections in this area of the pelvis.

Chlorhexidine is applied to the abdominal area extending from the nipple line to the pubic symphysis, and povidone iodine is used in the vagina from the pubic symphysis to the inner thighs. The patient is draped with leggings and a laparoscopy sheet. If extensive surgery is likely to be performed, and bowel manipulation or injury anticipated, as in the case of extensive adhesions or endometriosis, it is advisable to administer a mechanical bowel preparation prior to surgery. The use of a nasogastric or orogastric tube prior to the establishment of the pneumoperitoneum is suggested if the left upper quadrant insufflation technique is used to minimize the risk of gastric injury. Prophylactic antibiotics are not routinely used but can be administered if an increased risk of infection is plausible.

- LITHOTOMY POSITION WITH EXTENDED BUTTOCKS
- SHOULDER BRACES
- FOLEY CATHETER IN THE BLADDER
- UTERINE MANIPULATOR
- NASOGASTRIC TUBE
- RETURN ELECTRODE

CREATION OF PNEUMOPERITONEUM

Creation of a pneumoperitoneum and the insertion of a Veress needle and primary trocar are the most critical steps when performing laparoscopy. Common sites of Veress needle and trocar insertion are shown in Figure 5.3.

Extraperitoneal insufflation is one of the most common complications of laparoscopy regardless of body weight and is responsible for technical failures that frequently lead to abandonment of the procedure.

There are four subgroups of patients who can present problems during the development of the pneumoperitoneum during laparoscopy:

1. Obese patients
2. Very thin patients
3. Patients with scars from previous abdominal surgeries
4. Patients with failed insufflation

The abundant abdominal wall and intraabdominal fat of obesity decrease tactile sensation and pose difficulty

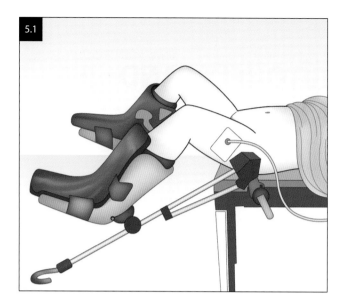

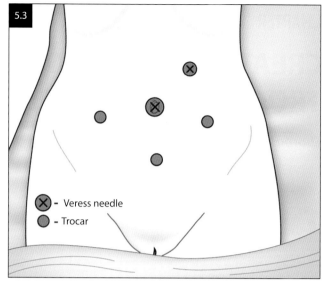

for the standard transumbilical Veress needle insertion and establishment of a pneumoperitoneum. Higher insufflation pressures may be encountered in these patients.

Extra caution is required with very thin patients, since the abdominal wall lies very close to the retroperitoneal vascular structures.

VERESS NEEDLE TECHNIQUES

- Transumbilical placement
- Left upper quadrant placement
- Palmer's point
- Ninth intercostal space
- Transuterine placement

The presence of abdominal scars increases the possibility of omental or bowel adhesions to the abdominal wall, which may interfere with the successful development of the pneumoperitoneum, and may lead to bowel injury. Bowel and other intraabdominal structures have great motility and are resistant to needle puncture unless they are fixed to the abdominal wall by some pathologic process.

In patients with failed insufflation or preperitoneal insufflation, it becomes difficult to enter the peritoneal cavity since the peritoneum is peeled off and an artificial space is created by trapped CO_2 gas that prevents reentry of the Veress needle into the peritoneal cavity (Figure 5.4). Therefore, in these cases, an alternative insufflation site should be chosen.

TRANSUMBILICAL INSUFFLATION

The umbilical area is the most common site for Veress needle placement. Carbon dioxide or nitrous oxide (N_2O) are most often used for insufflation, since room air is not very soluble in blood and may cause embolism if it

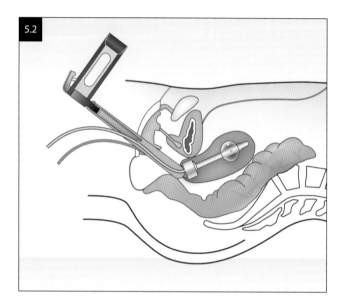

enters a blood vessel. CO_2 is preferred for most laparoscopic surgery, and N_2O is often used for laparoscopy under local anesthesia.

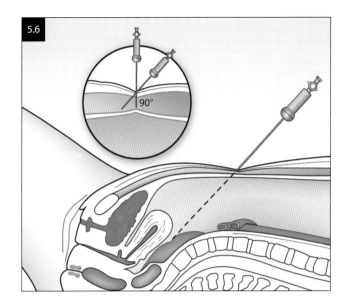

> CAREFUL SELECTION OF THE INSUFFLATION TECHNIQUE AND THE INSUFFLATION SITE SHOULD BE CHOSEN FOR EACH PATIENT.

A skin incision of about 1.2 cm may be made using a number 11 scalpel blade at the umbilical area (Figure 5.5). The Veress needle should be inspected and checked before insertion (make sure that all moving parts are freely mobile). The valve on the Veress needle should be placed in open position during insertion to allow the air to enter the abdominal cavity as the tip of the needle advances. This will prevent possible creation of negative pressure caused by lifting of the abdominal wall that may hold the bowel close to the abdominal wall. When the valve is open, it will also immediately alert the surgeon of a major blood vessel injury.

The operating table with the patient should be placed in an unaltered supine position. The needle is then typically inserted at a 45° angle (with respect to the patient and also to the floor when flat) at the midline and directed toward the uterine fundus (Figure 5.6). Placing the patient in Trendelenburg position prior to the insertion of the Veress needle and primary trocar changes the position of the major retroperitoneal vessels, and places them in the path of the needle and the trocar, which, in turn, places the patient at greater risk of major vascular injury. The 45° angle of Trendelenburg is added to the surgeons' perceived 45° angle of needle placement, making the position of the needle vertical to the retroperitoneal blood vessels (Figure 5.7).

Lifting the abdominal wall prior to needle insertion is favored by many surgeons (Figure 5.8), while some insert directly into the abdomen using gentle traction without abdominal wall elevation. Others use towel clips to grasp and lift the abdominal wall at the time of Veress needle insertion, especially for patients of both very low and higher BMIs. Depending on abdominal wall thickness, the angle of insertion may vary from 45° to 90°. In obese patients, the angle of insertion should be close to 90° to minimize the chance for preperitoneal insufflation. If proper intraperitoneal placement of the needle is not attained, one more attempt should be

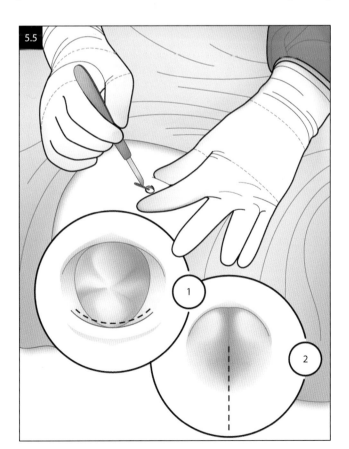

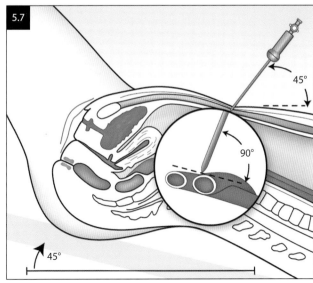

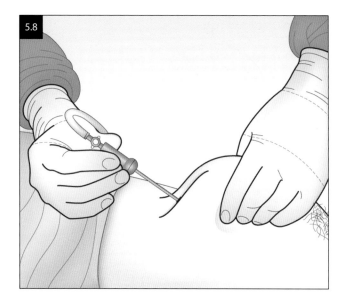

5.8

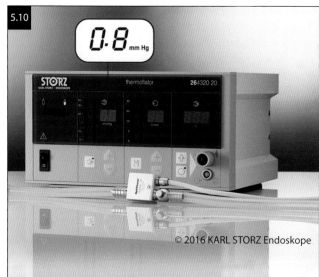

5.10

© 2016 KARL STORZ Endoskope

considered before choosing an alternative site. There are a number of tests that may help ensure proper needle placement and avoid possible complications during the insufflation procedure.

1. Hanging drop test: attaching an open syringe filled with saline to the Veress needle and observing the drop of saline while negative intraabdominal pressure is created by lifting the anterior abdominal wall (Figure 5.9)
2. Intraabdominal insufflation pressure (Figure 5.10)
3. Aspiration and sounding test, using an aspiration needle on the syringe (Figure 5.11)

Although these tests might be of some value in determining proper needle placement, many operators rely primarily on the intraabdominal insufflation pressure and flow volume to ensure proper intraperitoneal needle placement.

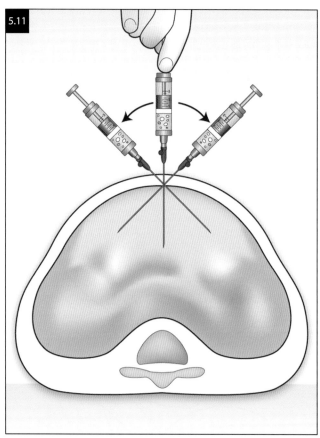

5.11

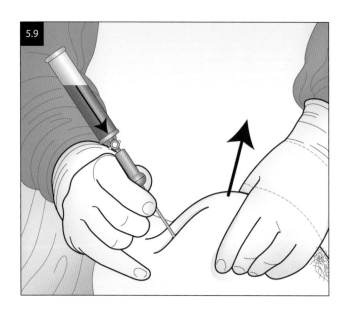

5.9

- CHECK THE VERESS NEEDLE BEFORE INSERTION
- CHECK THE STARTING PRESSURE IF MECHANICAL INSUFFLATORS ARE USED
- PLACE THE PATIENT IN FLAT POSITION
- MAKE THE SKIN INCISION OF ABOUT 1.5 CM
- INSERT THE NEEDLE IN MIDLINE POSITION AT A 45° ANGLE WHILE PULLING ON THE ABDOMINAL SKIN TO FORM A COUNTERTRACTION

- IF THE INSUFFLATION PRESSURE IS ABOVE
  10 MM HG WITHDRAW THE NEEDLE AND REPEAT
  THE SAME PROCEDURE AT THE PROXIMAL END OF
  THE UMBILICAL INCISION
- IF HIGH PRESSURE IS OBTAINED AGAIN,
  WITHDRAW THE NEEDLE AND CONSIDER AN
  ALTERNATIVE PUNCTURE SITE
- IF DEALING WITH A MORBIDLY OBESE PATIENT
  OR PATIENTS WITH SCARS FROM PREVIOUS
  ABDOMINAL SURGERIES, AN ALTERNATE PRIMARY
  INSUFFLATION SITE MAY BE CONSIDERED

Initial intraabdominal insufflation pressure should not exceed 10 mm Hg, and it is the most reliable parameter for monitoring insufflation and proper needle placement. If the initial insufflation pressure exceeds 10 mm Hg, the Veress needle is most likely in the preperitoneal space or has entered an intraabdominal viscus or omentum, and it should be repositioned or withdrawn. Since lateral movement of the needle tip may in fact widen an inadvertent laceration in an underlying blood vessel or loop of bowel, it should be withdrawn vertically. If the surgeon is uncertain that the needle is not placed intraperitoneally, the Veress needle should be withdrawn and reinserted before too much preperitoneal emphysema has developed. During insufflation, other clinical signs such as disappearance of liver dullness and symmetric distension of the lower abdomen can be observed. During the process of insufflation, the slow rise in the intraabdominal pressure compared with the insufflated volume of gas should be monitored. If the intraabdominal pressure rises quickly over 14 mm Hg, before 1.5–2 L of gas are insufflated, the suspicion of preperitoneal or viscus insufflation may be assumed. If the needle is properly placed, the peritoneal cavity is insufflated with 3–6 L of CO_2, depending on the patient's intraperitoneal volume. After insufflating about 1.5–2 L of CO_2, intraabdominal pressures will begin to rise. Insufflation should be continued until the pressures reach at least 20–25 mm Hg. Since the abdominal cavity is a closed space and its volume varies from patient to patient, insufflation pressure is a better indicator of adequate peritoneal insufflation and distension than the volume of gas used. When the insufflation pressure reaches 20–25 mm Hg, distension of the abdominal cavity should be adequate for safe insertion of the trocar, and the needle should be withdrawn. Using higher intraabdominal pressure at the outset provides greater proprioception for peritoneal entry and increases the underlying distance between the large vessels and viscera. Figure 5.12 represents the distance from the trocar tip as it pierces the abdominal wall to the retroperitoneal structures at 15 mm Hg and at 25 mm Hg. Notice that the distance from the tip to the retroperitoneal structures is much greater if the abdomen is insufflated to 25 mm Hg.

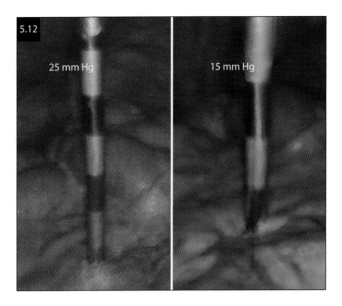

After the trocar is inserted, the pressure on the insufflator should be set at approximately 14–15 mm Hg.

ALTERNATIVE SITES AND TECHNIQUES

An alternative site for needle placement can be selected if the umbilical area is deemed unsuitable for insertion.

SUBCOSTAL INSUFFLATION TECHNIQUE

Insertion of the Veress needle through the subcostal space in the left midclavicular line is a safe alternative to transumbilical insufflation. A small stab skin incision is made in the left midclavicular line just beneath the rib cage. A Veress needle is placed at a 90° angle and pushed into the abdominal cavity. No abdominal wall elevation is performed. Three distinct pops of the needle can be felt as the needle advances toward the peritoneal cavity through the anterior and posterior layers of the rectus sheath as well as the peritoneum. Whereas the first two pops typically progress in rapid sequence, a notable delay in the third pop is not uncommonly encountered secondary to the stretching and final release of the parietal peritoneum. The abdominal wall is usually thin in this area, no more than 3–4 cm (Figure 5.13). If the initial intraperitoneal pressure is higher than 10 mm Hg, the needle should be slightly withdrawn 1–2 cm and the pressure rechecked, as the needle tip may be lodged against the underlying omentum.

SUBCOSTAL APPROACH

- MAKE A SMALL STAB INCISION IN THE
  MIDCLAVICULAR LINE, JUST BELOW THE COSTAL
  MARGIN, ON THE PATIENT'S LEFT SIDE.
- INSERT THE VERESS NEEDLE AT A 90° ANGLE.

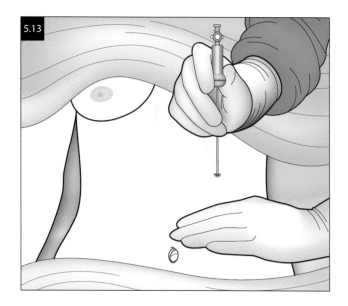

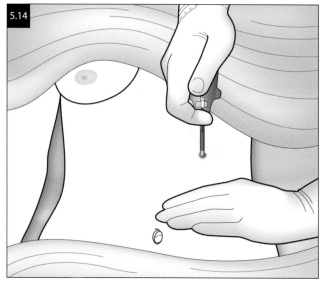

- THREE POPS OF THE NEEDLE ARE USUALLY FELT.
- IF INITIAL PRESSURES ARE TOO HIGH, PULL THE NEEDLE BACKWARD. IT MAY BE STUCK IN THE OMENTUM.

The left upper quadrant is easily accessible and is usually free of underlying intraabdominal adhesions. This area is generally safe for needle and trocar insertion, because the rib cage provides adequate tension and prevents the downward displacement of the abdominal wall. This approach works well for patients after failed transumbilical insufflation. It can be used as a primary route in obese patients, and for patients who have undergone previous abdominal surgeries with suspected adhesions below the umbilical area, regardless of type of prior incision.

Moreover, subcutaneous emphysema is rarely encountered when insufflating in this space. Spleen injury is unlikely during a midclavicular and subcostal insertion, whereas the left lobe of the liver may rarely be in harm's way. To help avoid liver injury, the Veress needle should be directed caudally, at an angle slightly less than 90°.

In a patient with suspected abdominal adhesions, upon successful insufflation, the Veress needle is withdrawn and a 5 mm trocar is inserted through the same space (Figure 5.14). Through this trocar sleeve, a 5 mm scope is introduced, and the umbilical area is inspected for the absence of adhesions. If the umbilical area is free of adhesions, a 10 mm trocar is inserted into the peritoneal cavity under direct vision.

OPEN TECHNIQUE

The majority of complications associated with a laparoscopic procedure occur at time of entry. There is currently no clear consensus on the safest mode of entry. A recently updated Cochrane review revealed a reduction in the incidence of failed entry with the use of an open-entry technique compared to closed entry. Further, a reduction in the incidence of failed entry, reduced risk of extraperitoneal insufflation, and reduced omental injury were seen with direct as compared to Veress needle entry. However, this review found no evidence that any single technique or instrument helped to reduce the occurrence of vascular and/or visceral injury. Ultimately, choice of entry should be based on surgeon preference, experience, and comfort level.

OPEN TECHNIQUE

- MAKE A 2–3 CM HORIZONTAL INCISION IN THE UMBILICAL AREA. USE KELLY CLAMPS AND "S" SHAPED RETRACTORS TO DISSECT TISSUE TO THE FASCIA. WHEN FASCIA IS VISUALIZED, USE A SCALPEL TO INCISE THE FASCIA.
- PLACE ONE "o" VICRYL SUTURE TO EACH SIDE OF THE FASCIAL INCISION.
- CONTINUE DISSECTION OF THE ABDOMINAL WALL LAYERS WITH KELLY CLAMPS AND SCISSORS UNTIL THE PERITONEAL CAVITY IS REACHED.
- ONCE THE PERITONEAL CAVITY IS ENTERED, PLACE THE BLUNT TROCAR WITH THE CONICAL OBTURATOR INTO THE ABDOMINAL CAVITY. THE LENGTH OF THE TROCAR CAN BE ADJUSTED BY SLIDING THE CONICAL OBTURATOR ALONG THE TROCAR.
- ANCHOR THE VICRYL SUTURES AROUND CLEATS ON THE CONICAL OBTURATOR, TO FIX IT TO THE ABDOMINAL WALL.
- ATTACH THE INSUFFLATION TUBING TO THE TROCAR INSUFFLATION PORT.
- REMOVE THE BLUNT TROCAR FROM THE TROCAR SLEEVE AND INSERT THE LAPAROSCOPE.

Open laparoscopy (Hasson technique) is a popular technique among many gynecologists and general surgeons. It is very useful for some patients, particularly those suspected of having adhesions from previous surgeries or who are pregnant. The open technique utilizes a small 2–3 cm umbilical skin incision (Figure 5.15). Peritoneal entry with this method is predicated on the sequential identification and separation of all fundamental layers of the abdominal wall including the peritoneum. The open laparoscopy trocar set contains a 10 mm cannula, blunt trocar, and a conical obturator that plugs off the abdominal skin incision (Figure 5.16). The dissection is performed into the abdomen with Kelly clamps and special "S"-shaped retractors. After the abdominal fascia is visualized and incised, two 0-Vicryl™ sutures are placed into the fascia to support and hold the blunt trocar that is inserted into the abdominal cavity after the incision is carried through the peritoneum. Gas is insufflated directly through the cannula, and a blunt trocar is replaced with the laparoscope (Figures 5.17 and 5.18).

Reported to have a comparatively lower risk for retroperitoneal vascular injury, this technique may be safer than using a blind, Veress needle or trocar insertion; however, its application may not similarly prevent bowel injuries. Open laparoscopy can be especially difficult to perform in a morbidly obese patient, because one must penetrate 8–10 cm of adipose tissue before reaching the fascia and then the peritoneal cavity through a small skin incision.

DIRECT TROCAR INSERTION

Some surgeons prefer to use direct trocar insertion as their preferred method for primary peritoneal access. This technique should ideally be reserved for thinner patients with a flaccid anterior abdominal wall, as it is difficult to grasp and elevate the abdominal wall sufficiently in more obese patients. Using this technique, a

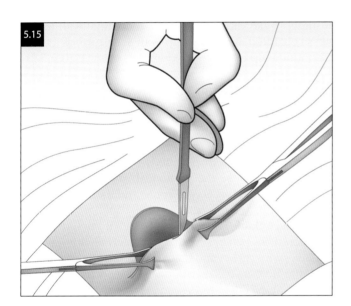

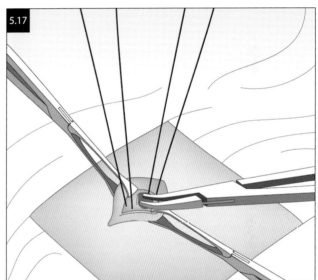

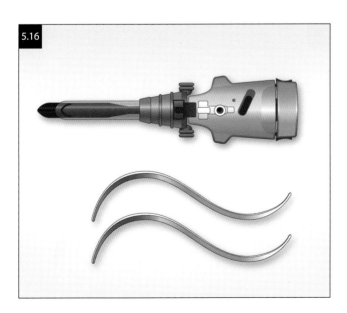

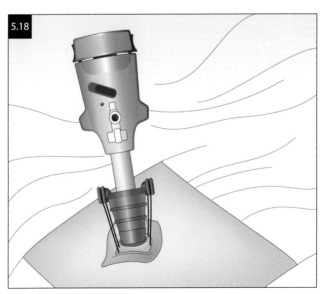

small incision is made in the umbilical area, the abdominal wall is lifted with one hand, and a trocar is pushed with the dominant hand into the potential space of the abdominal cavity. Insufflation tubing is attached to the trocar, and the laparoscope is inserted (Figure 5.19).

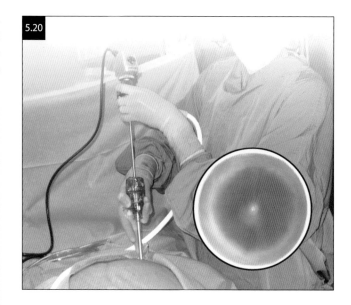

DIRECT TROCAR PLACEMENT

- Blind direct trocar placement
- Direct vision trocars

TECHNIQUE

- Make a 1.5 cm umbilical incision
- Lift the anterior abdominal wall with the left hand
- Insert the trocar with the right hand aiming toward the uterus
- Connect the tubing and begin the insufflation

Direct trocar insertion may also present a problem for surgeons with smaller hands because it requires significant strength and force to lift the abdominal wall and push the trocar into the peritoneal cavity. Although the availability of direct vision trocars may enhance the safety of insertion, it does not preclude proper technique. The disposable visual access (optical) trocars are used to gain peritoneal access either directly or after Veress needle insufflation. The 5 or 10 mm laparoscope is placed into the trocar sheath, and the trocar is pushed with twisting motion into the abdominal cavity (Figure 5.20). The layers of the abdominal wall are sequentially visualized as the trocar is advanced through the abdominal wall. Overall, the procedure is quite safe and reliable. A reusable trocar made by Karl Storz using the Archimedian principle to work like an auger can also be used to enter

the peritoneal cavity under direct vision. The trocar is simply screwed into the abdominal wall without any pushing. Under direct vision, the abdominal wall is progressively lifted and pulled up with each turn of the trocar until the tip enters the abdominal cavity (Figure 5.21).

TRANSUTERINE INSUFFLATION

This method enables easy and safe access to the peritoneal cavity, bypassing transabdominal entry of the Veress needle in obese patients. Transuterine insufflation is a useful modality in patients with a large abdominal panniculus, because the peritoneal cavity can be easily entered via the transcervical route and then through the uterine fundus (Figure 5.22).

This technique is simple and safe. It should not be considered in patients with large uterine fibroids and patients who are candidates for chromopertubation, since the hole in the uterine wall created by the Veress needle may facilitate the escape of the dye and prevent uterine distention.

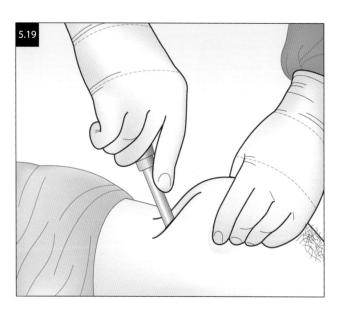

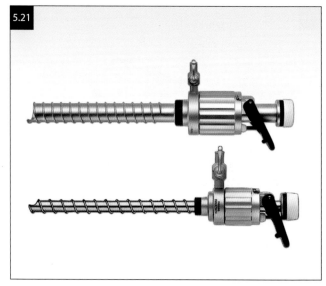

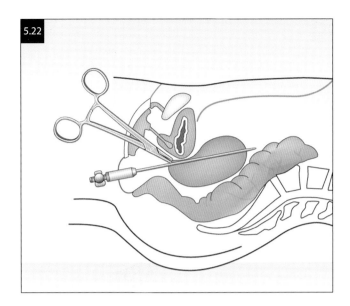

With the patient in a moderate Trendelenburg position, a speculum is placed in the vagina. The anterior cervical lip is grasped with an atraumatic grasper, and the uterus is pulled forward to straighten its axis. The uterine cavity is sounded to obtain information on the size and direction of the cavity. A long Veress needle is passed through the cervix into the uterine cavity until slight resistance is felt when the needle reaches the fundus. The needle is then pushed through the uterine fundus until it reaches the peritoneal cavity, detected by a pop of the needle as it advances through the uterus. The peritoneal cavity is then insufflated with CO_2. Somewhat higher initial insufflation pressures, up to 15 mm Hg, can be encountered initially with this method. As the abdominal cavity is being insufflated, the pressures begin to drop. After the abdomen has been successfully insufflated, the patient is placed in a flat position, and the trocar can then be inserted transumbilically or

TRANSUTERINE APPROACH:

- Insert the vaginal speculum.
- Grasp the anterior cervical lip with the tenaculum and pull it forward.
- Sound the uterine cavity using uterine sound.
- Grasp the long Veress needle with sponge forceps and introduce the needle through the cervix into the uterine cavity. Apply pressure to perforate the fundus.
- Connect the tubing, and turn the insufflation on. Higher pressure in the range of 15–20 mm Hg is expected.
- Insert the trocar and remove the Veress needle under direct laparoscopic vision.

through the left upper quadrant. This technique should be considered in obese patients and whenever failed transabdominal entry has resulted in significant preperitoneal insufflation.

INSERTION OF THE VERESS NEEDLE USING THE TOWEL CLIP TECHNIQUE

When using this technique, towel clips are placed into the umbilicus which is everted; a 10 mm incision is then made along the base. The Veress needle and the trocar are then inserted in the abdominal cavity at a 90° angle while elevating with the towel clips (Figure 5.23).

TROCAR PLACEMENT

Extra insufflation of the peritoneal cavity to 25 mm Hg will create enough elevation and resistance against the peritoneum for safe insertion of the trocar.

The trocar and sheath are held between the middle and index fingers with the hub of the trocar against the palm of the hand. With wrist motion, the trocar is usually advanced with the dominant hand at a 45° angle in midline position toward the hollow of the sacrum. The other hand rests on the abdomen, holding the trocar sheath between the index finger and the thumb to act as a safeguard to prevent excessive penetration of the trocar through the abdominal wall (Figure 5.24). The trocar sheath is slightly wider than the trocar tip, and it may

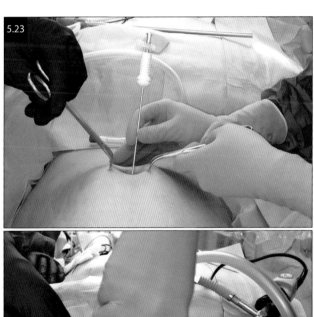

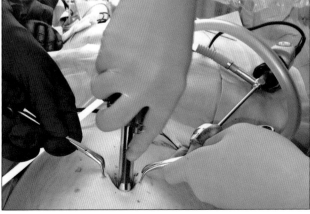

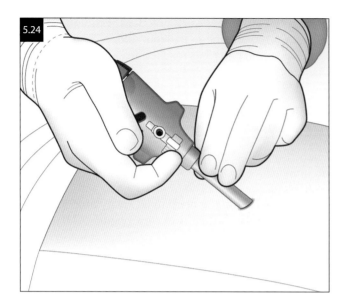

5.24

get caught in the fascia. As the force is applied to the trocar, its tip may be pushed too far into the abdomen, as the trocar sheath passes the resistance of the fascia. Therefore, some type of safeguard mechanism should be applied on the trocar to avoid its excessive penetration. Alternatively, the index finger is extended along the shaft of the trocar to act as a brake (Figure 5.25). Depending on the abdominal wall thickness, the angle of insertion may vary from 45° to 90°. In obese patients, the angle of insertion should be close to 90° (Figure 5.26).

There is no need to lift the abdominal wall during the trocar insertion after proper insufflation. If the abdominal cavity has been insufflated to a pressure of 25 mm Hg, the volume of gas is sufficient to stabilize the abdominal wall for safe insertion of the trocar. Once the trocar is inserted into the abdominal cavity, the obturator is removed, and the trocar sheath is held in place. The hiss of escaping gas can be heard by depressing the flap valve. This is a comforting sound as it assures the surgeon that the trocar is in the proper locale.

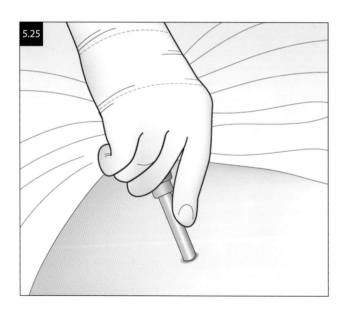

5.25

- EXTENSIVE INSUFFLATION OF THE PERITONEAL CAVITY—THE MORE THE BETTER.
- ANGLE OF INSERTION IS USUALLY 45°–60°.
- USE A SAFEGUARD MECHANISM DURING TROCAR PLACEMENT.
- BEFORE PLACING ANCILLARY TROCARS, INSPECT THE INSIDE ABDOMINAL WALL FOR THE PRESENCE OF ADHESIONS.
- GENTLY TAP THE AREA WITH THE INDEX FINGER, WHERE THE PUNCTURE IS PLANNED, AND LOOK FOR THE INDENTATION OF THE ABDOMINAL WALL THROUGH THE LAPAROSCOPE.
- LOOK FOR BLOOD VESSELS BY TURNING THE ROOM LIGHTS OFF AND ILLUMINATING THE AREA ON THE ABDOMINAL WALL WITH THE LAPAROSCOPE FROM INSIDE.
- MAKE A SMALL 5 MM SKIN INCISION IN THE AREA CLEAR OF BLOOD VESSELS.
- INTRODUCE THE TROCAR SLEEVE UNDER LAPAROSCOPIC VISION, AIMING TOWARD THE POSTERIOR CUL-DE-SAC.
- REPEAT THE SAME PROCEDURE FOR EACH ANCILLARY PORT.

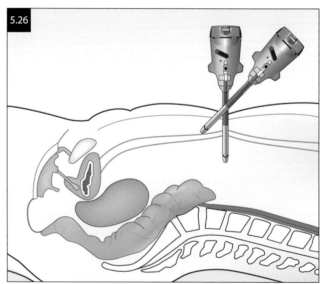

5.26

Most laparoscopic surgeries can be performed using 5 mm accessory trocar sleeves, but if a linear stapler or laparoscopic morcellator are to be used, a 12 mm trocar is inserted usually in the midline or umbilical position. Ancillary trocars should be inserted under direct vision (Figure 5.27). The upper margin of the bladder should be identified, and a Foley catheter should help avoid accidental bladder perforation. A suprapubic site in the midline is most commonly utilized, while right and left lower quadrant sites above the pubic hairline and lateral

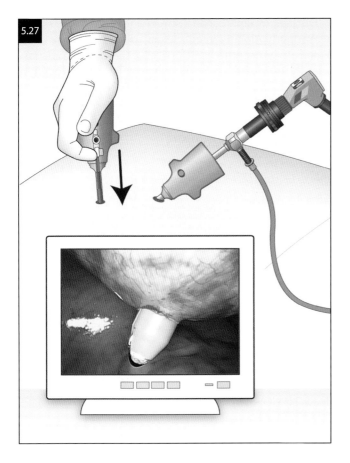

5.27

to the deep epigastric vessels are commonly added to perform more complex procedures. The abdominal wall may be transilluminated by the laparoscope at the site of the lateral secondary trocar placements in order to demarcate and avoid the superficial epigastric blood vessels. This technique is useful but cannot be relied on to locate the inferior epigastric vessels, especially in obese or dark-skinned patients. The authors prefer to place the ancillary 5 mm ports higher, approximately at the level of the umbilicus, about 8–10 cm lateral to the umbilicus. Placing the ancillary ports in higher positions provides a greater capacity to manipulate tissue, especially for removing a large fibroid uterus. Finger-tapping the skin from above can identify the area of trocar placement, and a small skin incision should be made before the trocar sleeve is inserted. The trocars should be placed perpendicular to the abdominal wall making sure that they do not slide tangentially along the abdominal wall. This is especially important in very obese patients where trocars often slide out of the peritoneum if they have not been placed properly at the 90° angle. If inadequate insufflation places the trocar tip close to the bowel, the pressure on this trocar should be intermittently released while it is twisted until reaching the peritoneal cavity. If an ancillary trocar is already placed, a grasper can be inserted into the peritoneal cavity and used to elevate the abdominal wall to assist placement of an additional trocar. If only one hand is used to insert a secondary trocar, the index finger should be extended along the shaft as a safeguard against deep penetration.

TERMINATION OF THE LAPAROSCOPIC PROCEDURE

At the end of the laparoscopic procedure, the abdominal cavity should be inspected for absence of bleeding or retroperitoneal hematoma during reduced intraperitoneal pressure. All ancillary trocars should then be sequentially withdrawn under direct laparoscopic vision to ensure hemostasis. The patient is placed in a flat position, as much gas as possible is allowed to escape, and the laparoscope is then removed. Typically, a certain amount of gas remains trapped in the peritoneal cavity, which can irritate the peritoneum, creating discomfort and minor pain referred to the shoulder area for up to 2 weeks postoperatively. Abdominal gas should be relieved by gentle pressure on the lower abdomen with the valve opened to allow escape. The surgeon may ask anesthesia at this time to give the patient two large breaths to facilitate more complete gas removal. The trocar sheath is removed with the valve open to prevent room air from entering the abdominal cavity, aided by keeping gentle pressure on the abdominal wall close to the trocar site while pulling the trocar sleeve with the other hand. If any difficulties were encountered during Veress needle or primary trocar placement and/or significant omental or bowel adhesions were noted during the laparoscopic procedure, the umbilical trocar should be withdrawn under direct laparoscopic guidance to ensure that the bowel was not injured during peritoneal access. Generally speaking, any fascial incision greater than 5 mm should be closed to prevent hernia formation. For routine trocar site closure, a 0 absorbable suture is used to approximate deep fascia, and 4-0 is used for the skin (Figure 5.28). Several devices are available for closure of the fascia and peritoneum under direct vision, such as the Endoclose (Tyco Healthcare, Norwalk, Connecticut, or Carter-Thomason, CooperSurgical, Trumbull, Connecticut) (Figure 5.29). In order to prevent the risk for small bowel obstruction from a Richter hernia, closure must include both fascial and peritoneal defects.

ALWAYS INSPECT THE ABDOMINAL CAVITY FOR THE ABSENCE OF BLEEDING, HEMATOMA, OR BOWEL INJURY BEFORE WITHDRAWING THE LAPAROSCOPE.

- CHECK FOR HEMOSTASIS BEFORE TERMINATING THE LAPAROSCOPIC PROCEDURE.
- WITHDRAW THE ANCILLARY TROCARS UNDER DIRECT LAPAROSCOPIC VISION TO CHECK FOR HEMOSTASIS.
- IF MORE ATTEMPTS WERE MADE BEFORE ESTABLISHING ADEQUATE PNEUMOPERITONEUM, OR IF UMBILICAL ADHESIONS ARE OBSERVED,

WITHDRAW THE TROCAR SLOWLY BEFORE RELEASING THE PNEUMOPERITONEUM TO CHECK FOR POSSIBLE BOWEL INJURIES. IF NO ABNORMALITIES ARE OBSERVED, REINSERT THE TROCAR SLEEVE, AND RELEASE THE PNEUMOPERITONEUM.

- CLOSE ALL FASCIAL INCISIONS OF 1 CM AND GREATER USING ABSORBABLE SUTURE.
- FOR 5 MM INCISIONS, ONLY SKIN CLOSURE IS PERFORMED.

During any laparoscopic surgery, the procedure should be properly documented. Visual documentation using digital image capture and prints at the outset and periodically thereafter serve to memorialize the procedure and provide invaluable reference for both the patient and future pelvic surgeons.

SUGGESTED READING

Ahmad G, Oflynn H, Duffy JM, Phillips K, Watson A. Laparoscopic entry techniques. *Cochrane Database Syst Rev.* 2012;15(2):CD006583.

Ballem RV, Rudomanski J. Techniques of pneumoperitoneum. *Surg Laparosc Endosc.* 1993;3:42–43.

Byron JW, Fujiyoshi CA, Miyazawa K. Evaluation of the direct trocar insertion technique at laparoscopy. *Obstet Gynecol.* 1989;74:423–425.

Childers JM, Brzechffa PR, Surwit EA. Laparoscopy using the left upper quadrant as the primary trocar site. *Gynecol Oncol.* 1993;50:221–225.

Dingfelder JR. Direct laparoscope trocar insertion without prior pneumoperitoneum. *J Reprod Med.* 1978;21:45–47.

Garry R. A consensus document concerning laparoscopic entry techniques. Middlesbrough, March 19–20, 1999. *Gynecol Endosc.* 1999;8:403–406.

Hasson HM. Open laparoscopy: A report of 150 cases. *J Reprod Med.* 1974;12:234–238.

Hurd WW, Bude RO, Delancey JO, Pearl ML. The relationship of the umbilicus to the aortic bifurcation; Implications for laparoscopic technique. *Obstet Gynecol.* 1992;80:48–51.

Mlyncek M, Truska A, Garay J. Laparoscopy without use of the Veress needle: Results in a series of 1600 procedures. *Mayo Clin Proc.* 1994;69:1146–1148.

Morgan HR. Laparoscopy: Introduction of pneumoperitoneum via transfundal puncture. *Obstet Gynecol.* 1979;54:260–261.

Mumford SD, Bhiwandiwala PP, Chi IC. Laparoscopic and minilaparotomy female sterilization compared in 15,167 cases. *Lancet.* 1980;ii(8203):1066–1070.

Palmer R. Safety in laparoscopy. *J Reprod Med.* 1974;13(1):1–5.

Penfield AJ. How to prevent complications of open laparoscopy. *J Reprod Med.* 1985;30:660–663.

Poindexter AN, Ritter M, Fahim A, Humprey H. Trocar introduction performed during laparoscopy of the obese patient. *Surg Gynecol Obstet.* 1987;165:57–59.

Reich H, Levie M, McGlynn F, Sekel L. Establishment of pneumoperitoneum through the left ninth intercostal space. *Gynaecol Endosc.* 1995;4:141–143.

Vakili C, Knight R. A technique for needle insufflation in obese patients. *Surg Laparosc Endosc.* 1993;3:489–491.

Wolfe WM, Pasic R. Transuterine insertion of Veress needle in laparoscopy. *Obstet Gynecol.* 1990;75:456–457.

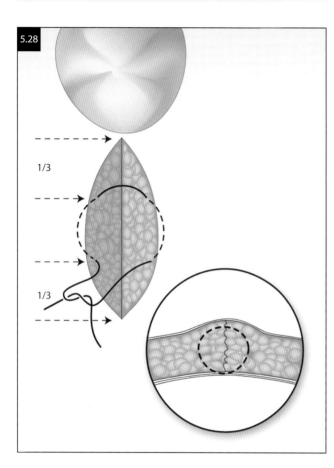

5.28

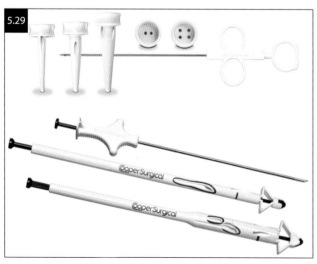

5.29

CHAPTER 6
ENERGY SYSTEMS IN LAPAROSCOPY

Andrew I. Brill

ELECTROSURGERY

Electricity is produced when valence electrons are freed from atoms of conductive materials. When these electrons are set in motion in the same direction an electric current (I) is produced, that is measured in amperes. Opposite charges on the ends of the conductor cause the electrons to flow in one direction toward the positive terminal. The difference in potential between the positive and negative poles provides the electromotive force (voltage) to drive the current through the conductor (Figure 6.1).

Current that flows in one direction through a circuit is called direct current (DC). When alternating current (AC) flows through a circuit, the movement of electrons reverses direction at regular intervals, which is expressed as cycles per second (Hertz). Since the effects of current on the load are all that is important, the periodic reversal of current flow does not undo its work.

The amount of current that flows through a circuit is determined by the electromotive force (voltage) across the circuit and the resistance that circuit provides to the current. Resistance (R) is the difficulty that a material presents to the flow of electrons and is measured in Ohms. Resistance of biologic tissues varies depending on the water content. It is very high in desiccated tissue, moderate in lipid-rich adipose tissue, and very low in vascular tissue. Resistance for alternating current is expressed as impedance due to the induction of additional resistive phenomena (inductance) that include the effects of imploding electrostatic fields and the oppositional electromotive force of out-of-phase magnetic fields.

Current is directly proportional to the voltage and inversely proportional to the resistance, as expressed by Ohm's law:

$$I = V / R$$

Therefore, greater resistance requires greater voltage, and with a fixed resistance, greater voltage creates greater current. When the switch of an electric circuit is left open (i.e., when the resistance is infinite), as when keying an electrosurgical electrode without tissue contact, it is logical that the energy source will work at maximum voltage. This means that an electrosurgical generator produces the highest voltage across the electrode when it is activated remotely from the tissue surface without current flow. In order to better understand the basic principles of the electric current, the analogy of the electric current to the water flow is presented in Figure 6.2.

Power is the rate of doing work and is expressed in watts (W). It represents the total quantity of electrons moved and the pressure gradient against which the movement occurred, as expressed by

$$W = I \times V$$

Inserting Ohm's law:

$$W = I2 \times R \text{ and } W = V2 / R$$

Therefore, power to tissue increases as a function of both the square of the voltage and the square of the current.

The ratio of voltage-to-current is primarily responsible for the electrosurgical effects on tissue.

Other important factors are time (duration of current application) and power density. The power density represents the amount of energy applied per unit of surface and time, and can be represented in the following way:

$$\text{Power density} = \frac{\text{Power output} / \text{Time}}{\text{Surface}}$$

This equation shows that if time is kept constant, power density depends on the wattage and surface of the active electrode. Change in power density can be achieved by changing the power output, or by changing the contact area. Indeed, to maximize power density, we use higher energy output and a small contact electrode (Figure 6.3).

GREATER VOLTAGE
↓
GREATER FORCE
↓
GREATER RISK

PRINCIPLES OF ELECTROSURGERY

CURRENT

Using current that reverses its direction periodically, electrosurgery is exclusively performed with high-frequency

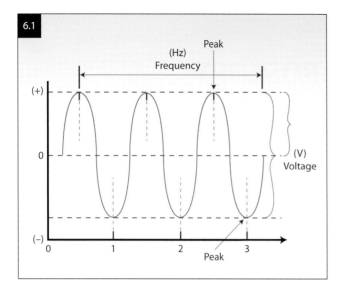

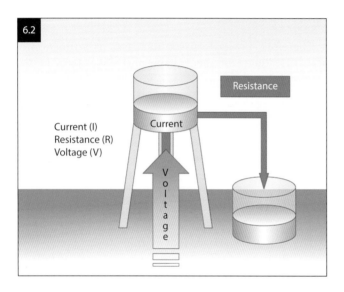

alternating current. The frequency with which current changes direction is measured in cycles per second or Hertz (Hz). Since electrosurgery relies only on the effects of current on the load (tissue), this periodic reversal does not undue the tissue effects. Normal household current has a frequency of 60 Hz (cycles per second). Low-frequency alternating current causes tetanic neuromuscular activity by rapidly reversing depolarization of neuromuscular tissue (faradic effects). These effects do not occur at frequencies greater than 100,000 cycles per second (Hz), where the net positional change of cellular ions is minimal. Justifiably then, electrosurgery is typically performed using alternating currents ranging between 500,000 Hz and 3 million Hz (Figure 6.4).

BIPOLAR AND MONOPOLAR MODES

Bipolar electrosurgery utilizes two terminals of equal size that are extremely close by virtue of being situated across from one another at the end of an electrosurgical instrument. Rather than the patient being part of the electric circuit, the current is only conducted by the tissue restricted between the distal electrodes (Figure 6.5). In monopolar electrosurgery, current is passed through the body by applying two differently shaped electrodes at distant locations of the body. Since the surgical electrode is much smaller than the return electrode, tissue effects are moderated by substantially different current densities (Figure 6.6).

WAVEFORMS

Although most contemporary electrosurgical generators have front panel controls that are labeled "cut," "blend," and "coag," these terms are not necessarily related to actual tissue effects. The variety of choices simply reflects different degrees of waveform modulation (damping) that can be incrementally produced by the generator's solid-state circuitry. Modulation is the periodic interruption of

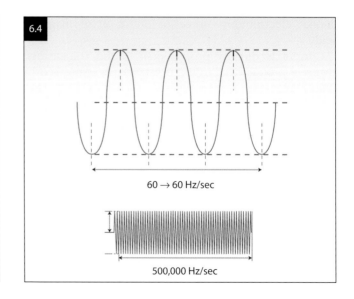

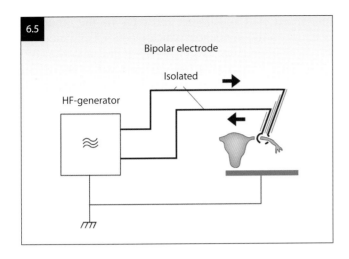

6.5

Bipolar electrode

Isolated

HF-generator

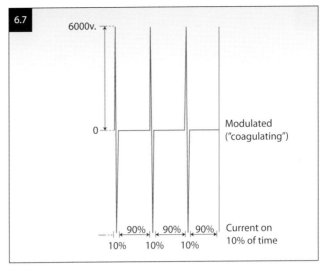

6.7

6000v.

0

Modulated
("coagulating")

90% 90% 90%

10% 10% 10%

Current on
10% of time

current flow (Figure 6.7). The "cut" mode of the generator produces an unmodulated (undamped) pure sine wave with a relatively low peak voltage. The "coag" mode produces the most modulated waveform that correspondingly has the highest peak voltage. Therefore, for equal power settings, increasing waveform modulation (i.e., switching from "cut" to "blend" to "coag") causes the peak voltage to proportionally increase, i.e., energy must be conserved (Figure 6.8).

GROUNDING

A fundamental understanding of grounding is necessary to practice monopolar electrosurgery with safety. A ground is any form of conductive connection between an electric circuit and earth. Since the earth has an infinite capacity to absorb electric charges, any electrically charged object connected to the earth will equalize its potential difference with the earth.

THE DISPERSIVE ELECTRODE PAD

Although the dispersive electrode pad provides a pathway of low impedance for returning current to the generator, its misapplication can result in catastrophic thermal insult that is usually undetected at the time of injury.

The rules for proper usage seek to minimize impedance while providing the greatest surface area for current return. Impedance is primarily minimized by choosing a site with adequate water content for conduction. Areas of skin with hyperkeratosis or hair and those that overlie dense fat deposits (e.g., buttocks) should be avoided, while hair-free or shaved skin over larger muscles is preferred (e.g., upper thigh). Impedance is further reduced by choosing a site as close as possible to the active electrode (Figure 6.9). The surface area of the return electrode must be large enough to permit the returning current to be widely dispersed. Tissue heating is intimately related to current density; current density is inversely related to the square of the surface area, and the rise in tissue temperature is directly proportional to the square of the current. Therefore, small decrements in the surface area between the dispersive pad and the skin can dramatically result in injurious thermal effects to the underlying tissues. A large surface area is guaranteed by a uniform and unalterable application. Areas with bony prominences are prone to movement on patient repositioning (such as the back and buttocks) and should be avoided. Since the edge of the dispersive electrode pad closest to the active electrode tends to concentrate the current, the longer edge of the pad should be placed toward the operative site.

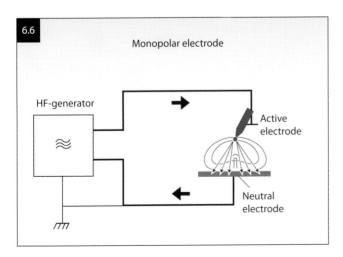

6.6

Monopolar electrode

HF-generator

Active
electrode

Neutral
electrode

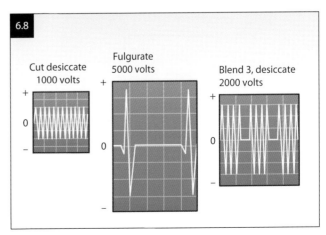

6.8

Cut desiccate
1000 volts

+

0

−

Fulgurate
5000 volts

+

0

−

Blend 3, desiccate
2000 volts

+

0

−

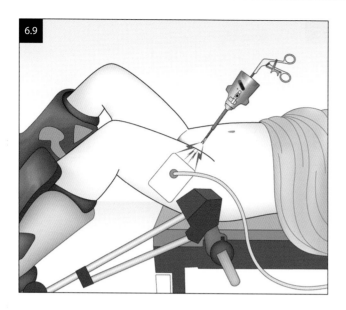

ELECTRODE MONITORING SYSTEMS

Contemporary electrosurgical generators are equipped with an automatic alarm and a shutdown mechanism that activates when the connection between the generator and the return electrode is not intact. However, this does not monitor the adequacy of contact between the surface of the grounding pad and the patient. Since the impedance to the flow of current via the dispersive electrode is quite small until most of the pad has peeled away, any drop in electrosurgical effectiveness should alarm the surgeon to check the application of the dispersive electrode.

Valleylab (Boulder, Colorado), originally introduced a return electrode monitoring (REM) system that monitors the dispersive pad's connection to the generator and the degree of contact with the patient. The dispersive pad is split into two functional halves; a small current is generated to flow through the first half, through the

contiguous skin and tissue, and then via the other half to return to the generator, which electronically monitors the local impedance (Figure 6.10). If the impedance is exceeded by separation from the skin, then the circuit is opened, and an alarm is sounded. This innovation in dispersive pad technology completely eliminates the risk of thermal damage from an unpeeled electrode.

TISSUE EFFECTS OF ELECTROSURGERY

Owing to the impedance, electric energy when applied to the tissue is transferred to thermal energy, and the tissue effect of this thermal energy directly depends on the temperature inside of the tissue and the time required to reach that temperature (Figure 6.11). Electrosurgical energy produces three distinct effects on tissue: cutting, fulguration, and desiccation.

By varying the rate and extent of the thermodynamic effects of electric current in biological tissue, high-frequency electrosurgery is used to cut and/or coagulate. Although the efficiency of hemostasis is related to the depth of coagulation, it is of paramount importance that no more tissue suffers thermal damage than is absolutely necessary. The art of electrosurgery is balancing between the need for absolute hemostasis and the least amount of deep coagulative necrosis.

CUTTING (ELECTROSECTION)

The cutting of tissue occurs when there is sufficient voltage (at least 200 V) between the electrode and the tissue to produce an electric arc, which concentrates the current to specific points along the tissue surface. The open circuit creates an electric field that ionizes the intervening air. An avalanche of colliding and accelerating charged ions forms a plasma cloud that gives off light and sound as the ions pass to lower energy states to produce an electric arc (Figure 6.12). The extremely high current density delivered

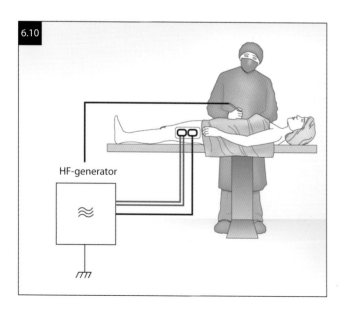

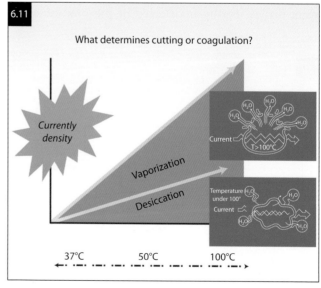

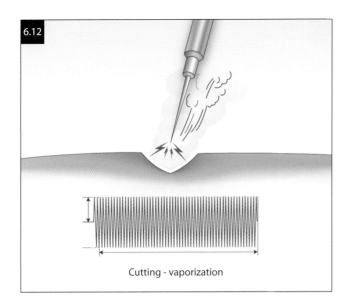

Cutting - vaporization

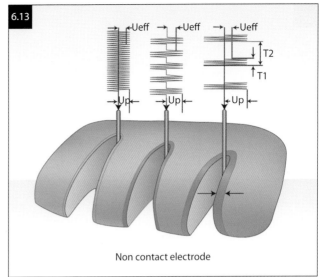

Non contact electrode

by the arc rapidly superheats the cellular water to temperatures greater than 6000°C. Explosive cellular vaporization ensues secondary to the production of highly disruptive pressure (steam occupies six times the volume of liquid water!) and acoustic forces. Arcing is then enhanced by an envelope of steam vapor that becomes instantly ionized. The use of the unmodulated "cut" waveform helps sustain this envelope by producing an uninterrupted current that continuously maintains the same pathways for arc formation. However, since the "cut," "blend," and "coag" outputs all provide peak voltages greater than 200 V, any generator setting can be utilized to perform electrosection. In any case, tissue contact eliminates the steam envelope and abolishes the cutting arc.

In general, the depth of coagulation along the cut edges increases with increasing voltage and length or intensity of the electric arcs. Therefore, an unmodulated "cut" waveform produces a cut with the least amount of coagulative necrosis, whereas waveforms with greater modulation and higher peak voltages (i.e., higher "blend" and the "coag" settings) result in substantially larger zones of coagulation (Figure 6.13).

When using conventional electrosurgical generators, the smallest volume of coagulation during electrosection is assured by employing the thinnest possible electrodes (i.e., edge rather than surface), using the unmodulated "cut" waveform with low peak voltage, and cutting as rapidly as possible using a single pass of the electrode. Deeper coagulation occurs when opposite parameters are applied. A higher "blend" (i.e., blend two or three) or the "coag" waveform may be selectively employed during the electrosection of highly vascular tissues (e.g., leiomyoma) to provide a significant measure of hemostasis along the cut margins.

A new breed of electrosurgical generators, such as the Force Triad (Medtronic) (Figure 6.14), incorporate automatic control circuits to ensure that the intensity of the electric arcs and the output voltage are kept constant (constant voltage generator). This makes the depth

of coagulation relatively independent of the cutting rate and depth, as well as the magnitude of the output current. Thus, the distance of coagulation remains constant regardless of the magnitude of the output current. With this type of equipment, the operator can move the electrode as quickly or slowly as desired and at any angle without significantly affecting the depth of coagulation.

DESICCATION AND COAGULATION

Contact of tissue with the surface of an active electrode leads to conduction of current with a low current density (Figure 6.15). Resistive heating is produced by the high-frequency agitation of intracellular ionic polarities. As the tissue is slowly heated to temperatures above 50°C and maintained, irreversible cellular damage is initiated by deconfiguration of regulatory proteins followed by the denaturation of cellular proteins (white coagulation). Further heating to 100°C leads to complete evaporation of cellular water (desiccation), hemostasis secondary to the contraction of blood vessels and the surrounding tissues, and conversion of collagens to glucose that has an adhesive effect between the tissue and electrode.

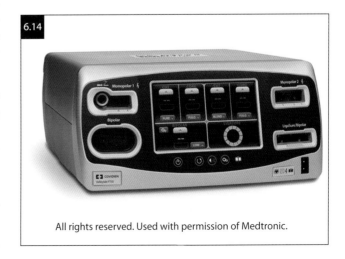

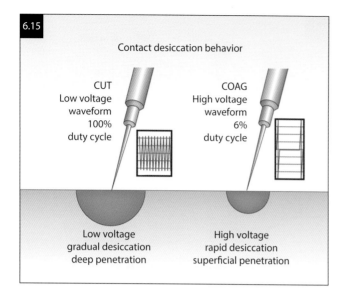

6.15 Contact desiccation behavior

CUT
Low voltage
waveform
100%
duty cycle

COAG
High voltage
waveform
6%
duty cycle

Low voltage
gradual desiccation
deep penetration

High voltage
rapid desiccation
superficial penetration

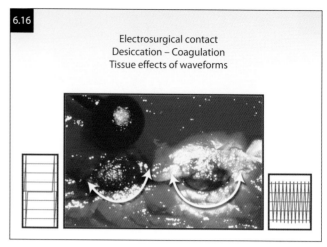

6.16 Electrosurgical contact
Desiccation – Coagulation
Tissue effects of waveforms

Temperatures above 200°C cause carbonization and charring. The prudent application of monopolar electrosurgery to tissue is continuously moderated by monitoring for the terminal evanescence of steam formation and tissue whitening; tissue charring and smoke are indicative of overzealous coagulation.

Until the tissue reaches a temperature of 100°C and is completely desiccated, the rise in tissue temperature is directly proportional to the tissue resistance (degree of desiccation), time of current flow, and the square of the current density. Therefore, temperature change is more rapid at superficial depths and evolves more gradually with larger surface electrodes.

As the tissue is progressively desiccated, current flow is moderated by a zone of electrically insulated steam vapor that forms between the electrode and tissue. The flow of current will eventually cease based on the output voltage. At lower voltages using the unmodulated "cut" waveform, the coagulative process continues until the tissue is entirely dried out (soft coagulation). Continued application of current after completion of the evaporative phase leads to tissue adherence. Therefore, soft coagulation should ideally be terminated at the time of vapor formation.

At higher voltages when using modulated waveforms (especially with smaller electrodes and higher current densities), the vapor layer and desiccated tissue are punctured by electric arcs (forced coagulation) causing further coagulation until the coagulum is so thick it cannot be penetrated. Tissue becomes carbonized, sticky, and precariously unstable. This results in deeper coagulation at the expense of greater force, intense arcing, and increased temperature generation (Figure 6.16).

During soft coagulation, the lower voltage of the "cut" waveform heats the tissue more slowly so heat can flow into deeper tissue layers. Hence, it can be said that soft coagulation is more effective coagulation. Since the reduction of abnormal uterine bleeding after endometrial ablation is related to the degree of destruction of the basalis layer and superficial myometrium, it can be formally argued that the

unmodulated "cut" waveform should be used during hysteroscopic electrocoagulation of the endometrium.

In consideration of all the physical parameters that govern the behavior and effects of high-frequency alternating electric current in biological tissue, laparoscopic monopolar electrosurgery should ideally be performed using the unmodulated "cut" waveform for cutting and deep coagulation of tissue. Any electrode configured with both a flat surface and an edge (e.g., spatula electrode or electrosurgical scissors) can be used as an all-purpose electrosurgical tool with this waveform. The concentration of current at the edge or tip of the electrode provides arcing and hemostatic cutting of tissue. Blunt dissection, tissue traction, coaptation of small blood vessels, and contact coagulation can all be effectively accomplished using the flat surface (Figure 6.17).

FULGURATION

Electric arcs generated by modulated waveforms with higher peak voltages (fulguration) can superficially coagulate a broad surface of tissue with open vessels as large as 2 mm (Figure 6.18). Current modulation allows the steam envelope to dissipate between the

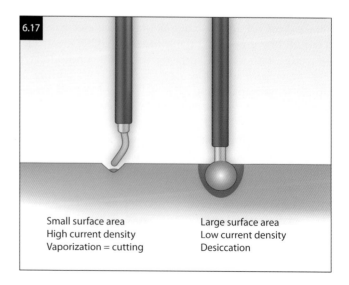

6.17

Small surface area
High current density
Vaporization = cutting

Large surface area
Low current density
Desiccation

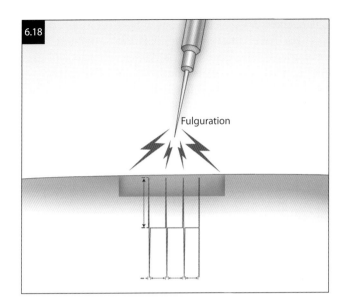

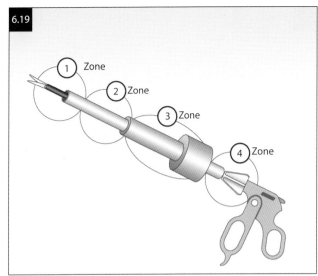

interruption of sparks, causing the electric arcs to strike the tissue surface in a widely dispersed and random fashion, thereby preventing tissue cutting. Although the higher voltage sparks are larger and create broad areas of charring (to >500°C) and tissue destruction, current flow is limited to the superficial tissue layers due to rapid desiccation and the buildup of tissue resistance. Fulguration is relatively useless in the presence of a wet surgical field due to the diffusion of current by saline-rich blood.

Teleologically then, the only selective indication for using the highly modulated "coag" waveform during monopolar electrosurgery is for the superficial coagulation of tissue along a large surface area. Exemplary needs for fulguration during laparoscopic surgery include the myometrial bed after myomectomy, the base of the ovarian cortex after cystectomy, and the oozing veins enwrapping Cooper ligament during colposuspension. Since thermal effects are kept quite superficial by the rapid surface desiccation, fulgurative current is the best choice to superficially electrocoagulate areas of endometriosis over vital structures such as the bladder and ureter.

The argon beam coagulator (ABC) is a true fulgurating electrosurgical device that utilizes the flow of argon gas through an electrode device to form a comparatively longer bridge of electric arcs to the tissue. This gas is easier to ionize than air, allowing the electric arcs to create a more uniform surface coagulation effect. The high flow of gas (4 L/min) displaces oxygen and nitrogen as well as pooled blood, which focuses the effective surface area, and reduces the formation of smoke, carbonization, and tissue buildup on the tip of the electrode.

PROBLEMS OF MONOPOLAR ELECTROSURGERY DURING LAPAROSCOPIC SURGERY

Contrary to the open surgical environment during laparotomy, the bulk of most instruments and nearly all surrounding intraabdominal structures are not visualized during any laparoscopic procedure. Furthermore, nearly all of the potential conductors during laparoscopic electrosurgery are also out of the surgeon's field of view. Intended and unintended couriers of direct or induced currents include the abdominal wall, metallic trocar sheaths and instruments, the operating laparoscope, contiguous visceral tissues, and the active electrode (which is the only part of the circuit under view!) (Figure 6.19). It comes as no surprise that most accidental electrosurgical burns during laparoscopic surgery are undetected at the time of injury.

INSULATION FAILURE

Insulation failure occurs secondary to breaks or holes in the insulation caused by physical abruption during use (such as during passage through an incompletely engaged trumpet cannula) or during normal reprocessing procedures. Completely intact insulation (especially on disposable instrumentation) can be breached by very high voltage (e.g., during open circuit activation or using a modulated "coag" waveform). Any break or breach in insulation may provide an alternate pathway for the flow of current. If the defective portion of insulation contacts tissue during electrode activation, an electric arc will bridge directly from the electrode through the defect to this tissue (Figures 6.20 and 6.21). Thermal damage will occur if the current density is high enough to significantly heat the tissue. Since these defects are usually out of the field of view, this type of injury usually occurs undetected at the time of insult.

Insulation failure can be minimized by periodically inspecting the insulation covering of all laparoscopic electrodes (especially at the shoulder) for small cracks and defects. Disposable monopolar electrodes should not be reused. The risk of high voltage can be eliminated by using the unmodulated "cut" waveform, and avoiding open circuit activation.

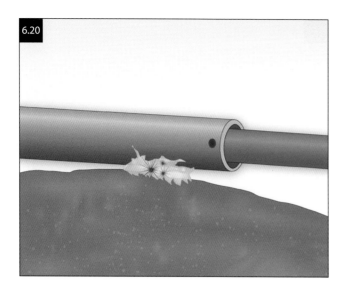

DIRECT COUPLING

Direct coupling of current occurs when an activated electrode makes unintended contact with another metal object in the area of the surgical field. Accidental electrode contact with a suction-irrigator probe, the operating laparoscope, or a metal cannula creates an alternate pathway that is normally conducted up through a metal trocar to the abdominal wall and back to the dispersive electrode. However, if any of these devices are isolated from direct contact with the abdominal wall by an insulator (e.g., plastic cannula or self-retaining device), the current may take an alternate pathway through a point of contact with adjacent tissue (Figure 6.22). Again, if the current density is high, thermal damage may occur.

Direct coupling can be avoided by never activating the generator when the electrode is touching or in near proximity to another metal object in the surgical field.

CAPACITIVE COUPLING

Capacitance is the property of an electric circuit to store energy. Any device that creates capacitance is called

a capacitor. A capacitor exists whenever two conductors that have different potentials are separated by an insulator. A difference of potential or voltage will exist between two conductors that have differing numbers of free electrons (an overall negative charge on the conductor with excess, and a positive charge on the electron-deficient conductor). Although separation by an insulator prevents the flow of electrons between these conductors, the potential difference nevertheless creates an attraction or electrostatic force between them. This force results in an electric field and creates a reservoir of stored energy. When an alternating current flows through a circuit, the applied voltage and flow of current periodically change direction. This means that a capacitor with alternating current is continuously "charged" in alternating directions. With each reversal of current flow, the energy of the stored electric field is discharged. Although no actual current flows through the capacitor, the charged current from capacitance completes the circuit and in essence conducts the alternating current. Since the amount of capacitance is directly proportional to the voltage, capacitance is greatest during open circuit activation and with a highly modulated current such as the "coag" waveform.

Capacitive coupling is the induction of stray current to a surrounding conductor through the intact insulation of an active electrode. In fact, all of the necessary ingredients for the localized genesis of capacitance are provided by an activated monopolar electrode that is passed through a conductive sheath.

Two conductors of differing potentials, the active electrode and the metal sheath (e.g., trocar sheath, working channel of an operating laparoscope, or irrigator-aspirator probe), are separated by the insulation of the electrode (Figures 6.23 and 6.24). On activation, up to 80% of the generator current is induced on the metal sheath by capacitance. Normally this stray current is safely returned to the dispersive electrode by conduction through the large area of contact between the metal trocar sheath

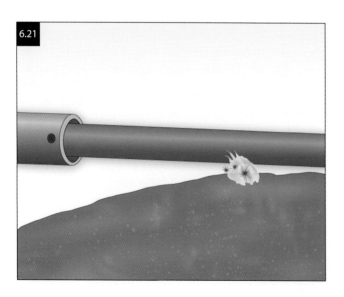

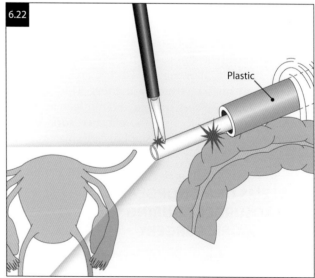

Plastic

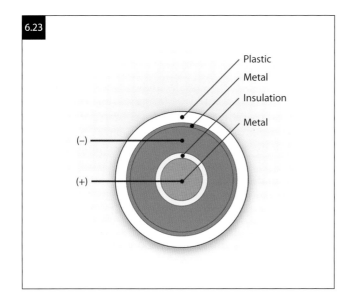

6.23

Plastic
Metal
Insulation
Metal

(−)
(+)

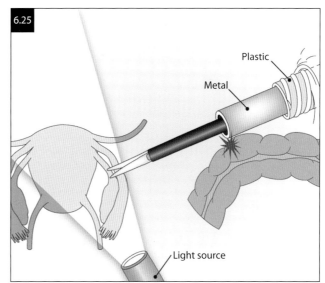

6.25

Plastic
Metal

Light source

and the abdominal wall. The magnitude of capacitance is greater with higher voltage, smaller cannulas, and longer electrodes. Furthermore, the induced current will persist until the electrode is deactivated or it is conducted via an alternate pathway.

If the metal trocar sheath is attached to the abdominal wall by a nonconductive plastic device (e.g., hybrid trocar [metal/plastic] or plastic self-retaining screw device), the induced current becomes electrically isolated from the abdominal wall. Contact between the cannula and a visceral structure provides an alternate pathway for the stray current to discharge (Figure 6.25). Significant thermal damage will occur if the current density is sufficiently concentrated by a small area of contact. A similar phenomenon of capacitive coupling and isolation of current may occur during activation of an electrode placed through the working port of an operating laparoscope that is isolated from the abdominal wall by an all-plastic cannula. In either case, the thermal injury is usually out of the surgeon's field of view.

Capacitance is minimized by using an unmodulated "cut" waveform and avoiding open circuit activation (i.e., minimizing voltage). An all-metal system will suffice for the safe conduction of capacitively coupled current back to the dispersive electrode. Hybrid cannula systems (mixtures of plastic and metal) should not be used to house monopolar electrosurgical devices.

BIPOLAR ELECTROSURGERY

During monopolar electrosurgery, a high density of electrons leave the active electrode and are ultimately dispersed over the broad surface of a return electrode pad. The current returns to the generator after the electrons pass through the patient via a myriad of variably conductive pathways.

Bipolar technology consolidates an active electrode and a return electrode into an electrosurgical instrument with two small poles (e.g., tines of forceps or blades of scissors) (Figure 6.26). Rather than coursing through the patient, the flow of alternating current is symmetrically distributed through the tissue between the poles, reversing direction every half cycle. This eliminates the risk

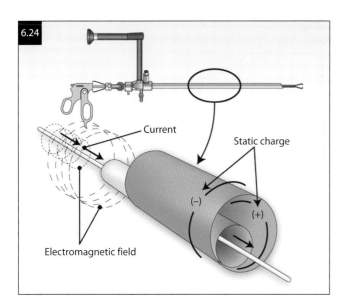

6.24

Current
Static charge

(−)
(+)

Electromagnetic field

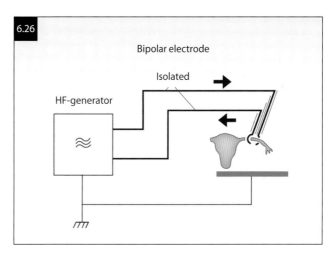

6.26

Bipolar electrode

Isolated

HF-generator

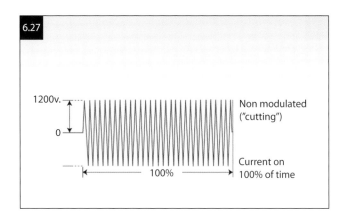

of capacitive coupling and alternate current pathways. Power requirements are significantly less than with monopolar surgery due to the current concentration between the poles. Therefore, an unmodulated "cut" waveform with low peak-to-peak voltage is the generator output during bipolar electrosurgery (Figure 6.27). These factors typically limit the thermal effects to desiccation and coagulation of tissue. Laparoscopic scissors and shears depicted as bipolar cutting devices are usually mechanical cutting devices that simultaneously desiccate at the edge of the cutting electrodes. Using advanced solid-state technology, true bipolar electrosurgical cutting can be accomplished using two more recently introduced bipolar cutting electrodes paired to a dedicated low-voltage electrosurgical generator. The 5 mm PK Cutting Electrode (Olympus America) consists of a retractable active needle electrode paired with a return electrode collar near the distal tip. Tissue cutting is generated when both electrodes are placed in contact with tissue and then drawn across the tissue surface during activation. More recently, a Plasmaspatula 5 mm cutting-coagulation spatula electrode and a J-hook were introduced that consist of conductive surfaces that can be manipulated and keyed to either cut or coagulate tissue (Figure 6.28). Using bipolar electric current, these devices deliver an ionized corona

of energy, which instantly vaporizes tissue entering its margins of active force. The low thermal mass of the ionized electrons contains the spread of tissue desiccation and coagulation. Since the PK electrosurgical generator produces a low-voltage output, the high impedance posed by very desiccated or fatty tissues may preclude vaporization by either of these novel bipolar electrodes.

Bipolar electrosurgery is used for laparoscopic tubal sterilization by sequentially grasping and desiccating the midportion of the fallopian tube and adjacent mesosalpinx with the Kleppinger forceps. Failure of this method usually results from incomplete destruction of the tubal lumen with persistent viability of the endosalpinx. Complete desiccation is best ensured by including the vascular portion of the tube in the forceps, coagulating at least 3 cm of contiguous areas along the ampullary portion of the tube, using relatively low power (25 W) and an inline ammeter to ensure that the tissue is completely desiccated (Figure 6.29).

The localization of current between the poles of the instrument during bipolar electrosurgery offers several distinct advantages. Thermal damage is generally limited to a discrete volume of tissue. The bipolar forceps can be used to coapt and thermally weld blood vessels. The concentrated current and small distance between the poles makes it possible to desiccate tissue that is immersed in fluid. The apparent disadvantages of this modality arise when open blood vessels are retracted or tissue pedicles are very thick.

Although the flow of current and primary thermal effects is restricted to the tissue between the poles, this does not remove the risk of thermal effects to tissue that is distant from the operative site. In fact, the net thermal effects are also governed by the physical parameters described during monopolar electrosurgery. The application of bipolar current leads to the gradual desiccation of the intervening tissue. The rate of tissue coagulation at any given power is moderated by the applied surface area of the poles, the thickness of the pedicle, the formation

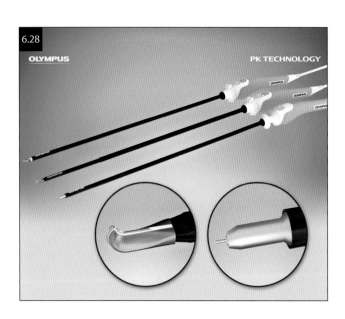

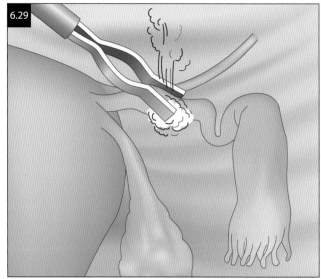

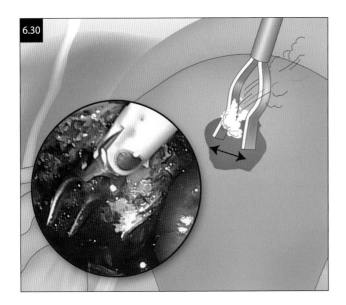

of a vapor layer between the poles and tissue, and the evanescing degree of tissue hydration. Impedance is maximal when the vapor phase is abolished as the tissue is completely desiccated. If the current is further applied and maintained more than several seconds, a secondary thermal bloom occurs to surrounding tissues from a correspondingly rapid rise in tissue temperature. Thus, tissues at some distance from the operative site may undergo subtle but irreversible thermal damage (e.g., the pelvic ureter during overzealous bipolar desiccation of the uterine artery).

During laparoscopic surgery, other than tubal sterilization, the spread of thermal damage during bipolar desiccation should be minimized by terminating the flow of current at the end of the vapor phase, cooling the surrounding tissues with irrigating solution, applying current in a pulsatile rather than continuous fashion, avoiding the use of an inline ammeter to determine the endpoint of desiccation, and securing vascular pedicles by using a stepwise process that alternates between partial desiccation and incremental cutting. The smallest depth of coagulative necrosis will occur when the sides or tips of a slightly open forceps are used to lightly "paint" the tissue surface for directed hemostasis (Figure 6.30).

TAKING THE JUDGMENT OUT OF BIPOLAR ELECTRODESICCATION

Rather than using the judgment of the surgeon to assess the thermal endpoint during bipolar desiccation, newer bipolar devices can now think for you. The latest advance in bipolar electrosurgery is the introduction of three novel ligating-cutting devices that minimize electromagnetic force by delivering electric energy as high-current and low-voltage output. Once tonal feedback from a dedicated generator confirms complete desiccation of the tissue bundle, the pedicle is cut by advancing a centrally set mechanical blade. By directly responding to incremental increases in tissue resistance during coaptive desiccation,

total energy delivery with these devices is dramatically less than conventional bipolar systems (300 V versus 1200 V!). Comparatively then, carbonization, tissue sticking, smoke, incomplete desiccation, and lateral thermal damage are all significantly reduced with these new devices. All produce sufficient energy and vascular coaptation to reliably seal both ovarian and uterine arteries.

Relying on the breakthrough that vessel wall fusion can be achieved using electric energy to denature collagen and elastin in vessel walls to reform into a permanent seal, the 5 and 10 mm LigaSure Laparoscopic Vessel Sealing Device (Medtronic) applies a high coaptive pressure to the compressed tissue bundle during the generation of tissue temperatures under 100°C; hydrogen cross-links are first ruptured and then denature resulting in a vascular seal that has high tensile strength. These laparoscopic instruments for vessel sealing and dividing come in a number of distal configurations including blunt, Maryland, dolphin, and multifunctional, which also provide electrosurgical cutting using conventional monopolar current (Figure 6.31).

The second device, the 5 and 10 mm PK Cutting Forceps (Olympus Surgical America, Orangeburg, New York), utilizes advanced solid-state generator software to deliver pulsed energy with continuous feedback control. The cycle stops once it senses that tissue response is complete; the cool-down phase ensures collagen, and elastin matrix reforms without tissue fragmentation. Electric energy delivery in this fashion results in more uniform tissue heating and in less average and total energy delivery when compared to conventional bipolar systems (Figure 6.32).

A third device, the 5 mm EnSeal Laparoscopic Vessel Fusion System (Ethicon Endosurgery, Cincinnati, Ohio) is an innovative bipolar instrument that for all practical purposes displaces the command of the electrosurgical generator into the 3 and 5 mm distal jaw materials available for this instrument.

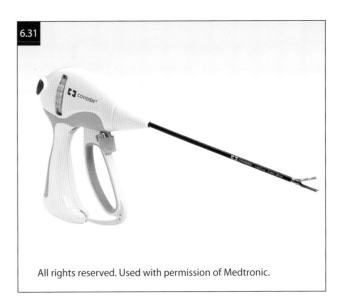

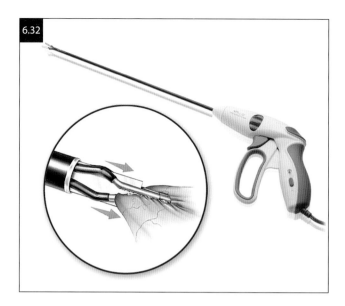

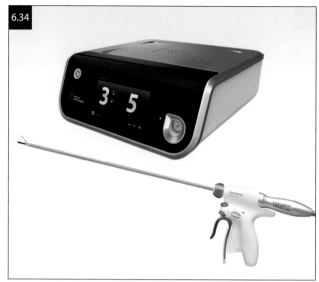

This "smart electrode" contains a set of plastic jaws embedded with nanometer-sized spheres of nickel that conduct a locally regulated current. Tissue temperatures never exceed 120°C due to the progressive generation of resistance in the plastic jaws. With this device, desiccation is facilitated by simultaneously advancing a mechanical blade that both cuts and squeezes the tissue bundle to eliminate tissue water. Reducing tissue water during heating at the coaptive interface further addresses lateral thermal spread by reducing the production of percussive steam during tissue desiccation and vaporization. The newest version of this device articulates up to 110°, facilitating a perpendicular approach to vessels and greater access to tissue in deep or tight spaces (Figure 6.33).

ULTRASONIC ENERGY

The Harmonic Scalpel (Ethicon Endosurgery, Cincinnati, Ohio) is an ultrasonically activated device that provides

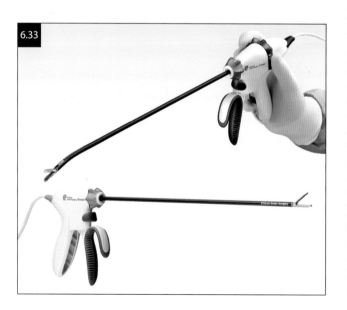

mechanical energy to cut and coagulate tissue. Connected to a dedicated generator, electric energy passes to the hand piece, which houses a piezoelectric crystal. The electric signal causes piezoelectric ceramics in the transducers to activate and convert the electric energy into mechanical or longitudinal motion, which is transferred to the blade extender. From the blade extender the ultrasonic wave is amplified as it travels down the shaft to the blade tip where it produces a maximum motion of 55,500 cycles/second. This permits simultaneous cutting and coagulation as ultrasound travels easily through cellular water. Tissue coagulation and cutting occur by two ultrasound wave effects. First, compression involves the transfer of mechanical energy to tissue. The internal mechanical friction breaks the hydrogen bonds of the collagen molecule that give it a tertiary structure resulting in protein denaturation. During this process, a sticky coagulum forms and seals the vessel at temperatures less than 100°C. Second, cavitation occurs with blade vibration, produced by a transient area of low atmospheric pressure at the tip. This causes fluid within the cells to vaporize and eventually rupture or cavitate. Moreover, vapor formation between the tissue planes facilitates surgical dissection by expanding and separating these layers. The surgeon can moderate tissue effects by varying tissue tension (density) and keying generator power settings to control blade excursion and frequency per cycle. Governed by the interaction between living tissue and ultrasound, cutting velocity is directly related to blade excursion, tissue traction, and blade surface area, and inversely related to tissue elasticity. The fastest cutting with the least amount of coagulation occurs when tissue is placed on tension and firmly compressed, lifted, or rotated with the sharpest side of the blade set at maximum excursion (power 5). Maximum coagulation is best achieved by relaxing tension, minimizing excursion (power 1), and using the blunt edge of the blade. Consequently, the surgeon must always be mindful of the potential for premature incision of a vascular

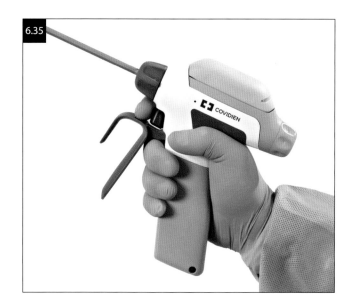

6.35

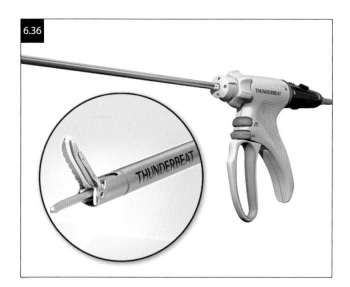

6.36

pedicle from applying too much tension or traction before complete desiccation. Now providing hemostasis similar to advanced bipolar devices for vessels up to 7 mm, the newest generator uses an adaptive technology that responds to changes in tissue impedance by regulating energy delivery to control temperature and improve the vascular seal (Figure 6.34).

More recently, several companies introduced new laparoscopic instrumentation that similarly employs ultrasonic energy to cut and coagulate tissue. The biophysical principles dictating the interaction between living tissue and ultrasound described above are the same for these devices. However, these devices lack impedance feedback to moderate ultrasound transmission and are only approved for sealing vessels up to 5 mm in diameter. Manufactured as a cordless ultrasonic device driven by a battery pack, Sonocision (Figure 6.35) (Medtronic, Minneapolis, Minnesota) has the added benefit of eliminating an associated power cord. More recently, a hybrid device, Thunderbeat (Olympus Surgical America,

Orangeburg, New York) (Figure 6.36), was introduced as a ligating-cutting device that provides both advanced bipolar vessel sealing along with the capacity to incise the tissue pedicle using ultrasonic energy.

SUGGESTED READING

Amaral JF, Chrostek C. Depth of thermal injury: Ultrasonically activated scalpel vs electrosurgery. *Surg Endosc.* 1995;9:226.

Corson SL, Unger M, Kwa D, et al. Laparoscopic laser treatment of endometriosis with the Nd:YAG sapphire probe. *Am J Obstet Gynecol.* 1989;160:718–723.

D'Arsonval MA. Action physiologique des courants alternaifs. *Soc Biol.* 1891;43:283–286.

Erbe Elcktromedzin. *Operating Instructions Manual.* Erbotom ACC 450. Tubingen, Germany; 1990.

Ewing J. *A Treatise on Tumors*, 2nd ed. Philadelphia, PA: WB Saunders; 1922:17.

Friedman J. The technical aspects of electrosurgery. *Oral Surg.* 1973;36:177–187.

Hambley R, Hebda PA, Abell E. Wound healing of skin incisions produced by ultrasonically vibrating knife, scalpel, electrosurgery, and carbon dioxide laser. *J Dermatol Surg Oncol.* 1988;14:1213–1217.

Honig WM. The mechanism of cutting in electrosurgery. *IEEE Trans Biomed Eng BME.* 1975;22:58–65.

Kelly HA, Ward GE. *Electrosurgery.* Philadelphia, PA: WB Saunders; 1932.

Lamberton GR, Hsi RS, Jin DH, et al. Prospective comparison of four laparoscopic vessel ligation devices. *J Endouro.* 2008;22(10):2307–2312.

Luciano A, Soderstrom R, Martin D. Essential principles of electrosurgery in operative laparoscopy. *J Am Assoc Gynecol Laparosc.* 1994;1:189–195.

Luciano M, Whitman G, Maier DB, et al. A comparison of thermal injury, healing patterns, and postoperative adhesion formation following CO$_2$ laser and electromicrosurgery. *Fertil Steril.* 1987;48:1025–1029.

McCarus SD. Physiologic mechanism of the ultrasonically activated scalpel. *J Am Assoc Gynecol Laparosc.* 1996;3:601–608.

Nduka C, Super P, Monson J, et al. Cause and prevention of electrosurgical injuries in laparoscopy. *J Am Coll Surg.* 1994;179:161.

Nezhat C, Crowgey SR, Garrison CP. Surgical treatment of endometriosis via laser laparoscopy. *Fertil Steril.* 1986;45:778–783.

Phipps JH. Thermometry studies with bipolar diathermy during hysterectomy. *Gynaecol Laparosc.* 1994;3:5–7.

Reich J, MacGregor T III, Vancaillie T. CO$_2$ laser used through the operating channel of laser laparoscopes: In vitro study of power and power density losses. *Obstet Gynecol.* 1991;77:40–47.

Ryder RM, Hulka JF. Bladder and bowel injury after electrodesiccation with Kleppinger bipolar forceps: A clinicopathologic study. *J Reprod Med.* 1993;3:595–598.

Semm K. Endocoagulation: A new field of endoscopic surgery. *J Reprod Med.* 1976;16:195–203.

Sigel B, Dunn MR. The mechanism of bleed vessel closure by high frequency electrocoagulation. *Surg Gynecol Obstet.* 1965;121:823–831.

Tucker RD, Benda JA, Sievert CE, et al. The effect of bipolar electrosurgical coagulation waveform on a rat uterine model of fallopian tube sterilization. *J Gynecol Surg.* 1992;8: 235–241.

Tulandi T, Chan KL, Arseneau J. Histopathological and adhesion formation after incision using ultrasonic vibrating scalpel and regular scalpel in the rat. *Fertil Steril.* 1994;61: 548–560.

Vaincaillie TG. Electrosurgery at laparoscopy: Guidelines to avoid complication. *Gynaecol Endosc.* 1994;3:143–150.

Wattiez A, Khandwala S, Bruhat MA. Electrosurgery. In: *Operative Endoscopy.* Oxford: Blackwell Science; 1995:81–92.

CHAPTER 7
LAPAROSCOPIC SUTURING

Joseph L. Hudgens and Resad Paya Pasic

INTRODUCTION

Laparoscopic suturing is an essential skill for any laparoscopic surgeon. The ability to suture laparoscopically allows a surgeon to manage inevitable complications and avoid conversion to laparotomy. Competent laparoscopic suturing is achieved by understanding the relationships between the tissue, equipment, ports, and suture. It is the systematic application of and manipulation of these relationships that allow a surgeon to become proficient at laparoscopic suturing. The goal of this chapter is to present the equipment, sutures, and port configurations utilized in laparoscopic suturing. The second part of this chapter focuses on a systematic approach to learning laparoscopic suturing and the current status of suturing technologies.

EQUIPMENT

A quality needle driver is the most important piece of equipment needed for laparoscopic suturing. An ideal needle driver is able to hold the needle firmly in place, has a ratcheting mechanism to avoid fatigue, and should be able to grasp the suture without causing damage. Needle drivers come in an assortment of styles and are made by a variety of manufacturers (Figure 7.1). The assisting instrument is often just as important and should have the ability to effectively grasp the tissue, the needle, and the suture. It is recommended to use two needle drivers for laparoscopic suturing. If extracorporeal knot tying is performed, then a knot pusher is necessary. Knot pushers come in both open and closed varieties and are discussed further in the knot tying section. Scissors are needed to cut the suture and come in straight, curved, and hook varieties. At least two trocars are needed, but often a third is utilized by a surgical assistant. The main consideration in trocar selection is the diameter of the trocar relative to the needle and the valve mechanism that will allow for easy insertion and removal of the needle.

SUTURE CHARACTERISTICS AND SELECTION

A variety of sutures can be used in laparoscopic suturing, and selection is often based on surgeon preference. Criteria for ideal suture selection for laparoscopic procedures are no different than for open surgery. The memory of the suture and the ability of the surgeon to handle the suture with the laparoscopic instruments are important. The memory of the suture can be used as an advantage in forming the loop for intracorporeal knot tying but can also hinder the process if the suture is not properly aligned. Monofilament sutures make it easier to throw sliding or cinch knots but are not as good at maintaining tension as braided suture. The ideal needle used for closure should be decided based on the type of defect being closed. Barbed suture has been recently introduced and is discussed in the "Suturing technologies" section of this chapter.

PORT PLACEMENT: UNDERSTANDING TRIANGULATION

Triangulation in laparoscopy refers to the relationship between the tissue, ports, and camera. When two ports are placed, a plane is created between the two instruments. The angle that is created between these two ports depends on the distance between the two ports. Understanding the relationship between the camera and this plane and the tissue is critical to efficient laparoscopic suturing. The configurations used in gynecologic laparoscopy include ipsilateral, suprapubic, and contralateral configurations. Examples of each of these configurations and their resulting triangulation are shown in Figures 7.2 through 7.4. The ideal port placement for suturing and knot tying for gynecology have been widely debated. There are currently no studies that directly compare different port placements and their effect on laparoscopic suturing. All the port placements that are presented have been used clinically and can be utilized with the proper understanding of the relationships, practice, and experience. Each port configuration has certain advantages and disadvantages.

The most important factor in deciding on a port configuration is ergonomics. Understanding the ergonomic relationship between the port configurations and the surgeon's positioning and the manipulation of the instruments is critical in avoiding surgeon fatigue and possible injury from prolonged surgery. Most surgeons will agree that a relaxed posture and wrist position are the most important factors in avoiding strain and fatigue, with the elbows near the body. The wrist should be positioned in a manner that avoids excessive extension, flexion, or rotation to avoid strain with prolonged suturing.

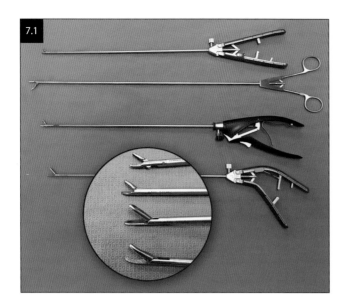

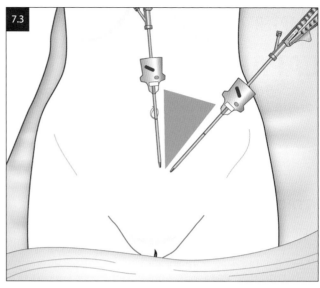

SYSTEMATIC METHOD

Laparoscopic suturing is a task that requires practice and repetition to become proficient. Proficient laparoscopic surgeons have mastered the ability to set the needle and pass it accurately through the tissue. It is the understanding of the relationships between the camera, instruments, needle, and tissue that leads to this proficiency. The use of different port configurations has hindered a universal technique from being adopted. By studying the cause-and-effect relationships between port placement, the camera, and the tissue, the surgeon can better recognize the critical steps and relationships that lead to efficient laparoscopic suturing. The goal of this section is to analyze the suturing process and to identify the critical elements that lead to successful tissue reapproximation and knot tying.

We broke down the suturing process into three main steps: (1) *setting the needle*, (2) *tissue reapproximation, and* (3) *knot tying.*

1. SETTING THE NEEDLE
2. TISSUE REAPPROXIMATION
3. KNOT TYING

By breaking down this process into these manageable steps, it allows the surgeon to learn each portion in an efficient manner. This avoids overloading the learning capacity, which can lead to frustration and inefficiency in the skill acquisition process. The following paragraphs present each segment in a step-by-step manner. This process can be followed to reproduce efficient suturing regardless of port configuration.

SETTING THE NEEDLE

The most critical relationship is the angle of the needle and the needle driver. The goal is to set the needle in a

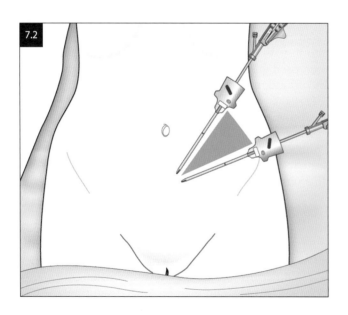

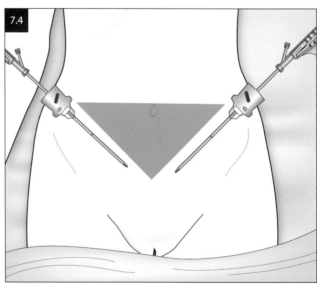

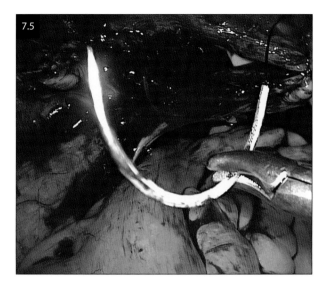

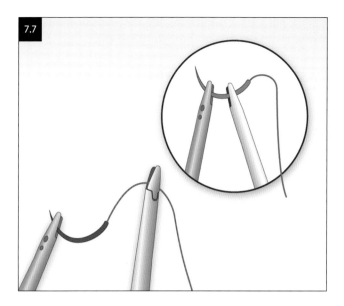

manner that allows for accurate placement of the needle through the tissue. A simple rotation of the needle driver around the axis of its shaft is the ideal way to drive the needle through the tissue. The most stable relationship between the needle and needle driver occurs when the needle is set in a perpendicular relationship to the shaft of the needle driver (Figure 7.5). This minimizes the torque or rotational force applied to the needle as it is passed through the tissue.

> SETTING THE NEEDLE IN A PERPENDICULAR RELA-
> TIONSHIP TO THE SHAFT OF THE NEEDLE DRIVER IS
> THE FIRST STEP IN EFFICIENT SUTURING.

In order to simplify the laparoscopic suturing and needle manipulation, we identify three points on the needle and the suture as points A, B, and C as well as the middle of the needle (Figure 7.6). For easier needle manipulation, it is important to remember that the left part of the needle belongs to the left hand, and the right part belongs to the right hand. The needle holders should not cross over to the other side (territory).

The needle is passed into the abdomen through the trocar by holding the suture at point "C" about 2 cm away from the needle hub with the dominant hand. With the suture in the right hand, the front half of the needle is grasped with the left hand (Figure 7.7). The suture is then manipulated with the nondominant hand until the plane of the needle is perpendicular to the shaft of the dominant needle driver. The right hand is then used to grasp the back half of the needle at point "C," about one-third distance from the hub of the needle as shown in Figure 7.8. The needle driver is then rotated so that the relationship and angle of the needle to the shaft of the needle driver are confirmed. If the needle is not in the proper orientation, the process is reversed, and the needle tip is grasped with the assisting instrument (left hand). The right hand then regrasps the suture, and the angle of the needle relative to the shaft is adjusted. The proper needle orientation is confirmed by rotating the needle driver, which allows us to establish the three-dimensional orientation on the two-dimensional screen. Once the needle lies in

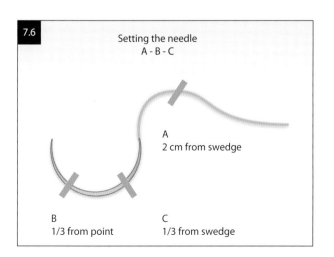

Setting the needle
A - B - C

A
2 cm from swedge

B
1/3 from point

C
1/3 from swedge

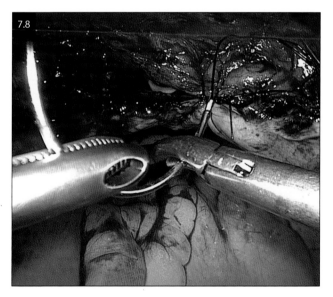

a perpendicular relationship with the shaft of the needle driver, it can be passed through the tissue.

TISSUE REAPPROXIMATION

The most reproducible way to pass the needle through the tissue is by simply rotating the needle driver around the axis of the shaft. The ultimate goal is to pass the needle through the tissue in a perpendicular relationship to the tissue suture line. The surgeon must understand the relationship between this tissue suture line and the needle driver. The left-hand or assistant instrument is used to grasp or place the tissue in an orientation so the needle can be easily passed. When the needle lies in a perpendicular relationship to the shaft of the needle driver, the tissue must be placed so that the tissue and the shaft of the needle driver lie in a parallel relationship (Figure 7.9). When this occurs, the needle can be passed through the tissue with a simple axial rotation of the needle driver. There are three requirements to successful laparoscopic suturing (the rule of 90°): (1) the needle should be grasped at a 90° angle to the needle holder; (2) the incision should be placed at a 90° angle to the needle; and (3) the needle tip should be placed at a 90° angle to the tissue.

---

1. NEEDLE SHOULD BE GRASPED AT 90° ANGLE TO THE NEEDLE HOLDER
2. INCISION SHOULD BE PLACED AT 90° ANGLE TO THE NEEDLE
3. NEEDLE TIP SHOULD BE PLACED AT 90° ANGLE TO THE TISSUE

Once the needle is passed through one side of the tissue, it is grasped with the assistant instrument and rotated through the tissue. The needle is reset as close to the tissue as possible to preserve the angle of the needle in relation to the needle driver. Once the needle is reset, the assistant instrument is used to grasp the other side of the tissue defect and place it in the proper orientation to allow passage of the needle with a simple axial rotation of the needle driver. If interrupted sutures are being placed, then the suture is ready to be tied. If a figure-of-8 suture is being performed, the suture is pulled through to allow for another passage of the needle through the tissue in a similar fashion, and then the knot is secured. If continuous suturing is being performed, such as in a myomectomy, the needle is passed through the tissue as described and then reset. The suture can be pulled through tissue using a nondominant hand—what is known as the pulley technique (Figure 7.10). The needle should be safeguarded from sticking vital structures by moving the needle toward the anterior abdominal wall in the midline. The assistant instrument can then be used to pull the suture through the tissue by pulling the suture cephalad. If a surgical assistant is being utilized, the assistant should be able to grasp the suture at the level of the tissue defect so that the surgeon can continue suturing. Efficient tissue reapproximation can be accomplished by repeating this simple process. The key to success lies in understanding the relationship of the needle, the shaft of the needle driver, and the orientation of the tissue defect. The role of the left-hand assisting instrument is vital to reliably passing the needle through the tissue, and it is more accurate to state that the left hand is utilized to place the tissue around the needle instead of imagining the needle being driven through the tissue.

THE USE OF THE LEFT HAND TO ORIENT THE TISSUE DEFECT IN A PARALLEL RELATIONSHIP IS CRITICAL TO EFFECTIVELY PASSING THE NEEDLE THROUGH THE TISSUE.

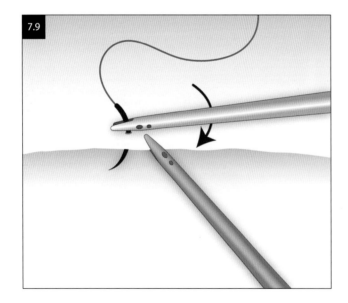

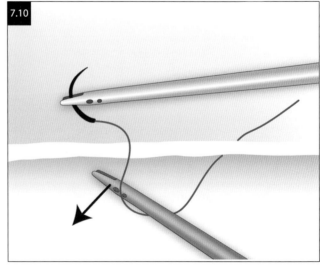

KNOT TYING

Once the suture has been placed through the tissue, the knot can be tied. This can be done by an extracorporeal or intracorporeal technique. Extracorporeal techniques are aided by the use of a knot pusher. Knot pushers are made by a variety of manufacturers and come in both open and closed models (Figure 7.11). The knot pusher is used like an extension of the surgeon's finger to secure the knot. The suture is threaded through the closed knot pusher, and a knot is thrown outside the patient's abdomen. The knot pusher is then used to push the knot down to the tissue. The knot is secured by pushing the suture past the knot, similar to the method used to secure knots in the pelvis during open surgery. Because tension can be difficult to maintain through the laparoscopic knot tying process, a second throw in the same direction is recommended to form a granny knot. This allows the second knot to be secure with the correct amount of tension. A monofilament suture such as PDS or Monocryl may be helpful in allowing the knot to slip down. A third throw in the opposite direction is then made to lock the previous knots. A total of four to six throws are made depending on the suture. When using an open-ended knot pusher, the steps are modified. The knot is first thrown, and then the knot pusher is slipped onto the suture. The knot pusher is then used to advance the suture down to the level of the tissue (Figure 7.12). The knot is then secured by placing tension on the suture past the knot, similar to the technique used with a closed knot pusher.

INTRACORPOREAL KNOT TYING

The ability to tie intracorporeal knots is an essential skill for the advanced laparoscopist. Although tying intracorporeal knots is more difficult than tying extracorporeal knots, once mastered it can be more efficient. The key to intracorporeal knot tying is understanding how to make

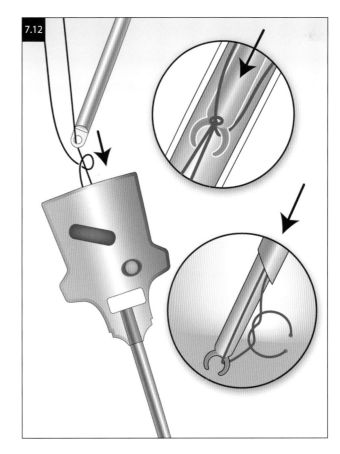

the loop and the common mistakes that are encountered with intracorporeal knot tying. By taking a systematic approach to learning the key relationships and these mistakes, difficulties in knot tying can be recognized and corrected. The loop can be formed with the assistance of the needle or simply by grasping the suture with the left hand to form the loop, which is referred to as expert knot tying. The use of the needle makes the loop easier to form but must be dropped in most instances to secure the knot. This facilitates additional steps that can be eliminated by learning expert knot tying.

The knot tying process can be divided into three parts: forming the loop, throwing the knot, and securing the knot. Forming the loop is the most important step and has three critical elements. Committing these steps to memory and understanding how they correspond to the common mistakes made by surgeons is essential in mastering efficient intracorporeal knot tying. Understanding the length of suture needed to form the loop is of great importance. The ideal length of suture used for intracorporeal knot tying is 15 cm or the length of a standard Mayo scissor. Once the suture is passed through the tissue, a short tail is made of about 2–3 cm. The left hand is then positioned on the suture so that the suture and the right hand are in a parallel or inline relationship. Once this parallel relationship is made between the suture and the right hand, the loop can be formed by moving the right hand over the tissue where the knot is to be secured (Figure 7.13). When expert knot tying is done, the rotation of the left hand has a critical role in establishing

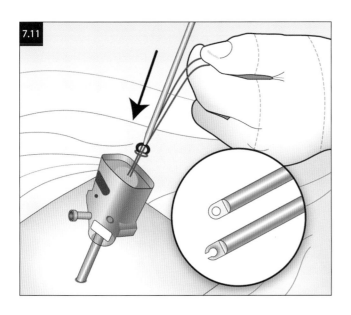

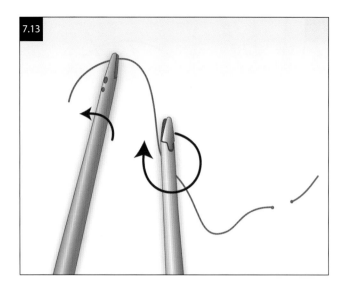

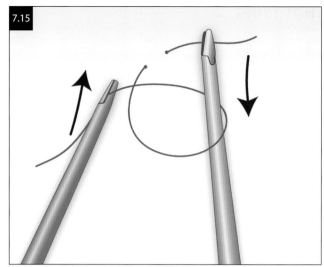

the orientation of the loop; understanding this relation-ship is the key to successful expert knot tying and loop formation. Once the loop is properly formed, the knot is thrown by wrapping the right instrument around the suture in the left hand (Figure 7.14). The short tail is then grasped, and the knot can be secured. The knot is secured by moving the left hand away from the knot, which removes the loop from the right hand and short tail. The right hand is then used to grasp and move the tail across the suture line. The left hand is then moved opposite the right hand and the knot laid flat (Figure 7.15). The left hand that is holding the loop is then moved back over the tissue and knot, while the right hand is kept in place, close to the knot (Figure 7.16). A second throw is then made in the opposite direction, by placing the dom-inant grasper underneath the suture, wrapping it around the dominant grasper to form the loop, and grasping the short tail. The short tail is grasped, and the knot is laid flat. This sequence is demonstrated in Figure 7.17. Care must be taken not to pull the right hand so much that a long tail is made. This creates a compound problem with

throwing the next knot, as the loop is shortened; even if the knot is able to be thrown, the long tail will often lead to the formation of a bowtie knot. The intracorporeal expert knot is much easier to tie around the needle, as shown in Figures 7.18 and 7.19, or if the needle holders are introduced from contralateral sides (Figure 7.20).

It is often difficult to maintain tension when tying intra-corporeal knots, and an air knot may occur. By learning to secure a cinch knot, this issue can be alleviated. To secure a cinch knot, you make your first throw and leave the knot loose. You then make a second throw in the opposite direction and complete an air square knot. The tail is released, and that hand is used to grab the por-tion of suture where the needle last exited the tissue. The right and left hands then pull the suture by apply-ing force in a 180° or opposite direction. The knot will snap and is converted to a sliding knot. The exit strand is released and the knot pushed down until it is secured (Figure 7.21). The tail is then grasped, and the knot is secured. A third throw is then made to lock the knot into place. This is a very versatile and important type of knot to learn to become proficient at laparoscopic suturing.

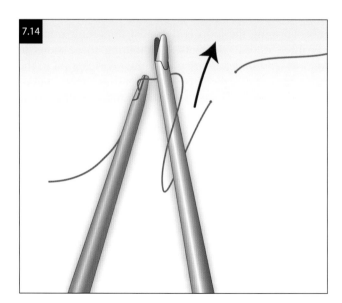

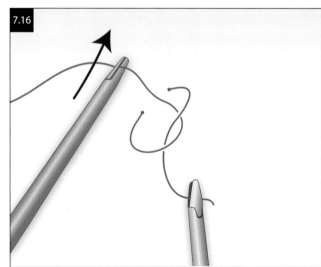

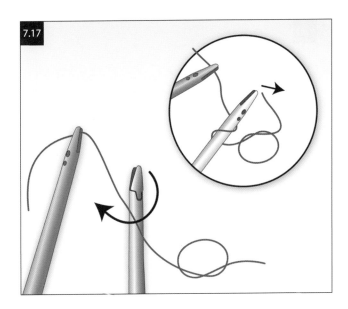

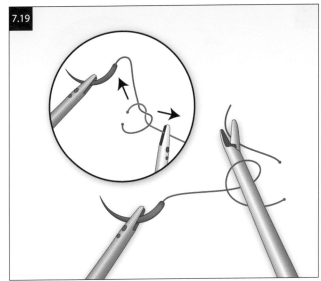

The most common mistakes are failure to maintain a short tail, lift and drift, and improper orientation of the loop. The surgeon must maintain a short tail. It is not maintaining the short tail that is the most common error and is the result of pulling the right hand too far from the knot. Difficulty throwing the knot comes from the suture not being in a parallel relationship with the right hand. Because the loop is not in the proper orientation, this leads the surgeon to the next mistake, which is lift and drift. To make throwing the knot easier, the surgeon lifts or drifts the suture away from the knot, which straightens the loop and makes knot tying difficult. It is only by understanding the relationship of loop length and avoiding lift and drift that the proper length of the loop is maintained. When the orientation of this loop is correctly aligned with the right hand, then intracorporeal knot tying becomes reproducible. By making a conscious effort to control the rotation of the left hand holding the suture, the proper orientation can be maintained for expert knot tying.

INTRODUCING ANY SIZE NEEDLE THROUGH 5 MM TROCAR

The technique of Drs. Courtney Clark and Harry Reich allows the placement of any size curved needle into the abdominal cavity by using a 5 mm incision. This technique is illustrated in Figures 7.22 through 7.25.

The ancillary trocar is withdrawn from the abdominal wall. The trocar hole is plugged with the assistant's finger to prevent the escape of gas from the peritoneal cavity (Figure 7.22).

The trocar is held in the surgeon's hand outside the abdominal cavity, and the needle holder or grasper is inserted through the trocar sleeve; the suture tail is grasped and pulled back through the trocar. The grasper is then reintroduced through the trocar along the suture, and the suture is grasped about 3–4 cm above the needle hub (Figures 7.23 and 7.24).

The needle holder is then introduced into the peritoneal cavity through the same incision, pulling the needle

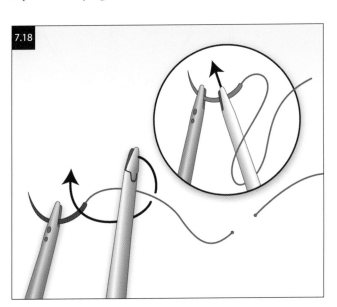

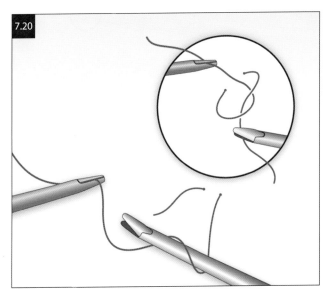

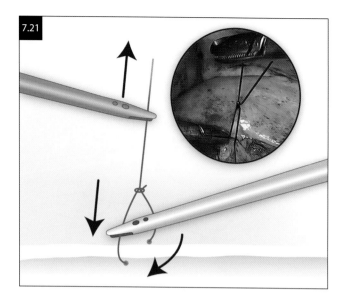

7.21

with it. When the needle is pulled into the abdominal cavity, the trocar sleeve is then pushed over the grasper, using it as a guide to seal the incision in the abdominal wall (Figure 7.25).

After introducing the needle into the abdominal cavity, a small clamp is placed at the suture tail to prevent the tail of the suture from being pulled into the trocar.

SUTURING TECHNOLOGIES

There are many products to aid with laparoscopic suturing. One of the first products was the Endoloop (Ethicon

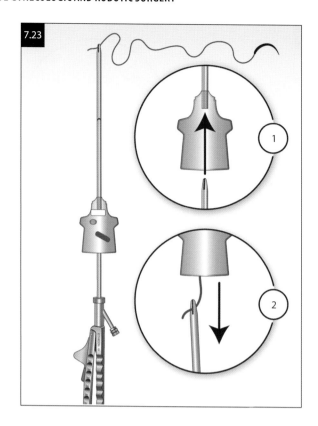

7.23

Endosurgery, Cincinnati, Ohio). The Endoloop is a loop ligature that can be passed through a trocar and placed around tissue. The Endoloop uses a pre-tied Roeder knot that is pushed down against the tissue and secured with a plastic knot pusher (Figure 7.26).

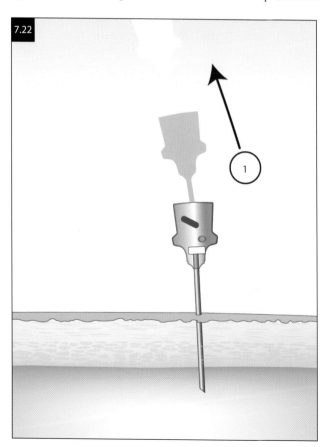

7.22

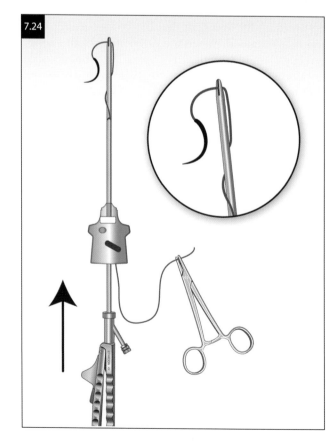

7.24

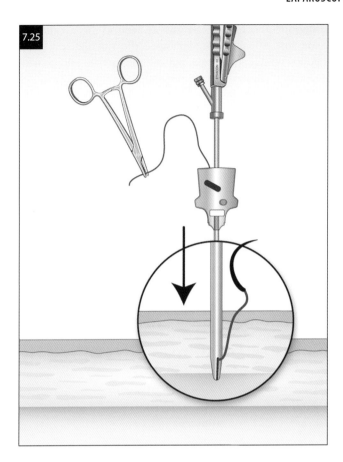

The Autosuture Endo Stitch (Medtronic, Boulder, Colorado) is the one-hand suturing device that allows an easy transfer of the straight needle between two arms. The wide-mouth jaws of the instrument open to 19 mm and allow for the grasping of a wide variety of tissue thickness with a 9 mm straight needle. The device uses a mechanical ratchet to pass the needle back and forth and eliminates the need to set and reset the needle. An integrated needle and suture allows for a wide variety of different suture combinations. However, this design limits the angle and depth at which the needle can be passed, and tissue manipulation with the assisting instrument is critical in obtaining adequate tissue bites (Figure 7.27). To overcome this limitation, another product, the SILS Endo Stitch (Medtronic) uses a similar mechanism on an articulating shaft. The articulating shaft design allows for more varied angles of approach and is often utilized in single-incision procedures. After the sutures have been placed through the tissue, the Endo Stitch can also be used for intracorporeal and extracorporeal knot tying. Other mechanical "sewing machine" devices include the Ethicon Suture Assistant and the RD 180 by LSI Solutions.

The Lapra-Ty by Ethicon is an absorbable PDS clip that is applied to the suture and prevents the suture from pulling through the tissue. A second clip can then be applied to the tail of the suture once it has been passed through the tissue to secure the suture line, avoiding any knot tying (Figure 7.28). Although these devices can improve surgical efficiency, the cost of these devices must be taken into account given their disposable nature.

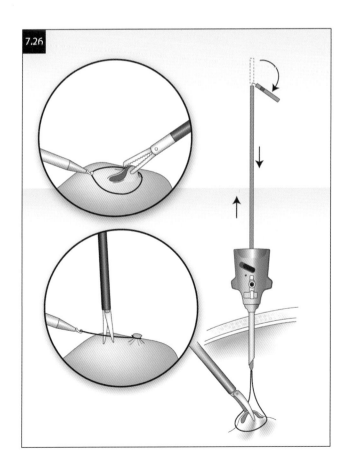

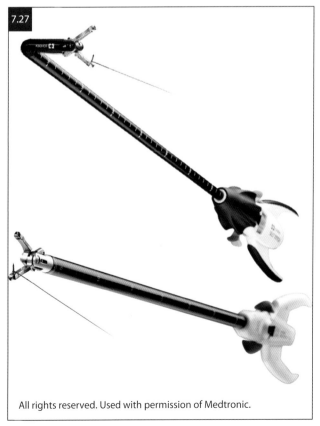

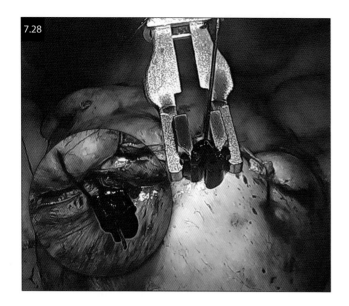

7.28

Barbed sutures have been introduced by Angiotech (Quill) and Covidien (V-Loc). They are able to maintain the tension of the suture in the tissue by utilizing a barbed pattern that anchors the suture in a unidirectional path. This often eliminates the need to anchor the suture with a knot.

The most advanced suture technology developed recently is arguably robotics. By utilizing a three-dimensional video system, depth perception is greatly improved. Additionally, robotic technology scales down movements and incorporates articulating instruments, thereby facilitating microsurgical suturing. This can be advantageous in procedures such as tubal reanastomosis. Specifically, the additional articulation allows the surgeon to move the instruments around the needle and tissue instead of having to move the needle and tissue around fixed instruments. Setting the needle and passing the needle through the tissue thus becomes much easier for some surgeons. The surgeon is also able to pass the needle through the tissue at angles that may be difficult to accomplish with fixed instrumentation.

Suturing technologies and robotics have all been developed to aid the surgeon in reapproximating tissue. No matter if using conventional instruments or suturing devices, the fundamentals that lead to efficient suturing are the same. A fundamental understanding of the geometric relationships between the instruments, tissue, needle, and camera is the real key to becoming proficient at laparoscopic suturing. Developing a systematic approach to suturing and breaking down each process into manageable and key parts will allow the laparoscopic surgeon to become successful at laparoscopic suturing.

SUGGESTED READING

Hudgens JL, Pasic R, eds. *Fundamentals of Geometric Laparoscopy and Suturing*. Tuttlingen, Germany: Endo Press; 2015.

Koh CH. *Laparoscopic Suturing in the Vertical Zone*. Tuttlingen, Germany: Endo Press; 2010.

Mencagilia L, Minelli L, Wattiez A. *Manual of Gynecologic Laparoscopic Surgery*, 11th ed. Tuttlingen, Germany: Verlag Endo Press; 2008.

Pasic R. All you need to know about laparoscopic suturing. In: Pasic R and Levine RL, eds. *A Practical Manual of Laparoscopy: A Clinical Cookbook*. 2nd ed. Taylor & Francis Group; 2007, Chapter 7, pp. 97–108.

CHAPTER 8
LAPAROSCOPIC TUBAL STERILIZATION

Ronald L. Levine and Thomas G. Lang

Laparoscopic sterilization is the most common type of female sterilization surgery performed in the United States. There are essentially four major methods. There is currently only one available U.S. Food and Drug Administration (FDA)-approved hysteroscopic sterilization device. This approach has been increasing in popularity over the past decade.

1. ELECTROSURGICAL USING BIPOLAR INSTRUMENTATION
2. CLIPS:
   a. HULKA
   b. FILSHIE
3. BANDS (FALLOPE RING)
4. SALPINGECTOMY
5. HYSTEROSCOPIC STERILIZATION—ESSURE

All of the laparoscopic methods that will be described may be performed through either a single-puncture technique using an operating laparoscope (Figure 8.1), or through a double-puncture technique using a 5 mm second puncture trocar that is typically placed in the midline suprapubic area. The double-puncture technique uses a 5 or 10 mm laparoscope that is inserted through an umbilical port (Figure 8.2). If the single-puncture technique is the method of choice, it is very important that a well-functioning uterine manipulator be employed. By moving the manipulator, it is possible to stretch the tube laterally. The surgeon can control the operative field by moving the laparoscope in and out, to obtain close-up or panoramic view, and by moving the instrument inserted through the operative channel.

One of the greatest causes of sterilization failure is the misidentification of either the round ligament or the uteroovarian ligament for the fallopian tube. Therefore, it is vital to identify all three structures and to trace the tube to the fimbriae if at all possible, prior to performing the sterilization (Figure 8.3).

Although many of our laparoscopic sterilization procedures are performed under general anesthesia, they can also be done under local anesthesia. When local is the method, the skin and deeper tissues are blocked using lidocaine (Figure 8.4). The art, however, is to instill a mixture of 10 cc Carbocaine and lidocaine transcervically via the uterine manipulator (Figure 8.5). The tubes can almost be seen to blanch. Prior to using the desired technique, we drip another 10 cc of lidocaine along the length of the tube (Figure 8.6). Another tip is to insufflate with NO_2 (nitrous oxide), which is less irritating to the peritoneal surface.

BIPOLAR COAGULATION

The technique of bipolar coagulation, as originally described by Dr. Richard Kleppinger, is still the most popular form of laparoscopic sterilization and is our suggested form of electrosurgical management.

The bipolar Kleppinger-type forceps have been described in Chapter 6. The tips of the forceps are where the energy is distributed from one tong to the other. It is therefore important that the tips enclose the tube as much as possible by opposing along the underlying mesosalpinx (Figure 8.7).

Bipolar coagulation provides a localized area of tubal and mesosalpingeal burn, thus requiring at least 2–3 cm to be coagulated. The tube is grasped in the ampullary portion of the tube at least 2 cm from the cornua (Figure 8.7). If applied too close to the uterus, there is some risk of creating a uteroperitoneal fistula with subsequent pregnancy in the distal segment. The tips of the tongs should minimally meet in the mesosalpinx to avoid excessive damage to the blood supply of the tube and its anastomotic branches to the ovary. The electrosurgical generator should be set to deliver a power of 25 W switched to a cut mode in order to desiccate the tissue sufficiently. If higher voltage is used by switching to the coag mode, the tube will rapidly coagulate just on its periphery, potentially leading to a sterilization failure. Optimally, the fallopian tube should be coagulated using two to three contiguous burns to provide a net area of 2–3 cm of coagulation. The endpoint of coagulation is the cessation of current flow as evidenced by use of an inline ammeter or by the end of water vapor emission and tissue whitening. After completing the coagulation, some surgeons also sever the tube in the middle of the burn area using laparoscopic scissors (Figure 8.8). However, many surgeons do not cut the tube, believing that it may lead to a higher failure rate from fistula formation. The failure rate at 10 years with the bipolar method according to the largest multicenter prospective study, the CREST study, was 2.48%. This number is lower, however, when current techniques are employed, when compared to techniques used in the late 1970s and early

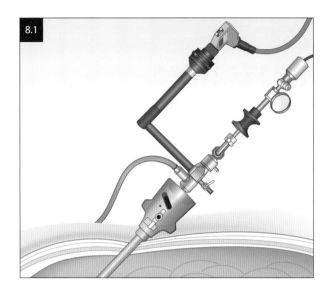

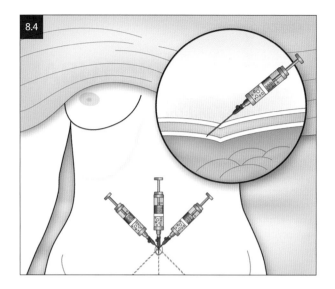

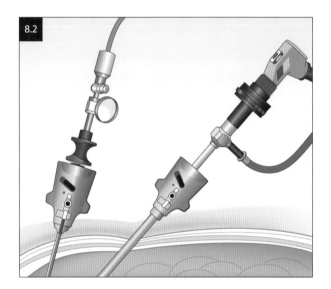

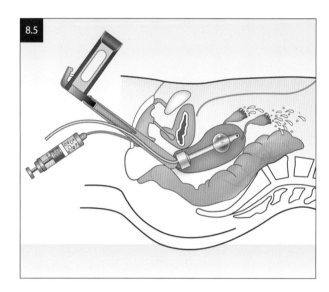

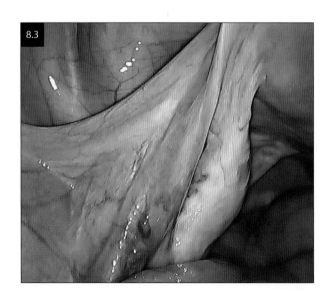

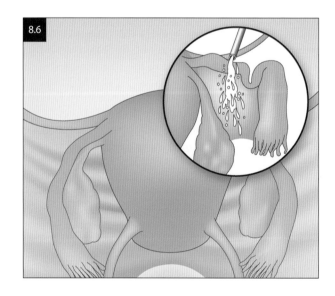

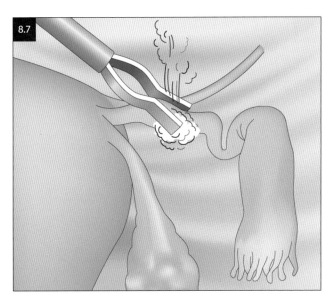

1980s. A secondary analysis of data for 5-year failure rates between 1985 and 1987 showed a 0.63% failure, while 5-year failure rates from 1978 to 1982 were 1.95%.

IMPORTANT NUMBERS

2 CM FROM FUNDUS

2–3 CM OF TUBE

2–3 CONTIGUOUS BURNS

25 W POWER USING CUT MODE

CLIPS

Mechanical occlusion of the tube is most commonly performed using a surgical clip. Although first described in 1976 and used in the United Kingdom for many years, the Filshie clip (CooperSurgical, Trumbull, Connecticut) was not approved in the United States until 1996. This clip is made of titanium with a silicone rubber lining that expands to keep the tube compressed as it flattens. This clip also requires a special applicator and an 8 mm trocar. It may also be advanced into the abdomen through the operating channel of the single-puncture operating laparoscope by half closing the upper jaw. When the finger bar is released, the clip opens and is then placed and locked around the fallopian tube (Figure 8.9). The Filshie clip must be applied to the isthmic portion of the tube to maximize efficacy. The bar is then squeezed to its limit, thus closing the clip and releasing it from the applicator. The clip locks around the tube and cannot be removed. Tubal occlusion is ultimately created by the combined actions of mechanical ischemia and swelling of the hydrophilic silicone lining. If misapplied, another clip may be placed. Since a small area of the tube is crushed, this method may yield a high success rate for surgical reversal. Data show that a properly applied Filshie clip has a relatively low failure rate of 0.23% with follow-up of 6–15 years.

When applying a clip through the operative scope, it is important to keep the clip applicator with the loaded clip close to the tip of the laparoscope and at a 45° angle toward the camera (Figure 8.10a,b). (Figure 8.10b demonstrates how not to hold the clip applicator.) If the clip applicator is pushed too far from the tip of the operative laparoscope, the perspective is lost, and the operator cannot get adequate magnification and visualization of the fallopian tube. Once the clip applicator is introduced with full view of the clip, the whole scope is pushed down toward the tube, and the clip is applied across the isthmic portion of the tube (Figure 8.11).

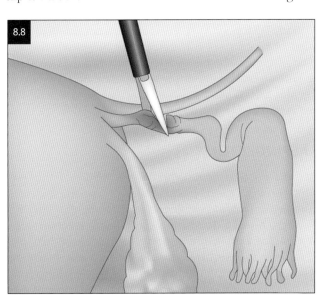

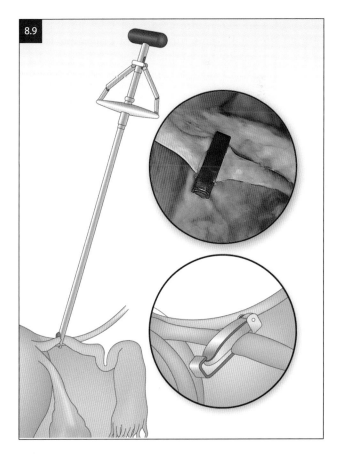

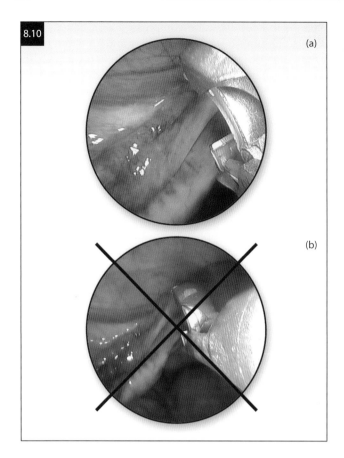

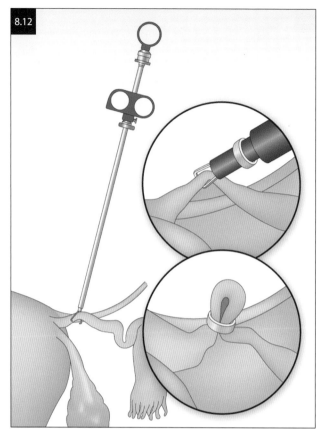

BANDS

Yoon and associates introduced the silastic band in 1974. This small silastic band is applied to the tube by use of a special 8 mm applicator that may be used through the single-puncture 12 mm operating laparoscope. The bands are preloaded onto the instrument using a special plastic loading device. The applicator is then passed down the channel, and grasping hooks are deployed from the end of the applicator (Figure 8.12). The tube is grasped in the isthmic area about 3 cm from

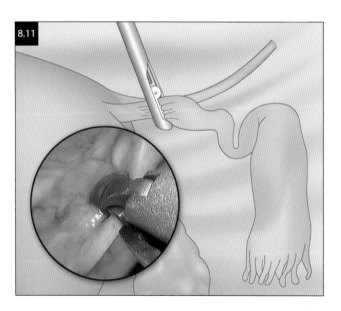

the cornua of the uterus. The tube is then drawn up into the inner cylinder of the applicator by the grasping hooks, and the silastic band is applied by moving the outer cylinder forward. It is important that a sufficient knuckle of tube is brought back into the applicator to assure that two complete lumens have been occluded. After application of the band, the grasping tongs are moved forward out of the inner cylinder to release the occluded tube.

Several problems have been described with the bands. There have been a significant number of complications secondary to tears in the mesosalpinx. Bleeding from this problem can usually be controlled by bipolar coagulation. Postoperative pain is more frequent than with clips or bipolar coagulation, presumably from the volume of tubal ischemia. A large number of these patients require an oral analgesic for several days postoperatively. Per the CREST study, the 10-year failure rate with this device was 1.77%.

SALPINGECTOMY

In the event that tubal pathology (i.e., hydrosalpinx) prevents proper placement of a clip or occluding device, complete or partial salpingectomy can achieve the following: not only does it provide a highly effective form of contraception, it also removes the pathology, may prevent some types of ovarian cancer, and serves to eliminate confounding findings on future pelvic sonography. This method is best performed using an energy-based

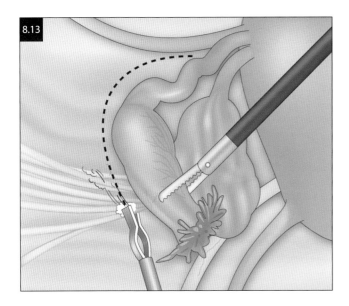

surgical device to sequentially coagulate and cut the mesosalpinx. It is important to avoid the ovary during dissection to minimize possible effects on ovarian function (Figure 8.13) (see Chapter 10).

HYSTEROSCOPIC STERILIZATION

There is currently one FDA-approved device for hysteroscopic tubal sterilization, the Essure device (Bayer Healthcare Pharmaceuticals, Leverkusen, Germany) (Figure 8.14). Hysteroscopic sterilization with this device offers a low-cost and low-risk approach that can also be performed in the office setting under paracervical block, with or without sedation. A hysteroscope with a 5Fr working channel is used with a 30° angled lens. The inserts are placed into the proximal section of each fallopian tube and then deployed. The microinserts then anchor themselves to the endosalpingeal mucosa. The microinserts are 4 cm long and 0.8 mm in diameter, but expand to 1.5–2 mm in diameter when

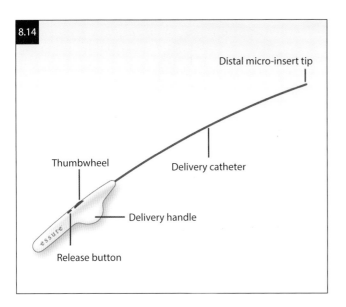

deployed (Figure 8.15). The microinserts contain two coils. The outer coil is made of a nickel titanium alloy, Nitinol (Nickel Titanium Naval Ordnance Laboratory), which is known for its unique properties of shape memory and superelasticity. Since 2011, nickel is no longer considered an absolute contraindication to having an Essure done. The inner coil is made of stainless steel that is wound with polyethylene terephthalate (PET) fibers. Once placed, the microinsert causes tissue ingrowth, and the tube is permanently occluded. Three months after the procedure, an Essure conformation test (ECT) is performed, which is a specific type of hysterosalpingogram that confirms complete tubal occlusion. Clinical trials involving 643 women revealed that no pregnancies occurred once bilateral tubal occlusion was confirmed with the ECT. It is important to place the patient on contraception until tubal occlusion is confirmed. Between the years of 1997 and 2005, 50,000 Essure procedures were performed, of which only 64 unintended pregnancies were reported to the manufacturer, and most of these were secondary to nonadherence of contraception during this window. Intramuscular Depo-Provera is a commonly used contraceptive because it may be given at the preoperative visit. This offers the advantage of thinning the endometrial lining, thereby easing the visualization of the ostia, and provides contraception for 12 weeks. Another helpful tip is to give preoperative nonsteroidal anti-inflammatory drugs (NSAIDs) such as Toradol 1 hour prior to the procedure to decrease tubospasm and uterine cramping. The 5-year failure rate of the Essure procedure has been reported by Babinski in 2010 at 0.17%. The potential disadvantage of the hysteroscopic sterilization method is that it is not reversible, and once the inserts are applied, they cannot be pulled back, and the entire tube may have to be removed.

Steps to proper placement are as follows:

1. Place the 30° hysteroscope with a 5 mm working channel through the cervix into the uterine cavity. Dilation is not always necessary and should be minimized to maintain uterine distention (Figure 8.16).

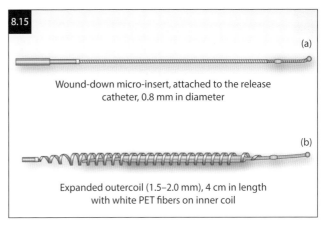

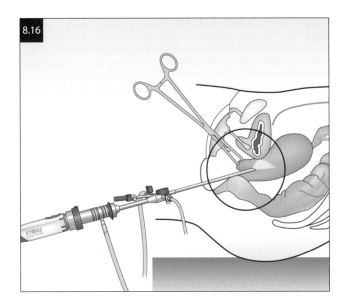

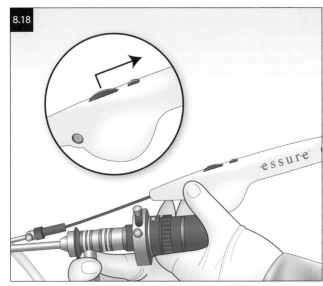

2. Survey the uterine cavity and identify both tubal ostia. Open the Essure system packing only after bilateral tubal ostia are identified.

3. Choose the more difficult ostium first. If you are unable to perform the cannulation, you do not have to waste the second device. Position the ostium into the center view of the video screen with the aid of the fore-oblique view of the hysteroscope. Advance the hysteroscope close to the ostium to add column strength to the device.

4. With the hysteroscope steady to avoid drifting, place the introducer through the working channel. It is important to avoid damaging the introducer during advancement, as this can also cause damage to the Essure device. Carefully insert the Essure catheter through the introducer using a gentle and constantly forward movement, while aligning the introducer and hysteroscope to prevent bending during insertion.

5. Advance the catheter tip into the ostium so that the black positioning marker is at the internal border of the ostium (Figure 8.17).

6. While the hysteroscope and catheter are held steady, roll the wheel back to a hard stop (Figure 8.18).

7. With gentle traction, pull back the entire device until the gold band "notch" is just outside the ostium. Adjust as necessary (Figure 8.19).

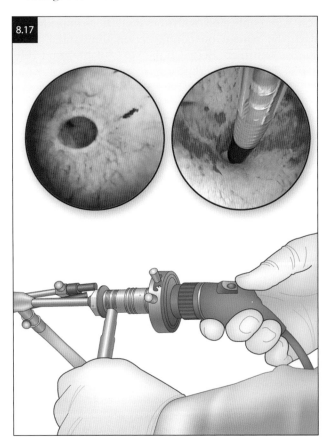

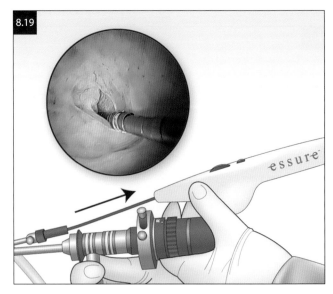

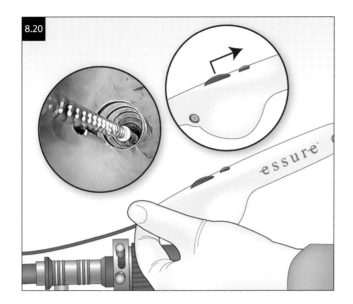

1. ROLL THE THUMBWHEEL BACK TO A HARD STOP ONCE THE BLACK POSITIONING MARKER IS AT THE OSTIUM
2. PRESS THE BUTTON ON THE HANDLE TO INITIATE THE DEPLOYMENT
3. ROLL THE THUMBWHEEL BACK TO A HARD STOP—THE MICROINSERT WILL EXPAND

Since complete tubal occlusion from fibrotic ingrowth after placement of the Essure device may take as long as 3 months, additional contraception should be used during this interval. Moreover, present guidelines in the United States require the use of a low-pressure hysterosalpingogram to confirm bilateral tubal occlusion.

SUGGESTED READING

American College of Obstetricians and Gynecologists. 2013. Reaffirmed 2107. ACOG practice bulletin. Benefits and risks of sterilization #133, Washington, DC: The College.

Grimes D. Update on female sterilization. *Contracept Rep.* 1996;7(3):1–2.

Ouzounelli M, Reaven LN. Essure hysteroscopic sterilization versus interval laparoscopic bilateral tubal ligation: A comparative effectiveness review. *J Minim Invasive Gynecol.* 2015;22:342–352.

Peterson HB, Xia Z, Hughes JM, et al. The risk of pregnancy after tubal sterilization: Findings from the U.S. Collaborative Review of Sterilization. *Am J Obstet Gynecol.* 1996;174:1161–1170.

8. Once the gold notch is at the correct position, press the button on the handle to initiate the deployment of the microinsert. Be sure to press firmly to ensure proper deployment.
9. Roll the thumbwheel back to a hard stop. At this point, the microinsert will expand and detach from the catheter (Figure 8.20).
10. Take a photograph of the number of coils, and slowly withdraw the catheter.
11. Repeat steps 3–10 on the contralateral ostium with a new catheter/device.

CHAPTER 9

LAPAROSCOPIC SURGERY FOR ADHESIONS

Harry Reich, Baruch S. Abittan, Mark Dassel, and Tamer Seckin

INTRODUCTION

Adhesions may be defined as abnormal tissue attachments between tissues and organs. They can be either congenital or acquired in nature. Acquired adhesions develop in response to trauma to the peritoneum as a result of either surgery or inflammation. Postoperative adhesions commonly occur after pelvic inflammatory disease or peritoneal cavity surgery and are the leading cause of intestinal obstruction. In one study, 93% of patients who had undergone at least one previous open abdominal operation had postsurgical adhesions. This is not surprising, given the reactive nature of the peritoneum and the fact that apposition of two injured peritoneal surfaces promotes adhesion formation. For most, intraperitoneal adhesions remain asymptomatic. Adhesions have been correlated with infertility related to tuboovarian involvement and pelvic pain. It is generally accepted that adhesions may impair organ motility, resulting in visceral pain transmitted by peritoneal innervation. Although nerve fibers have been demonstrated in pelvic adhesions, their presence has not been shown to be more common in women with chronic pelvic pain. Moreover, there does not appear to be an association between the severity of the adhesions and the amount of pain.

Surgery to treat intraperitoneal adhesions for pelvic pain should be undertaken only in those women whose symptoms have been correlated with a reasonable degree of certainty. The effectiveness of adhesiolysis in treating chronic pain is unclear. One recent study suggested that adhesiolysis is no more effective than diagnostic laparoscopy. Although many women may experience resolution of their symptoms after adhesiolysis, the results may be transient by virtue of a significant placebo effect. One study reported no difference in pain scores between patients who were prospectively followed after being randomized to adhesiolysis versus expectant management. Moreover, adhesiolysis surgery itself is associated with a high risk of adhesion reformation. Good results have been achieved with ovarian adhesiolysis in improving fertility in women. Division of adhesions around the ovary in this population has been demonstrated to increase pregnancy rates by over 50%. Regardless, it is clearly better to prevent adhesions rather than to treat them.

This chapter reviews the pathophysiology and epidemiology of adhesion formation, the equipment and techniques employed for adhesiolysis, and the various measures available for adhesion prevention.

EPIDEMIOLOGY OF ADHESIONS

The Scottish National Health Service Morbidity Record (SMR1) studied a cohort of patients who underwent open abdominal or pelvic surgery in 1986. The publication of this data from the Surgical and Clinical Adhesions Research (SCAR) study in 1999 suggests viewing adhesions as an iatrogenic disease, requiring further research to be better understood.

Adhesion-related readmissions were identified over a 10-year period and were categorized as being:

1. Directly related to adhesions (adhesiolysis and nonoperative readmissions for adhesions)
2. Possibly related (selected gynecologic operations, selected abdominal surgery)
3. Selected nonoperative readmissions, or readmissions potentially complicated by adhesions (leading to open or laparoscopic procedures)

Over the 10 years of this study, over one-third of the 29,790 patients who underwent open surgery were readmitted a mean of 2.1 times for complications directly or possibly related to adhesions. Of the total number of readmissions (21,347), 5.7% were directly related to adhesions. Readmissions occurred within the first year in 22.1%.

One of the most important aspects of the SCAR study is the long-term perspective, providing information on the timing of adhesion-related complications. In all groups, after a rapid increase in adhesion-related readmissions the first 1 or 2 years, the rate of readmission continued to increase steadily in a linear fashion with time. Previous studies have similarly shown that adhesion-related complications can occur 10 years after the initial surgical procedure.

The SCAR study was the first study to analyze the clinical burden of postoperative adhesions following open surgery on the female reproductive tract in an *entire population*. While previous studies were limited to following clinical outcomes following surgeries on small groups of patients, or investigating patients presenting with a complication of adhesions (such as bowel obstruction), due to the relatively small and stable population in Scotland, coupled with the comprehensive Scottish National Health Services Medical Record Linkage Database, the SCAR study was able to examine *all* readmissions to hospitals in Scotland over a 10-year period.

Laparoscopic surgery was not widely used in 1986. SCAR-2 (Surgical and Clinical Adhesions Research Study 2) was a follow-up study that assessed the burden of adhesion-related readmissions during a period 10 years later than that used in the original SCAR study and compared the overall extent of adhesion-related readmissions following laparoscopic gynecologic surgery with open gynecologic surgery. Gynecologic laparoscopy as well as open surgery was shown to carry significant risks of adhesion-related readmissions.

These epidemiologic data show that adhesion formation results in a significant number of readmissions following both laparoscopic and open surgery and that the risk of adhesion-related complications extends for many years after the initial procedure. There is, therefore, a need for clinical and cost-effective strategies to help reduce the development of adhesions.

PATHOPHYSIOLOGY OF ADHESION FORMATION

Adhesion formation is initiated following localized injury to the mesothelial layer of the peritoneum. Bleeding and leakage of plasma proteins lead to fibrin deposits at the injury site, which is augmented by posttraumatic inflammation. Within hours at the site of injury, inflammatory cytokines, predominately interleukins and tumor necrosis factor, attract and activate macrophages to release vascular permeability factor. Simultaneous release of histamine and kinins increases the level of vascular permeability leading to inflammatory exudation with fibrin deposition on the peritoneal surface. By day 2, the wound surface is covered by macrophages, islands of primitive mesenchymal cells and mesothelial cells. The enlarging fibrin mesh may attach to an adjoining surface, a process that is counteracted by locally synthesized fibrinolytic factors. Depending on the local peritoneal conditions, the fibrin mesh can either be degraded, resulting in scarless repair, or transformed into an adhesion consisting of connective tissue. If the fibrin is degraded within a few days, the defect heals without scarring. If it is allowed to enlarge for a sufficient period of time, it will reach other tissue surfaces and form a bridge between them, transforming the initially reversible fibrous adhesion into a fibrous, collagen-containing structure. The adhesion continues to mature as collagen fibrils organize into bands covered by mesothelium that contains blood vessels and connective tissue fibers.

LAPAROSCOPIC PERITONEAL CAVITY ADHESIOLYSIS

"Cold scissors dissection with focused bipolar backup" or use of ultrasound energy is the methodology for adhesiolysis with the least potential for adhesion reformation. It is better to avoid the time-honored technique of "grasp, coagulate, then cut." Substitute the concept of "cutting where bleeding is least likely." Magnification and close inspection through the laparoscope make this possible, remembering that tissue ischemia caused by thermal energy is the enemy.

Adhesiolysis can be time consuming and technically difficult. More complex procedures are best performed by an experienced surgeon. Despite undergoing a lengthy laparoscopic surgery, most patients are discharged on the day of the procedure, have avoided a large abdominal incision, experience minimal complications, and rapidly return to full activity. Moreover, symptom relief can be dramatic.

In this section, general adhesiolysis, enterolysis, pelvic adhesiolysis, ovariolysis, salpingo-ovariolysis, and salpingostomy are described. The laparoscopic treatment of acute adhesions is covered in a separate section, describing early laparoscopic treatment of acute pelvic infection, including abscesses to prevent the adhesive sequelae from sexually transmitted disease. Acute adhesiolysis in this setting can prevent chronic adhesion formation.

INSTRUMENTATION

Laparoscopes

Five different types of laparoscopes are useful for adhesiolysis: a 5 mm and a 10 mm 0° laparoscope; a 10 mm operative laparoscope with 5 mm operating channel; and a 5 and 10 mm oblique-angled laparoscope (30°) for upper abdominal and pelvic procedures (Figure 9.1). Other than its small bore, a 5 mm laparoscope can be very versatile by providing multiple visual ports (port hopping) and by enabling visualization and access to the entire abdominal cavity.

Scissors

Scissors are the preferred instrument to cut adhesions, especially if they are avascular or congenital (Figure 9.2). Using the magnification afforded by the laparoscope, most anterior abdominal wall, pelvic, and bowel adhesions can be carefully inspected and divided with minimal bleeding, using mechanical dissection alone.

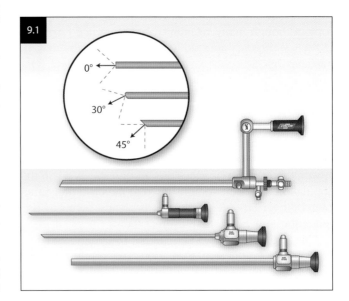

9.1

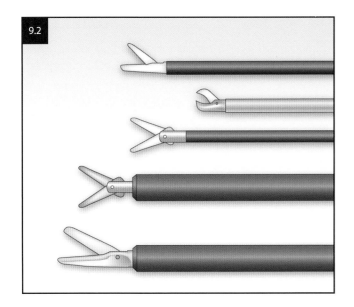

Loose fibrous or areolar tissue is separated by inserting a closed scissors and withdrawing it in the open position (Figure 9.3). Tissue is then pushed with the partially open blunt scissors tip to develop natural planes. Reusable 5 mm blunt-tipped sawtooth scissors and curved scissors (Richard Wolf Medical Instruments, Vernon Hills, Illinois, and Karl Storz Endoscopy, Culver City, California) cut well without the use of energy. Hook scissors are best for cutting suture and are not useful for adhesiolysis. Any scissors used should feel comfortable and not too long or encumbered by an electrical cord or rotation device, which can inhibit direction changes. Blunt or rounded-tip 5 mm scissors with one stable and one movable blade are used to divide thin and thick bowel adhesions sharply. Sharp mechanical dissection is the primary technique used for adhesiolysis to diminish the potential for adhesion formation; electrosurgery, ultrasonic energy, and lasers are usually reserved for hemostatic dissection of adhesions where anatomic planes are not evident and/or vasculature are anticipated. Thermal modalities should be avoided to help reduce adhesion recurrence.

Electrosurgery

Since monopolar *coag* current requires voltage over 10 times that of *cut* current and is associated with arcing to adjacent tissue, unintended thermal damage is more apt to occur. Thus, the use of *coag* current should be minimized during adhesion surgery. *Cut* current can be utilized to both cut and/or coagulate (desiccate) tissue simply by varying the surface area (current density) of the electrode in contact with tissue. Whereas tissue cutting is best achieved using the edge or tip of an electrode, the wider body (increased surface area) is best employed for tamponade and coagulation.

Electrosurgical injury to the bowel can occur beyond the surgeon's field of view during laparoscopic procedures from electrode insulation defects or capacitive coupling (see Chapters 6 and 38). Bipolar desiccation using cutting current between two closely opposed electrodes is safe and efficient for large vessel hemostasis. Large blood vessels are compressed and bipolar cutting current passed until complete desiccation is achieved, i.e., the current depletes the tissue fluid and electrolytes and fuses the vessel wall (Figure 9.4). *Coag* current should not be used for vessel sealing as it may rapidly desiccate the outer layers of the tissue, producing superficial resistance and thereby preventing deeper penetration. Small vessel hemostasis necessary for adhesiolysis is best achieved by using focused bipolar electrosurgery with an advance bipolar after precisely identifying and lavaging the vessel with electrolyte solution irrigation (Figure 9.5).

Ultrasonic devices

The use of the ultrasonic energy with the harmonic scalpel (Ethicon Endosurgery, Cincinnati, Ohio), Thunderbeat (Olympus Surgical America, Orangeburg, New York), or Sonicision (Medtronic Minneapolis, Minnesota) for laparoscopic adhesiolysis continues to gain popularity. The

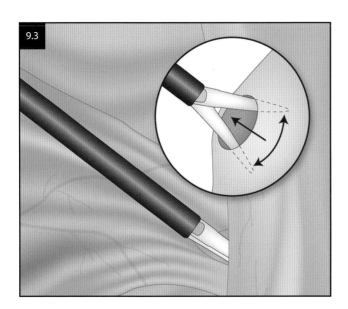

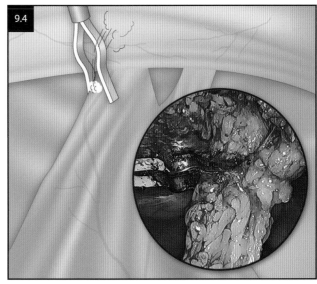

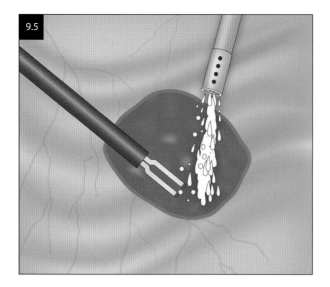

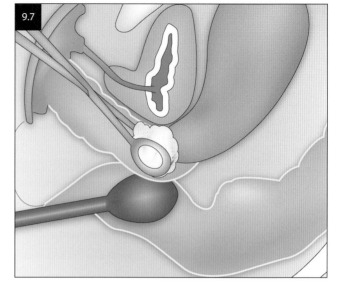

mechanical energy used to cut (cavitate) and coagulate tissue with potentially less lateral thermal spread to tissue such as the bowel make it more attractive than conventional electrosurgery for many surgeons. This is not to say, however, that injury cannot happen with this thermal modality. Thermal injury can occur from incidental contact with a superheated ultrasonic blade from direct friction with the opposing tissue jaw. Temperatures in excess of 230°C have been recorded, taking over 40 seconds to decrease to 60°C. Inadvertent tissue burning from direct conduction is prevented by always keeping the activated blade in the surgical view and tailoring operative maneuvers to avoid direct contact with unintended tissue until the blade has sufficiently cooled.

For adhesiolysis with ultrasonic energy, tissue is first grasped between the active blade and the inert tissue–holding jaw and is then steadily compressed, while the device is activated. Tissue cutting occurs by cavitational forces generated ultrasonically within the tissue pedicle, while coagulation is simultaneously attained for vessels up to 3 mm from secondary tissue heating (Figure 9.6).

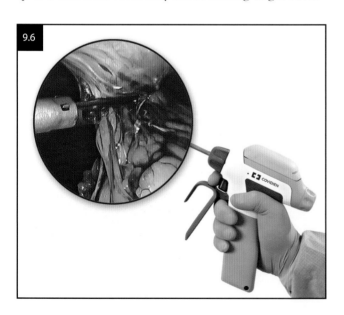

Elucidating the cul de sac

When there is a significant degree of cul-de-sac obliteration and the precise location of the rectum is in doubt, a sponge on a ring forceps, EEA sizer, or rectal probe can be inserted into the vagina or the posterior vaginal fornix, to anatomically define the rectum and posterior vagina to facilitate lysis of pelvic adhesions and/or excision of endometriosis (Figure 9.7).

Aquadissection and hydrodissection

Aquadissection is the use of hydraulic energy from pressurized fluid to aid in the performance of surgical procedures. Contrary to the unidirectional force applied with a blunt probe, the vector is multidirectional within the volume of expansion of the uncompressible fluid. Instillation of fluid under pressure displaces tissue, creating cleavage planes in the least resistant spaces (Figure 9.8). Aquadissection into closed spaces made up of adhesions produces edematous, distended tissue on tension with loss of elasticity, making further division easy and safe using blunt dissection, scissors dissection, laser, or electrosurgery. Instillation of fluid under pressure into closed spaces behind the peritoneum is called *hydrodissection*.

Suction-irrigators with the ability to dissect using pressurized fluid should ideally have a single channel to maximize suctioning and irrigating capacity. This permits the surgeon to perform atraumatic suction-traction-retraction, irrigate directly, and develop surgical planes (aquadissection). The distal tip should not have side holes as they impede these actions, spray the surgical field without purpose, and cause unnecessary tissue trauma when omentum, epiploic appendices, and adhesions become inadvertently caught during aspiration. The shaft should have a dull finish to prevent CO_2 laser beam reflection, allowing it to be used as a backstop.

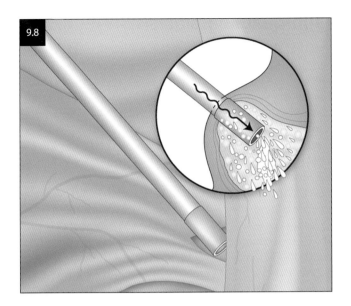

CLASSIFICATIONS

Peritoneal adhesiolysis has been classified into bowel enterolysis including omentolysis and female reproductive reconstruction (salpingo-ovariolysis and cul-de-sac dissection with excision of deep fibrotic endometriosis).

Bowel adhesions are divided into upper abdominal, lower abdominal, pelvic, and combinations. Adhesions surrounding the umbilicus are upper abdominal as they require an upper abdominal laparoscopic view for division.

The extent, thickness, and vascularity of adhesions vary widely. Intricate adhesive patterns exist with fusion to parietal peritoneum or various meshes.

Extensive small bowel adhesions are not a frequent finding at laparoscopy for pelvic pain or infertility. In these cases, the fallopian tube is usually adhered to the ovary, the ovary is adhered to the pelvic sidewall, and the rectosigmoid may cover both. Rarely, the omentum and small bowel are involved. Adhesions may be the result of an episode of pelvic inflammatory disease or endometriosis, but most commonly are caused by previous surgery.

Adhesions cause pain by entrapment of the organs they surround or traction on these organs. The surgical management of extensive pelvic adhesions is one of the most difficult problems facing surgeons today.

SURGICAL PLAN FOR EXTENSIVE ENTEROLYSIS

A well-defined strategy is important for small bowel enterolysis. Time frequently dictates that all adhesions cannot be lysed. From the history, the surgeon should conceptualize the adhesions most likely to be causing the pain (i.e., upper or lower abdomen, left or right) and clear these areas of adhesions. Almost always, the anterior abdominal wall adhesions must be released to adequately visualize the peritoneal cavity.

INCISIONS

Alternate sites for peritoneal access and techniques are employed whenever there is suspicion for periumbilical adhesions, especially in patients who have undergone laparoscopy or laparotomy, have lower abdominal incisions traversing the umbilicus, or have been noted to have extensive adhesions by prior operative report. Open laparoscopy at the umbilicus assumes similar risk for bowel laceration if the viscera is fused to the undersurface of the umbilicus.

The left ninth intercostal space near the anterior axillary line can be used for peritoneal access (Figure 9.9). This is the lowest anterior intercostal space, as ribs 11 and 12 are floating posteriorly. Adhesions are rare in this area, and the peritoneum is tethered to the undersurface of the ribs, making peritoneal tenting away from the needle unusual. A 5 mm skin incision is made over the lowest intercostal space (the ninth) near the anterior axillary line. The Veress needle is grasped near its tip, like a dart, between thumb and forefinger, while the other index finger spreads this intercostal space. The needle tip is inserted at a right angle to the skin (a 45° angle to the horizontal) between the ninth and tenth ribs. A single pop is felt on penetration of the peritoneum. Pneumoperitoneum to a pressure of 30 mm Hg is obtained. A 5 mm trocar is then inserted through this same incision that has migrated downward to below the left costal margin because of abdominal wall distension from the pneumoperitoneum. The peritoneal cavity is visualized through a 5 mm scope.

More widely employed, the left upper quadrant can also be used to safely access the peritoneal cavity. Called "Palmer point" after its initial description, this site of entry is located 1 cm inferior to the subcostal arch in the left midclavicular line (Figure 9.10). Choosing a site at least 8 cm lateral to the midline will help avoid inadvertent injury to the superior epigastric vessels as they travel within the rectus sheath. Here, the layers of the abdominal wall are separable, as the Veress needle or trocar successively traverses

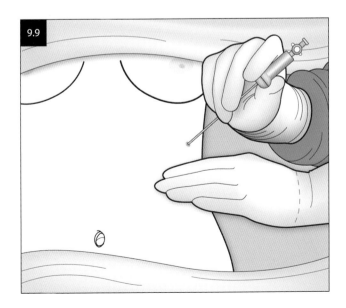

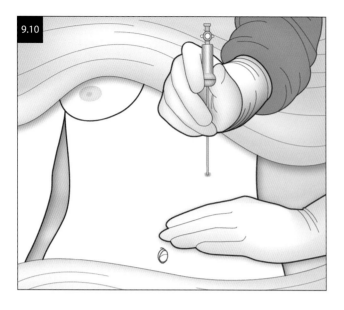

three perceivable layers including the subcutaneous tissue, rectus fascia, and then the parietal peritoneum after a relative delay (Figure 9.11) (see Chapter 5).

If extensive adhesions are initially encountered that surround the umbilical puncture, a higher insertion site can be expeditiously created. Thereafter, these adhesions can be freed down to and just beneath the umbilicus, and the surrounding bowel inspected for possible injury or perforation. If this higher insertion site cannot meet the remaining technical needs, an umbilical port site is then created to complete the surgery. Other laparoscopic puncture sites are placed as needed, usually lateral to the rectus abdominis muscles and always under direct laparoscopic vision. If an umbilical insertion is possible and extensive adhesions are present close to, but below the umbilicus, the operating laparoscope with scissors in the operating channel is the first instrument used. If a left upper quadrant 5 mm incision is necessary, there is usually room for another puncture site nearby to insert scissors for initial adhesiolysis.

ABDOMINAL ADHESIOLYSIS

Anterior abdominal wall adhesions involve the parietal peritoneum stuck to the omentum, transverse colon, and small bowel with varying degrees of fibrosis and vascularity. Adhesions may be filmy and avascular, filmy and vascular, or dense, fibrous, and vascular. All of these adhesions to the anterior abdominal wall should be released. If adhesions extend from above the level of the laparoscope in the umbilicus, another trocar is inserted above the level of the highest adhesion and the laparoscope is inserted there (Figure 9.12). Adhesions are easier to divide when working above them, instead of within them.

Adhesiolysis is performed using scissors alone if possible. Electrosurgery, CO_2 laser, and ultrasonic energy can also be judiciously used. In most cases, the initial adhesiolysis is performed with scissors. CO_2 laser through the laparoscope on adhesions close to the trocar insertion often results in reflection with loss of precision. Electrosurgery (cut current) is used only when the surgeon is confident that the small bowel is not involved in the adhesion.

If the patient has an abdominal scar and history of laparotomy, initial left upper quadrant entry and 5 mm laparoscope placement are advisable. Adhesions are rarely encountered at this site. After careful inspection of the abdominal cavity, the site that is free from adhesions is selected for the placement of the secondary trocar. The scissors or the grasper are introduced through the secondary site to free up the adhesions around the umbilical area in order to place the 10 mm trocar with the laparoscope (Figure 9.13).

Frequently, adhesions can be bluntly divided through the operating channel of the operating laparoscope by grasping the adhesion in the partially closed scissors, and gently pushing the tissue (Figure 9.14). If the plane of adhesions cannot be reached with the tip of the scissors, the abdominal wall can be pressed from above with the surgeon's or assistant's fingers to make it accessible to the scissors (Figure 9.15).

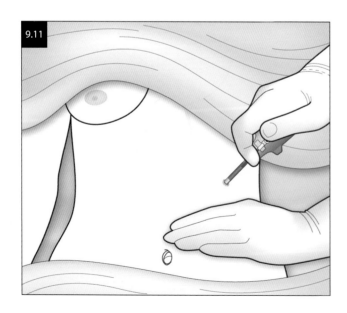

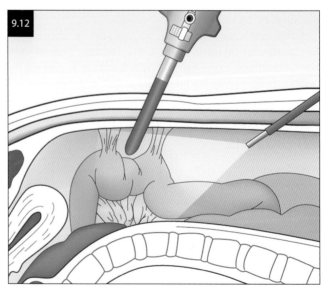

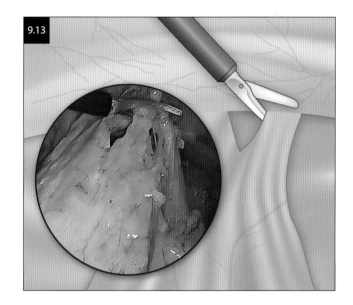

After initial adhesiolysis, visualization is improved allowing better access and exposure for further adhesiolysis. Secondary trocar sites can now be placed safely. After their insertion, the remainder of the adhesions can now be lysed using scissors with focused bipolar backup for rare arterial bleeders. Small venous bleeders are left alone as they will become hemostatic. On occasion, in operations in which symptomatic bowel adhesions are not the main problem, an electrosurgical spoon or knife is used to divide the remaining omental adhesions if the bowel is not involved. If the bowel is involved, dissection proceeds with scissors, without electrosurgery, through the second puncture site, aided by traction on the bowel from an opposite placed puncture site (Figure 9.16). If the adhesions are vascular and involve just the omentum without the bowel, they can be best managed with ultrasonic energy (Figure 9.17). The CO_2 laser may be used through the operating channel of the operating laparoscope. When using the CO_2 laser for adhesiolysis, aquadissection is performed to distend the adhesive

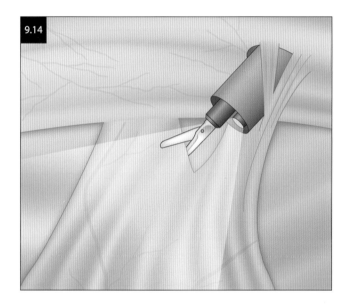

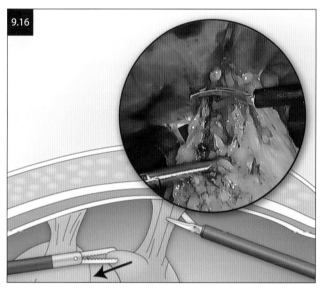

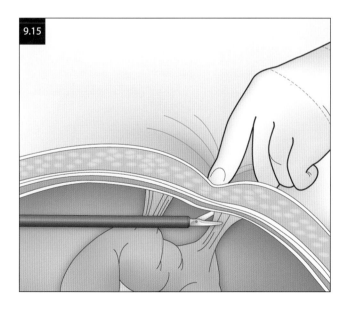

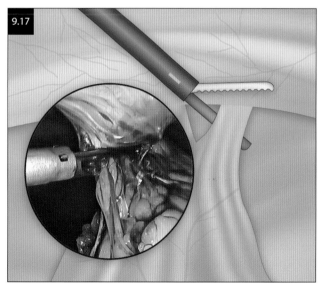

surface with fluid before vaporizing the individual adhesive layers. The suction-irrigator can also be used for suction traction and as a backstop to prevent thermal damage to other structures. The suction irrigator is also used to clean the laparoscopic optic, which is then wiped on the bowel serosa before continuing. Denuded areas of bowel muscularis are repaired transversely using a 3-0 or 4-0 absorbable seromuscular stitch. Denuded peritoneum is left alone. Minimal oozing should be observed and not desiccated unless this bleeding hinders the next adhesiolysis step or persists toward the end of the operation. With perseverance, all anterior abdominal wall parietal peritoneum adhesions can be released.

PELVIC ADHESIOLYSIS

The next step is to free all bowel loops in the pelvis. Small bowel attached to the vesicouterine peritoneal fold, uterus or vaginal cuff, and the rectum is liberated. There are three key points when performing intestinal adhesiolysis within the pelvis: scissors dissection without electrosurgery, countertraction, and blunt dissection. The bowel is gently held with an atraumatic grasper and lifted away from the structure to which it is adhered, exposing the plane of dissection. When adhesive interfaces are obvious, scissors are used. The blunt-tipped scissors are used to sharply dissect the adhesions in small, successive cuts taking care not to damage the bowel serosa. Countertraction will further expose the plane of dissection and ultimately free the attachment. Electrosurgery and laser are generally not used for adhesiolysis involving the bowel due to the risk of thermal damage and recurrent adhesion formation. However, when adhesive aggregates blend into each other, initial incision can be made very superficially with laser, and aquadissection distends the layers of the adhesions, facilitating identification of the involved structures. Division of adhesions continues with the CO_2 laser at 10–20 W in pulsed mode. The aqua-dissector and injected fluid from it are used as a backstop behind adhesive bands that are divided with the CO_2 laser.

DEEP PELVIC ADHESIOLYSIS

Especially in cases of severe endometriosis, the rectosigmoid may be adhesed to the left pelvic sidewall, obscuring visualization of the left adnexa and ovarian vessels. If full exposure of the left pelvic sidewall is required, or if uretero-lysis needs to be performed, the rectosigmoid reflection should be mobilized first. Dissection starts well out of the pelvis at the left iliac fossa. Scissors are used to develop the space between the sigmoid colon and the psoas muscle to the iliac vessels, and the rectosigmoid is then reflected toward the midline. Thereafter, with the rectosigmoid placed on traction, the rectosigmoid and any rectal adhesions to the left pelvic sidewall are systematically divided starting cephalad and continuing caudad. This dissection can be performed with scissors or with ultrasound energy

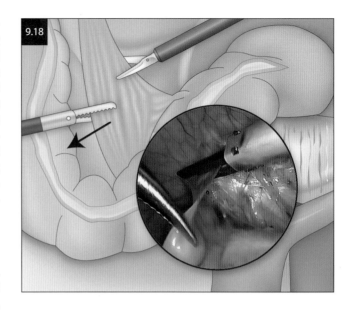

(Figure 9.18). Cul-de-sac adhesions can cause partial or complete cul-de-sac obliteration from fibrosis between the anterior rectum, posterior vagina, cervix, and the uterosacral ligaments (Figure 9.19). The technique of freeing the anterior rectum down to the loose areolar tissue of the rectovaginal septum before excising and/or vaporizing visible and palpable deep fibrotic endometriosis is used. Attention is first directed to complete dissection of the anterior rectum throughout its area of involvement until the loose areolar tissue of the rectovaginal space is reached. Using a rectal probe as a guide, the rectal serosa is opened at its junction with the cul-de-sac lesion. Careful dissection ensues using aquadissection, suction-traction, ultrasound or laser, and scissors until the rectum is completely freed and identifiable below the lesion. Keep in mind that fat belongs to the rectum during the resection in the recto-vaginal space. A sponge gauze can be placed in the abdomen through a 10 mm trocar port and grasped with the laparoscopic grasper to facilitate the dissection of the recto-vaginal space.

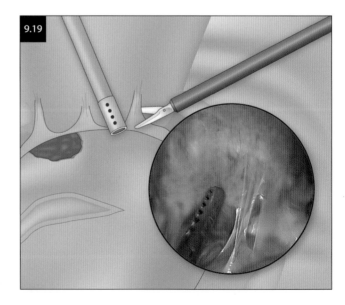

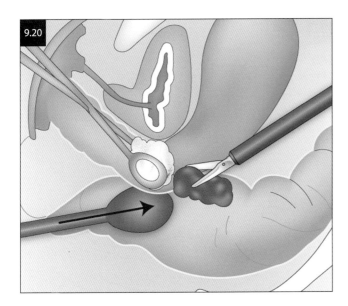

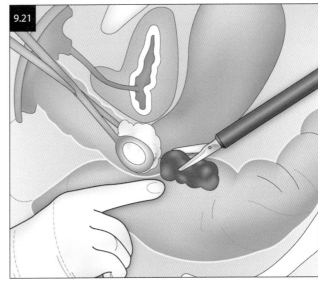

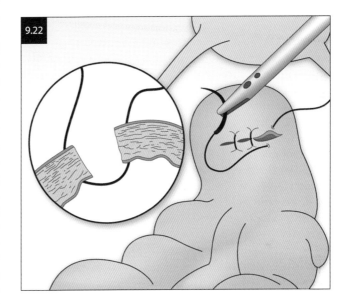

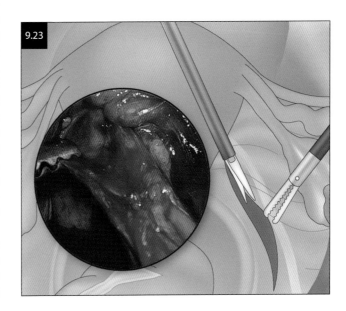

Excision of the fibrotic endometriosis is done only after rectal dissection is completed. Deep fibrotic, often nodular, endometriotic lesions are excised from the uterosacral ligaments, the upper posterior vagina (the location of which is confirmed by a manipulator such as a Valtchev retractor or a sponge in the posterior fornix), and the posterior cervix (Figure 9.20). The dissection on the outside of the vaginal wall proceeds using laser, scissors, or ultrasound energy, until the soft pliable upper posterior vaginal wall is uncovered. It is frequently difficult to distinguish fibrotic endometriosis from the cervix at the cervicovaginal junction and above. Frequent palpation using rectovaginal examinations helps identify occult lesions. When the lesion infiltrates through the vaginal wall, an *en bloc* laparoscopic resection from cul-de-sac to posterior vaginal wall is done, and the vagina is repaired laparoscopically with the pneumoperitoneum maintained by inserting a 30 cc Foley balloon or surgical glove with a sponge in the vagina. Another option is to first mobilize a vaginal lesion vaginally, close the vagina over the mobilized portion, and then complete this en bloc excision laparoscopically. Occasionally, a fibrotic cul-de-sac lesion encompassing both uterosacral ligament insertions and the intervening posterior cervix-vagina and anterior rectal lesion can be excised as one en bloc specimen. Endometriotic nodules infiltrating the anterior rectal muscularis are excised, usually with the surgeon's or the assistant's finger in the rectum just beneath the lesion (Figure 9.21). Deep rectal muscularis defects are always closed with suture. These defects are detected by filling the rectum and rectosigmoid with a blue dye solution. Full-thickness rectal lesion excisions are suture-repaired laparoscopically (Figure 9.22) or incorporated in an anterior discoid resection using a #29 or 33 EEA stapler as shown in Chapter 15.

When a ureter is close to the lesion, its course in the deep pelvis is traced by opening its overlying peritoneum with scissors or a laser (Figure 9.23) as shown in Chapters 15 and 20. On the left, this often requires scissors reflection of the rectosigmoid, as previously described, starting at the pelvic brim. Focused bipolar energy can be diligently used to control arterial and unabated venous bleeding.

ADNEXAL ADHESIOLYSIS (SALPINGO-OVARIOLYSIS)

Ovarian adhesions to the pelvic sidewall can be filmy or fused. Initially, adhesions between the ovary and fallopian tubes and other peritoneal surfaces are identified. It is imperative to establish the surrounding anatomy prior to cutting any tissue to avoid damage to vital structures. The plane of dissection is identified and followed to avoid damage to other structures. The utero-ovarian ligament may be held with an atraumatic grasper to facilitate countertraction and expose the line of cleavage. During ovariolysis, it is important to preserve as much peritoneum as possible while freeing the ovary. Dissection starts either high in the pelvis just beneath the infundibulopelvic ligament or deep on the pelvic sidewall below the ureter in the pararectal space. In each case, scissors are used both bluntly and sharply to mobilize the ovary from the sidewall (Figure 9.24). Alternatively, aquadissection may be used to facilitate identification of adhesion layers and to provide a safe backstop for a CO_2 laser. Once an adhesion layer is identified, the aquadissector can also be placed behind this ridge and used as a backstop during CO_2 laser adhesiolysis.

Adhesiolysis is performed sharply and bluntly in a methodical manner working caudad until the cul-de-sac is reached.

If fimbrioplasty is to be performed, the tube is distended by transcervical injection of dilute indigo carmine through a uterine manipulator (Figure 9.25). This distends the distal portion of the tube, which is stabilized, and the adhesive bands are freed using scissors, laser, or micropoint electrosurgery. If necessary, the fimbriated end can be progressively dilated using 3 mm alligator-type forceps. The closed forceps are placed through the aperture, opened, and removed (Figure 9.26). This is repeated one or more times. If the opening does not remain everted on its own, the intussusception salpingostomy method of

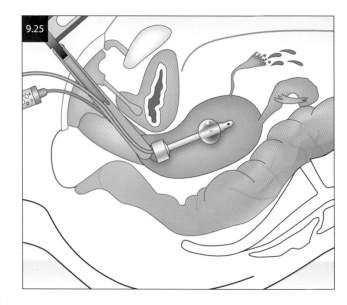

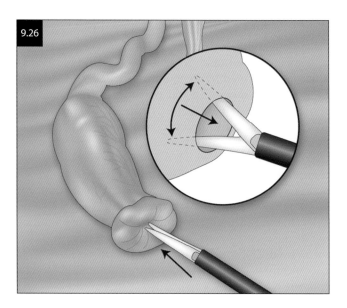

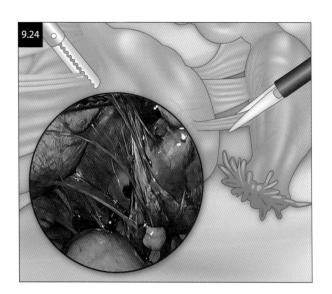

McComb is used to avoid thermal damage to the ciliated tubal epithelium from CO_2 laser or electrosurgery. The tip of the aquadissector is inserted approximately 2 cm into the newly opened tube, suction applied, and the tube fimbrial edges pulled around the instrument to turn the tube end inside-out. The borders of the incision act as a restrictive collar to maintain the mucosa in this newly everted configuration (Figure 9.27). In some cases, the ostial margin should be sutured to the ampullary serosa with 6-0 suture (Figure 9.28).

FINALIZING THE PROCEDURE

At the close of each operation, hemostasis can be confirmed by inspecting the dissected surfaces with the tip of the laparoscope submerged below the irrigant. Since intraperitoneal pressure is not transmitted through fluid, any bleeders controlled by the compressive force of the pneumoperitoneum will be detected. Any active bleeders are then controlled using mechanical pressure with a

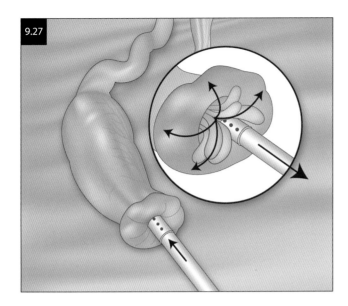

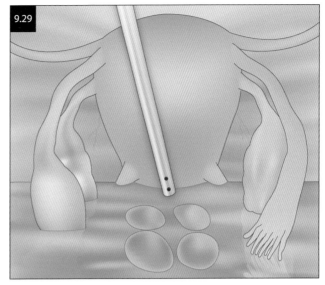

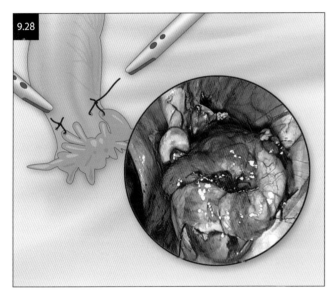

laparoscopic grasper or with focused bipolar electrosurgery. Moreover, the integrity of the rectum and rectosigmoid are often checked at this time as well by instillation of dilute indigo carmine solution through a 30 cc Foley catheter or air transanally using a proctoscope. A final copious lavage with Ringer lactate solution is undertaken and most clots directly aspirated; at least 2 L of lactated Ringer solution are left in the peritoneal cavity to displace CO_2 (Figure 9.29) and help prevent adhesions.

HAND-ASSISTED LAPAROSCOPY

Primarily in the field of solid organ surgery and bowel surgery, hand-assisted laparoscopy or "handoscopy" has recently become more popular. The main advantage of handoscopy is that it allows the surgeon to regain the tactile feel of surrounding tissues previously lost to laparoscopists while permitting a more purposeful manipulation of larger organs, especially the small bowel. Often, the use of handoscopy for tissue palpation enables a successful laparoscopic adhesiolysis. At times, during

laparoscopic procedures, visualization can be poor due to dense adhesions and the inability to determine tissue planes. With the placement of the operator's hand inside the peritoneal cavity, the surgeon is usually able to palpate surrounding organs and allow for a better tissue dissection plane that otherwise may not have been possible through direct visualization only. Not only can the use of a hand port facilitate an otherwise tedious procedure, it effects a safer operation for the patient with less chance of bowel injury. If bowel resection should become necessary, the use of the hand port allows for exteriorization of the segment that requires resection, once again making the procedure easier and less time consuming. A handoscopy incision is usually only 6–8 cm and is placed in the left, right lower portion, or center of the abdomen with insertion of the operator's nondominant hand. The entire peritoneal cavity can be examined through any of these incisions with the operator's hand, and it can be used for organ extraction as well (Figure 9.30). Several different types of handoscopy ports are available, and all provide equal access to the peritoneal cavity (Figure 9.31).

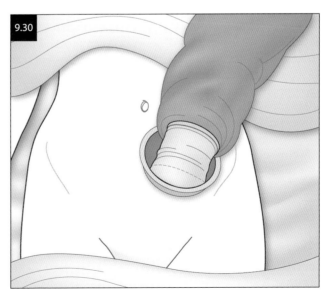

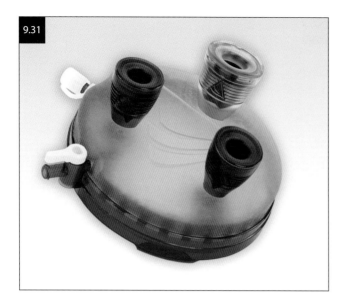

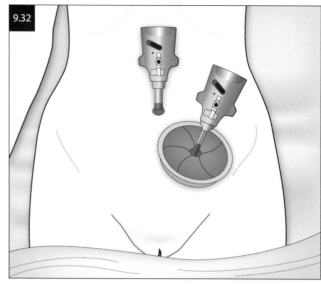

When placing a handoscopy port for adhesiolysis, the operator must first choose a location on the abdominal wall that will allow optimal access to the point where adhesions are greatest. After the hand port location is chosen, a marking pen should be used to outline the area of the abdominal wall where the hand port is to be placed. The area for the incision should be anesthetized with a local anesthetic agent for postoperative pain control, and an incision should then be made into the skin. The size of the incision should be the same size as the operator's glove size. After this is completed, a muscle splitting technique should be used to enter the peritoneal cavity just as the operator would in performing an open appendectomy if the incision is placed laterally. Once the peritoneal cavity is entered, the hand port can then be placed. All of the hand port devices require that any adhesions on the peritoneal side of the incision be lysed prior to inserting the handoscopy device. Additionally, these devices should not be placed over any bony prominences (i.e., iliac crest) or encompassing any bowel in the peritoneal ring surface as to injure any bowel in the abdomen. If the handoscopy port is placed in the upper abdomen, the falciform ligament may require division prior to inserting the ring. Once the handoscopy device is in place, the lysis of adhesions can proceed in an orderly fashion by identifying the tissue planes by feel with the operator's fingers and additionally being able to provide appropriate traction and countertraction to allow for a safe adhesiolysis. Incidental enterotomies can be sutured with conventional suture and then tied using a one-hand knot-tying technique with the intraabdominal hand. Should any bowel resections be required, the hand port can be used as a mini laparotomy site for extraction of any specimens and for exteriorizing any bowel that may require resection and or repair. Additionally, all handoscopy devices that are placed through the abdominal wall act as a wound protector and may minimize postoperative wound infections as well as protect from any potential tumor seeding if the operation is for malignancy. The opening of the Ethicon Lap-Disc is like a camera shutter that can be reduced to

seal the pneumoperitoneum around any size trocar (Figure 9.32). Similarly, gel ports can also accommodate 5 or 10 mm trocars.

Once the procedure is completed, the hand port device is removed, anterior and posterior rectus sheath muscle fascia are closed with either 0 or 2-0 absorbable suture, and the skin is then closed in a subcuticular manner. Additionally, a variety of "pain buster" catheters are now available for insertion into the suprafascia layer of the wound, which allow for excellent postoperative analgesia. These help to minimize postoperative narcotic requirements, thereby facilitating an earlier return of bowel function and more expedient discharge from the hospital. It has been the author's personal experience that patients undergoing a handoscopy type of operation parallel their recovery in the same manner as a conventional laparoscopic case with a delay of only 1 day in recovery. If a bowel resection should be required, the patient usually only requires fasting overnight, and clear liquids may be started on the first postoperative day. The patient is maintained on clear liquids until passing flatus and moving bowels. Most patients are discharged home on the second postoperative day if a bowel resection has been required.

OPEN ADHESIOLYSIS

In certain situations an open adhesiolysis is best for the patient. It is usually performed after an attempted laparoscopic approach has been abandoned. A Pfannenstiel incision is rarely adequate. A midline incision is usually required if the entire peritoneal cavity is encased in dense fibrotic adhesions. Open adhesiolysis is reserved for the worst possible cases where laparoscopic adhesiolysis has failed, where there have been several incidental enterotomies made, or adhesiolysis cannot be performed secondary to encasement of the bowel. Open adhesiolysis should be considered in patients unable to tolerate CO_2 insufflation.

Open adhesiolysis is performed in the same way as a laparoscopic adhesiolysis. All adhesions are taken down from the abdominal wall usually with the Metzenbaum scissors. All loops of bowel are extracted out of the pelvis. Finally, all interloop adhesions are lysed from the ligament of Treitz to the ileo-cecal valve. Incidental enterotomies are repaired at the time of discovery to avoid intraperitoneal contamination and development of infection. Hemostasis must be meticulous during the entire dissection as in a laparoscopic procedure. An abundant amount of warm irrigation fluid is used as well. It is extremely important to keep the tissues moist to prevent desiccation from atmospheric air as this can stimulate adhesion reformation.

ACUTE ADHESIOLYSIS FOR PELVIC INFLAMMATORY DISEASE

LAPAROSCOPIC TECHNIQUE

Redness and hyperemia along with slight serous exudate in the cul-de-sac are typically seen in uncomplicated cases of pelvic inflammatory disease. These minor cases require a bacteriologic diagnosis by sampling the exudate without further surgical treatment. In more advanced cases, a thorough surgical treatment may be achieved laparoscopically, according to the skills of the surgeon.

Adhesiolysis is the first step of treatment. The approach is from simple to complex, from outside to inside. But the infected tissues are very friable and bleed easily. They can also tear easily, creating false planes. The choice of instrument is very important. In our experience, blunt dissection with aquadissection is the major atraumatic and safe technique in such patients. Aquadissection is performed by placing the tip of the suction-irrigation cannula against the adhesive interface between bowel-adnexa, tube-ovary, or adnexa-pelvic sidewall, then using both the cannula tip and the pressurized physiologic solution to develop a dissection plane. Grasping of organs must be avoided and gentle mobilization of adnexa may be obtained with an atraumatic forceps holding the round ligament or the ovarian ligament. To avoid blind dissection, hemostasis should be achieved using warm saline and focused bipolar coagulation. The magnification provided by the laparoscope should help avoid bowel injuries. Electrosurgery is rarely used on acute adhesions. It is used to remove dense chronic adhesions between tube and ovary, preferentially with a cut current. Arteriolar bleeding is controlled with focused bipolar coagulation.

TUBOOVARIAN ABSCESS DRAINAGE AND TUBAL SURGERY

Following the basic rule of surgery, all abscesses should be drained. Through the ancillary puncture site, a grasping forceps is introduced and used for traction and retraction. A suction-irrigation cannula is then used to mobilize omentum, small bowel, rectosigmoid, and tuboovarian adhesions until the abscess cavity is entered (Figure 9.33). Purulent fluid is aspirated while the operating table is partially returned to a 10° Trendelenburg position to

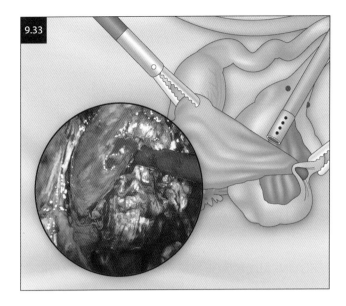

minimize spread into the upper abdomen. After the abscess cavity is aspirated, aquadissection is used to separate the bowel and omentum completely from the reproductive organs and to lyse any tuboovarian adhesions. The grasping forceps is then used to place tissue to be dissected on tension so that the surgeon can accurately identify the distorted tissue planes prior to aquadissection. When the dissection is completed, the abscess cavity (necrotic inflammatory exudate) is excised in pieces using a 5 mm biopsy forceps. Cultures should be taken from the aspirated fluid, the inflammatory exudate excised with biopsy forceps, and the exudate near the tubal ostium. Under laparoscopic vision, friable adhesions and purulent collections are broken up with a blunt probe and the purulent discharge completely drained.

After ovulation, purulent material from acute salpingitis may gain entrance into the inner ovary by inoculation of the corpus luteum, which may then become part of the abscess wall. Thus, after draining the abscess cavity and mobilizing the entire ovary, a gaping hole may be noted in the ovary that had been intimately involved in the abscess cavity. This area should be well irrigated; it will heal spontaneously.

Tubal lavage with indigo-carmine dye through a uterine manipulator is attempted. With early acute abscess, the tubes are rarely patent due to interstitial edema. However, when the abscess process has been present for more than 1 week and/or the patient was previously treated with an antibiotic, lavage frequently documents tubal patency, and inspissated necrotic material may be pushed from the tube. In cases of complete distal occlusion, injecting dye from below to stretch the filmy distal adhesions causing the early hydrosalpinx may sometimes open the tube.

Drainage of a pyosalpinx depends on the location of the occlusion. When the tube is becoming acutely obstructed at its end, the agglutinating fimbriae may be opened gently with blunt dissection (fimbrioplasty). Further widening of the ostium with grasping forceps is done by introducing a blunt forceps in closed position into the ampulla, then opening it slightly and withdrawing it while in an open position. Retrograde irrigation of the tube through the fimbriated end is performed with the aquadissector to remove infected debris and diminish the chance of recurrence. The fimbrial endosalpinx is visualized at this time and its quality assessed for future prognosis.

Rarely a longitudinal incision is necessary to drain the pyosalpinx. Using a fine monopolar electrode at the antimesenteric border, a salpingostomy is made. This incision must be at least 1.5 cm long. Pus is aspirated and the lumen of the tube thoroughly rinsed. Electrosurgery for tubal fimbrial eversion should be avoided as it deeply burns the tissues.

PERITONEAL LAVAGE FOR ABSCESS SURGERY OR BOWEL SPILLAGE SURGERY

Copious rinsing with warm solution followed by gentle aspiration is an essential part of pelvic abscess surgery after bowel spillage. The peritoneal cavity is irrigated thoroughly with Ringer lactate solution until the effluent is clear. The total volume of irrigant may exceed 20 L. As part of this procedure, two liters of Ringer lactate solution are flushed into the upper abdomen, one on each side of the falciform ligament, to dilute any purulent material that may have gained access to these areas during the initial 30° Trendelenburg positioning. Reverse Trendelenburg position is then used for the "underwater" exam. The laparoscope and the aquadissector are manipulated into the deep cul-de-sac beneath floating bowel and omentum, and this area is alternately irrigated and suctioned until the effluent is clear. An underwater examination is then performed to observe the completely separated tubes and ovaries and to document complete hemostasis. No drains, antibiotic solutions, or heparin are used. At the close of each procedure, at least 2 L of Ringer lactate can be left in the peritoneal cavity to prevent fibrin adherences from forming between raw surfaces during the early healing phase and to dilute any remaining bacteria. Given that the absorption rate of fluid from the adult peritoneum cavity is 35 mL/h, the typical 2–3 L volume of crystalloid used for hydroflotation should be absorbed in 70–80 hours.

ADHESION PREVENTION

Despite abundant evidence of the high rates of adhesion formation following abdominal and pelvic surgeries, steps are rarely taken by surgeons to prevent adhesions. A number of explanations have been posited, including ignorance among both patients and physicians about adhesions and their prevention, and the likelihood of adhesion-related complications being managed by a physician other than the surgeon who performed the initial operation.

To investigate the extent of patient ignorance regarding adhesion formation, the International Adhesions Society surveyed patients with a history of abdominal or pelvic surgeries. The 570 patients who responded to the survey had undergone 952 procedures. Patients had been informed about adhesions before only 27% of their surgeries, and before only 55% of adhesiolysis procedures. The risk of adhesion formation was included as part of the formal informed consent in only 12.8% of the time. While the author notes the limitations involved in interpreting a study of this nature, the findings highlight the rarity of postoperative adhesions as a topic of discussion between the surgeon and patient. This is surprising in light of the common practice during the consent process to discuss risks of laparoscopic surgery complication including pain, bleeding, infection, and damage to the bowel/bladder/urethra (1:1000 in sterilizations and 1:500 for other procedures), as well as risks of general anesthesia (<1:100). Comparatively, the risk of a directly adhesion-related (adhesiolysis) readmission in the first year following a therapeutic laparoscopic surgery (1:70, except tubal sterilizations) or open surgery on the fallopian tubes (1:120) or ovaries (1:170) is much more significant. Adhesion-related readmissions are even greater following high-risk laparoscopic surgery (1:80) and open ovarian surgery (1:50).

APPROACHES TO ADHESION PREVENTION

There are essentially two major adhesion prevention strategies: good Halstedian surgical technique and the utilization of antiadhesion adjuvants.

GOOD SURGICAL TECHNIQUE

Good surgical technique is theoretically important for adhesion prevention. All the techniques employed in microsurgery should be adopted, including:

1. Gentle tissue handling (minimal use of forceps, retractors, and clamps on tissue not intended for removal)
2. Meticulous hemostasis to minimize blood in the peritoneal cavity
3. Irrigation to minimize serosal drying
4. Prevention of intraperitoneal infection (copious irrigation to dilute peritoneal bacteria count and blood products)
5. Minimization of foreign bodies
6. Use of fine nonreactive sutures
7. Minimal use of thermal energy to limit peritoneal ischemia

A meta-analysis and systematic review were performed on all randomized controlled trials (RCTs) correlating surgical techniques used in abdominal and pelvic operations with adhesion-related outcomes. Although one RCT pointed toward a decrease in adhesion formation based on surgical techniques, the meta-analysis established that none of the specific techniques that were compared reduced the incidence of small bowel obstruction and infertility, the two main adhesion-related clinical outcomes. They concluded that little evidence exists that using less invasive techniques, causing less ischemia, or introducing fewer foreign bodies, reduced the extent and/or severity of adhesion formation.

ADHESION PREVENTION AGENTS

Meticulous surgical technique should be the first defense against the formation of postoperative adhesive disease. However, adequate treatment of intraabdominal pathology frequently results in significant denudation of peritoneal surfaces. Despite the application of Halstedian technique, operative procedures may often result in significant adhesiogenesis. For these situations, a plethora of adhesion preventative agents have been examined in both human and animal models. The perfect adhesion barrier agent must meet certain criteria. It must be nonreactive and easily applied. It must have delayed absorption lasting through the postsurgical adhesiogenic inflammatory period. It must be adherent to target tissues, and functional when blood is present (Table 9.1). To date, no agent has met all of these criteria. Current adhesion prevention adjuvants fall into three categories: (1) pharmacologic, (2) direct application liquids, or (3) direct application solids.

In a 10-year period between 2005 and 2014, manuscripts detailing over 150 antiadhesion treatments in animal models have been published. Fewer than 25 have resulted in RCTs in humans. As of 2015, Cochrane meta-analyses have identified seven agents from randomized controlled clinical trials that show efficacy in decreasing intraabdominal and pelvic adhesion formation (Table 9.2). Of the nine studies evaluating these seven agents, only one was of high quality according to the GRADE scale, a tool that evaluates the strength of RCTs. Despite evidence of associated decrease in adhesion formation, an important point to consider is the tenuousness of the data linking intraperitoneal adhesions to relevant clinical outcomes such as pain and fertility. No RCT has demonstrated the efficacy of any adhesion preventative agent in improving pain scores or fertility outcomes. As a result, adhesion barrier studies are designed to evaluate the presence of intraperitoneal adhesions as the primary outcome measure.

Some of the difficulty in evaluating agents for prevention of adhesions is the variety of outcome measures used in manuscripts. Some studies examine the prevention of *de novo* adhesions; some examine the prevention of reformation of existing adhesions. Still other studies examine the change in adhesion score. The variety of outcome measures makes meta-analysis and interpretation of findings more difficult.

Pharmacologic agents

Pharmacologic agents have been extensively studied in animal models for the prevention of intraabdominal and pelvic adhesions. Studied agents include corticosteroids, antihistamines, antioxidants, calcium channel blockers, nonsteroidal anti-inflammatory drugs, anticoagulants, and more. The majority of these medications are designed to decrease the inflammatory response or target fibrinolytic pathways. Many have shown efficacy in animal models; however, few have made it into human RCTs.

Corticosteroids in the form of intravenous dexamethasone followed by oral prednisone have shown modest benefit in adhesion prevention in an RCT; however, this has not been extensively studied. Both heparin and promethazine did not show any benefit in terms of adhesion prevention; GnRH agonists and reteplase plasminogen activators also did not show any benefit. Like liquids, solid and semisolid antiadhesion agents have shown no pharmacologic antiadhesion efficacy in trials regarding increasing fertility or decreasing pain outcomes.

Liquid agents

Liquid agents are primarily used for their ability to physically separate peritoneal surfaces by hydroflotation. The theory behind these agents is that they prevent physical apposition of inflamed surfaces until the adhesiogenic inflammatory process has had time to resolve. This time period is typically 48–72 hours, when most postoperative adhesions are thought to initiate formation. This means that a large amount of fluid needs to be present in the intraabdominal and pelvic space for this period of time. At a clearance rate of approximately 30–50 mL/h, this means that upward of 2–3 L of fluid needs to be instilled into the peritoneal cavity to be present the requisite amount of time to separate adhesiogenic surfaces. Stressing the importance of adequate volume in liquid agents, a meta-analysis of 23 trials using crystalloid solution demonstrated no improvement in adhesions when less than 500 mL of crystalloid was infused intraperitoneally. In an attempt to increase absorption time, liquid agents for adhesion prevention tend to be large osmotic molecules, which are theoretically less readily absorbed intraperitoneally.

Among liquid antiadhesion agents, dextran, icodextrin, and hyaluronic acid have all been studied by RCT. Dextran is a complex branched polysaccharide composed of multiple glucose molecules. The dextran solution widely used for adhesion prevention was Dextran 70 (marketed as Hyskon, Medisan pharmaceuticals Inc. Parsippany, New Jersey). This solution was shown to mildly decrease

---

TABLE 9.1

THE PERFECT ADHESION PREVENTION AGENT

1. NONREACTIVE
2. DELAYED ABSORPTION
3. EASILY APPLIED
4. ADHERENT TO TARGET TISSUE
5. FUNCTIONAL WHEN BLOOD IS PRESENT

TABLE 9.2

ADHESION BARRIER AGENTS WITH SHOWN BENEFIT IN RANDOMIZED CONTROLLED CLINICAL TRIALS

INTERVENTION VERSUS CONTROL	ODDS RATIO (CI)	NUMBER OF CASES	NUMBER OF STUDIES	QUALITY OF EVIDENCE (GRADE SCORE)	STUDY OUTCOME MEASURE
CORTICOSTEROIDS	0.27 (0.13–0.58)	187	2	Low	WORSENING OF ADHESION SCORE AT SECOND-LOOK LAPAROSCOPY
	4.83 (1.71–13.65)	75	1	Low	IMPROVEMENT OF ADHESION SCORE AT SECOND-LOOK LAPAROSCOPY
HYDROFLOTATION AGENTS	0.34 (0.22–0.55)	566	4	HIGH	ADHESIONS AT SECOND-LOOK LAPAROSCOPY
GEL AGENTS	0.25 (0.11–0.56)	134	4	HIGH	ADHESIONS AT SECOND-LOOK LAPAROSCOPY
	0.16 (0.04–0.57)	58	2	MODERATE	WORSENING ADHESION SCORE AT SECOND-LOOK LAPAROSCOPY
OXIDIZED REGENERATED CELLULOSE	0.50 (0.30–0.83)	360	3	VERY LOW	*DE NOVO* ADHESIONS IN LAPAROSCOPY
	0.38 (0.27–0.55)	554	7	MODERATE	*DE NOVO* ADHESIONS IN LAPAROTOMY
	0.16 (0.07–0.41)	100	3	LOW	REFORMATION ADHESIONS IN LAPAROSCOPY
POLYTETRAFLUORETHYLENE	0.17 (03–0.97)	42	1	LOW	*DE NOVO* ADHESIONS IN LAPAROTOMY MYOMECTOMY
SODIUM HYALURONATE AND CARBOXYMETHYLCELLULOSE	0.49 (0.45–0.53)	127	1	MODERATE	MEAN DIFFERENCE IN ADHESION SCORES
FIBRIN SHEET	1.2 (0.42–3.41)	62	1	VERY LOW	ADHESIONS AT SECOND-LOOK LAPAROSCOPY

HEAD-TO-HEAD	ODDS RATIO (CI)	NUMBER OF CASES	NUMBER OF STUDIES	QUALITY OF EVIDENCE (GRADE SCORE)	STUDY SPECIFICATIONS
POLYTETRAFLUOROETHYLENE VERSUS OXIDIZED REGENERATED CELLULOSE	−0.379 (−5.12 TO −2.46)	62	2	VERY LOW	
ANTIADHESION GEL (AS INSTILLANT) VERSUS HYDROFLOTATION AGENT	0.36 (0.19–0.67)	342	2	HIGH	ADHESIONS PRESENT
	0.28 (0.12–0.66)	342	2	HIGH	ADHESION SCORE

pelvic adhesions; however, there was associated fluid overload-related side effects including vulvar/leg edema, and pleural effusion. In addition, severe reactions such as disseminated intravascular coagulation, hypotension, and anaphylaxis were attributed to Hyskon use. As a result, Hyskon as an adhesion barrier has been discontinued.

Icodextrin 4% (marketed as Adept, Baxter, Deerfield, Illinois) is a carbohydrate polymer as well. Like Hyskon, large amounts are instilled into the peritoneal cavity, and rare adverse events such as sepsis, impairment of anastomotic healing, and disseminated intravascular coagulation have been linked to icodextrin. Both a 2002 and 2007 RCT indicated a nonsignificant trend toward adhesion prevention.

Dilute hyaluronic acid solution (marketed as Sepracoat, Genzyme Corporation, Cambridge, Massachusetts) showed moderate efficacy in reducing *de novo* adhesions. Not approved in the United States, it was used in Europe for a short time but was ultimately discontinued due to adverse effects.

Solid and semisolid agents

Different from liquid-based agents, solid and semisolid agents are limited in that they work only in site-specific locations. This site specificity can also be advantageous in that a lesser amount of the agent is needed to target adhesiogenic surfaces such as denuded tissue beds or damaged serosal surfaces. The goal period of time before absorption of the material is 5–7 days after surgery. A series of Cochrane reviews identified one gel agent and four solid membrane agents as having efficacy in preventing *de novo* or reformation adhesions. No agent has proven effective for improving fertility or decreasing pain.

As a group (of four RCTs), gel agents were found to be effective against adhesion formation. However, of these studies, only one statistically significantly found fewer cases with adhesions on second-look laparoscopy. This study examined the use of auto-cross-linked hyaluronic acid and found that significantly fewer adhesions

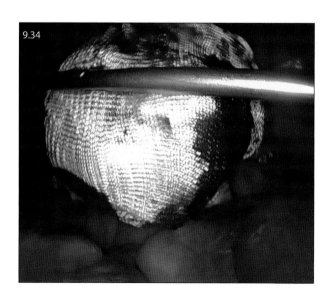

9.34

developed with its use. A series of other RCTs showed a trend toward efficacy using other gel-based agents including a polyethylene glycol (PEG)-based agent (Spraygel, Confluent Surgical, Waltham, Massachusetts) available in Europe, and auto-cross-linked hyaluronan gels (marketed as Hyalobarrier, Fidia Advanced Biopolymers, Abano Terme, Padova, Italy). No gel agent has been found to be more effective than any other; however, when compared with lactated Ringer solution, Intergel (Lifecore Biomedical Inc., Chaska, Minnesota), a now discontinued ferric hyaluronate gel, was found to be significantly more effective. It was discontinued due to associated tissue reactions and abscess-like pelvic infections.

Solid membrane agents are the best studied, most used, and most efficacious of the adhesion prevention agents. Of these, oxidized regenerated cellulose (Interceed, Ethicon Inc., Somerville, New Jersey) (Figure 9.34) is perhaps the best studied. It has been shown to be statistically better than controls at halting reformation adhesions, as well as *de novo* adhesions at laparoscopy. Similarly at laparotomy, oxidized regenerated cellulose prevents reformation adhesions but has not been shown to statistically reduce *de novo* adhesions. Oxidized regenerated cellulose is a cloth-like mesh sheet that can be placed laparoscopically (off-label) or through a laparotomy incision. Its greatest weakness is its loss of efficacy when bleeding is present, when a stabilized fibrin clot may actually promulgate adhesion formation.

Expanded polytetrafluoroethylene surgical membrane (Gore-Tex, W.L. Gore and Associates, Flagstaff, Arizona) is a nonreactive and nonabsorbable membrane that has been shown to result in fewer adhesions when compared with controls or oxidized regenerated cellulose. Since it is nonabsorbable and must be secured in place by laparoscopic sutures or staples, its usefulness in laparoscopy is somewhat limited.

Sodium hyaluronate/carboxymethylcellulose (Seprafilm, Genzyme, Cambridge, Massachusetts) has been U.S. Food and Drug Administration (FDA)-approved for antiadhesion use since 1996 and has been generally found to be safe and efficacious; however, there is not an abundance of data supporting its efficacy. It comes as a translucent, brittle sheet, 5 by 6 inches, that sticks to wet surfaces when freed of its paper sheath. This makes its placement laparoscopically technically challenging. Surgeons have placed it in solution to make a slurry in order to introduce it laparoscopically; however, its efficacy in this route of delivery is not supported by good data.

Many of the newer antiadhesion agents tend to be gels or synthetic copolymers that form barriers when combined and applied to tissues. Some of the agents have small studies supporting their efficacy, but no larger data. Still others show promise, but their producers have been using them in other capacities and have not yet sought approval for use in adhesion prevention.

European guidelines for the prevention of postoperative adhesions in gynecologic surgery are listed in Table 9.3.

TABLE 9.3

EUROPEAN GUIDELINES

IN RECENT YEARS, EUROPEAN "FIELD GUIDELINES" FOR THE PREVENTION OF POSTOPERATIVE ADHESIONS IN GYNECOLOGIC SURGERY HAVE BEEN PROPOSED BY THE ANTI-ADHESIONS IN GYNECOLOGY EXPERT PANEL (ANGEL). ALTHOUGH SEVERAL SIMILAR RECOMMENDATIONS HAVE BEEN MADE BY OTHER CONSENSUS STATEMENTS ON ADHESIONS, THE "FIELD GUIDELINES" WERE SPECIFICALLY ORGANIZED WITH THE GOAL TO "PROVIDE SURGEONS WITH A QUICK REFERENCE GUIDE TO ADHESION PREVENTION ADAPTED TO THE CONDITIONS OF THEIR DAILY PRACTICE." CONSTRUCTED FROM THE RESEARCH DONE BY THE EXPERT ADHESIONS WORKING PARTY OF THE EUROPEAN SOCIETY OF GYNAECOLOGICAL ENDOSCOPY (ESGE), THEIR RECOMMENDATIONS ARE ORGANIZED INTO SIX BASIC RULES:

1. THE RISK OF POSTOPERATIVE ADHESIONS SHOULD BE SYSTEMATICALLY DISCUSSED WITH ANY PATIENT SCHEDULED FOR OPEN OR LAPAROSCOPIC ABDOMINAL SURGERY PRIOR TO OBTAINING HIS OR HER INFORMED CONSENT
2. SURGEONS NEED TO ACT TO REDUCE POSTOPERATIVE ADHESIONS IN ORDER TO FULFILL THEIR DUTY OF CARE TOWARD PATIENTS UNDERGOING ABDOMINAL SURGERY
3. SURGEONS SHOULD ADOPT A ROUTINE ADHESION REDUCTION STRATEGY AT LEAST FOR PATIENTS UNDERGOING HIGH-RISK SURGERY, INCLUDING
   A. OVARIAN SURGERY
   B. ENDOMETRIOSIS SURGERY
   C. TUBAL SURGERY
   D. MYOMECTOMY
   E. ADHESIOLYSIS
4. GOOD SURGICAL TECHNIQUE IS FUNDAMENTAL TO ANY ADHESION REDUCTION STRATEGY:
   A. CAREFULLY HANDLE TISSUE WITH FIELD ENHANCEMENT (MAGNIFICATION) TECHNIQUES
   B. FOCUS ON PLANNED SURGERY AND, IF ANY SECONDARY PATHOLOGY IS IDENTIFIED, QUESTION THE RISK:BENEFIT RATIO OF SURGICAL TREATMENT BEFORE PROCEEDING
   C. PERFORM DILIGENT HEMOSTASIS AND ENSURE DILIGENT USE OF CAUTERY
   D. REDUCE CAUTERY TIME AND FREQUENCY AND ASPIRATE AEROSOLIZED TISSUE FOLLOWING CAUTERY
   E. EXCISE TISSUE—REDUCE FULGURATION
   F. REDUCE DURATION OF SURGERY
   G. REDUCE PRESSURE AND DURATION OF PNEUMOPERITONEUM IN LAPAROSCOPIC SURGERY
   H. REDUCE RISK OF INFECTION
   I. REDUCE DRYING OF TISSUES
   J. USE FREQUENT IRRIGATION AND ASPIRATION IN LAPAROSCOPIC AND LAPAROTOMIC SURGERY WHEN NEEDED
   K. LIMIT USE OF SUTURES AND CHOOSE FINE NONREACTIVE SUTURES
   L. AVOID FOREIGN BODIES WHEN POSSIBLE—SUCH AS MATERIALS WITH LOOSE FIBERS
   M. AVOID NONPERITONIZED IMPLANTS AND MESHES
   N. LIMIT USE OF DRY TOWELS OR SPONGES IN LAPAROTOMY
   O. USE STARCH- AND LATEX-FREE GLOVES IN LAPAROTOMY
5. SURGEONS SHOULD CONSIDER THE USE OF ADHESION REDUCTION AGENTS AS PART OF THE ADHESION REDUCTION STRATEGY
   A. GIVE SPECIAL CONSIDERATION TO AGENTS WITH DATA SUPPORTING SAFETY IN ROUTINE SURGERY AND EFFICACY IN ADHESION PREVENTION
   B. CONSIDER PRACTICALITY, EASE OF USE, AND COST OF AGENTS WHEN SELECTING AGENTS FOR ROUTINE PRACTICE
6. GOOD MEDICAL PRACTICE IMPLIES THAT ANY SERIOUS OR FREQUENTLY OCCURRING RISKS BE DISCUSSED BEFORE OBTAINING THE PATIENT'S INFORMED CONSENT PRIOR TO SURGERY

WHILE GUIDELINES ARE CURRENTLY AVAILABLE ONLY FOR ADHESION PREVENTION IN GYNECOLOGIC SURGERY, A RECENT META-ANALYSIS ASSESSED THE USE OF ADHESION BARRIERS FOR NONGYNECOLOGIC ABDOMINAL SURGERIES; THE AUTHORS OF THIS STUDY HOPE TO USE THE DATA COLLECTED TO DEVELOP GUIDELINES FOR USE OF THESE ADHESION BARRIERS IN NONGYNECOLOGIC ABDOMINAL SURGERY.

CONCLUSION

Adhesion formation after gynecologic surgery is common. When compared to laparotomy, laparoscopy has been shown to result in less *de novo* adhesion formation, but adhesion reformation continues to be a problem for both surgical approaches. Sequelae of intraabdominal adhesion formation can be fatal, result in infertility, and may be a source of chronic pelvic pain. Minimally invasive surgical management of adhesion formation affords the patient all of the known benefits of laparoscopic surgery including less postoperative analgesics, shorter hospital stays, less infection, and more rapid convalescence and return to normal activities. Unfortunately, recurrence after adhesiolysis for intestinal obstruction is not uncommon (8%–32%). Thus, for some patients, adhesiolysis may become a repeat surgical procedure. No longer can the surgeon ignore the benefits of minimally invasive surgery for adhesiolysis. While these techniques and procedures are not without risk, patients should not be denied their inherent advantages. Astute clinicians must work together to discern the most appropriate uses for this therapy. To date, no antiadhesion agent has proven globally efficacious. Part of the difficulty in finding a suitable adhesive barrier is in establishing pain and fertility outcomes in an incompletely understood cause-and-effect relationship between adhesions and these practical outcomes. Though many antiadhesion agents have been shown to decrease *de novo* and reformation adhesions, establishing superiority is difficult given the heterogencity in studies and surgeon skill. In order to determine the optimal adhesion-preventing agent, more high-quality studies will need to be performed with attention to meaningful outcomes such as fertility and pain scores.

SUGGESTED READING

Ahmad G, Mackie FL, Iles DA et al. Fluid and pharmacological agents for adhesion prevention after gynaecological surgery. *Cochrane Database System Rev.* 2014;7:CD001298.

Ahmad G, O'Flynn H, Hindocha A, Watson A. Barrier agents for adhesion prevention after gynaecological surgery. *Cochrane Database System Rev.* 2015;4:CD000475.

Ahrenholz DH, Simmons RL. Fibrin in peritonitis. I. Beneficial and adverse effects of fibrin in experimental E. coli peritonitis. *Surgery.* 1980;88:41.

An expanded polytetrafluoroethylene barrier (Gore-Tex Surgical Membrane) reduces post-myomectomy adhesion formation. The Myomectomy Adhesion Multicenter Study Group. *Fertil Steril.* 1995;63(3):491–493.

Azziz R. Microsurgery alone or with INTERCEED Absorbable Adhesion Barrier for pelvic sidewall adhesion re-formation. The INTERCEED (TC7) Adhesion Barrier Study Group II. *Surg Gynecol Obstet.* 1993;177(2):135–139.

Broek RPG, Kok-Krant N, Bakkum EA, Bleichrodt RP, van Goor H. Different surgical techniques to reduce post-operative adhesion formation: A systematic review and meta-analysis. *Hum Reprod Update.* 2013;19:12–25.

Broek RPG, Stommel MWJ, Strik C, van Laarhoven CJHM, Keus F, van Goor H. Benefits and harms of adhesion barriers for abdominal surgery: A systematic review and meta-analysis. *Lancet.* 2014;383:48–59.

Brown CB, Luciano AA, Martin D et al. Adept (icodextrin 4% solution) reduces adhesions after laparoscopic surgery for adhesiolysis: A double-blind, randomized, controlled study. *Fertil Steril.* 2007;88(5):1413–1426.

Bryant T. Clinical lectures on intestinal obstruction. *Med Tim Gaz.* 1872;1:363–365.

Burns JW, Skinner K, Yu LP et al. An injectable biodegradable gel for the prevention of postsurgical adhesions: Evaluation in two animal models. In *Proceedings of the 50th Annual Meeting of the American Fertility Society*, San Antonio, TX, November 5–10, 1994.

Close MB, Chistensen NM. Transmesenteric small bowel plication or intraluminal tube stenting. *Am J Surg.* 1979;138:89–91.

Coddington CC, Grow DR, Ahmed MS, Toner JP, Cook E, Diamond MP. Gonadotropin-releasing hormone agonist pretreatment did not decrease postoperative adhesion formation after abdominal myomectomy in a randomized control trial. *Fertil Steril.* 2009;91(5):1909–1913.

Correia A. Adhesion prevention in gynecologic surgery. *J Gynecol Surg.* 2014;30(4):8.

De Wilde RL, Brolmann H, Koninckx PR et al., and the Anti-Adhesions in Gynecology Expert Panel (ANGEL). Prevention of adhesions in gynaecological surgery: The 2012 European field guideline. *Gynecol Surg.* 2012;9:365–368.

DeWilde RL, Trew G. Postoperative abdominal adhesions and their prevention in gynaecological surgery. Expert consensus position. Part 2—Steps to reduce adhesions. *Gynecol Surg.* 2007;4:243–253.

Diamond MP. Reduction of adhesions after uterine myomectomy by Seprafilm membrane (HAL-F): A blinded, prospective, randomized, multicenter clinical study. Seprafilm Adhesion Study Group. *Fertil Steril.* 1996;66(6):904–910.

Diamond MP. Reduction of *de novo* postsurgical adhesions by intraoperative precoating with Sepracoat (HAL-C) solution: A prospective, randomized, blinded, placebo-controlled multicenter study. The Sepracoat Adhesion Study Group. *Fertil Steril.* 1998;69(6):1067–1074.

Diamond MP, Linsky CB, Cunningham TC et al. Synergistic effects of Interceed (TC7) and heparin in reducing adhesion formation in the rabbit uterine horn model. *Fertil Steril.* 1991;55:389–394.

DiZerega GS. Contemporary adhesion prevention. *Fertil Steril.* 1994;61(2):219–235.

Farquhar C, Vandekerckhove P, Watson A, Vail A, Wiseman D. Barrier agents for preventing adhesions after surgery for subfertility. *Cochrane Database Syst Rev.* 2005;3.

Fox Ray N, Denton WG, Thamer M, Henderson SC, Perry S. Abdominal adhesiolysis: Inpatient care and expenditures in the United States in 1994. *J Am Coll Surg.* 1998;186(1):1–9.

Franklin RR. Reduction of ovarian adhesions by the use of Interceed. Ovarian Adhesion Study Group. *Obstet Gynecol Sep* 1995;86(3):335–340.

Fu-Hsing Chang, Hung-Hsueh Chou, Chyi-Long Lee et al. Extraumbilical insertion of the operative laparoscope in patients with extensive intraabdominal adhesions. *J Amer Assoc Gynecol Laparosc.* 1995;2(3):335–337.

Group AS. Reduction of postoperative pelvic adhesions with intraperitoneal 32% dextran 70: A prospective, randomized clinical trial. *Fertil Steril.* 1983;40(5):612–619.

Hellebrekers BW, Trimbos-Kemper TC, Boesten L et al. Preoperative predictors of postsurgical adhesion formation and the Prevention of Adhesions with Plasminogen Activator (PAPA-study): Results of a clinical pilot study. *Fertil Steril.* 2009;91(4):1204–1214.

Jansen RP. Failure of intraperitoneal adjuncts to improve the outcome of pelvic operations in young women. *Am J Obstet Gynecol.* Oct 15 1985;153(4):363–371.

Kligman I, Drachenberg C, Papdimitriou J et al. Immunohistochemical demonstration of nerve fibers in pelvic adhesions. *Obstet Gynecol.* 1993;82:566–568.

Lower AM, Hawthorn RJ, Clark D, Boyd JH, Finlayson AR, Knight AD, Crowe AM. Surgical and Clinical Research (SCAR) Group. Adhesion-related readmissions following gynaecological laparoscopy or laparotomy in Scotland: An epidemiological study of 24,046 patients. *Hum Reprod.* 2004;19(8):1877–1885.

Mais V, Ajossa S, Piras B, Guerriero S, Marongiu D, Melis GB. Prevention of de-novo adhesion formation after laparoscopic myomectomy: A randomized trial to evaluate the effectiveness of an oxidized regenerated cellulose absorbable barrier. *Hum Reprod.* 1995;10(12):3133–3135.

Mettler L, Audebert A, Lehmann-Willenbrock E, Schive K, Jacobs VR. Prospective clinical trial of SprayGel as a barrier to adhesion formation: An interim analysis. *J Am Assoc Gynecol Laparosc.* 2003;10(3):339–344.

Operative Laparoscopy Study Group. Postoperative adhesion development after operative laparoscopy: Evaluation at early second look procedures. *Fertil Steril.* 1991;55:700–704.

Peters A, Trimbos-Kemper G, Admiraal C et al. A randomized clinical trial on the benefit of adhesiolysis in patients with intraperitoneal adhesions and pelvic pain. *Br J Obstet Gynaecol.* 1992;99:59–62.

Reich H. Laparoscopic treatment of extensive pelvic adhesions including hydrosalpinx. *J Reprod Med.* 1987;32:736.

Reich H. Endoscopic management of tuboovarian abscess and pelvic inflammatory disease. In: Sanfilippo JS and Levine RL, eds. *Operative Gynecologic Endoscopy.* New York, NY: Springer-Verlag; 1989:118.

Reich H. Laparoscopic excision of deep fibrotic endometriosis of the cul-de-sac and rectum (extensive endometriosis). *Operative Tech Gynecol Surg.* 2000;5:13–19.

Reich H, Fazel A. Laparoscopic management of pelvic inflammatory disease (including abscess). *Operative Tech Gynecol Surg.* 2000;5:41–47.

Reich H, Levie M, McGlynn F, Sekel L. Establishment of pneumoperitoneum through the left ninth intercostal space. *Gynaecol Endosc.* 1995;4:141–143.

Reich H, McGlynn F. Laparoscopic treatment of tubo-ovarian and pelvic abscess. *J Reprod Med.* 1987;32:747.

Reich H, McGlynn F, Salvat J. Laparoscopic treatment of cul-de-sac obliteration secondary to retrocervical deep fibrotic endometriosis. *J Reprod Med.* 1991;36:516.

Reich H, Vancaillie T, Soderstrom R. Electrical techniques. Operative laparoscopy. In: Martin DC, Holtz GL, Levinson CJ, Soderstrom RM, eds. *Manual of Endoscopy.* Cypress, CA: American Association of Gynecologic Laparoscopists; 1990:105.

Sekiba K. Use of Interceed(TC7) absorbable adhesion barrier to reduce postoperative adhesion reformation in infertility and endometriosis surgery. The Obstetrics and Gynecology Adhesion Prevention Committee. *Obstet Gynecol.* 1992;79(4):518–522.

Shear L, Swartz C, Shinaberger JA, Barry KG. Kinetics of peritoneal fluid absorption in adult man. *N Engl J Med.* 1965;272:123–127.

Singhal V, Li T, Cooke I. An analysis of the factors influencing the outcome of 232 consecutive tubal microsurgery cases. *Br J Obstet Gynaecol.* 1991;98:628–636.

Skau T, Nystrom P, Ohman L, Stendahl O. The kinetics of peritoneal clearance of *Escherichia coli* and *Bacteroides fragilis* and participating defense mechanisms. *Arch Surg.* 1986;121:1033.

Steege JF, Stout AL. Resolution of chronic pelvic pain after laparoscopic lysis of adhesions. *Am J Obstet Gynecol.* 1991;165:278–281.

Sutton C. ed. New techniques in advanced laparoscopic surgery. In: *Bailliere's Clinical Obstetrics and Gynecology. Laparoscopic Surgery.* London: Bailliere Tindall/W.B.Saunders; 1989, Chapter 13, 3.3:655–681.

Swank DJ, Swank-Bordewijk SCG, Hop WCJ et al. Laparoscopic adhesiolysis in patients with chronic abdominal pain: A blinded randomised controlled multi-centre trial. *Lancet.* 2003;361:1247–1251.

Ten Broek RP, Kok-Krant N, Verhoeve HR, van Goor H, Bakkum EA. Efficacy of polyethylene glycol adhesion barrier after gynecological laparoscopic surgery: Results of a randomized controlled pilot study. *Gynecol Surg.* 2012;9(1):29–35.

Tinelli A, Malvasi A, Guido M et al. Adhesion formation after intracapsular myomectomy with or without adhesion barrier. *Fertil Steril.* 2011;95(5):1780–1785.

Tulandi T, Closon F, Czuzoj-Shulman N, Abenhaim H. Adhesion barrier use after myomectomy and hysterectomy: Rates and immediate postoperative complications. *Obstet Gynecol.* 2016;127(1):23–28.

Wallwiener D, Meyer A, Bastert G. Adhesion formation of the parietal and visceral peritoneum: An explanation for the controversy on the use of autologous and alloplastic barriers? *Fertil Steril.* 1998;69(1):132–137.

Watson A, Vandekerckhove P, Lilford R. Liquid and fluid agents for preventing adhesions after surgery for subfertility. *Cochrane Database Syst Rev.* 2000;2:CD001298.

Welch JP. Adhesions. In: Welch JP, ed. *Bowel Obstruction.* Philadelphia, PA: WB Saunders; 1990:154–165.

Wiseman DM, Trout JR, Diamond MP. The rates of adhesion development and the effects of crystalloid solutions on adhesion development in pelvic surgery. *Fertil Steril.* 1998;70(4):702–711.

CHAPTER 10

ECTOPIC PREGNANCY

Sukrant Mehta and Jonathon Solnik

INTRODUCTION

Ectopic pregnancy occurs when the developing blastocyst becomes implanted at a site other than the endometrial cavity. It occurs in approximately 1.5%–2% of pregnancies and accounts for 9% of pregnancy-related mortality and less than 1% of overall mortality in women.

The prevalence of ectopic pregnancy among women who present to an emergency department with first trimester bleeding, pain, or both ranges from 6% to 16%. Significant hemorrhage resulting from ectopic pregnancy is the leading cause of maternal mortality in the first trimester and accounts for 9% of all pregnancy-related deaths in the United States. The overall incidence of ectopic pregnancy has increased during the mid-twentieth century, plateauing at approximately almost 20 per 1000 pregnancies in the early 1990s, the last time national data were reported by the Centers for Disease Control and Prevention. This rising incidence is strongly associated with an increased incidence of pelvic inflammatory disease and advanced reproductive technologies. This likely represents an underestimation of what is actually occurring due to the underreporting of women treated in physician offices.

RISK FACTORS AND PROTECTIVE INFLUENCES

Identifiable risk factors for ectopic pregnancy are fairly intuitive, well described, and include previous ectopic pregnancy, tubal pathology and surgery, and *in utero* diethylstilbestrol (DES) exposure. Previous genital infections, intrauterine device (IUD) use, infertility, multiple sexual partners, smoking, *in vitro* fertilization, and young age at time of first sexual encounter are also associated with this phenomenon. If a nulliparous woman is diagnosed with an ectopic pregnancy, her likelihood of carrying a pregnancy to term is much lower than another who had a preceding or interval intrauterine pregnancy.

Women who are using a reliable form of contraception (hormonal or intrauterine) are somewhat protected

---

SIGNS AND SYMPTOMS SUGGESTIVE OF ECTOPIC PREGNANCY

- Nausea, breast fullness, fatigue, amenorrhea
- Lower abdominal pain, heavy cramping, shoulder pain
- Uterine bleeding/spotting
- Pelvic tenderness; enlarged, soft uterus
- Adnexal mass, tenderness
- Positive pregnancy test
- Serum levels of hCG <6000 mIU/mL at 6 weeks
- Less than 66% increase in hCG titers in 48 hours
- Serum progesterone <25 ng/mL
- Aspiration of nonclotting blood on culdocentesis
- Absence of gestational sac in the uterus (by ultrasound) when the hCG titer exceeds 2500 mIU/mL
- Gestational sac outside the uterus (by ultrasound)

MAJOR CONTRIBUTING FACTORS AND ASSOCIATED RELATIVE RISK FOR ECTOPIC PREGNANCY[a]

RISK FACTOR	RELATIVE RISK
Current use of IUD	11.9
Use of clomiphene citrate	10.0
Prior tubal surgery	5.6
Pelvic inflammatory disease	4.0
Infertility	2.9
Induced abortion	2.5
Adhesions	2.4
Abdominal surgery	2.3
T-shaped uterus	2.0
Myomata	1.7
Progestin only oral contraceptive pills (OCPs)	1.6

[a] Adapted from Marchbanks PA et al. Risk factors for ectopic pregnancy: A population based study. *JAMA* 1988;259:1823–1827.

against an extrauterine pregnancy simply because they are less likely to conceive. However, if they do conceive, the probability of an ectopic pregnancy becomes relatively higher in comparison.

DIAGNOSIS

Abdominal pain, amenorrhea, and vaginal bleeding represent the classic symptoms of ectopic pregnancy, which should be suspected in women of reproductive age with these symptoms, especially those at risk. The diagnosis is typically based on clinical impression, with transvaginal ultrasound (TVS) findings and beta-human chorionic gonadotropin hormone (β-hCG) values. Confirmation by exploratory surgery or histopathologic examination of tissue is not necessary and no longer represents the gold standard as it did before these tools were readily available. However, in their absence, it may not be possible to differentiate between a failed intrauterine or extrauterine pregnancy.

Suspicion for an extrauterine pregnancy is raised when the β-hCG concentration is greater than 1500 IU/L (discriminatory zone threshold) and TVS examination reveals a complex adnexal mass separate from the ovary and no intrauterine pregnancy. The diagnosis becomes more blurred when TVS shows no evidence of pathology. Interpretation of the endometrial complex may be of use; a thin stripe suggests lack of intrauterine development, but a thickened stripe may also result from the influence of estrogen regardless of where the pregnancy lies.

A serum β-hCG concentration less than 1500 IU/L with a negative TVS examination remains inconclusive and should be followed by repetition of both of these tests in 2–3 days to follow the rate of rise of the β-hCG in a hemodynamically stable patient.

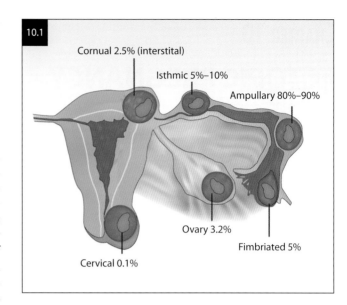

10.1

Cornual 2.5% (interstital)

Isthmic 5%–10%

Ampullary 80%–90%

Ovary 3.2%

Fimbriated 5%

Cervical 0.1%

5% in the fimbriated portion, and about 2.4% in the interstitium (cornua). Other sites include the ovary (3.2%), the cervix (less than 0.15%), and elsewhere in the abdomen (1.3%) (Figure 10.1).

ANATOMY OF THE FALLOPIAN TUBE

The oviduct or tube is approximately 10–12 cm long. The tube can be functionally and anatomically divided into four parts. The intramural or interstitial portion of the tube is approximately 1 cm long and traverses through the myometrium and opens in the endometrial cavity. This is the "valve" where the sperm line up to start their journey up the oviduct. It is also a highly vascular area and makes conservative surgical management more difficult.

This isthmus of the tube is approximately 4–6 cm in length. It is composed of a double layer of muscle and inner lumen. The outer muscle layer runs longitudinal to the axis of the tube and is thicker than the inner muscle layer, which is oriented in a circular fashion. The lumen of the isthmus is approximately 1–2 mm until it gets to the ampulla where it enlarges.

The ampulla is the longest segment of the tube and makes up approximately two-thirds of the total length. Beneath the mucosa of the ampullary portion of the tube, there is a series of large blood vessels, mostly veins originating from the utero-ovarian supply to the tube. These become engorged at the time of ovulation to bring the fimbriae closer to the ovary. They can also be problematic during surgical treatment for an ectopic pregnancy, because these vessels travel in a thick longitudinal muscle layer. The lumen of the tube is wider in this segment, and the mucosa has more rugae, which are covered with ciliated and secretory cells. These cells may be damaged with infection, previous ectopic pregnancy, or surgery, predisposing patients to a greater risk of tubal pregnancy.

DIFFERENTIAL DIAGNOSIS IN CASES OF SUSPECTED ECTOPIC PREGNANCY

- SPONTANEOUS ABORTION
- RUPTURED OVARIAN CYST
- CORPUS LUTEUM HEMORRHAGICUM
- ADNEXAL TORSION
- PELVIC INFLAMMATORY DISEASE
- ENDOMETRIOSIS
- UROLITHIASIS
- URINARY TRACT INFECTION
- APPENDICITIS
- OTHER LOWER GASTROINTESTINAL TRACT DISEASE

LOCATION

The majority of ectopic pregnancies occur in the fallopian tube (over 90%), with 80%–90% of these occurring in the ampullary portion, 5%–10% in the isthmic portion,

The final portion of the tube is the infundibulum of the oviduct. It is funnel shaped, and its most distal end is called the fimbriae. There are greater concentrations of ciliary cells here that facilitate transportation of the ovum into the ampulla.

The blood supply to the tube arises from a cascade of vessels originating from an arcuate formed by a branch of the ovarian artery and a tubal branch of the uterine artery. This arcuate is located in the mesosalpinx, between the fallopian tube and ovary. Vessels then perforate the medial side of the tube and travel in the intimal layer.

MANAGEMENT

Women diagnosed with an ectopic gestation are typically offered either medical or surgical treatment rather than being managed expectantly because of the potential risk for resultant morbidity or mortality. Immediate surgical indications include hemodynamic instability, impending or ongoing ectopic mass rupture, inability or unwillingness to comply with medical therapy and follow-up requirements, lack of timely access to a medical institution for management of subsequent rupture, and failed medical therapy. Notwithstanding the above, medical therapy with methotrexate remains a viable option and likely represents a larger proportion of women treated who are not accounted for by epidemiologic means.

MEDICAL MANAGEMENT

The use of methotrexate has enabled treatment of ectopic pregnancy to be even more conservative than laparoscopy. It can be used in all types of ectopic gestation either intramuscularly or directly into the gestation. Not all patients are candidates for medical management. Table 10.1 shows some of the criteria used to delineate the appropriate patients. If the criteria are met, then

---

TABLE 10.1

INDICATIONS FOR USE OF METHOTREXATE IN ECTOPIC PREGNANCY

- PATIENT IS RELIABLE, COMPLIANT, HEALTHY, AND HEMODYNAMICALLY STABLE
- ULTRASOUND NOTES DEFINITE ECTOPIC GESTATION
- PREGNANCY SAC IS LESS THAN 4 CM
- hCG TITERS <10,000 IU/mL
- PROGESTERONE LEVELS <10 ng/mL
- ABSENT FETAL CARDIAC ACTIVITY
- NORMAL LIVER FUNCTION TEST, COMPLETE BLOOD COUNT (CBC)
- GIVE RhoGAM IF Rh NEGATIVE

---

50 mg/m^2 (body surface area) is given in a single intramuscular (IM) dose. Quantitative hCG is checked on days 4 and 7. Weekly titers are then obtained until the titer is negative. A drop in titers of 15% should be seen from the day 4 value to the day 7 value. Less than 10% of patients need a second injection of methotrexate. This method is 80%–90% effective but runs the risk of emergent surgical correction for rupture. Therefore, the patient must be reliable, compliant, and aware of this risk. A study by Dudly et al. looked at characteristics of ectopic pregnancies that ruptured while being treated with methotrexate. An hCG that increased by >66% every 48 hours or a persistent increase in hCG after treatment were found to be independent predictors of tubal rupture and should perhaps lower one's threshold for surgical intervention.

Reproductive potential after an ectopic pregnancy has been studied comparing medical and endoscopic surgical treatment. Cumulative intrauterine pregnancy (IUP) rates following both laparoscopy and conservative therapy range from 36% to 58%, with a cumulative ectopic recurrence rate of approximately 25% for both treatment groups. Reproductive outcome seems to depend more on the patient's medical/surgical history than on the treatment modality used.

A systematic review of several observational studies reported a failure rate of 14.3% or higher with single-dose methotrexate when pretreatment β-hCG levels were higher than 5000 mIU/mL, compared with a 3.7% failure rate for β-hCG levels less than 5000 mIU/mL. If β-hCG levels are higher than 5000 mIU/mL, multiple doses may be appropriate, as an inpatient or at least overnight observation.

LAPAROSCOPIC TREATMENT

High-resolution ultrasound, early diagnosis, microsurgical techniques, and nonsurgical management suggest that many, if not most women may be offered a more conservative approach in an attempt to preserve the affected tube. Readily available anesthesia, advanced cardiovascular monitoring, the ability to convert to laparotomy, and superior magnification provided by laparoscopy make this minimally invasive option a more desirable approach. Laparoscopy resulted in shorter operative times, less blood loss, fewer analgesic requirements, shorter hospital stays, and decreased costs when compared to laparotomy in three prospective studies that compared the two modalities. A Cochrane review of the surgical management of ectopic pregnancy also supported laparoscopy as the treatment of choice for eligible patients, as did a meta-analysis that evaluated effectiveness of surgery, medical treatment, and expectant management of tubal ectopic pregnancy in terms of treatment success, financial costs, and future fertility. The authors also concluded that systemic methotrexate was a good alternative in selected patients with low serum β-hCG concentrations.

SALPINGECTOMY VERSUS SALPINGOSTOMY

If the contralateral fallopian tube appears normal, then salpingectomy is a reasonable treatment option that avoids the 5%–8% risk of persistent or recurrent ectopic pregnancy in the affected tube. Salpingectomy is selectively chosen in the presence of uncontrolled bleeding, tubal destruction from a massive ectopic with or without rupture, recurrent ectopic in that tube, patient desire, severe adhesion, or hydrosalpinx. A hemodynamically stable woman who strongly desires to preserve fertility is an appropriate candidate for salpingostomy. Based on current yet limited data, there appears to be no difference in the rate of subsequent intrauterine pregnancy in women who undergo salpingostomy compared to salpingectomy.

SURGICAL MANAGEMENT BASED ON LOCATION

The location, size, and extent of the tubal pregnancy are observed laparoscopically, and the appropriate management is then based on these factors. All surgical approaches start by identification and mobilization of the involved fallopian tube and inspection of the uninvolved side (Figure 10.2).

Ampullary ectopic: If the pregnancy is in the mid-ampullary segment, a 5–7 mL dilute solution of vasopressin is injected with a relatively fine needle (we prefer a 22 G spinal needle inserted directly through the abdominal wall) into the mesosalpinx just below the pregnancy and over the antimesenteric surface of the segment containing the gestation (Figure 10.3). Although there is no standard recommended solution, we have had good success with a dilution of 20 U in 100 mL of normal saline. It is extremely important to make sure that the vasopressin is not injected directly into a vessel, as it can cause arterial hypertension, bradycardia, and death. Using a laser, microelectrode, scissors, or

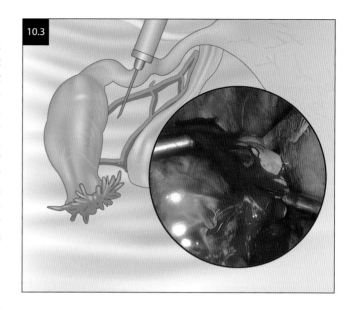

harmonic scalpel, a linear incision is made over the pregnancy approximately 1–2 cm in length, but this can vary based on the size of the ectopic. Typically, the incision should be slightly smaller than the visualized affected portion of the tube. This minimizes surgical injury to an already damaged tube and is usually sufficient for removal of the gestational tissue. We recommend use of a low-voltage current at 60 W power setting, using a fine electrode (needle point or scissors) if using monopolar electrosurgery. These techniques also reduce inadvertent damage to the tube, which may help to preserve function and reduce subsequent adhesion formation. As the incision is created, the contents of the pregnancy usually begin to extrude (Figure 10.4). This can be completed with hydrodissection techniques by placing the irrigator tip between the presumed implantation site and mucosal surface of the oviduct or using gentle traction with laparoscopic forceps (Figure 10.5). In some cases, more

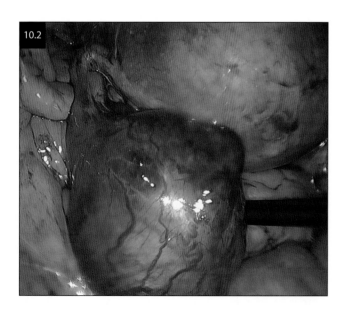

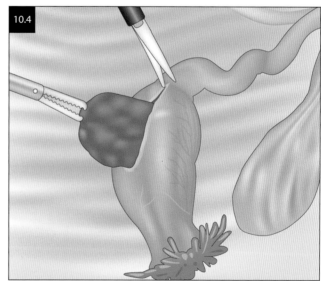

forceful irrigation in the salpingostomy incision may be required to dislodge the pregnancy from its implantation sites. In our experience, grasping at tissue tends to fragment the pregnancy, making it more difficult to remove all contents without creating more bleeding. At times, simply being patient and allowing for passive expulsion will provide the best results.

Regardless of technique, the surgeon should carefully inspect the bed to ensure complete removal of gestational tissue. Occasionally, brief bursts of bipolar energy may be needed to desiccate more briskly bleeding edges. Oozing from the tubal bed is common and will usually stop without intervention. Copious irrigation is used to dislodge trophoblastic tissue and remove blood from the peritoneal cavity. The tubal opening is left to heal by secondary intention, unless the defect is wide and the edges do not come together spontaneously. For such cases, the edges may be approximated with a single 4-0 absorbable suture.

If the pregnancy is located in the distal ampullary segment of the tube, the surgeon may consider grasping the more proximal tubal segment and "milking" the pregnancy toward and out of the fimbriated edges of the tube (Figure 10.6). This can also be performed for partially extruded tubal pregnancies and infundibular pregnancies. Implementing microsurgical techniques, such as gentle tissue handling and maintaining moisture of serosal tissues, will likely result in a better outcome with formation of fewer *de novo* adhesions.

Isthmic ectopic: If this scenario is encountered, linear salpingostomy is not as successful because these pregnancies typically grow through the lumen of the tube and erode into the tubal muscularis. Since isthmic ectopic pregnancies are more likely to result in persistent disease and tubal patency is seldom preserved, segmental tubal resection should be performed. This can be accomplished by various means, with a relatively

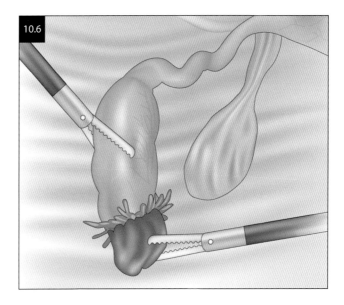

bloodless resection with use of bipolar forceps, grasping both proximal and distal to the gestation and desiccating from the antimesenteric surface to the mesosalpinx. This segment is then incised and the mesosalpinx sequentially desiccated and incised in a similar fashion (Figure 10.7). Depending on the size of the ectopic, some patients may be able to undergo successful microsurgical tubal reanastomosis at a later date.

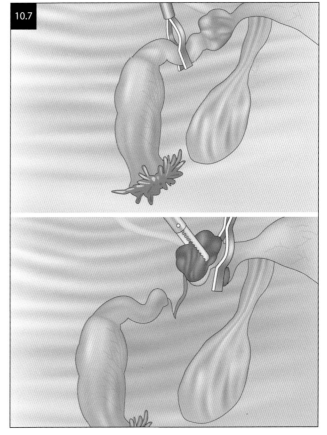

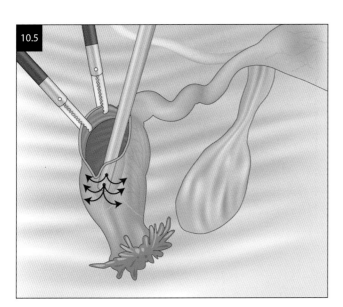

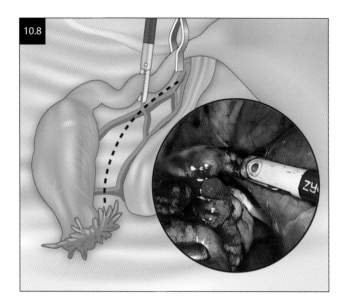

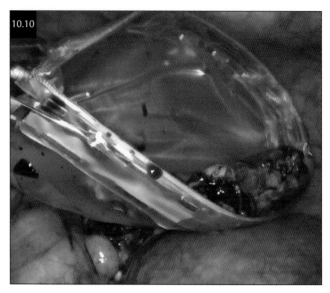

When performing salpingectomy for an isthmic ectopic pregnancy, the tube is removed from its anatomical attachments by one of various methods including bipolar energy, laser, endoscopic stapling devices, ultrasonic energy, or endoloops (Figures 10.8 and 10.9). The mesosalpingeal incision begins at the proximal isthmus of the tube and progresses to the fimbriated end. The products of conception are most easily removed through a 10 mm trocar sleeve with or without the use of an endo-bag (Figure 10.10).

Interstitial/cornual ectopic: These types of ectopic pregnancies are rare with a prevalence of 1:5000 live births (Figure 10.11). The vascular nature of the cornua accounts for a mortality rate of 2%–2.5%. The traditional management of this type of ectopic gestation is by laparotomy with extended salpingectomy and/or cornual resection. Hysterectomy was the preferred means of surgical management historically; however, with improved techniques and innovations, most patients can be managed more conservatively. If the diagnosis is made early and the patient is stable, nonsurgical approaches may be considered, including locally or systemically administered methotrexate. If medical management is not possible, surgical treatment options include immediate laparotomy, laparoscopy, or a combined laparoscopic and hysteroscopic approach.

If the overlying myometrium is thin, a laparoscopic resection may be possible. Bipolar coagulation on the thinnest portion of the interstitium should be used with caution, but monopolar scissors are readily used to enter the gestational sac. The fetus and gestation are then removed from this incision, and bleeding is controlled

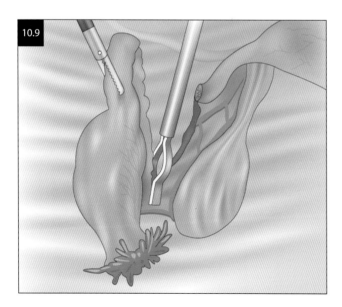

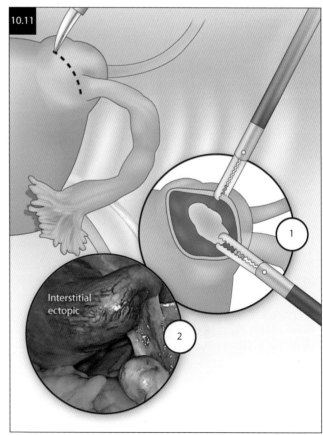

Interstitial ectopic

with bipolar coagulation. The uterus is then closed using absorbable suture. The cornua are extremely vascular, and profuse bleeding can occur rapidly. Therefore, it is always prudent to have blood products readily available and consent for more invasive procedures if emergently indicated, such as hysterectomy. Use of vasoactive agents to constrict local vasculature and purse-string tourniquets have been described to minimize blood loss during these at-risk procedures.

A hysteroscopic approach to the interstitial ectopic has also been described. During that particular case, an interstitial ectopic was diagnosed and persisted despite multiple doses of methotrexate. The gestational sac was directly visualized via real-time sonography, and through the hysteroscope, the gestational sac was ruptured, and the placental tissue was removed from the left cornu under sonographic guidance. Two weeks postoperatively, the patient's β-hCG level became undetectable and her ultrasound showed no evidence of pregnancy.

Ovarian pregnancy: The incidence of an ovarian ectopic is 0.7 per 100 ectopic gestations. Surgical management of ovarian pregnancy can be achieved via oophorectomy. The ovarian ligament is grasped with bipolar forceps, cauterized, and then cut. The mesoovarium is then taken down in a progressive fashion. This can also be performed using an Endoloop or with the harmonic scalpel.

Cervical pregnancy: This is also a rare form of ectopic pregnancy, with a rate of less than 0.15%, and in the past was treated by hysterectomy. Currently, the most common surgical approach for cervical pregnancy is curettage, although successful hysteroscopic resection of a cervical pregnancy has also been reported. Medical management with methotrexate, whenever possible, is preferred, due to the severe hemorrhage that can occur if appropriate precautions are not taken, given the rich blood supply to the cervix and its inability to reduce hemorrhage by contraction. The risk of postevacuation hemorrhage can be minimized with vascular occlusive techniques, which has been successfully reported by both transvaginal ligation of the cervical branches of the uterine arteries or uterine artery embolization, which offers the advantage of being less invasive. Another option is using a Foley balloon for tamponade, which has been shown to be more effective than vaginal packing.

RUPTURED ECTOPIC PREGNANCY

Patients who present with ruptured ectopic pregnancy, large hemoperitoneum or a surgical abdomen notwithstanding, are not necessarily excluded from a laparoscopic approach. There are several factors to keep in mind when performing laparoscopy in these patients.

Establishment of the pneumoperitoneum and placement of the trocars may be just as timely as performing an exploratory laparotomy. When placing the insufflation needle in the abdomen filled with blood, the surgeon may encounter higher initial insufflation pressures, since

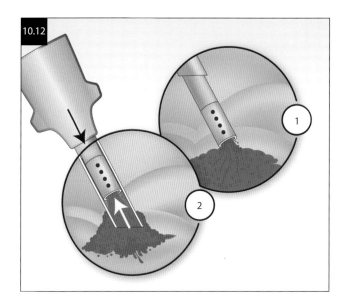

10.12

the tip of the needle may be immersed in blood. Hasson (open laparoscopic) entry should also be considered, especially since a larger fascial defect in the umbilicus may facilitate retrieval of the specimen.

Typically, a four-port technique is utilized. For most ectopic pregnancies, an umbilical trocar is placed first, but left upper quadrant entry can be done if the patient has had multiple previous surgeries, similar to other appropriate indications. After entering the abdomen and inserting the laparoscope, the patient should be placed in Trendelenburg position, and a high suprapubic port and two lower quadrant ports should be inserted. We prefer four-port placement so that two surgeons can use both hands to expedite the case. During situations where there is a large amount of blood in the abdomen or pelvis, a 10 mm suction irrigator tip should be used. Irrigating more mature clots will help lyse the solid portions, also facilitating removal of obscuring blood. A large collection of blood clots can also be effectively removed using a standard 5 mm suction tip attached to wall suction to pull clots up and evacuate against the trocar sleeve (Figure 10.12).

Only enough blood should be suctioned to allow for visualization of the affected portion of the tube and accomplish the task at hand. Typically, the tube is extensively damaged and salpingectomy is required, which can be accomplished quite efficiently. Good communication with the anesthesia team is paramount to a successful operation and should be had prior to entering the operating room. A grasper can also be introduced for quick localization of the ruptured tube and to tamponade the bleeding site.

ACKNOWLEDGMENTS

We would like to thank Drs. Gerard Roy and Anthony Luciano for their contribution to the original publication, and Drs. Sony Singh and Jay Goldberg for providing images for current illustrations.

PEARLS

- KNOWN RISK FACTORS FOR ECTOPIC PREGNANCY INCLUDE PREVIOUS INSULTS TO THE TUBE SUCH AS INFLAMMATORY/INFECTIOUS PROCESSES OR EXPOSURES, PELVIC OR TUBAL SURGERIES, AND MÜLLERIAN ANOMALIES.
- THE MAJORITY OF ECTOPIC PREGNANCIES OCCUR IN THE AMPULLARY PORTION OF THE FALLOPIAN TUBE.
- THE DIAGNOSIS OF ECTOPIC PREGNANCY MADE CLINICALLY AND SUSPICION FOR AN ECTOPIC PREGNANCY ARE HEIGHTENED WHEN THE B-HCG CONCENTRATION IS GREATER THAN 1500 IU/L AND TVS EXAMINATION REVEALS A COMPLEX ADNEXAL MASS WITH NO EVIDENCE OF INTRAUTERINE PREGNANCY.
- EXPECTANT MANAGEMENT CAN BE OFFERED TO A SELECT FEW WHO HAVE BEEN COUNSELED APPROPRIATELY.
- SURGICAL MANAGEMENT IS INDICATED FOR UNSTABLE PATIENTS, THOSE WHO DO NOT MEET DESCRIBED CRITERIA FOR MTX (ACTIVE KIDNEY/LIVER DISEASE, B-HCG LEVELS >5000, MASS >3.5 CM, FETAL POLE WITH CARDIAC ACTIVITY) OR ARE UNABLE TO COMPLY WITH CONSERVATIVE MANAGEMENT.
- REPRODUCTIVE OUTCOME APPEARS TO BE SIMILAR FOR WOMEN WHO RECEIVE METHOTREXATE AND SURGICAL MANAGEMENT.
- ALTHOUGH NO DEFINITIVE CONCLUSIONS HAVE YET BEEN REACHED, SALPINGOSTOMY SHOULD BE CONSIDERED OVER SALPINGECTOMY IN STABLE PATIENTS WHO DESIRE FUTURE CHILDBEARING.
- PATIENTS WITH LARGE HEMOPERITONEUM ARE NOT NECESSARILY EXCLUDED FROM A LAPAROSCOPIC APPROACH IF THE SURGEON AND FACILITY ARE CAPABLE OF PROCEEDING WITH EXPEDITED SURGICAL MANAGEMENT.

SUGGESTED READING

Alleyassin A, Khademi A, Aghahosseini M, Safdarian L, Badenoosh B, Hamed EA. Comparison of success rates in the medical management of ectopic pregnancy with single-dose and multiple-dose administration of methotrexate: A prospective, randomized clinical trial. *Fertil Steril.* 2006;85:1661–1666.

Ankum W, Mol B, Van de Veen F, Bossuyt P. Risk factors for ectopic pregnancy: A meta-analysis. *Fertil Steril.* 1996;65:1093–1099.

Barnhart KT, Simhan H, Kamelle SA. Diagnostic accuracy of ultrasound above and below the beta-hCG discriminatory zone. *Obstet Gynecol.* 1999;94:583–587.

Bouyer J, Coste J, Fernandez H et al. Sites of ectopic pregnancy: A 10-year population-based study of 1800 cases. *Hum Reprod.* 2002;17:3224–3230.

Budnick SG, Jacobs SL, Nulsen JC, Metzger DA. Conservative management of interstitial pregnancy. *Obstet Gynecol Surv.* 1993;48:694.

Centers for Disease Control and Prevention (CDC). Ectopic pregnancy—United States, 1990–1992. *MMWR Morb Mortal Wkly Rep.* 1995;44:46.

Chang J, Elam-Evans LD, Berg CJ et al. Pregnancy-related mortality surveillance—United States, 1991—1999. *MMWR Surveill Summ.* 2003;52:1–8.

Condous G, Okaro E, Khalid A et al. The accuracy of transvaginal ultrasonography for the diagnosis of ectopic pregnancy prior to surgery. *Hum Reprod.* 2005;20:1404–1409.

Gun M, Mavrogiorgis M. Cervical ectopic pregnancy: A case report and literature review. *Ultrasound Obstet Gynecol.* 2002;19:297–301.

Hajenius PJ, Mol F, Mol BW et al. Interventions for tubal ectopic pregnancy. *Cochrane Database Syst Rev.* 2007;CD000324.

Hardy TJ. Hysteroscopic resection of a cervical ectopic pregnancy. *J Am Assoc Gynecol Laparosc.* 2002;9(3):370–371.

Lundorff P, Thorburn J, Hahlin M et al. Laparoscopic surgery in ectopic pregnancy. A randomized trial versus laparotomy. *Acta Obstet Gynecol Scand.* 1991;70:343.

Menon S, Colins J, Barnhart KT. Establishing a human chorionic gonadotropin cutoff to guide methotrexate treatment of ectopic pregnancy: A systematic review. *Fertil Steril.* 2007;87:481–484.

Mol F, Mol BW, Ankum WM et al. Current evidence on surgery, systemic methotrexate and expectant management in the treatment of tubal ectopic pregnancy: A systematic review and meta-analysis. *Hum Reprod Update.* 2008;14:309–319.

Mol F, Strandell A, Jurkovic D, Yalcinkaya T, Verhoeve H. The ESEP study: Salpingostomy versus salpingectomy for tubal ectopic pregnancy: The impact on future fertility: A randomised controlled trial. *BMC Women's Health.* 2008;8:11.

Murray H, Baakdah H, Bardell T, Tulandi T. Diagnosis and treatment of ectopic pregnancy. *CMAJ.* 2005;173:905.

Senterman M, Jibodh R, Tulandi T. Histopathologic study of ampullary and isthmic tubal ectopic pregnancy. *Am J Obstet Gynecol.* 1988;159:939.

Soriano D, Vicus D, Mashiach R et al. Laparoscopic treatment of cornual pregnancy: A series of 20 consecutive cases. *Fertil Steril.* 2008;90:839.

CHAPTER 11

LAPAROSCOPIC MANAGEMENT OF THE ADNEXAL MASS

Sukhpreet Singh Multani, Resad Paya Pasic, and Joseph L. Hudgens

The management of an adnexal mass combines the need for appropriate workup and sound judgment to ensure the optimal outcome.

Whereas the laparoscope is an essential tool in the surgical armamentarium, it should only be employed in an appropriate fashion, relegating some patients to be best managed by laparotomy.

The adnexa includes the ovary, fallopian tube, broad ligament, blood vessels, and fascia contained within. Acknowledging there are many causes for a pelvic mass, this chapter only considers gynecologic conditions.

Once an adnexal mass is identified, fundamental questions that must be addressed include the following: What is the origin of the mass? Are there additional laboratory or radiologic studies that would be useful? Does it require surgical removal, and if so, what type of surgery would be most appropriate?

GYNECOLOGIC PROBLEMS CAUSING ADNEXAL MASSES

OVARY
  FOLLICULAR CYSTS
  NEOPLASM
    BENIGN
    MALIGNANT
    METASTATIC
FALLOPIAN TUBE
  ECTOPIC PREGNANCY
  HYDROSALPINX
  PYOSALPINX
  NEOPLASM
UTERINE
  PEDUNCULATED MYOMA
  MÜLLERIAN ANOMALY
  CORNUAL PREGNANCY
OTHER
  PARATUBAL CYST
  PERITONEAL CYST
  PELVIC ABSCESS

NONGYNECOLOGIC CAUSES OF AN ADNEXAL MASS

BOWEL
  FECES
  DIVERTICULAR DISEASE
  ILEITIS
  APPENDICITIS
  MUCINOUS TUMOR OF APPENDIX
  SMALL BOWEL STROMAL SARCOMA
  COLON CANCER
URINARY
  DISTENDED BLADDER
  PELVIC KIDNEY
  URACHAL CYST
  URINOMA
  URETERAL NEOPLASM
MISCELLANEOUS
  RETROPERITONEAL NEOPLASM
  RETROPERITONEAL HEMATOMA
  MESOTHELIAL TUMORS
  PERITONEAL CYST
  INTERNAL ILIAC ARTERY ANEURYSM

HISTIOLOGIC DIFFERENTIAL FOR OVARIAN NEOPLASM

EPITHELIAL TUMORS
  SEROUS
  MUCINOUS
  ENDOMETRIOMA/ENDOMETRIOID
  CLEAR CELL
SEX CORD/STROMAL TUMORS
  GRANULOSA
  FIBROMA/THECOMA
  SERTOLI-LEYDIG
  GONADOBLASTOMA

GERM CELL
  TERATOMA
  DYSGERMINOMA
  ENDODERMAL SINUS (YOLK SAC)
  CHORIOCARCINOMA
  EMBRYONAL

DIAGNOSIS OF ADNEXAL MASS

Most commonly, the diagnosis of a gynecologic cause for an adnexal mass can be secured using a combination of a targeted history, pelvic examination, radiologic studies, and laboratory testing. Developing a systematic approach to establish a differential diagnosis using an assiduous evaluation is essential.

Using both anatomic and histologic frameworks can help organize this process (see boxes).

The possibility of an ectopic pregnancy should always be excluded by drawing a serum β-hCG in any woman of childbearing age who is sexually active.

RADIOLOGIC STUDIES

Following the exclusion of pregnancy, the most fruitful investigation of an adnexal mass is transvaginal ultrasound. If an ovarian cyst/mass is identified, sonographic features concerning for an underlying malignancy, especially in a postmenopausal woman, include increased volume, internal septations larger than 3 mm, papillations, excrescences, indistinct margins, solid elements, and thickening of the wall (Figure 11.1). Scoring systems have been developed to help better determine the risk of malignancy based on ultrasonic features. Whereas there was concern about the presence of persistent simple ovarian cysts in postmenopausal women, it is now established that they are extremely common, and not only is the risk of malignancy low especially for unilocular cysts <10 cm in diameter, but most will resolve spontaneously when followed by serial sonography.

Although there are several sonographic scoring systems that have been proposed to quantify the overall risks associated with ovarian sonomorphology, none has been universally accepted. The American College of Obstetricians and Gynecologists (ACOG) in 2002 proposed one scoring system based on three criteria: (1) ovarian tumor volume, (2) cyst wall structure, and (3) septa structure. In this proposed scoring system, a score of 5 or more (indicating volume of >500 cm³ and a structure that was complex and solid, displaying cystic areas with extratumoral fluid) had 89% sensitivity in identifying a malignant mass.

Ancillary tests have been applied to help better differentiate benign from malignant ovarian cysts. Despite initial enthusiasm, color-flow Doppler demonstrating blood flow within and around the cyst has not achieved a pivotal role in the workup of adnexal masses. The waveform shape obtained by Doppler imaging provides a rough indication of the type of blood flow within a blood vessel. Tumor vessels typically have continuous high diastolic flow with low pulsatility due to the lack of a muscular layer in the vessel wall; this is associated with a low resistance index. Normal arterioles have a muscular layer that helps regulate parenchymal perfusion. This is associated with a lack of continuous diastolic flow, high pulsatility, a resistance index higher than 0.7, and the presence of a diastolic notch (Figure 11.2). Unfortunately, some benign lesions including hemorrhagic luteal cysts, dermoid cysts, and inflammatory masses such as tuboovarian abscesses may all demonstrate low impedance or high diastolic flow similar to cancers.

More accurate methods of ultrasonography have been, and are being developed, including three-dimensional (3D) ultrasound as well as the use of intravenous contrast agents with the ultrasound.

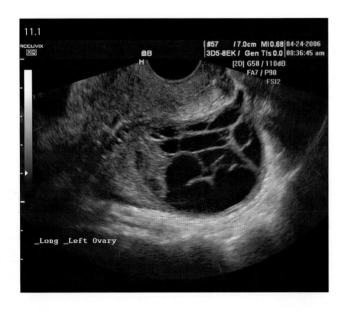

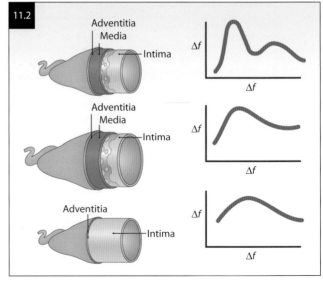

While an adnexal mass can be seen on computed tomography (CT) scanning of the abdomen or pelvis, this modality is not as helpful for the workup. Magnetic resonance imaging (MRI) has a higher sensitivity and specificity for the diagnosis of an adnexal mass, but at a considerable increase in cost. It may be particularly helpful in determining whether a solid mass such as pedunculated fibroid is arising from the uterus and for adnexal masses in obese patients, where ultrasound imaging may be suboptimal. Fat suppression sequencing can be used to confirm the diagnosis of a dermoid cyst in instances of complex adnexal masses, where conservative management may be preferred over surgery because of a patient's desire to be simply followed radiographically, and for those with significant medical comorbidities.

LABORATORY STUDIES

Although the antigenic marker CA125 plays a significant role in the management of epithelial ovarian cancer, it may not be useful for differentiating an adnexal mass as benign or malignant. First, it is only elevated in up to 50% of all stage 1 epithelial carcinomas of the ovary; second, it is nonspecific and can be elevated by many benign and other malignant lesions. Many of these benign causes for an elevated CA125 will resolve after menopause, making CA125 a more predictive tool for evaluating a postmenopausal woman for ovarian cancer.

Tumor marker panels that combine CA125 seem to improve sensitivity by 5%–10% in the detection of malignancy, but specificity decreases. Most recently, OVA1, a panel that includes five immunoassays (CA-125, transferrin, prealbumin, apolipoprotein A1, β2-microglobulin) using a proprietary algorithm, produces a single-digit result that is meant to stratify a female's risk of malignancy. Premenopausal patients with a score >5 and postmenopausal patients with a score >4.4 were determined to be at higher risk. The addition of OVA1 may aid in detecting advanced-stage ovarian cancers. A particular advantage of this panel is a higher sensitivity in comparison to CA-125 for all histologic subtypes, premenopausal women, and early stage disease. In a multi-institutional OVA1 trial, the panel correctly identified more than 70% of malignancies missed by the ACOG criteria. Sensitivity improved from 77% to 94%, including an increase in premenopausal women from 58% to 91%, when OVA1 was used in conjunction with the ACOG criteria. The overall specificity of the ACOG criteria with OVA1 was 35%.

Other tumor markers that may be tested, particularly prior to surgery in young females under the age of 30 with a mainly solid adnexal mass, include α-fetoprotein raised in endodermal sinus (yolk sac tumors), LDH (raised in dysgerminoma), β-hCG (raised in choriocarcinoma), and alpha subunit of inhibin (raised in granulosa cell tumors).

Elevated serum levels of carcinoembryonic antigen (CEA) can be found in a variety of benign diseases and cancers, including mucinous ovarian carcinoma. Although the sensitivity of CEA and positive predictive value of this tumor marker are poor, 25% and 14%, respectively, it has utility in assessing disease response to treatment. Similarly, CA 19-9, which is predominantly noted in pancreatic cancer, can be detected in ovarian cancer, however, is not a marker for detection but rather when elevated can aid in monitoring disease response.

SURGERY

Once the decision is made that laparoscopic surgery is appropriate, the surgical procedure should only be performed by a surgeon with skill, experience, and understanding of the underlying disease.

One of the main concerns for a patient undergoing surgery for an adnexal mass is whether or not it may be a cancer. If the mass could represent an early ovarian cancer, then further surgery should be performed expeditiously in conjunction with a gynecologic oncologist. The ACOG has issued guidelines on which patients should be referred to a gynecologic cancer specialist prior to surgery.

The referral decision can be stratified based on whether the patient is post- or premenopausal. If physical examination and imaging point toward a pelvic mass, referral to a gynecologic oncologist is warranted in the presence of one of these additional findings. In postmenopausal women, these findings include an elevated CA125 level (>35 U), evidence of abdominal or distant metastasis, ascites, family history of ovarian/breast cancer, or a nodular/fixed pelvic mass. In the premenopausal woman, findings include a very elevated CA125 level (>200 U), ascites, family history of ovarian/breast cancer, or evidence of abdominal or distant metastasis.

PREOPERATIVE PREPARATION

Patients should be counseled about the possible findings at the time of surgery, and the procedures that might be necessary. All patients undergoing laparoscopy should be warned that conversion to a laparotomy may be necessary. Those with known, or suspected, severe adhesions and those in whom cancer might be detected should undergo preoperative bowel preparation. Collaboration with other specialties including colorectal surgery and urology may be warranted in patients with complex presentations.

SURGICAL APPROACH

All patients undergoing surgery for an adnexal mass should have appropriate prophylactic measures taken that address thromboembolism, antibiotics, and the need for beta-blockers. The surgery should normally be performed under general anesthetic. The whole of the abdominal skin should be prepared in case a laparotomy is needed, and all patients should have a vaginal prep.

A Foley catheter should be placed to reduce the chance of bladder injury, to improve the operative view, and to track the patient's urine output. If the patient has a uterus and is not pregnant, then a uterine manipulator can be placed to allow manipulation of the uterus in order to facilitate the adnexal dissection. If the uterus is absent, a sponge-on-a-stick in the vagina may be very helpful.

When operating on a patient with a large adnexal mass, care should be taken not to rupture the mass on initial trocar insertion. A left upper quadrant approach is useful in these patients as well as in those with previous surgery involving a midline incision. This approach is also helpful in the case of specimen removal. The patient should have a nasogastric or orogastric tube placed to empty and decompress the stomach when entering the left upper quadrant.

An open-entry technique either at the umbilicus or above the level of the midline scar is also useful with regard to specimen removal. Whichever route is used, a camera is placed through the initial port, and once enough CO_2 has been insufflated, an assessment is made of the abdominopelvic cavity. A 0° diagnostic laparoscope is often adequate, but one that is 30° may be useful in case of a large mass or extensive adhesions. Three 5–12 mm ancillary ports are utilized as needed (Figure 11.3), and the port configuration is dependent on the surgeon's preference and the pathology present. The laparoscope is rotated around to inspect the peritoneum, liver, gallbladder, omentum, appendix, and at least the surface of the stomach and small and large bowel. Gross disease may be visible with the camera port alone, but if not, then a second port is placed and a grasper is passed to facilitate this inspection.

In the pelvis it is necessary to assess all pelvic structures, including the peritoneum, uterosacral ligaments, round ligaments, tubes, ovaries, and ureters. Careful attention is made to check for peritoneal nodules that would need to be biopsied. Adhesions may greatly impede visibility and should be cleared with great care using systematic dissection.

If a gynecologic cancer is found, either by the initial findings or on frozen section, management should be continued with the involvement of a gynecologic cancer specialist so that the patient's outcome is optimized. In this situation, the laparoscopist's role is to make the diagnosis in the least morbid fashion.

If preoperative preparation has been made, and provided that the cancer is macroscopically confined within the ovary, a full laparoscopic staging operation can be performed including hysterectomy, bilateral salpingo-oophorectomy, peritoneal washings, peritoneal biopsies, subcolic omentectomy, and bilateral para-aortic and pelvic node dissection.

An ovarian mass in an adolescent is more likely to be malignant when compared to one in an adult, mandating a heightened concern by a proper workup and orchestrated management.

Moreover, extra caution should always be exercised in a woman with an adnexal mass who has previously undergone hysterectomy. Removal of adnexal structures may be difficult under these circumstances due to adhesions, especially if the mass arises from the left adnexa after previous abdominal surgery.

ADNEXAL MASS REMOVAL

Once preliminary inspection has been completed, peritoneal washings are obtained, and a determination has been made that the mass can be safely removed, an adnexal mass involving the ovary or fallopian tube can be extirpated in two fundamental ways: First, remove the adnexal mass by identifying and coagulating the infundibulopelvic ligament and following the incision toward the origin of the fallopian tube and uteroovarian ligament, as shown in Figure 11.4. Choosing this methodology requires a keen knowledge of the course of the ureter in relationship to the adnexa, especially if the ovary is adherent to the pelvic sidewall and lies on top of the ureter. In these situations, the ovary should be freed from the pelvic sidewall by pushing it from below and freeing the adhesions with scissors, while maintaining

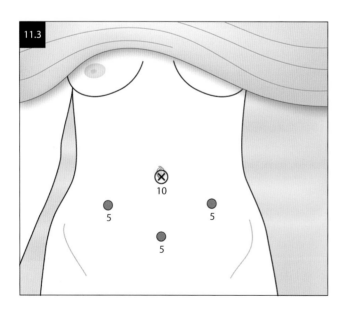

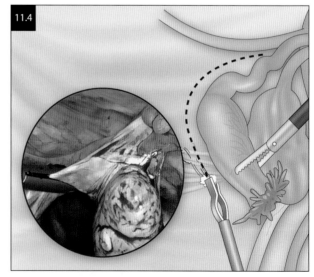

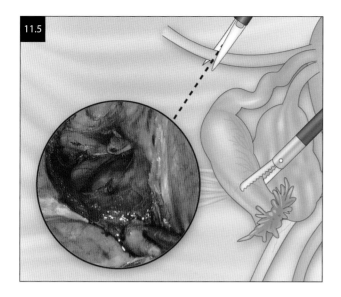

traction on the ovary with a suction-irrigator. Once the ovary is free, the incision can be carried as shown.

The second approach is to first gain entry into the retroperitoneum by dividing the ipsilateral round ligament or the peritoneum just lateral to the infundibulopelvic ligament (Figure 11.5). The fallopian tube is grasped gently and pulled away from the sidewall as the opening in the lateral peritoneum is extended cranially. The ureter is then identified through the peritoneum or in the retroperitoneum. A window created in the posterior leaf of the broad ligament above the ureter can be extremely helpful in isolating the infundibulopelvic vessels (Figure 11.6). There are several instruments available to coagulate and transect the ovarian vessels, including the bipolar forceps, Harmonic scalpel (Ethicon Endosurgery, Cincinnati, Ohio), Ligasure (Valley Lab, Boulder, Colorado), Gyrus cutting forceps (Gyrus/Acmi, Maple Grove, Minnesota), and EnSeal (Ethicon Endosurgery, etc.). Sutures may also be used to ligate the ovarian vessels. When employing an energy-based surgical device, it is important to avoid heat damage to the ovarian or mass capsule to prevent rupture.

Once the infundibulopelvic pedicle has been ligated, the attachments of the ovary to the sidewall can be transected. Finally, the uteroovarian vessel can be coagulated and transected similar to the infundibulopelvic vessels.

Throughout the adnexal resection, ovarian manipulation should be minimized to avoid rupture and the dissemination of malignant cells, which has been shown to adversely affect prognosis in such patients. If a dermoid cyst ruptures, the pelvis should be irrigated copiously with saline until clear of fatty debris and hair in order to avoid possible chemical peritonitis. Cyst rupture at the time of laparoscopy has been noted to be 15%–100% compared to 4%–13% at the time of laparotomy, per Nezhat et al. in a review of 10 years of surgical cases. The incidence of chemical peritonitis in this review was noted to be only 0.2%, representing 1 patient in 370 cases of spillage.

Not uncommonly, an adnexal mass may be adherent to the large or small bowel. Bowel serosa should not be forcefully held with graspers. The bowel edges should be carefully defined, and the laparoscopic scissors should be used to cut the adhesions. Thermal devices should not be used close to the bowel. And, cutting parallel to the surface can reduce the risk for damaging the bowel wall. Once the bowel is freed, it should be carefully inspected for serosal damage.

When an adherent mass is resected, oozing and bleeding can occur. Hemostasis can be attained by direct pressure, the use of surgical energy, suture, surgical clip, or the use of hemostatic agents. A 4 × 4 gauze can be placed through a 10–12 mm port and adjacent to the bleeding areas (Figure 11.7). A suction-irrigator can be applied to allow more efficient identification and application of bipolar or other energy. Identification and, in some cases, mobilization of the ureter and bowel before the application of energy are important steps to avoid thermal damage to these structures.

There are several hemostatic agents available on the market; however, all of them come in one of two

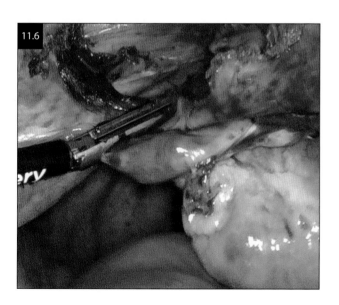

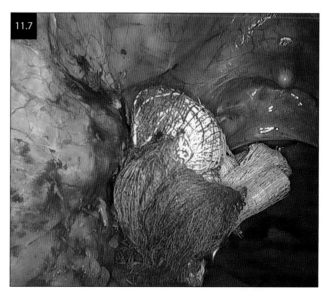

varieties. They are either physical agents or biologically active agents. Physical agents provide a scaffold for local clot formation to provide hemostasis. Biologically active agents activate the coagulation cascade with conversion of either prothrombin or fibrinogen to their active component. Each agent has its advantages and disadvantages, which include onset of action, postoperative duration, cost, risk of infection, and allergic response.

OVARIAN CYSTECTOMY

Aspiration of a simple ovarian cyst at laparoscopy in an attempt to treat is usually unsuccessful and risks the dissemination of an occult carcinoma. As far as diagnostic aspiration is concerned, cytologic analysis of aspirated cyst fluid has a high false-negative rate and is therefore not helpful for the management of adnexal masses.

Whereas cystectomy is never indicated for potentially malignant cysts, it is the procedure of choice for benign ovarian cysts including dermoid, endometrioma, and complicated functional types.

While the ovary is supported using a grasper placed beneath, an incision is made on the border between normal ovarian tissue and the cyst. This allows the cyst wall to be identified and facilitates dissection of the normal ovarian tissue (Figures 11.8 and 11.9). The surgeon should ideally try to remove the entire cyst without rupture. If an ultrasonically simple cyst appears benign at laparoscopy and appears to be too large to remove intact, the wall may be decompressed by puncturing with a needle attached to suction tubing, which minimizes spillage of the cyst fluid. In order to minimize the spill of the cyst fluid into the abdominal cavity, an Endoloop may be placed on the area where the cyst puncture is going to be performed. The aspiration needle is inserted through the Endoloop, and the fluid is then aspirated. The ovary is grasped, and the loop

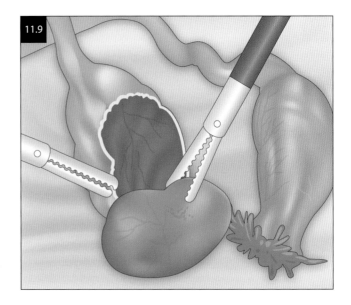

is constricted around the puncture site while the needle is removed (Figure 11.10). If the cyst fluid appears serous, the cyst can be elevated with two graspers and the incision slightly extended with laparoscopic scissors, allowing the remainder of the fluid to be removed (Figure 11.11). The interior wall of the cystic cavity is then inspected laparoscopically. Any suspicious areas discovered during surgery should be biopsied and sent for frozen section. If benign, resection of the entire cyst wall should be performed.

Endometriomas can be very difficult to enucleate from normal ovarian tissue, and in those cases, the cyst should be opened and part of the ovary resected as shown in Figure 11.11. The cyst wall is identified and peeled off the ovary with the help of a traumatic grasper by holding the capsule. Another grasper is used on the ovarian capsule. Countertraction in a linear fashion is used to separate the cyst wall from the remainder of the ovary (Figure 11.12). Bleeding from the ovary is usually

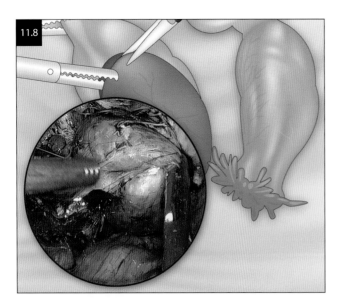

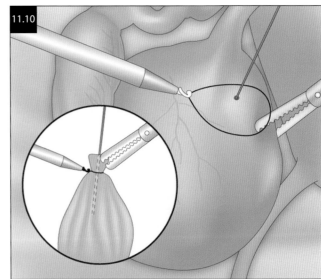

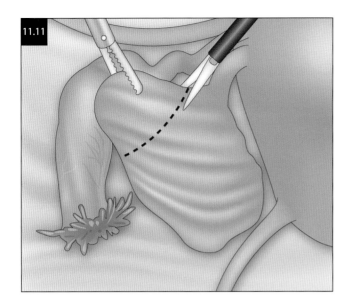

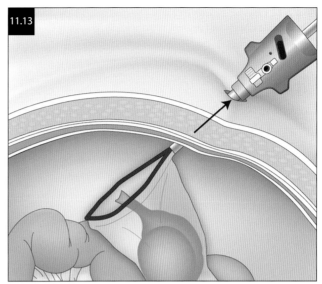

self-limited, or it can be controlled with a spot coagulator or bipolar forceps. The resected tissue and the ovarian capsule are removed through a laparoscopic port by rotating the grasper and pulling it through the port. If the cyst cannot be removed directly, then it should be placed into a laparoscopic bag for removal. Bags come in a variety of sizes and may be self-deployed (Figure 11.13). Tissue extraction techniques from the peritoneal cavity are presented in Chapter 14.

SURGERY IN PREGNANCY

Laparoscopic removal of an adnexal mass in pregnancy is sometimes necessary, and several factors should be considered. Depending on the gestational age, preoperative consultation should be made with an obstetrical specialist. Patients in the second trimester should be placed in the dorsal supine position with left lateral tilt, and antithromboembolic stockings and sequential compression devices should be applied. The placement of the

laparoscope and the operating trocars should be modified depending on the uterine size. An open technique or left upper quadrant technique should be used for initial placement. The pneumoperitoneal pressure should be limited to 12 mm Hg or less to ensure adequate venous return to the heart. This will maximize maternal cardiac output and minimize fetal acidosis. However, brief elevations at the beginning of the procedure can be well tolerated. During the operative procedure, it is a good idea to minimize uterine manipulation.

SUGGESTED READING

ACOG Committee Opinion: number 280, December 2002. The role of the generalist obstetrician-gynecologist in the early detection of ovarian cancer. *Obstet Gynecol.* 2002;100:1413–1416.

Bast RC Jr, Badgwell D, Lu Z et al. New tumor markers: CA125 and beyond. *Int J Gynecol Cancer.* 2005;15(suppl 3):274–281.

Bristow RE, Smith A, Zhen Z et al. Ovarian malignancy risk stratification of the adnexal mass using a multivariate index assay. *Gynecol Oncol.* 2013;128(2):252–259.

Chan L, Lin WM, Uerpairojkit B, Hartman D, Reece EA, Helm W. Evaluation of adnexal masses using the new 3D ultrasound technology: A preliminary report. *J Ultrasound Med.* 1997;16:349–354.

Childers JM, Lange J, Surwit EA. Laparoscopic surgical staging in ovarian cancer. *Gynecol Oncol.* 1995;59:25–33.

Daoud E, Bodor G. CA-125 concentrations in malignant and nonmalignant disease. *Clin Chem.* 1991;37:1968–1974.

Jacobs I, Bast RC Jr. The CA 125 tumour-associated antigen: A review of the literature. *Hum Reprod.* 1989;4(1):1–12.

Kohler C, Tozzi R, Klemm P, Schneider A. Laparoscopic paraaortic left-sided transperitoneal infrarenal lymphadenectomy in patients with gynecologic malignancies: Technique and results. *Gynecol Oncol.* 2003;91:139–148.

Maiman M, Seltzer V, Boyce J. Laparoscopic excision of ovarian neoplasms subsequently found to be malignant. *Obstet Gynecol.* 1991;77:563–567.

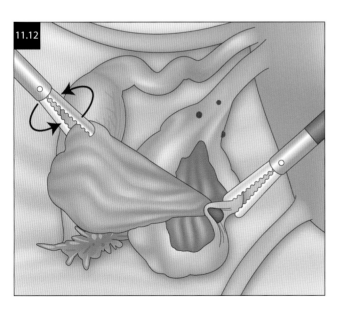

Miralles C, Orea M, Espana P et al. Cancer antigen 125 associated with multiple benign and malignant pathologies. *Ann Surg Oncol.* 2003;10:150–154.

Nezhat C, Kalyoncu S, Nezhat C et al. Laparoscopic management of ovarian dermoid cysts: Ten years' experience. *JSLS.* 1999;3(3):179–184.

Reich HF, McGlynn F, Wilkie W. Laparoscopic management of stage I ovarian cancer. A case report. *J Reprod Med.* 1990;35:601–605.

Sassone AM, Timor-Tritsch IE, Artner A et al. Transvaginal sonographic characterization of ovarian disease: Evaluation of a new scoring system to predict malignancy. *Obstet Gynecol.* 1991;78:70.

Sunoo CS. Laparoscopic removal of a large adnexal mass. *Obstet Gynecol.* 2004;103(5 Pt 2):1087–1089.

Wolf SI, Gosink BB, Feldesman MR, Lin MC, Stuenkel CA, Braly PS, Pretorius DH. Prevalence of simple adnexal cysts in postmenopausal women. *Radiology.* 1991;180:65–71.

Chapter 12

LAPAROSCOPIC MYOMECTOMY

Linda Shiber and Thomas G. Lang

INTRODUCTION

Uterine leiomyoma are exceedingly common, and the incidence increases with age. In addition, the incidence of fibroids varies between ethnic groups with a higher prevalence among African American women. Though many women with fibroids are asymptomatic, large leiomyoma or those impinging on the uterine cavity often cause bothersome symptoms and may warrant surgical intervention. Myomectomy is the surgical treatment of choice when approaching symptomatic uterine leiomyoma in women desiring future fertility. Minimally invasive techniques for myomectomy have been developed in more recent decades and have afforded reproductive-aged women suffering from fibroids an opportunity for symptom relief with added benefits over laparotomy of shorter hospital stay, rapid recovery from surgery, decreased adhesion formation, improved cosmesis, and pregnancy outcomes that are equivalent to those observed after laparotomy.

PREOPERATIVE ASSESSMENT

The symptoms reported by women with symptomatic uterine leiomyoma vary according to the size and location of these masses. Symptoms commonly include prolonged or heavy menses, mass effect complaints such as urinary frequency or pelvic pain, recurrent miscarriage, and infertility.

After obtaining a detailed history, performing a physical exam, and obtaining routine screening such as Papanicolaou smear, workup for fibroids begins with ultrasonographic assessment of the uterus. Conventional pelvic ultrasound is the typical imaging study ordered and is very cost effective. However, for ideal imaging of not only the overall size and shape of the uterus but also the contours of the uterine cavity, saline infusion sonography is more helpful. If the uterus is too large to be imaged via ultrasound, magnetic resonance imaging (MRI) may be used to aid with fibroid mapping and surgical planning.

IMAGING MODALITIES

Ultrasound
Saline enhanced ultrasound
MRI

Depending on the patient's age, comorbidities, and symptomatology, endometrial biopsy may be performed to rule out malignancy. Hemoglobin should be checked to evaluate for anemia. In women who are specifically being evaluated for infertility, other contributing factors must also be ruled on or out—for example, ovulatory function, tubal patency, or presence of müllerian anomalies—before attributing difficulty becoming/remaining pregnant to fibroids that do not have an intracavitary component.

Management of leiomyoma depends on the patient's age, therapeutic goals, size and location of her fibroids, and plans for future fertility. Management options can be classified into four categories:

1. *Medical management*: Oral contraceptives, nonsteroidal anti-inflammatory medications, intrauterine device, gonadotropin-releasing hormone agonists
2. *Conservative surgical management—patient not desirous of future fertility*: Endometrial ablation, uterine fibroid embolization, radiofrequency fibroid ablation, uterine artery ligation
3. *Conservative surgical management—patient is desirous of future fertility*: Myomectomy
4. *Definitive surgical management*: Hysterectomy

Preoperative counseling is extremely important. The patient must understand the risks of laparoscopy (including risk of leiomyosarcoma and tissue morcellation, damage to bowel, bladder, and blood vessels), as well as the risk of conversion to laparotomy and hysterectomy. She must also understand that a myomectomy may not improve her symptoms, and with regard to infertility, she may not become pregnant after surgery. The risk of uterine rupture and a discussion of route of delivery (i.e., requiring cesarean section) with future pregnancies must be addressed and documented in the medical record.

For the purpose of this chapter, we focus on women desiring fertility preservation and surgical management with myomectomy. After imaging has been obtained, recommendations can be made regarding the route of surgery. Intracavitary fibroids can often be treated hysteroscopically, while intramural, subserosal, and pedunculated fibroids must be treated abdominally, whether in a minimally invasive fashion or via laparotomy.

SELECTING ROUTE OF SURGERY: MINIMALLY INVASIVE APPROACH VERSUS LAPAROTOMY

Once it is determined that myomectomy is the treatment plan for a patient, care must be taken to choose the route of surgery most appropriate for a particular patient's pathology. Generally, the upper limits for attempting laparoscopic myomectomy are a uterine size less than 16–18 weeks, fewer than five leiomyoma, and/or largest myoma less than 15 cm. Myomectomy for leiomyoma that are located within the broad ligament, abutting the cervix, or proximal to the cornua, can be exceedingly challenging, and this must also be taken into consideration when selecting a surgical approach. Competent suturing skills are a must for a surgeon attempting laparoscopic myomectomy.

In addition, any patient with rapid fibroid growth or a suspicion of malignancy on imaging, history, or exam, should undergo laparotomy, not laparoscopy, so tissue may be removed *en bloc*. Last, a plan for tissue removal must be discussed with the patient. Many hospitals have removed power morcellators from their shelves in the wake of the controversy surrounding this technique and its potential to disseminate occult malignancy throughout the peritoneal cavity. Most women undergoing laparoscopic myomectomy are young, reproductive-aged women, making their risk of occult leiomyosarcoma much lower than the 1/300 incidence quoted by the U.S. Food and Drug Administration in 2014. With appropriate patient counseling, however, power morcellation is still a viable option for tissue removal if performed within a bag to contain any small tissue fragments. Alternate techniques that can be offered for tissue removal include mini-laparotomy for morcellation at the level of the skin, use of a SILs port at the umbilicus or suprapubically to access the myoma(s) for removal, or creation of a posterior colpotomy with transvaginal tissue morcellation.

OTHER CONSIDERATIONS PRIOR TO SURGERY

Anemia should be improved prior to surgery both by addressing red blood cell stores and decreasing losses during menses. Oral iron should be initiated as soon as possible. In women with severe anemia, preoperative blood transfusion (at least 24 hours prior to surgery) versus intravenous iron infusions can be administered. To decrease menstrual losses prior to surgery, women can be placed on oral contraceptive pills or gonadotropin-releasing hormone agonists such as LupronDepot. While a GnRH agonist can temporarily decrease the size of the myoma, improve anemia, and decrease the need for transfusion, it can make surgical planes more difficult to identify intraoperatively.

Obtaining informed consent is of great importance. The patient must understand the risks of laparoscopy (including damage to bowel, bladder, and blood vessels), as well as the risk of conversion to laparotomy and hysterectomy. The rare risk of occult malignancy must be addressed. It must be emphasized that myomectomy may not improve symptoms. With regard to infertility, the patient must be advised that the data about pregnancy outcomes with myomectomy for any type of fibroid aside from those that are submucosal are lacking, and no definitive information exists on whether myomectomy affords a net fertility benefit. The risk of uterine rupture and a discussion of route of delivery (i.e., requiring cesarean section) with future pregnancies needs to be addressed and documented in the medical record. Risk of recurrence of fibroid tumors, especially in younger women, should also be discussed.

SURGICAL TECHNIQUE

POSITIONING

After induction of anesthesia, attention to correct patient positioning is key to facilitating surgery as well as preventing untoward complications. Basic thromboembolism prophylaxis is observed by ensuring the patient has bilateral sequential compression devices on the calves. Preoperative antibiotics are generally *not* administered; however, if entry into the endometrial cavity occurs, a dose is given.

The patient is positioned in dorsal lithotomy with the arms tucked at her sides in a neutral fashion, and hands, wrists, and elbows are padded with foam. To prevent sliding cephalad while in Trendelenburg position, a large beanbag is strapped to the operating room bed and is beneath the patient. Legs are placed in stirrups, taking care not to hyperflex or hyperextend the hips or knees. Once positioning has been optimized, the beanbag is attached to suction while assistants secure it around the patient, especially superior to the shoulders, creating a sort of cocoon.

After sterile preparation of the abdomen and perineum, the patient is draped. A Foley catheter is placed, followed by a uterine manipulator that allows for chromotubation, such as Rumi. The manipulator is helpful for optimizing the position of the uterus during laparoscopic dissection and suturing as well as evaluating the patency of the fallopian tubes and recognizing entry into the endometrial cavity. We routinely perform diagnostic hysteroscopy to evaluate the uterine cavity and make sure that there are no fibroids present in the uterine cavity.

PORT PLACEMENT

Primary port entry may be either infraumbilical or at Palmer point if the uterus is very large or if the patient has had prior abdominal surgery. Various accessory port configurations can be used for laparoscopic myomectomy, depending primarily on surgeon's preference as well as the planned suturing and tissue extraction techniques. Generally, a 10 mm port versus a SILs port (for later tissue extraction) is placed at the umbilicus, followed by left and right lower quadrant ports superior

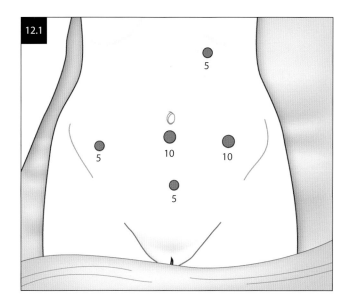

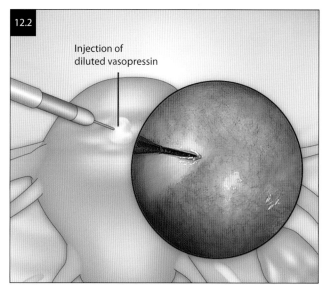

Injection of diluted vasopressin

and lateral, taking care to avoid the inferior epigastric vessels (Figure 12.1). A suprapubic port may be placed for later suturing or to pass a myoma screw or tenaculum for aiding with visualization and retraction.

TECHNIQUE

After peritoneal entry, a careful survey of the abdomino-pelvic organs is performed. In patients who are undergoing myomectomy for infertility, the pelvis is inspected for evidence of endometriosis or stigmate of pelvic inflammatory disease, the ovaries are visualized, the fallopian tubes are inspected for adhesions, and chromotubation is performed to assess tubal patency.

First, a 20-gauge spinal needle or a laparoscopic needle with a syringe attached is introduced and dilute vasopressin is injected into the myometrium overlying the myoma (Figure 12.2). A dilution of 20 units vasopressin in 100–200 mL normal saline is used. This practice decreases blood loss and provides hydrodissection, which allows easier dissection. If vasopressin is not available, or is contraindicated based upon patient comorbidities, bilateral uterine artery clipping using vascular clips can be performed to decrease surgical blood loss (Figure 12.3). These clips can be removed at the end of the procedure.

Next, using a monopolar hook or ultrasound energy, the myometrium overlying the fibroid is incised (Figure 12.4). The length and axis of the incision depend on the location and size of the fibroid. Suturing a horizontal incision may be easier than suturing a vertical incision; however, a vertical incision may be necessary to avoid injury to the fallopian tube or the uterine vessels. If possible, an incision should be made that will allow for removal of multiple fibroids, thereby decreasing the number of cuts on the uterus and later adhesion formation. The incision is then extended deeply until the myoma is visualized. The myoma is then grasped with a laparoscopic tenaculum or myoma screw, and the myometrium surrounding it is placed on countertraction to facilitate enucleation

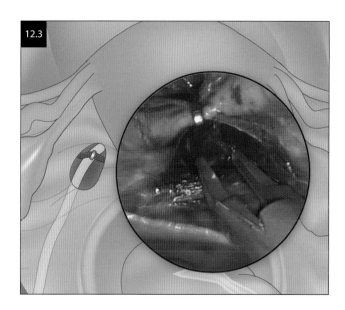

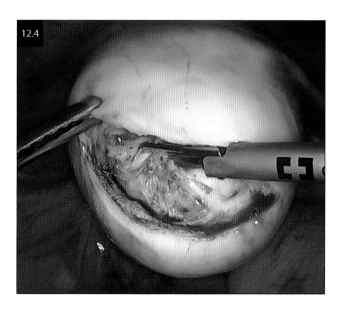

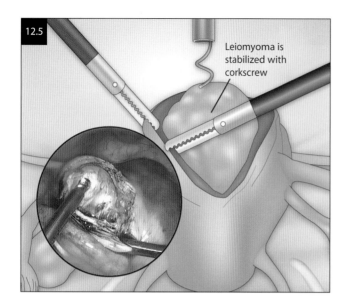

Leiomyoma is stabilized with corkscrew

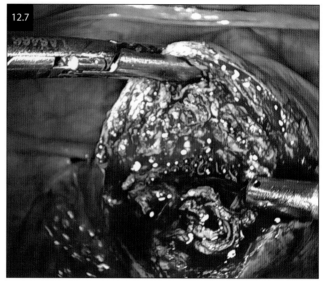

(Figure 12.5). Placing the tenaculum or myoma screw through the left upper quadrant trocar may provide better traction than using the lateral ports. A combination of blunt and monopolar/ultrasonic dissection is used until the myoma is completely separated (Figure 12.6). Care is taken to avoid entry into the endometrial cavity; evaluation of its integrity can be assessed with chromotubation with blue dye (Figure 12.7).

CLOSURE

Before beginning closure of the defect, hemostasis should be assured. If the endometrium was entered, the defect can be repaired with single or interrupted sutures of 3–0 or 4–0 Monocryl on an SH needle. Intracorporeal knot tying is preferred given the delicate nature of this repair (Figure 12.8). Additionally, effort is taken to skim the endometrium, avoiding placing exposed suture in the cavity, which may contribute to subsequent intrauterine adhesive disease.

Next, the myometrium is reapproximated with one or two layers of continuous running suture. Various suture materials may be used, including 0-vicryl on a CT1 needle or barbed suture such as VLoc or Stratafix. We commonly use barbed suture for this closure as the barbs help maintain consistent tension and eliminate the need for knot tying, increasing efficiency (Figure 12.9).

After the myometrium is reapproximated and hemostatic, the serosa is closed. 3–0 Monocryl suture on a CT1 needle is generally used, and this layer is closed in a continuous, running fashion versus the "in-to-out" baseball stitch technique (Figure 12.10). Once the serosa is closed, final inspection for hemostasis is performed. Any areas with persistent bleeding are managed using either bipolar energy or by placing additional figure-of-8 sutures. The pelvis is irrigated, and when no further bleeding is noted, an adhesion barrier, such as Interceed, may be placed over the suture line to decrease adhesion formation (Figure 12.11).

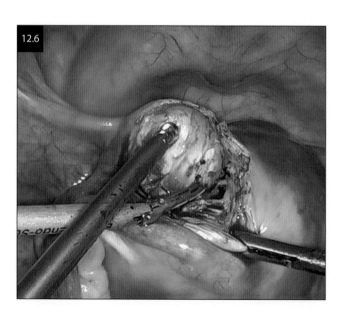

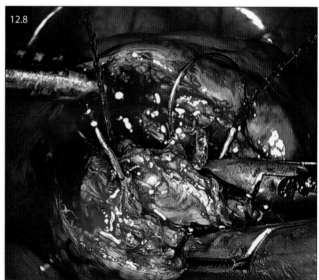

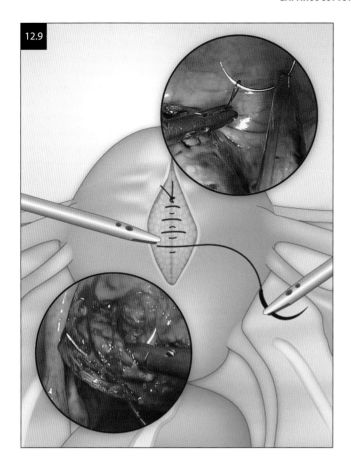

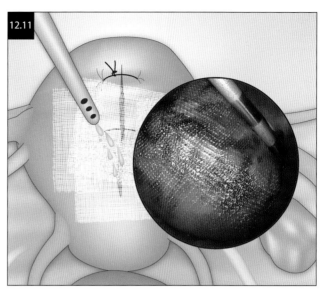

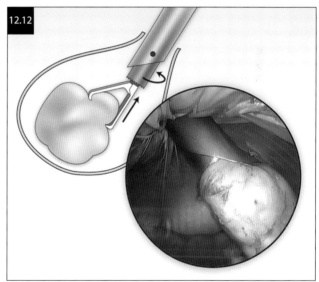

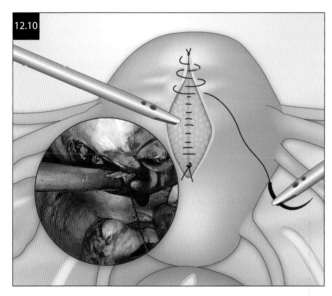

TISSUE REMOVAL

Once the uterine defect is closed and hemostasis is attained, the myoma(s) must be removed from the peritoneal cavity. Again, options for tissue removal that minimizes theoretical spread of microscopic tissue fragments include the following: (1) contained power morcellation using a laparoscopic specimen bag (Figure 12.12); (2) creation of a mini-laparotomy incision suprapubically or using a SILs port—both allow insertion of a bag, manipulation of the tissue into the bag, and then sharp morcellation with

the scalpel (Figure 12.13); and (3) creation of a posterior colpotomy so that the tumor can be removed/morcellated vaginally. Regardless of the tissue removal technique, the peritoneal cavity must be thoroughly inspected to ensure that no residual fragments of myoma remain. Please refer to Chapter 14 on tissue extraction techniques.

LAPAROSCOPICALLY ASSISTED MYOMECTOMY

Laparoscopically assisted myomectomy (LAM) is a safe alternative to laparoscopic myomectomy and is less difficult and less time consuming. The general criteria for LAM are as follows: myoma greater than 8 cm; multiple fibroids requiring extensive morcellation; and deep, large, intramural or transmural fibroids requiring uterine repair in multiple layers. Using a combination of laparoscopy and a 3–5 cm abdominal incision may enable more gynecologists to apply this technique (Figure 12.14). This technique may decrease the time required

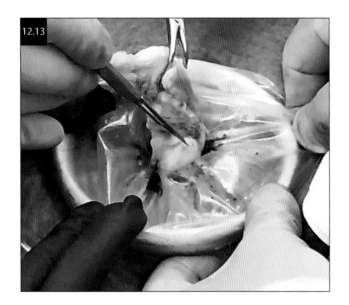

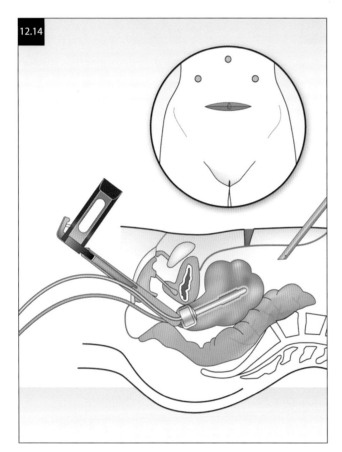

for enucleation of the fibroid and closure of the myometrial defect. A conventional suturing technique is used to suture the uterus in two or three layers, thereby reducing the chances of uterine dehiscence and adhesions.

The three major objectives of LAM are as follows:

1. Reduction of blood loss by quicker enucleation of the fibroid
2. Maintenance of myometrial integrity by applying conventional suturing technique
3. Quicker morcellation and removal of the fibroid

LAM reduces the duration of the operation and the need for extensive laparoscopic experience when performed with morcellation and conventional suturing.

LAM TECHNIQUE

Laparoscopy is performed, and laparoscopic ports are placed. The most prominent myoma is liberally injected at the base with dilute vasopressin solution. A laparoscopic incision is made over the uterine serosa and then into the surface of the fibroid. The incision is extended until the capsule is reached. A corkscrew manipulator or tenaculum is used to grasp the leiomyoma and to move the uterus toward the midline suprapubic trocar site in order to enlarge it to a 4 cm transverse skin incision. Once the incision of the fascia is made transversely, the rectus muscle is divided using a monopolar electrode. This typically provides excellent access to the abdominal cavity (Figure 12.15). The peritoneum is entered transversely, and the leiomyoma is observed. Using the corkscrew manipulator, the leiomyoma is then brought to the mini-laparotomy incision. The corkscrew manipulator is replaced by two Lahey Tenacula, and the tumor is extracorporeally shelled and then morcellated (Figure 12.16). If uterine size allows, the uterus is exteriorized to complete the repair. As many leiomyomas as possible should ideally be removed through one uterine incision. When other leiomyomas are present and cannot be removed through the initial uterine incision, the abdominal opening is approximated with two or three Allis clamps or an inflated latex glove. The remaining leiomyomas are then removed in the same manner under laparoscopic control. The uterus is then exteriorized again through the abdominal incision and the myometrium is closed in layers using 2-0 and 0 polydioxanone sutures (Figure 12.17). The uterus is palpated to ensure that no small intramural leiomyomas remain, and it is returned to the peritoneal cavity. The fascia is closed with number 0 polyglactin suture, and the skin is closed in a subcuticular manner.

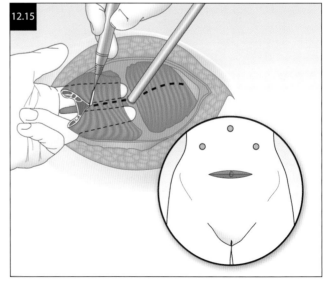

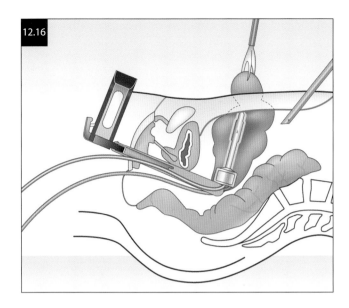

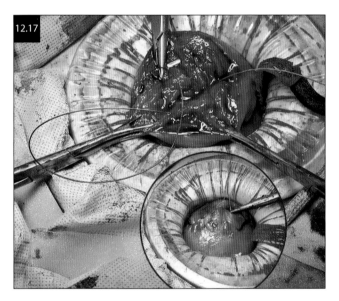

The laparoscope is then used to evaluate for complete hemostasis, and the pelvis is observed to detect and treat any pathology that may have previously been obscured by myomas. Copious irrigation is used, blood clots are removed, and Interceed may be applied over the uterus to help prevent adhesions.

POSTOPERATIVE CONSIDERATIONS

Depending on the extent of the surgery and the patient's medical comorbidities, she may be discharged home from the postanesthesia care unit or kept for observation overnight. Our practice is to admit these patients for 23 hour observation. This allows us to assess postoperative hemoglobin, to monitor pain control, and to ensure immediate postoperative milestones are met. Combination pain control with nonsteroidal anti-inflammatory drugs and oral narcotics along with ice packs to the abdomen seem to improve patient pain scores and satisfaction.

Patients are seen for follow-up in the office at 2 weeks and 6 weeks postoperatively. Attempts at pregnancy should be deferred for at least 3 months after laparoscopic myomectomy.

SUGGESTED READING

American College of Obstetricians and Gynecologists. ACOG practice bulletin. Alternatives to hysterectomy in the management of leiomyomas. *Obstet Gynecol* 2008;112(2 Pt 1):387.

Buttram VC, Reiter RC. Uterine leiomyomata: Etiology, symptomatology, and management. *Fertil Steril* 1981;36:433.

Donnez J, Dolmans M-M. Uterine fibroid management: From the present to the future. *Hum Reprod Update* 2016;22(6):665–86.

Donnez J, Tatarchuk TF, Bouchard P et al. Ulipristal acetate versus placebo for fibroid treatment before surgery. *N Engl J Med* 2012;366(5):409–20.

Freidman AJ, Rein NS, Harrison-Atlas D et al. A randomized, placebo-controlled, double blind study evaluating leuprolide acetate depot treatment before myomectomy. *Fertil Steril* 1989;52:728.

Goldberg J, Pereira L, Berghella V, Diamond J, Darai E, Seinera P, Seracchioli R. Pregnancy outcomes after treatment for fibromyomata: Uterine artery embolization verses laparoscopic myomectomy. *Am J Obstet Gynecol* 2004;191:18–21.

Hald K, Langbrekke A, Klow NE, Noreng HJ, Berge AB, Istre O. Laparoscopic occlusion of uterine vessels for the treatment of symptomatic fibroids: Initial experience and comparison to uterine artery embolization. *Am J Obstet Gynecol* 2004;190:37–43.

Nezhat C, Nezhat F, Bess O, Nezhat CH, Mashiach R. Laparoscopically assisted myomectomy: A report of a new technique in 57 cases. *Int J Fertil Menopausal Stud* 1994;39(1):39–44.

Pron G, Mocrski E, Bennet J et al. Pregnancy after uterine embolization for leiomyomata: The Ontario multicenter trial. *Obstet Gynecol* 2005;105:67–76.

Vilos GA, Allaire C, Laberge P-Y et al. The management of uterine leiomyomas. *J Obstet Gynaecol Can* 2015;37(2):157–78.

Chapter 13

NONSURGICAL OPTIONS FOR TREATMENT OF UTERINE FIBROIDS

David J. Levine

To date, the most common treatments for uterine fibroids are myomectomy and uterine artery embolization for women who are interested in uterine preservation, and may have failed more conservative therapy.

Myomectomy is performed traditionally through a relatively large abdominal incision but in selected cases can be performed laparoscopically by a physician with advanced laparoscopic skill. In either case, the fibroids are removed by incisions made through the uterine wall, which are then methodically closed by suturing in a layered fashion. Unless very superficial in depth, myomectomy potentially weakens the integrity of the gravid uterine wall, which may have significant implications for the conduct of subsequent pregnancies. However, at this moment, myomectomy is the only treatment approved by the U.S. Food and Drug Administration (FDA) for uterine fibroids in women who are interested in future pregnancy.

UTERINE ARTERY EMBOLIZATION

Uterine artery embolization (UAE) is performed by an interventional radiologist placing polyvinyl alcohol particles (355–500 mm) into the uterine vasculature, with its endpoint being occlusion of the perifibroid plexus (Figures 13.1 and 13.2). Most patients experience moderate to severe pain from ischemia. This ischemic pain may last for up to 24 hours and frequently requires parenteral narcotic analgesia. Recovery is usually 4–5 days with intermittent cramping and constitutional (flu-like) symptoms. Long-term studies with follow-up of 3–6 years reveal a treatment failure and subsequent invasive treatment rate of 13%–28%. The significant failure rate, based on return of symptoms such as heavy menstrual bleeding and pelvic pressure, is multifactorial, including the appearance and growth of new myomas, incompletely infarcted myomas, and concurrent adenomyosis.

The effect of UAE on ovarian function based on follicle-stimulating hormone (FSH) as a determinate of ovarian failure appears to be age related and is more apt to occur after age 45. Critical loss of the follicular cohort is presumably caused by misembolization of the occlusive particles into the ovarian circulation.

ACESSA PROCEDURE

The Acessa procedure is a novel system that performs laparoscopic, ultrasound-guided, volumetric thermal ablation of uterine fibroids using radiofrequency energy. The procedure has the capability to treat all visible fibroids regardless of location or size. It is typically performed on an outpatient basis, promising rapid return to normal activity. Its capacity to thermally spare the surrounding myometrium, isolate the fibroids for specific treatment, and minimize postoperative adhesion formation differentiates it from previous coagulation treatments that employed a bipolar needle or fiber laser under laparoscopic guidance.

PATIENT SELECTION

The ideal patient has a history of symptomatic uterine fibroids that have never been treated surgically. She has become progressively symptomatic from pelvic pressure or pain and/or heavy menstrual bleeding. Moreover, she has affirmed her strong interest to conserve her uterus and ameliorate her symptoms while accepting that in all likelihood they will not be eliminated completely. Preoperative evaluation typically includes an endometrial biopsy for irregular or heavy menstrual bleeding, and uterine imaging using either pelvic ultrasound or magnetic resonance imaging (MRI) to determine the size, location, and number of fibroids to be treated. The ultimate treatment plan will be determined while mapping the uterus with intraabdominal ultrasound at the time of surgery.

OPERATING ROOM PREPARATION

The basic laparoscopic equipment including an insufflator, light source, and camera are arranged in the usual fashion. However, an ultrasound monitor is placed adjacent to the laparoscopic screen. Both screens are typically situated at the patient's feet so that the surgeon and assistant have an unimpeded and comfortable view of both images.

PROCEDURE

General endotracheal anesthesia is administered; the patient is intubated, and an orogastric tube is placed. A forced air-warming blanket (Bair hugger) is not utilized

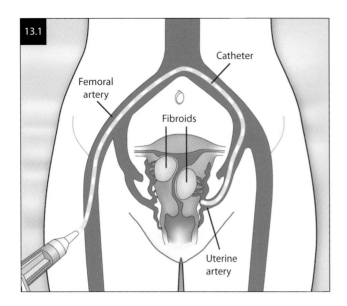

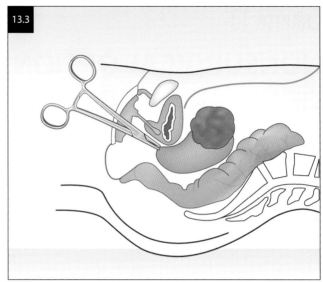

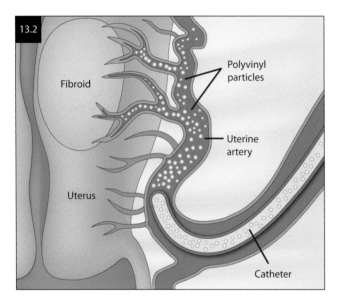

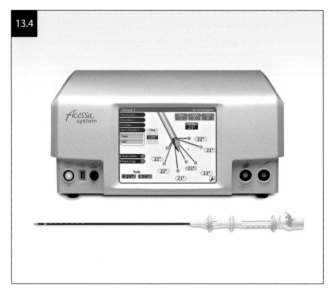

because it may cause the patient to sweat and interfere with the specially designed return electrodes. Before the patient is prepped, all lotion is removed from the skin superior to the patellas using rubbing alcohol. The return electrode pads are placed symmetrically just above both patellas. The patient is frog legged, and a Foley catheter is inserted into the bladder. Next, a single-tooth tenaculum is placed on the cervix at 12 and 6 o'clock, respectively (Figure 13.3). This will be utilized to anteflex and retroflex the uterus. A uterine manipulator is not used because it will distort the ultrasound image, and a metal manipulator may conduct heat and damage the endometrial cavity. The patient is then adequately draped, and all laparoscopic cables and instruments are arranged in their routine positions. The return electrode cables are attached to the Acessa generator, and the intraabdominal ultrasound transducer is attached for use (Figures 13.4 and 13.5).

Abdominal entry is entirely dependent on the surgeon's preference; however, with a large fibroid uterus, a supraumbilical laparoscopic port may be necessary to maintain adequate visualization. This may be facilitated by first using a left upper quadrant entry using a 3 or 5 mm scope, which allows the surgeon to simultaneously evaluate placement of the midline camera port (superior) and the midline fundal port (inferior). The midline fundal port must be 10 mm to accommodate the ultrasound wand, and its fundal location is necessary for adequate scanning and retraction (Figure 13.6).

MAPPING THE UTERUS AND FORMULATING A TREATMENT PLAN

Uterine mapping is performed to evaluate the uterus from all planes. It is wise to use a consistent mapping technique, so that all fibroids are identified. The intraabdominal ultrasound images are always oriented so that the surface of the uterus being scanned is at the top of the screen (Figures 13.7 and 13.8). As an example, starting from the patient's right, serially scan with the ultrasound from the fundus to the cervix, identifying all

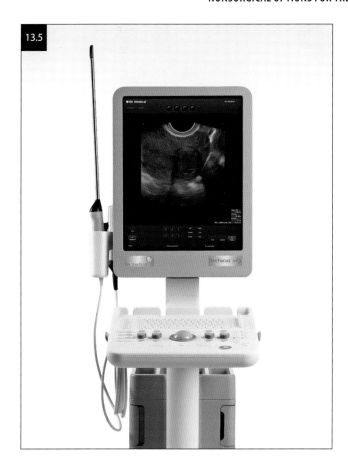

13.5

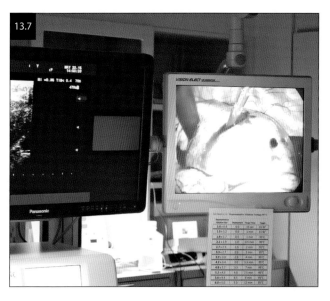

13.7

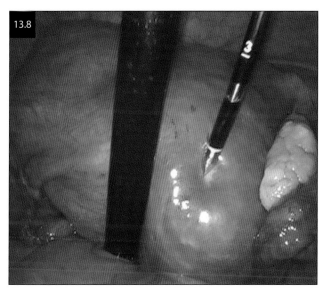

13.8

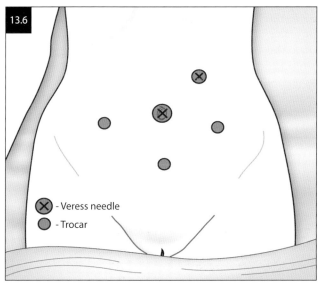

13.6

$\bigotimes$ - Veress needle

$\bullet$ - Trocar

fibroids are not round but rather oblong, which risks that a single treatment in the center of the fibroid will not suffice. Larger fibroids 6–8 cm will require multiple smaller treatments. These may cross one another or be arranged in quadrants to treat the entire volume of the fibroid.

TREATMENT

The treatment is usually begun with the most fundal or easily visualized fibroid. Based on the size of the fibroid, one or multiple locations are visualized on the fibroid for placement of the Acessa handpiece. The uterus is stabilized with the ultrasound probe, and a location 1–2 cm from the ultrasound port is chosen for introduction of the handpiece into the abdomen. A 2 mm puncture is made, and by rotating the handpiece it can be slowly introduced under direct vision into the abdominal cavity (Figure 13.9). If the fibroid can be treated with a single puncture (usually 3–4 cm at most), the ideal placement

fibroids. This procedure is then repeated on the patient's left. Next, identify the endometrial stripe. Fibroids that are intramural and lie adjacent to the cavity need to be identified. These may be responsible for excessive menstrual bleeding; thus, their identification is of extreme importance. It is imperative to formulate a treatment plan prior to deploying any radiofrequency energy. Once treatment has been started, the effect of heating may confuse the orientation of the fibroids. It is also helpful to measure all the fibroids in two planes. Most

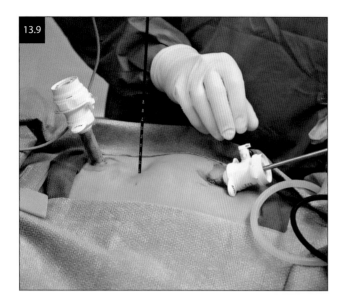

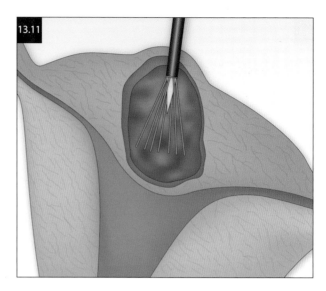

would be directly in the center of the fibroid. This can be accomplished by visualizing the midline of the fibroid sonographically from a sagittal and transverse view. Once midline is confirmed, a spot is chosen on the serosa which corresponds to the sonographic midline, and the sharp handpiece is slowly rotated into the fibroid until it is 1 cm through the capsule of the fibroid (Figure 13.10). To confirm the location of the tip of the handpiece, transverse and sagittal views are repeated. If the handpiece is found to be in the midline, the array is deployed (Figure 13.11). To deploy the array, maintain downward pressure while simultaneously sliding down the handpiece ring. If both of these maneuvers are not simultaneously performed, the arms will not be deployed adequately, and treatment will fail. In the event of deployment failure, simply retract the array and repeat the procedure using the proper technique. The tips of the array should be 1 cm from the periphery of the capsule, as confirmed by ultrasound (Figure 13.12). If the deployment was too deep or too shallow, it can be easily

adjusted. However, care should be taken to fully retract the array prior to adjusting the depth, as failing to do so will damage the handpiece, making it unusable. The handpiece displays the length of array deployment, and in accordance with the treatment chart, a time for treatment will be determined (Figure 13.13).

It is not unusual to have a dense fibroid that prevents adequate opening of the array. It this case, it is acceptable to treat the accessible area of the fibroid (usually 1–1 1/2 cm), which will soften the fibroid. Once softened, the fibroid will allow the array to open freely, and a greater area can then be treated in the usual manner. Once the treatment of the fibroid is complete, the array is retracted and the coagulation setting is selected on the generator. The handpiece is then slowly removed while coagulating the tissue to prevent any bleeding. The above procedure is repeated until all of the fibroids have been treated. In fact, there is no limit to the size or depth of a fibroid that may be treated. Nevertheless, treating a pedunculated or type O submucosal fibroid should be avoided. When a fibroid is not round but rather oblong,

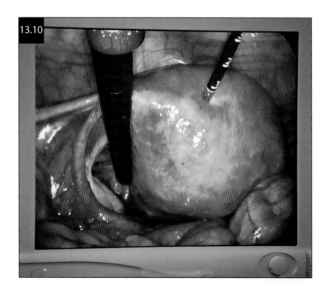

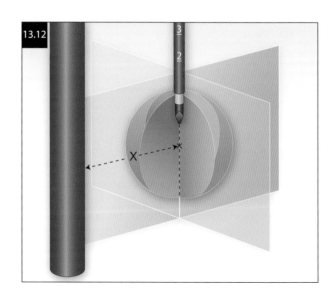

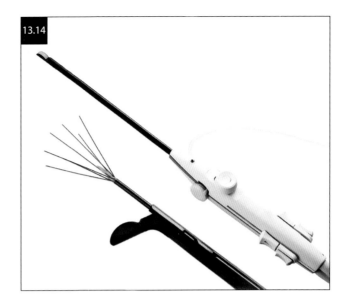

13.13

Representative ablation settings

Ablation (cm)	Deployment	Time	Power
1.0 × 0.8	—	15 sec	15 W
1.5 × 1.2	—	1 min	15 W
1.9 × 1.7	0.5	1 min	95°C
2.1 × 1.9	1.0	30 sec	95°C
2.7 × 2.3	1.5	2 min	95°C
3.3 × 2.7	2.0	3 min	95°C
3.9 × 3.0	2.5	4 min	95°C
4.2 × 3.4	3.0	5.5 min	95°C
4.8 × 3.7	3.5	7 min	95°C
5.2 × 4.3	4.0	7.5 min	95°C
5.6 × 4.4	4.5	8 min	95°C
6.0 × 5.0	5.0	12 min	95°C

13.14

multiple treatments through multiple sites with multiple punctures are frequently necessary. Larger fibroids may require an overlapping technique to access the entire circumference of the fibroid. Retreating the same area is permissible and of no clinical consequence. The most challenging fibroids are deeply set in the myometrium and lie next to the endometrial cavity. To access deeper fibroids, it is best to start by measuring the distance from the serosa to the fibroid using the ultrasound. Taking care to stabilize the uterus with the ultrasound probe, insert the handpiece slowly. Using the ultrasound, monitor the course of the handpiece every few centimeters to ensure it is following the projected course. Once the predetermined depth has been reached, and ultrasound confirms that the handpiece is at the desired location within the fibroid, the array may be deployed in the usual manner.

Once all of the fibroids have been treated, the surgeon should rescan the uterus to confirm a complete treatment. A suction irrigator can now be used to lavage the uterine surface and identify any bleeding sites. The trocar sites are then closed in the usual manner, and the patient can return home once the usual discharge criteria after laparoscopic surgery are realized.

The Acessa procedure provides a number of realized and potential benefits. The 36-month data showed a significant decrease in symptoms related to fibroid bulk and a 45% decrease in menstrual bleeding. From a patient's perspective, it is a minimally invasive outpatient procedure with an average recovery of 2–3 days. Gynecologists can adapt their existing surgical skills to perform the procedure. Moreover, the structural integrity of the uterus is not compromised, providing safety for women interested in future conception. This may allow women to deliver vaginally instead of by cesarean section. One of the major benefits of this technology is the utilization of an intraabdominal ultrasound probe to target and treat uterine fibroids. Postclinical trial data demonstrated a 50% increase in the number of fibroids

identified using intraabdominal ultrasound as compared to preoperative transvaginal ultrasound or MRI, promising more complete treatment than either myomectomy or UAE.

Utilizing similar radiofrequency (RF)-based technology, VizAblate is a nonincisional transcervical approach to the treatment of fibroids (Figure 13.14). The technology utilizes real-time intrauterine ultrasound in combination with an RF energy probe. The treatment device is deployed directly through the ultrasound handle making it easier for the operator to control the application of the treatment probe. Once the fibroid has been identified via ultrasound, the probe is deployed directly into the fibroid, and the treatment is monitored using a graphic interface that automates treatment parameters (Figure 13.15). The software is designed to control the depth and extent of treatment, avoiding myometrium and serosa. In October 2014 the FDA granted the technology an Investigational Device Exemption (IDE), which allowed it to begin a pivotal trial to demonstrate its efficacy and safety.

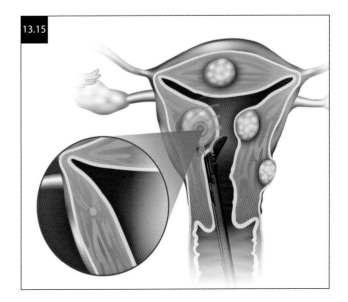

13.15

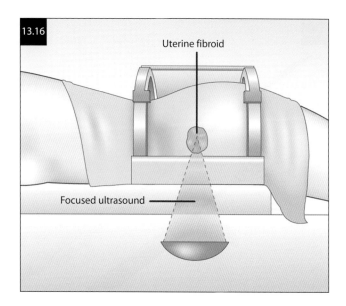

13.16

Uterine fibroid

Focused ultrasound

MAGNETIC RESONANCE IMAGING–FOCUSED ULTRASOUND THERAPY

This treatment utilizes high dosages of focused ultrasound waves (high-intensity focused ultrasound [HIFU]) to destroy uterine fibroids while sparing the surrounding myometrium. The procedure is conducted under the guidance of magnetic resonance (MRI). A small volume of fibroid is heated to 85°C, causing coagulative necrosis (Figure 13.16).

The treatment of each fibroid involves creating a grid from which the treatment is designed and followed. The average length of treatment is 3 hours, and the patient must remain still during that time. Though totally noninvasive, patient selection is limited to those women who have fibroids along the anterior abdominal wall. There can be no intervening bowel or previous scars to interfere with the ultrasound beam. Though of growing popularity abroad, this technology has yet to receive widespread use in the United States.

SUGGESTED READING

Berman JM, Guido RS, Garza Leal JG et al. Three-year outcome of the Halt trial: A prospective analysis of radiofrequency volumetric thermal ablation of myomas. *J Minim Invasive Gynecol*. 2014;21(5):767–774. PMID 24613404.

Brolmann H, Bongers M, Garza-Leal JG et al. The FAST-EU trial: 12 month clinical outcomes of women after intrauterine sonography-guided transcervical radiofrequency ablation of uterine fibroids. *Gynecol Surg*. 2016;13:27–35.

Brucker SY, Hahn M, Kraemer D et al. Laparoscopic radiofrequency volumetric thermal ablation of fibroids versus laparoscopic myomectomy. *lnt J Gynaecol Obstet*. 2014;125(3):261–265. PMID 24698202.

Chudnoff SG, Berman JM, Levine DJ et al. Outpatient procedure for the treatment and relief of symptomatic uterine myomas. *Obstet Gynecol*. 2013;121(5):1075–1082. PMID 23635746.

CHAPTER 14

TISSUE RETRIEVAL IN LAPAROSCOPIC SURGERY

Linda Shiber and Resad Paya Pasic

Uneventful access into the peritoneal cavity without the use of a significant laparotomy is the raison d'être for laparoscopic surgery. Minimally invasive techniques have now been adopted by all areas of surgery, and continued advancements have reached levels thought unimaginable even a decade ago. Yet, the advantage of a skillfully performed laparoscopic procedure is greatly diminished if the surgery culminates in a large incision created for the removal of an extirpated organ or tissue. This tactical challenge led one of the first pioneers of laparoscopic surgery to declare that the creation of effective, minimally invasive techniques for laparoscopic tissue retrieval is the "Holy Grail" of the discipline. Such techniques must be intrinsically safe and both time and cost efficient if they are to enhance the inherent benefits of laparoscopic surgery.

CLASSICAL TECHNIQUES

Prior to the introduction of specialized instrumentation, laparoscopic tissue retrieval was limited to simple techniques derived from open surgery. Benign specimens up to 8 mm in diameter, such as an oviduct, can be directly retrieved up through lateral 5 mm incisions. The tissue is drawn up into the cannula using gentle rotation while opening the flapper valve as the specimen is removed. For specimens too broad to fit entirely into the sleeve, the tissue is grasped at its narrowest aspect and drawn partially into the port. Provided there is no infection or possible malignancy, the cannula, grasping instrument, and specimen can be withdrawn from the abdominal cavity all together in one smooth motion (Figure 14.1). To help replace the trocar, a blunt probe can be placed into the peritoneal cavity via the trocar tract to act as a guidepost as the cannula is then advanced in place over it.

For slightly larger specimens such as postmenopausal ovaries without malignant features, decompressed adnexal cysts, or the appendix, a 10–12 mm umbilical cannula is often adequate for tissue removal. Removal of larger and firmer masses may be facilitated by using a 10 mm spoon or claw forceps for their tenacity. Grasping forceps may be placed through an operative laparoscope and the specimen extracted under direct vision by drawing the laparoscope along with the grasped specimen up through the sleeve. This method is well suited to the appendix, as it minimizes the likelihood of wound contamination. Alternatively, the instrument with the specimen may simply be removed together with the sleeve in

a manner similar to that described above using a 5 mm sleeve. If the surgeon is not using an operative (10 mm) laparoscope, a 5 mm laparoscope may be introduced through one of the lateral ports and the tissue recovered with a grasping forcep under direct vision using either of the above techniques. It is important to grasp and hold onto the specimen while changing to a 5 mm laparoscope in order to avoid losing it within the upper abdomen.

The removal of larger specimens such as benign, premenopausal ovaries, small myomas, or the gallbladder often requires enlargement of the umbilical incision. This can be accomplished using a classical open Hasson technique but may be technically difficult and require an exaggerated skin incision in order to approach the rectus fascia in obese patients. Reich described a technique that greatly facilitates extension of the fascial incision in these cases by using laparoscopic scissors passed through an operative laparoscope (Figure 14.2). The peritoneum and fascia are clearly visualized under laparoscopic magnification and opened with laparoscopic scissors. The specimen is then removed through this incision using a grasper as described above, and the fascia is reapproximated in the traditional fashion using permanent or delayed absorbable suture. Extension of the fascial incision may be avoided by use of a 10 mm laparoscopic scissor placed through a 10 mm sleeve. Laparoscopic graspers are used to stabilize the specimen while manually morcellating it into pieces small enough to be recovered via the 10 mm port sleeve (Figure 14.3). This is done under direct vision with a 5 mm laparoscope placed through the other 5 mm port, and this works well for smaller myomas. Alternatively, the surgeon can perform manual morcellation by using a laparoscopic scalpel manufactured by Storz that fits through a 10 mm port (Figure 14.4). The specimen is then securely held safely distant from the vital structures of the pelvic sidewall, and cut into small pieces for retrieval. In experienced hands, this technique works well for such specimens as small myomas, but it is time consuming and not without significant risk of penetrating injury to the bowel or major vessels.

Using a posterior colpotomy is another approach to facilitate specimen removal. This type of incision in the posterior vaginal fornix is well suited to the recovery of large ovaries, cysts, and myomas from the peritoneal cavity. The anatomic relationship of the rectum to the posterior vagina must be defined prior to performing

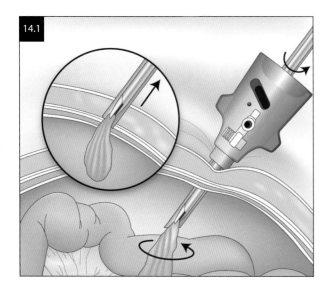

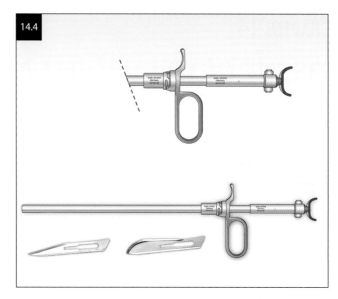

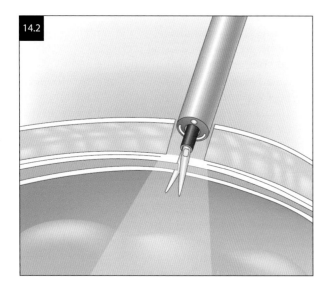

laparoscopic culdotomy. This is facilitated by placement of a uterine manipulator, and elevating the uterus anteriorly to expose the posterior cervicovaginal junction. A probe is placed into the rectum to provide additional assistance when difficulty is encountered opening a scarred posterior cul-de-sac. Once normal anatomy is established, the upper vagina is delineated with a moist sponge on a ring forceps or the bulb end of a rubber infant nasal suction (the suction tip cut off) with a ring forceps inside. Either of these implements will highlight the proper incision site slightly above and between the uterosacral ligaments, while maintaining pneumoperitoneum once the incision is made. A transverse culdotomy incision is then made laparoscopically using either a monopolar electrode tip set at 80–100 W of cutting current, with laser energy at a comparable power setting, or with ultrasonic energy (Figure 14.5). Laparoscopic grasping or traditional ring forceps may then be carefully passed through this incision into the pelvis and the specimen withdrawn vaginally under direct laparoscopic

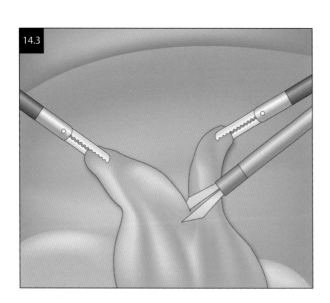

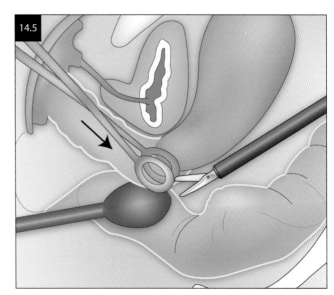

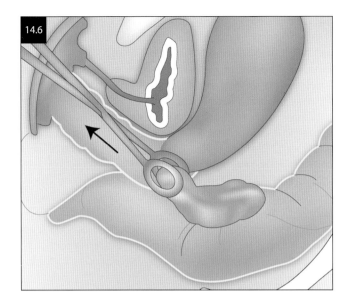

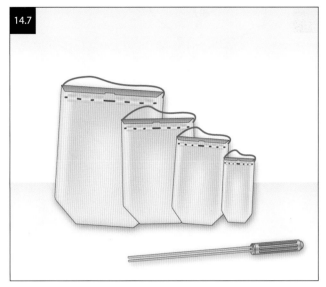

view (Figure 14.6). The culdotomy incision is then vaginally or laparoscopically sutured ligated. When using this technique, trauma to vital structures is avoided by direct laparoscopic vision and the maintenance of sufficient pneumoperitoneum with a moist vaginal sponge or the cut infant suction bulb described above. If the surgeon prefers, a 5 mm instrument can be used to deliver the specimen from above into the vagina where it may be grasped with the fingers and removed. In cases of tissue suspicious for malignancy, a specialized laparoscopic tissue retrieval bag (see next section) may, likewise, be passed into the vagina for specimen removal.

SPECIALIZED BAGS FOR LAPAROSCOPIC TISSUE RETRIEVAL

The need to collect the gallbladder during a laparoscopic cholecystectomy was the first impetus to innovate instrumentation for the safe and efficacious laparoscopic removal of larger tissues. "Bagging" the specimen with a sterile glove initially allowed for more traction with less fear of rupture and spillage while removing an enlarged specimen via a small incision. Today, the laparoscopic surgeon may choose from numerous products designed expressly for laparoscopic tissue retrieval.

Modern retrieval systems are of varying degrees of sophistication ranging from small plastic bags to large, self-opening pouches contained within an introducer sheath. These devices must be easy to see and maneuver within the abdomen, strong, and, most importantly, impermeable to infectious or malignant tissue.

Made by a variety of companies, the extraction bags can have a drawstring and are rolled tightly, customarily inserted into the abdomen via a 10–15 mm port, and then manipulated so tissue can be loaded and then securely contained. The drawstring is then exteriorized through the port, bringing the edges of the bag outside the skin incision so the specimen can then be extracted through the open mouth of the exteriorized bag. Although helpful

for larger volumes of tissue, these bags can be exceedingly difficult to manipulate in the pelvis. Efficiency and success rely on *in vitro* rehearsal, logistics, and teamwork.

Nylon bags are another option currently available for tissue removal. These consist of heavier sheets of nylon that are stitched or welded together. The seams are treated with a polyurethane coating to prevent leakage of tissue or fluid. The Lapsac (Cook Women's Health, Spencer, Indiana) is approved by the U.S. Food and Drug Administration (FDA) for tissue morcellation and comes in 50, 200, 750, and 1500 mL sizes (Figure 14.7). The sac is rolled and introduced through a 10–12 mm port by pushing it with a laparoscopic grasper placed through a 10–5 mm reducer. A specialized reusable Lapsac Introducer may be used as well. The larger sizes of this bag can be unwieldy to manipulate intraabdominally. Tabs at the top edges of the sac facilitate a triangular opening, and a polypropylene drawstring secures the specimen inside. A larger specimen may be easier to contain if the bag is first partially filled with irrigation fluid to stabilize its base and expand its lumen. Once the specimen is inside the sac, the drawstring is pulled with a grasper and brought out through a 10–15 mm port. The port is then withdrawn from the abdomen, and the bag edges are drawn up through the skin, bringing the specimen as near to the incision as possible. The specimen can then be recovered using firm, gentle, traction. Large cystic masses can be decompressed within the bag using a suction device prior to retrieval. Larger solid masses can be carefully morcellated manually using either crushing forceps or scalpel (Figure 14.8). Enlargement of the umbilical incision or a small low transverse abdominal incision or minilaparotomy may be required to safely recover the specimen. Direct laparoscopic observation via the umbilicus or via a laterally placed 5 mm laparoscope facilitates difficult retrievals and helps minimize the risk of bag rupture.

Derived from technology used to make hot air balloons, Espiner E-Sacs (Espiner Medical Products,

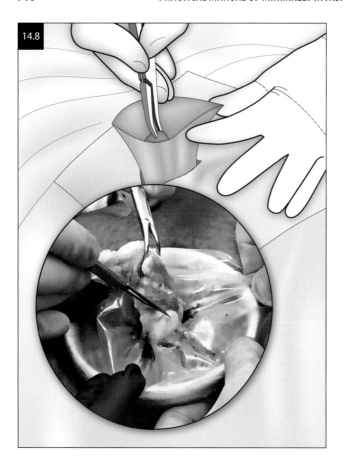

and incorporates a nitinol wire into the mouth of the sac. This wire serves both to hold open the mouth of the sac and to draw it closed for tissue capture. For improved handling, the Master E-Sac (150–2000 mL) uses an introducer rod to deploy and control the sac and to close it securely around the specimen.

Improving on the difficulty often encountered by trying to manipulate a free-floating bag within the abdomen, "plunger-style" tissue retrieval systems were innovated by two manufacturers. These bags are self-opening and, thus, more stable for easy tissue deposition. Endo Catch Gold (Autosuture, Inc., Norwalk, Connecticut) consists of a disposable pouch of impermeable polyurethane 15 cm deep whose mouth is 6 cm in diameter. The 10 mm instrument is introduced into the abdomen and the plunger advanced to deploy the pouch. Once the specimen is inside, the pouch is cinched closed by pulling on the green ring, and the pouch is pulled slightly to free it completely from the introducer cannula. The introducer and port are then withdrawn and the string used to draw the bag edges up through the skin where the specimen can be recovered. For larger specimens, the Endo Catch II is 23 cm deep with a 12.5 cm opening and must be introduced via a 15 mm port. The Endopouch Retriever (Ethicon Endo-Surgery, Cincinnati, Ohio) is a similar self-opening system that employs an impermeable 224 mL polyurethane pouch. Like the Endo Catch products, it uses a plunger-type introducer via a 10–12 mm port. The Inzii retrieval system (Applied Medical, Rancho Santa Margarita, California) is a similar product with a self-opening, "plunger-style" design that comes in 5, 10, and 12/15 mm diameter (Figure 14.10).

The Alexis Contained Extraction System (Applied Medical) is a 17 cm in diameter polyurethane bag that is used in combination with gel point or gel point mini-ports. It is designed for manual morcellation of large specimens and features a large bag that comes with a plastic guard ring that protects the bag from sharp instrumentation.

Clevedon, United Kingdom) (Figure 14.9) are made using polyurethane-lined Nylon 66 fabric. Nylon 66 is notable for its lightness and strength. It handles well and is quite easily seen within the abdomen. The Standard E-Sac comes in various sizes, ranging from 60 to 900 mL, and is designed for deployment through 10–12 mm trocars. The addition of tabs on the mouth and bottom facilitate handling and opening. Like the Cook product above, it is introduced into the abdomen using a 5 mm instrument and the specimen recovered similarly. The Super E-Sac is similar to the Standard E-Sac but is larger (1050–3500 mL)

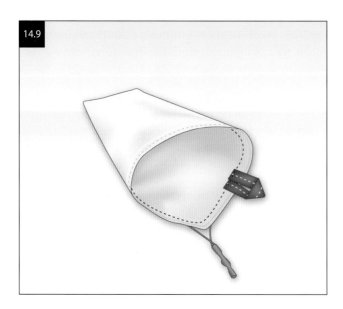

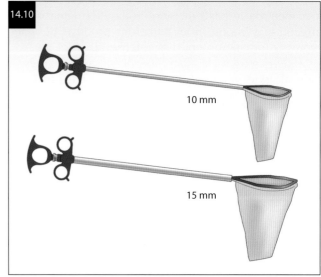

Both of these systems use bags of good tensile strength and provide added convenience in that they can be deployed for specimen recovery using one hand.

There are limited data comparing the handling characteristics, strength, and permeability of the systems described above. Surgeons should use clinical judgment and preference to select the product that will permit him or her to safely and most effectively recover specimens laparoscopically.

ELECTROMECHANICAL MORCELLATION

The expansion of minimally invasive surgery to include the extirpation of increasingly large organs created the need to render masses of solid tissue into smaller pieces for endoscopic retrieval. This was addressed with invention of the power morcellator. The first electromechanical morcellators became commercially available in 1995 after minimal "vetting" of their safety profiles and validation of safe techniques/guidelines for usage.

In 2014, after a well-publicized case of dissemination of occult leiomyosarcoma following electromechanical morcellation of a presumed benign fibroid uterus, the FDA issued a statement advising against usage of these devices for women with fibroid uteri.

Following the ensuing media and legal frenzy, national societies, including the American Congress of Obstetricians and Gynecologists (ACOG), AAGL, and the Society of Gynecologic Oncology (SGO), called for a balanced review of the literature. Innovation of techniques to improve the safety of these devices was encouraged rather than abandonment of the minimally invasive surgical techniques they facilitated.

Prior to and following this polarizing debate, it is important to recognize that the principles of safe electromechanical morcellation are the same and encompass three major points:

1. Ensure careful patient selection and thorough preoperative workup to eliminate the chance of morcellating a malignancy. This includes avoiding the use of this technology in older/postmenopausal women with enlarging masses or in those patients with other risk factors for malignancy.
2. Avoid serious injury due to lack of visualization, incorrect positioning of the device/blade, and uncontrolled tissue handling. Because morcellation involves the risk of potentially serious injury to vital structures of the abdomen and pelvis, safety is of the utmost importance. Most importantly, the morcellator must be visualized *at all times*. This is accomplished using a 5 mm laparoscope placed through either a lateral or a left upper quadrant (Palmer point) port while the morcellator is introduced through the umbilical port (Figure 14.11). The morcellator can also be introduced through the low lateral abdominal port while the 10 mm laparoscope with the camera is kept in the

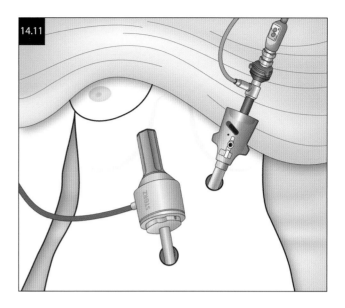

umbilical port (Figure 14.12). Morcellation should be performed within the pelvis and with the patient in the steep Trendelenburg position in order to provide the activated blade with the greatest possible clearance from surrounding structures. The 45° tip of the morcellator sheet helps feed the tissue into the morcellator shaft and allows for cutting longer tissue specimens. Finally, safe technique includes having an assistant use a laparoscopic grasper to draw the tissue into the morcellator and stabilize the specimen while the surgeon holds the activated instrument motionless and distant from the bowel and pelvic sidewalls (Figure 14.13). The activated morcellator should *never* be driven toward the tissue, as this creates the greatest risk of accidental injury. Ideally, the top portion of the circular blade should be in view to avoid coring the specimen. When the blade begins to dive into the tissue, the surgeon should adjust the angle of the blade and redirect its upper edge to the tissue

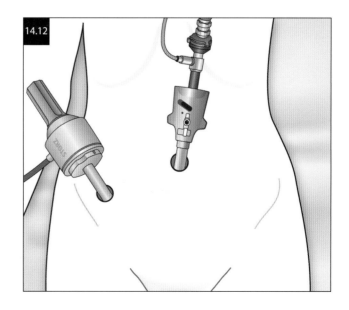

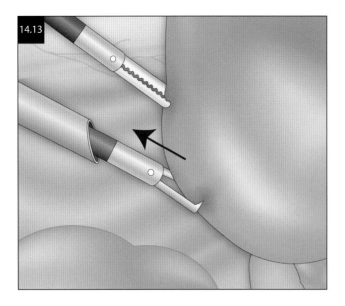

14.13

surface. The correct technique involves, "skinning" the specimen by removing strips of tissue from the outside edges (Figure 14.14) rather than creating a "Swiss cheese" effect that is unsafe and makes the specimen difficult to handle. Adherence to these principles is essential to safe and efficient tissue extraction.

3. Prevent dissemination of tissue throughout the abdomen, ensure retrieval of tissue, and evaluate containment.

More recently, much effort has been put toward designing systems that enable electromechanical morcellation in a contained fashion to prevent the inadvertent spread of tissue fragments within the peritoneal cavity, which can result in spread of both occult malignancy or benign conditions such as leiomyomatosis peritonei. These are discussed in detail in the following section.

SYSTEMS FOR TISSUE MORCELLATION

Multiple manufacturers have produced power morcellator devices, though in light of recent controversy, not all are currently available for purchase and use. All of these instruments incorporate a proprietary intrinsic or extrinsic motor drive unit that is used to power a rapidly rotating cylindrical blade. They differ in design characteristics and power but function in the same manner by cutting cylindrical strips of tissue.

The LiNA Xcise (Lina Medical, Norcross, Georgia) battery-powered, cordless laparoscopic morcellator is a 15 mm instrument that requires no port sleeve and employs a blunt plastic obturator for insertion into the abdomen (Figure 14.15). A blade guard covers the blade for abdominal entry and while the instrument is not in use. The operator may activate the unit in a simple on/off (all or none) fashion and may select to operate the blade in a clockwise or counterclockwise direction by means of a toggle switch on the external motor drive. A pneumoseal mechanism within the instrument maintains pneumoperitoneum while preventing the backsplash of tissue and blood while morcellating. The entire instrument is disposable.

The Rotocut G1 (Karl Storz GmbH & Co. KG, Tuttingen, Germany) represents the newest generation of morcellators (Figure 14.16). This instrument is notable for its power and versatility due to an internal hollow shaft motor unit that interchangeably accepts both 12 and 15 mm blades. It requires no port sleeve and is introduced into the abdomen using a blunt metal obturator. The instrument incorporates a metal sleeve whose tip is obliquely shaped and designed to facilitate the proper specimen "skinning" technique while protecting surrounding structures. The system is activated by means of a foot pedal and is unique in that an external microcontroller unit (Unidrive Gyn) allows the operator to vary the blade speed (not unlike the "gas pedal" of an automobile) for the efficient morcellation of tissues of different

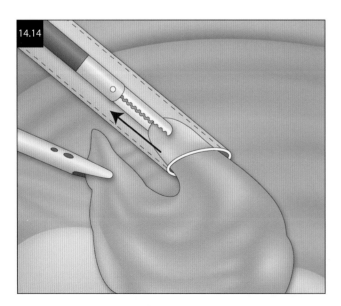

14.14

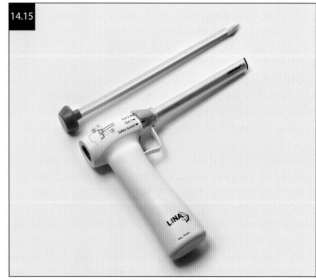

14.15

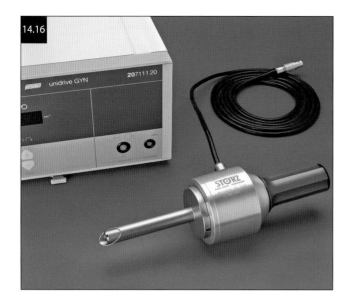

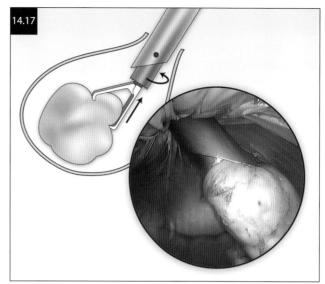

densities. The unit and its parts are fully autoclavable, and its blades are reusable.

For all of these units, blade sharpness is essential to efficient tissue cutting and directly related to the time needed to morcellate a large specimen. Therefore, it is important to ensure that the jaws of the tenaculum forceps are completely closed on the tissue when drawing it into the morcellator so that the activated blade is not damaged by contact with the metal instrument.

CONTAINED ELECTROMECHANICAL MORCELLATION

Techniques for performing electromechanical morcellation in a contained fashion to eliminate the spread of tissue fragments are being developed in an ongoing fashion. One technique involves inserting a large Lahey bag into the abdomen via a single-site laparoscopic port. The specimen is placed within the bag, the bag edges are exteriorized around the base of the access port, and then the bag is insufflated, conforming to the peritoneal cavity. The morcellator is then placed through the SILS port and in-bag morcellation performed (Figure 14.17).

A multiport technique has also been proposed in which the same procedure is performed to "bag" the specimen and insufflate the containment bag. The bag is then punctured with a lateral 5 mm port through which the laparoscope is placed. This risks contamination of the peritoneal cavity on extraction of the bag. Both techniques are challenging and can result in difficult visualization or destruction of the bag and retained plastic fragments; therefore, the importance of practicing these techniques prior to using them in a patient cannot be overstated.

Recently the FDA approved the PneumoLiner device (Advanced Surgical Concepts Ltd., Bray, Ireland, marketed by Olympus America). This is the first tissue containment system for use with certain laparoscopic

power morcellators to isolate the uterine tissue that is not suspected to contain cancer. The device consists of a containment bag and a tube-like plunger to deliver the device into the abdominal cavity where the tissue to be removed is placed into the bag and the bag is sealed and inflated. The morcellator and the laparoscope are placed through the same opening on the bag, requiring the use of a flexible 5 mm or 30° laparoscope (Figures 14.18 and 14.19). The FDA also requires that each physician attend the official training provided by Olympus in order to start using this containment device.

MINILAPAROTOMY CONTAINED TISSUE EXTRACTION

The addition of a SILS port to an infraumbilical, true minilaparotomy incision allows for improved visualization and more room to maneuver tissue with excellent cosmesis. Several companies are marketing new systems

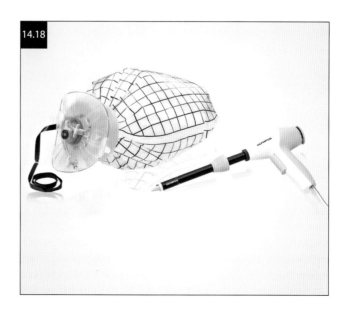

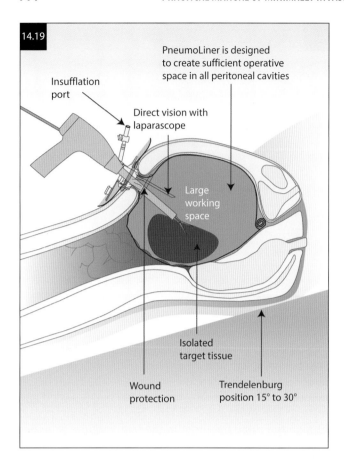

14.19

Insufflation port

Direct vision with laparoscope

PneumoLiner is designed to create sufficient operative space in all peritoneal cavities

Large working space

Isolated target tissue

Wound protection

Trendelenburg position 15° to 30°

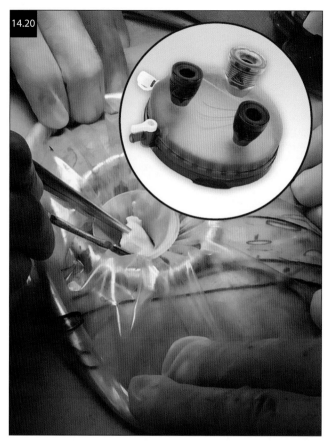

14.20

specifically for extraperitoneal contained manual morcellation; Applied Medical now offers a Gelpoint port (Figure 14.20) combined with Alexis Contained extractor bag that is inserted into the abdomen. The upper portion of the bag contains a flexible Alexis ring that is inserted in the abdomen and keeps the bag open for easier specimen placement. Once the specimen is placed into the bag, the Alexis ring is exteriorized, and a protective plastic collar is placed inside the bag to protect the bag and surrounding abdominal wall during manual morcellation (Figure 14.21). The specimen is then grasped with a tenaculum, and a continuous semi-circular cutting technique is employed to remove tissue in long strips.

NEWER VAGINAL TECHNIQUES

In addition to transabdominal tissue extraction, approaches to expediting vaginal tissue extraction and enhancing safety are being developed. A "coring" technique involves bringing the specimen into the vagina, using a scalpel to cut the central portion of the tissue, leaving serosa intact, and causing the specimen to collapse on itself. The "paper-roll" technique, tested in uteri >500 g, utilizes constant tension and rotation with counterclockwise incisions, removing the entire specimen in one continuous piece, making pathologic diagnosis easier. Finally, use of an Alexis retractor placed transvaginally has been described as helpful for aiding

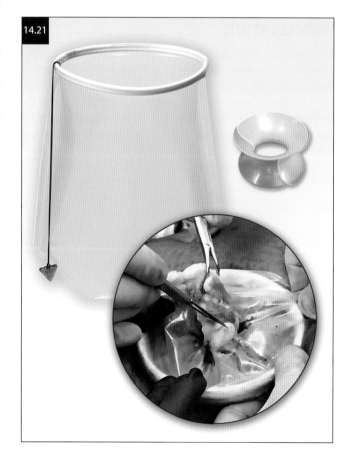

14.21

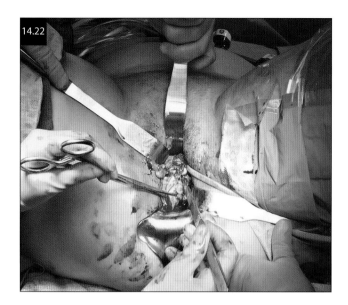

transvaginal tissue morcellation when the vaginal vault is narrow or relaxed. Transvaginal morcellation can be facilitated by using a long weighted speculum posteriorly, a curved Deaver placed anteriorly into the abdominal cavity, and right angle retractors placed into the lateral vaginal fornixes to achieve better exposure and to protect the vagina (Figure 14.22).

SUMMARY

Mastery of the different methods and systems for laparoscopic tissue retrieval is essential to the safe and successful practice of advanced laparoscopic surgery. Ongoing innovations in this integral part of minimally invasive surgery aim to optimize both patient safety and surgical efficiency. It is the surgeon's responsibility to stay abreast of these different products and techniques and employ those that consistently perform well in a variety of operative circumstances.

SUGGESTED READING

AAGL Advancing Minimally Invasive Gynecology Worldwide. AAGL practice report: Morcellation during uterine tissue extraction. *J Minim Invasive Gynecol.* 2014;21(4):517–530.

American College of Obstetricians and Gynecologists. May 2014. *Power Morcellation and Occult Malignancy in Gynecologic Surgery.* http://www.acog.org/Resources-And-Publications/Task-Force-and-Work-Group-Reports/Power-Morcellation-and-Occult-Malignancy-in-Gynecologic-Surgery. Accessed 9/20/2014.

Brown J. *AAGL Statement to the FDA on Power Morcellation.* American Association of Gynecologic Laparoscopists, 2014. http://www.aagl.org/aaglnews/aagl-statement-to-the-fda-on-power-morcellation/ Accessed 9/20/2014.

Cohen SL, Einarsson JI, Wang KC et al. Contained power morcellation within an insufflated isolation bag. *Obstet Gynecol.* 2014;124(3):491–497.

Cohen SL, Greenberg JA, Wang KC et al. Risk of leakage and tissue dissemination with various contained tissue extraction (CTE) techniques: An in vitro pilot study. *J Minim Invasive Gynecol.* 2014;21(5):935–939.

Ghezzi F, Cromi A, Uccella S, Bogani G, Serati M, Bolis P. Transumbilical versus transvaginal retrieval of surgical specimens at laparoscopy: A randomized trial. *Am J Obstet Gynecol.* 2012;207(2):112.e1–e6.

Kho KA, Anderson TL, Nezhat CH. Intracorporeal electromechanical tissue morcellation: A critical review and recommendations for clinical practice. *Obstet Gynecol.* 2014; 124(4): 787–793. doi:10.1097/AOG.0000000000000448.

Kho KA, Nezhat CH. Evaluating the risks of electric uterine morcellation. *JAMA.* 2014;311(9):905–906.

Kho KA, Shin JH, Nezhat C. Vaginal extraction of large uteri with the Alexis retractor. *J Minim Invasive Gynecol.* 2009;16(5):616–617.

Milad MP, Milad EA. Laparoscopic morcellator-related complications. *J Minim Invasive Gynecol.* 2014;21(3):486–491.

Miller CE. Methods of tissue extraction in advanced laparoscopy. *Curr Opin Obstet Gynecol.* 2001;13:399–405.

Montella F, Riboni F, Cosma S et al. A safe method of vaginal longitudinal morcellation of bulky uterus with endometrial cancer in a bag at laparoscopy. *Surg Endosc.* 2014;28(6):1949–1953.

Pritts EA, Parker WJ, Brown J et al. Outcomes of occult uterine leiomyosarcoma after surgery for presumed uterine fibroids: A systematic review. *J Minim Invasive Gynecol.* 2014;22(1):26–33.

Reich H. Specimen removal during laparoscopic surgery. In: Soderstrom RM, ed. *Operative Laparoscopy: The Masters' Techniques in Gynecologic Surgery,* 2nd ed. Philadelphia, PA: Lippincott-Raven; 1998:167–174.

Statement of the Society of Gynecologic Oncology to the Food and Drug Administration's Obstetrics and Gynecology Medical Devices Advisory Committee Concerning Safety of Laparoscopic Power Morcellation. Society of Gynecologic Oncology. 2014. www.sgo.org/newsroom/position-statements-2/morcellation/. Accessed 9/20/2014.

Uccella S, Cromi A, Bogani G, Casarin J, Serati M, Ghezzi F. Transvaginal specimen extraction at laparoscopy without concomitant hysterectomy: Our experience and systematic review of the literature. *J Minim Invasive Gynecol.* 2013;20(5):583–590.

Wong WS, Lee TC, Lim CE. Novel vaginal "paper roll" uterine morcellation technique for removal of large (>500 g) uterus. *J Minim Invasive Gynecol.* 2010;17(3):374–378.

Wright JD, Tergas AI, Burke WM et al. Uterine pathology in women undergoing minimally invasive hysterectomy using morcellation. *JAMA.* 2014;312(12):1253–1255. doi: 10.1001/jama.2014.9005.

CHAPTER 15

SURGERY FOR ENDOMETRIOSIS

Lidia Hyun Joo Myung, Luiz Flávio Cordeiro Fernandes, and Mauricio Simões Abrão

INTRODUCTION

Surgical treatment for endometriosis is a great challenge for surgeons in training, especially the deep infiltrating forms, and requires a long learning curve and study of important anatomical correlations.

Endometriosis is currently one of the most prevalent and studied diseases in gynecology and is defined as the presence of endometrial stromal or glandular cells outside the uterine cavity. It affects between 10% and 15% of women of reproductive age, and its exact pathogenetic mechanisms remain unclear to date. The symptoms are variable and not necessarily related to the extent of disease. The most frequent symptoms are dysmenorrhea, deep dyspareunia, chronic pelvic pain, intestinal and/or urinary symptoms that are cyclic, and infertility, impacting physical, mental, and social well-being. It is often under-diagnosed and takes an average of 10 years before the proper diagnosis is established. Simoens et al. calculated that annual health-care costs and lost productivity associated with endometriosis can be as high as $2801 and $1023 per patient, respectively. Extrapolating these findings to the U.S. population in 2002, the calculated annual costs of endometriosis were as high as $22 billion, assuming a 10% prevalence rate among women of reproductive age.

In 1990, Cornillie et al. defined deep endometriosis as lesions >5 mm of infiltration. In 1997, Nisolle and Donnez suggested that endometriosis could manifest as superficial implants in the pelvic peritoneum, as ovarian chocolate cysts referred to as endometriomas, and/or as deeply infiltrated lesions (depth >5 mm) in the bladder, ureters, retrocervical regions of the uterus, rectovaginal septum, and bowel. This differentiation was a landmark in the therapeutic management of the disease because it led to the perception that its deep infiltrative form should be considered a severe type of endometriosis requiring extremely specialized treatment to achieve optimal clinical results.

In 1996, the American Society for Reproductive Medicine (ASRM) revised an established surgical classification, categorizing the disease in four different stages, which are defined by a point system according to the surgical findings.

PREOPERATIVE EVALUATION

Diagnosing endometriosis remains a challenge because the symptoms are nonspecific, and laparoscopy is still the gold standard for definitive confirmation.

Although digital vaginal examination may provide evidence of thickening and/or painful nodules as points of tenderness at the posterior cul-de-sac or along the utero-sacral ligaments in cases of deep endometriosis, the clinical examination may appear as normal or nonspecific.

The success of the surgical treatment of endometriosis depends on establishing the specific site of the lesions prior to the procedure, especially for deep endometriosis. Magnetic resonance imaging (MRI), virtual colonoscopy, transvaginal ultrasonography (TVUS), and transrectal ultrasonography (TRUS) are noninvasive methods used to diagnose endometriosis. A TVUS performed according to a specific protocol, which consists of taking an oral laxative on the eve and a rectal enema 1 hour prior to the exam, and carried out by a trained professional has a sensitivity of 98% in the case of lesions affecting the rectosigmoid and 95% for the retrocervical disease, with a specificity of 100% and 98%, respectively. In cases of rectosigmoid endometriosis, this approach results in a positive predictive value of 93%–100%, and a negative predictive value of 96%–98% (Figure 15.1). MRI and virtual colonoscopy are becoming a useful adjunct to ultrasound scanning, especially in predicting severe endometriosis, whereas there seems to be a role for the use of additional endocavitary coils placed in the vagina together with the conventional pelvic-phased array coil.

SURGICAL MANAGEMENT

Method of access

Laparoscopy not only offers magnification of the image during the procedure but is also a more precise technique, being definitely the chosen access for endometriosis surgery. It is mandatory to respect the surgeon's ergonomic position, especially during lengthy operations, to avoid muscular strain and fatigue, which may cause errors and slowness. The preparation and positioning of the patient, as well as the creation of pneumoperitoneum and trocar insertion techniques, have already been described in Chapter 5.

MAPPING ENDOMETRIOSIS

The first step consists of exploring the abdominal anatomy and mapping out the extent of the disease, based on the preoperative image findings: perihepatic and epigastric regions, diaphragm, small intestine, cecum, appendix, rectal and sigmoid colon, ureters and bladder, peritoneal

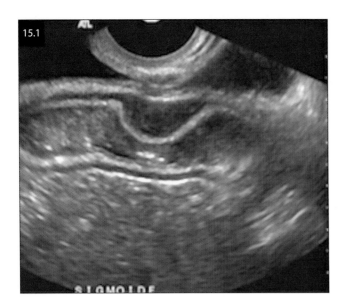

implants, ovaries, ovarian fossa, fallopian tubes, retrocervical and uterine regions, and pouch of Douglas.

PERITONEAL AND SUPERFICIAL ENDOMETRIOSIS

The surgical treatment of peritoneal endometriosis lesions (Figure 15.2) can be performed via

1. Excision preferentially using a pure cut mode monopolar electrode or scissors, or with an ultrasonic device such as the harmonic scalpel
2. Electrosurgical fulguration using a coag mode, as well as coagulation or vaporization using a pure cut mode

In the hands of surgeons with the requisite skills, the excision technique is preferred because it allows the removal of the entire lesion and thereby helps prevent recurrence.

OVARIAN ENDOMETRIOSIS

The indication for surgical treatment depends on a constellation of factors including the patient's age, symptoms, preoperative diagnosis, decisions regarding future fertility, and potential for malignant transformation.

The European Society of Human Reproduction and Embryology instructs that histology specimens should be obtained from cysts >3 cm in diameter with characteristics of endometriomas (Figure 15.3).

There is evidence that excisional surgery using a laparoscopic stripping technique to remove the pseudocapsule provides a more favorable outcome for the follicular cohort than drainage and thermal ablation with regard to the recurrence of the endometrioma and pain symptoms, and subsequent spontaneous pregnancy in women who were previously infertile. Consequently, this argues for surgical removal. However, in women who may subsequently undergo fertility treatment, there is insufficient evidence to determine the best option.

Excisional surgery for an endometrioma is predicated on restoration of normal anatomy and clarification of the ureter followed by a careful stripping to remove the cyst wall:

1. Dense adhesions and endometriotic implants are typically found between the ovary, the pelvic sidewall, and the peritoneum. These adhesive bands must be excised along with careful ureterolysis to avoid thermal or mechanical damage to the ureter.
2. First, the adhesions from the posterior leaf of the broad ligament to the ovary are mobilized.
3. The ovarian cyst frequently ruptures during this maneuver, and the chocolate-colored fluid should be irrigated and aspirated.
4. The cyst capsule is first identified and then systematically removed by grasping the margin of the

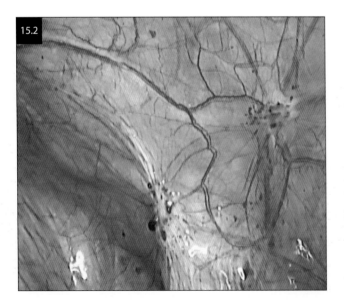

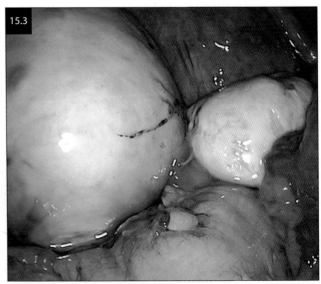

fenestration and then stripping off the ovarian stroma while tracted using countertension (Figure 15.4).

5. After stripping, hemostasis is attained using bipolar coagulation that is carefully applied to help preserve the ovarian follicular reserve and future fertility.

6. For cysts >4 cm in diameter, the edges of the ovarian defect should be reapproximated using intracorporeal suturing preferable with a small monofilament suture material.

ENDOMETRIOSIS OF THE URINARY TRACT

Involvement of the urinary tract occurs in approximately 1% of the patients with endometriosis. The bladder is affected in approximately 84% of cases, followed by ureter in 15%, kidney in 4%, and urethra in 2%. The disease originates in the outermost layers of the affected structures, typically up to the muscular layer. Bladder involvement usually presents with variable painful symptoms, including suprapubic pain, dysuria, hematuria, and recurrent urinary infections. Since medical treatment rarely provides satisfactory clinical improvement in these cases, surgical treatment is the preferred treatment option. This is especially true for ureteral endometriosis in order to avoid and/or treat urinary tract obstruction threatening renal compromise.

BLADDER ENDOMETRIOSIS

Ideally, surgical treatment should be carried out in a specialized center with a multidisciplinary team including a competent urologist, as described below:

1. A cystoscopy before the procedure permits better planning of the surgical approach and provides ureteral catheterization if indicated.

2. Transurethral resection is discouraged because most bladder lesions are transmural, which may lead to

the risk of bladder injury and incomplete excision of the lesion.

3. Bladder endometriosis is managed by performing partial cystectomy (Figures 15.5 and 15.6). The nodule can be removed using a laparoscopic grasper with a monopolar electrode or scissors using a pure cut mode or with a harmonic scalpel to minimize damage to the surrounding tissue (Figure 15.6).

4. Suture repair of the bladder defect is then performed in two layers using 3-0 Vicryl continuously for the inner layer and then in an interrupted fashion for the outer layer (Figure 15.7).

5. To identify any leakage after the procedure, blue dye solution is used in a retrograde fashion to distend the bladder. A Foley catheter is finally placed in the bladder for 7–14 days. Antibiotics are prescribed during this period.

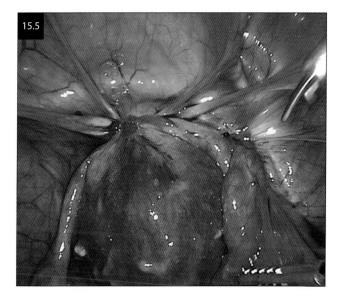

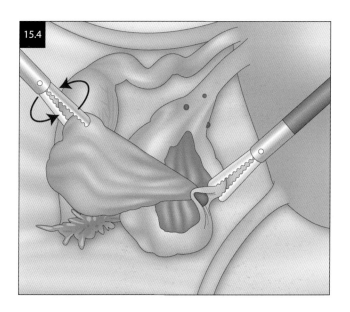

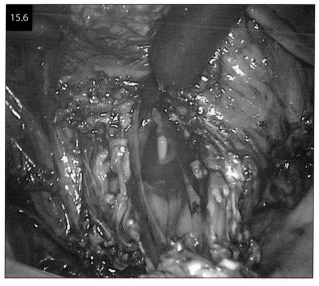

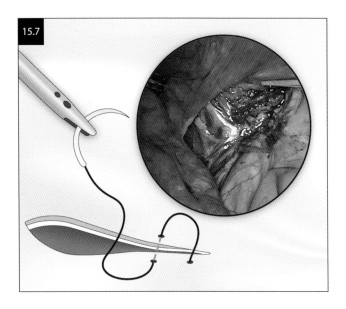

URETERAL ENDOMETRIOSIS

Ureteral endometriosis can be classified in two histologic types: extrinsic and intrinsic. Intrinsic ureteral endometriosis is histologically defined when deeply infiltrating lesions reach the muscularis of the ureteral wall. Ureteral endometriosis is considered extrinsic when the deeply infiltrating endometriosis causes ureteral obstruction, without involvement of the ureteral muscularis (Figure 15.8). The latter is more frequent than the former. The surgery consists of the following steps:

1. The ureters are carefully identified. Placement of illuminated ureteral stents may facilitate their identification.
2. Ureterolysis and adhesiolysis are preferably performed with careful use of sharp scissors without energy to help avoid thermal injury and fistula. In these situations, adhesions between ovarian endometriosis and ovarian fossa are commonly encountered.

3. In cases of extrinsic lesions, surgical excision is done carefully with scissors without energy and an atraumatic grasper. The ureterolysis is performed by grasping the peritoneum close at the pelvic brim and incising it with sharp scissors or a harmonic scalpel (Figure 15.9). The carbon dioxide helps dissect the surgical plane as a blunt grasper is used to dissect parallel to the ureter. Once the ureter is identified, it can be followed all along the pelvic sidewall (Figure 15.10).
4. In cases of intrinsic lesions infiltrating the muscle layer, the treatment option involves segmental resection of the affected ureteral portion, using scissors without energy and a ureteral stent catheter to perform an end-to-end anastomosis using a 5-0 absorbable monofilament suture (Figure 15.11). It is advisable to pass the ureteral stent before the ureteral resection if possible. If the stent cannot negotiate the point of stricture, it can certainly be passed into the proximal part of the ureter after the stricture is resected.

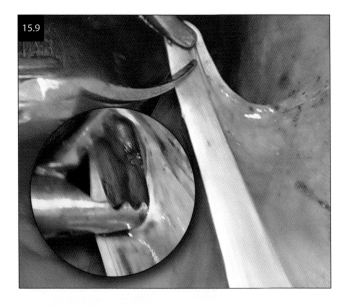

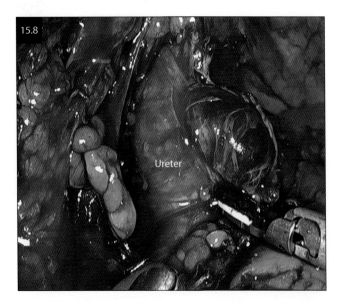

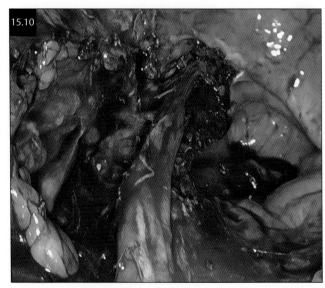

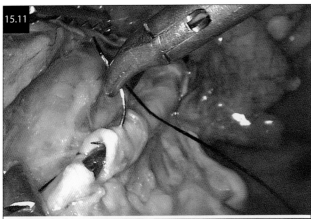

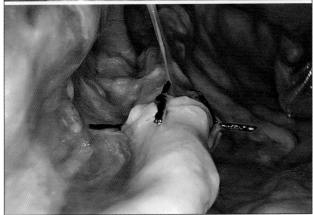

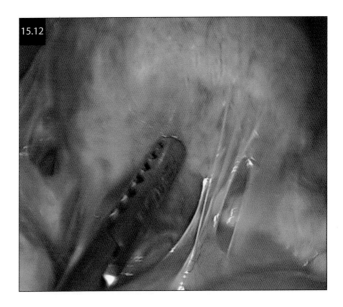

In rare cases, when the segmental resection is extensive and the end-to-end anastomosis is not possible, reimplantation of the ureter into the bladder is performed using the Boari flap or psoas hitch technique. Most studies demonstrate that ureterolysis is the treatment of choice, and radical surgery is the exception.

RETROCERVICAL AND VAGINAL ENDOMETRIOSIS

One of the greatest challenges in the treatment of deep endometriosis is the surgical treatment of lesions located in the pouch of Douglas, including the retrocervical region, the vagina, and the rectovaginal septum. In deep endometriosis associated primarily with pain, most of the studies demonstrate that the treatment of choice is surgical.

The management of such cases is associated with complicated surgical access and the proximity of important structures such as the rectum, the ureters, and the pelvic vessels and nerves. Injuries of the complex innervation of the pelvic region may lead to prolonged and incapacitating postsurgical disorders. These include bladder, bowel, and sexual disorders, such as urinary retention and incontinence, atonic bladder, fecal incontinence, and sexual dysfunction. This issue is made even more complex since these lesions may occur in young women as a result of the characteristics of the disease. In cases of retrocervical, posterior vaginal fornix, and rectovaginal septum lesions, the rectal wall may be adhered to the retrocervical region (Figure 15.12).

1. First, the anatomy of the ureters must be elucidated. After adhesiolysis and ureterolysis, the retrocervical region is accessed by dissecting lateral to the rectal wall in order to enter the pararectal space. This dissection is performed close to the side of the rectal wall up its anterior portion, where it typically comes into contact with the retrocervical region. The dissection is made using a bipolar coagulation grasper along with a sharp scissors, or with ultrasonic energy. It is important to remember the dictum that fat belongs to the rectum when dissecting into this space. This dissection can be readily achieved by placing gauze into the abdominal cavity through a 10 mm trocar with an atraumatic forceps to systematically push and open the tissue planes (Figure 15.13).

2. The dissection should continue in the direction of the rectovaginal septum if the lesion has invaded deeply into the vaginal fornix or the rectovaginal septum while exercising extreme care to avoid injury to the hypogastric nerve. The second assistant surgeon plays an important role in manipulating the uterus forward, manipulating the rectum backward with the help of a rectal probe, and performing a digital vaginal examination to confirm the location of the lesion and normal tissue (Figure 15.14).

3. After the ureters and rectum have been isolated, the lesions should be completely excised using a pure cut mode monopolar electrode or harmonic scalpel.

4. Lesions of the rectovaginal septum and vaginal fornix are removed in a single block, and repair of the culdotomy is performed using 2-0 absorbable suture by laparoscopy or the vaginal route. The lesions that have not infiltrated into the vagina are removed without any need for suture repair.

5. Laparoscopic repair of the culdotomy may need gas-containing vaginal occlusion to maintain pneumoperitoneum.

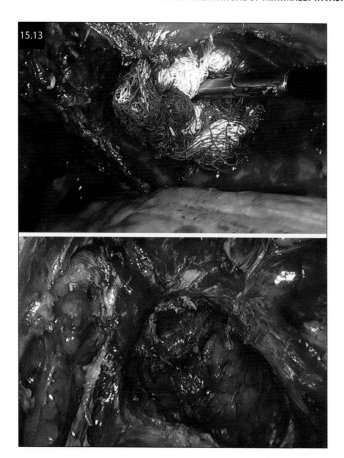

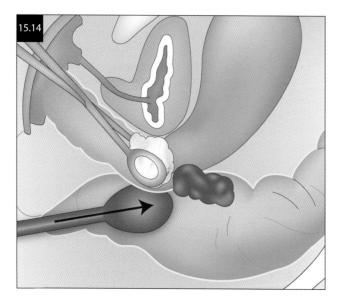

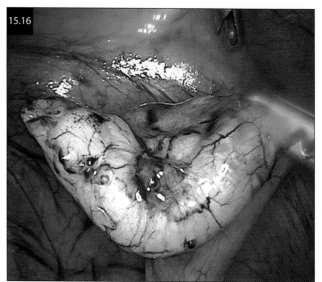

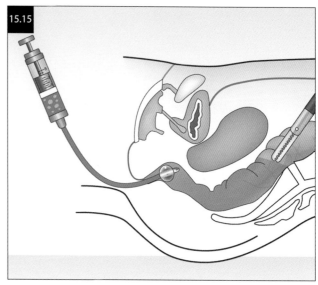

6. When the procedure is finalized, a safety test is performed by introducing 200 cc of methylene blue into the rectum, after placing a Foley catheter and inflating the balloon while the bowel above any concern is mechanically occluded with an atraumatic bowel grasper (Figure 15.15).

BOWEL ENDOMETRIOSIS

The bowel is involved in approximately 10% of endometriosis cases, of which 90% affect the rectum and/or the sigmoid. Other segments are less frequently affected, such as the appendix, ileum, and cecum in 7% of the cases and the jejunum and small intestine in 3% of the cases. Surgery is necessary when the small intestine is affected because of the risk of obstruction and in symptomatic rectosigmoid disease, because medical therapy is either temporarily effective or ineffective. Endometriosis of the appendix is found in 2.8% (Figure 15.16) of all cases of endometriosis and should be investigated when deeply infiltrating endometriosis is suspected, especially those who present with right iliac fossa pain. The carcinoid tumor of the appendix is part of the differential diagnosis, as this tumor has a prevalence of 0.3%–0.9% in the general population. Endometriosis of the appendix is usually present when associated disease is in the rectosigmoid, is retrocervical, or invades the bladder.

The success of the surgical treatment of endometriosis depends on accurately characterizing all significant lesions prior to the procedure. Transvaginal ultrasound, as previously described, can predict the size and site of the lesion and the layers of the organ affected by the disease. MRI also has an important role when a trained ultrasonographer is not available. MRI is less accurate than TVUS.

Several types of surgery have been indicated for rectosigmoid endometriosis. Whereas shaving seems to have lost popularity, it remains unclear whether and when discoid or segmental bowel resection should be performed. The argument in favor of segmental bowel resection is the completeness of endometriosis removal, especially if the affected area is >3 cm, whereas for smaller nodules a discoid resection could be considered.

Studies have demonstrated the feasibility of the laparoscopic approach to deep infiltrating endometriosis (DIE) with segmental or mechanical discoid colorectal resection. In our experience, if the rectosigmoid lesion is <3 cm in diameter and compromises less than 35% of the circumference, the discoid resection is feasible; otherwise, we perform the segmental resection with endoscopic stapler.

All patients are given a mechanical bowel preparation on the day before the procedure. Their legs are placed in stirrups. Pneumoperitoneum is created according to the Veress technique. A 10 mm port is placed through the umbilicus for a 0° camera and three other 5 mm ports are placed in the right iliac fossa, suprapubic, and left iliac fossa regions, respectively.

The shaving technique is as follows:

1. Adhesiolysis, ureterolysis, and retrocervical region dissection are performed as described above for retrocervical endometriosis.
2. The bowel is then grasped with atraumatic forceps for traction to allow blunt dissection and excision of the superficial bowel lesion using sharp scissors. The enteric defect is then sutured in two layers (Figure 15.17).

3. After this procedure, 120 mL of air is injected into the rectum while submerged in irrigation fluid to ensure that there is no leakage. A dilute solution of methylene blue is then introduced into the rectum to confirm visceral integrity.

To perform a discoid resection, the following steps are utilized:

1. Adhesiolysis, ureterolysis, and dissection of the retrocervical region are sequentially performed as described above.
2. The lateral and anterior wall of the bowel is systematically dissected in order to anatomically surround the lesion.
3. The lesion is then directly incised in order to free it from the posterior aspect of the uterus and/or the vagina. As needed, residual lesions are left and can then be removed separately.
4. A suture is then placed into the endometriotic lesion, which helps identify the areas to be excised.
5. An open circular stapler is inserted, positioning the endometriotic lesion into the gap between the anvil and the stapler (Figure 15.18).
6. Two instruments are used to hold each thread of the suture in order to provide downward traction on the bowel. This helps imbricate the affected area into the hollow, while the stapling device is being closed (Figure 15.19).
7. The stapler is activated.
8. The excised area is inspected to ensure that it contains both the endometriotic lesion as well as the suture.
9. After the procedure, 120 mL of air is injected into the rectum while submerged in irrigation fluid to ensure that there is no leakage. A dilute solution of methylene blue is then introduced into the rectum to confirm the integrity of the anastomosis.

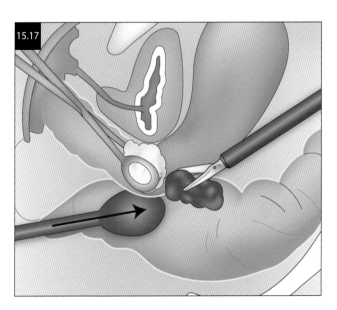

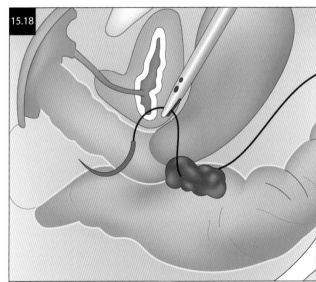

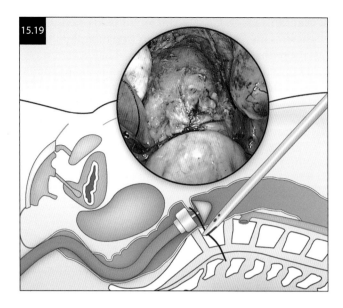

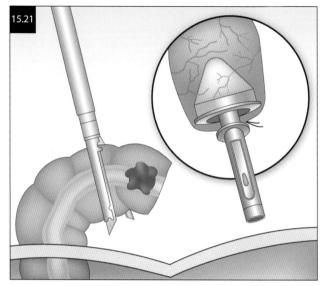

The surgical technique for laparoscopic segmental resection of the rectum, lesions >3 cm or multifocal, follows the following steps:

1. Adhesiolysis is performed to restore normal anatomical relationships affecting the adnexa, uterine fundus, posterior cul-de-sac, uterosacral ligaments, and bowel.
2. The sigmoid is then released from the left lateral abdominal wall, opening the retroperitoneum with identification of the left ureter while opening the mesosigmoid.
3. The anterior wall of the rectum is dissected free from the posterior surface of the cervix. The healthy part of the distal rectum-sigmoid is skeletonized. A linear stapler is applied distally to the area affected by the disease (Figure 15.20).
4. The divided bowel enclosing the disease portion is exteriorized through a right iliac or suprapubic ±4 cm incision and transected proximal to the lesion.

5. The anvil of the circular stapler is then placed inside the stump, and a purse-string suture is secured (Figure 15.21).
6. The bowel containing the anvil is reintroduced into the abdominal cavity and a 33 mm circular stapler is introduced through the anus and connected to the anvil (Figure 15.22).
7. The stapler is activated to form the end-to-end anastomosis.
8. After this procedure, 120 mL of air is injected into the rectum, while submerged in irrigation fluid to ensure that there is no leakage (Figure 15.23). Also, a dilute solution of methylene blue can be introduced into the rectum to confirm the integrity of the anastomosis.

CONCLUSION

The success of a surgery for endometriosis depends on assiduous preoperative evaluation, including mapping

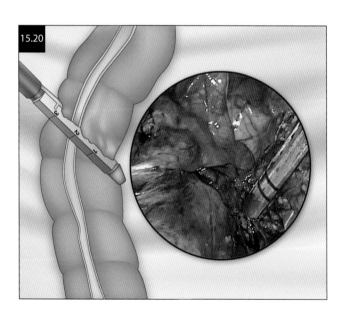

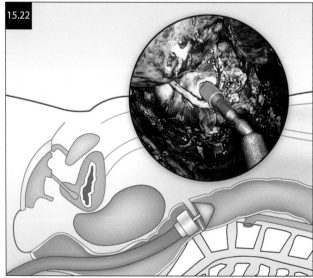

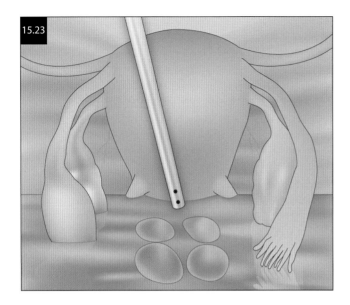

the exact locations of lesions using proper imaging techniques. Surgical treatment should ideally involve a multidisciplinary team of trained surgeons operating in harmony. The learning curve in laparoscopic surgery for endometriosis requires intensive training. Postoperative quality of life is directly related to complete resection of deep lesions.

SUGGESTED READING

Abrao MS, Dias Jr JA, Bellelis P, Podgaec S, Bautzer CR, Gormatsky C. Endometriosis of the ureter and bladder are not associated diseases. *Fertil Steril.* 2009;91:1662–1667.

Abrao MS, Dias Jr JA, Rodini GP, Podgaec S, Bassi MA, Averbach M. Endometriosis at several sites, cyclic bowel symptoms, and the likelihood of the appendix being affected. *Fertil Steril.* 2010;94(3):1099–1101.

Abrao MS, Goncalves MO, Dias Jr JA, Podgaec S, Chamie LP, Blasbalg R. Comparison between clinical examination, transvaginal sonography and magnetic resonance imaging for the diagnosis of deep endometriosis. *Hum Reprod.* 2007;22(12):3092–3097.

Abrao MS, Neme RM, Averbach M, Petta CA, Aldrighi JM. Rectal endoscopic ultrasound with a radial probe in the assessment of rectovaginal endometriosis. *J Am Assoc Gynecol Laparosc.* 2004;11:50–54.

Abrão MS, Podgaec S, Fernandes LFC. Surgical therapies: Pouch of Douglas and uterovaginal pouch resection for endometriosis. In: Giudice LC, Evers JLH, Healy DL, eds. *Endometriosis: Science and Practice.* Oxford, UK: Blackwell Publishing Ltd.; 2012:402–409.

Abrao MS, Sagae UE, Gonzales M, Podgaec S, Dias JA Jr. Treatment of rectosigmoid endometriosis by laparoscopically assisted vaginal rectosigmoidectomy. *Int J Gynaecol Obstet.* 2005;91(1):27–31.

American Society for Reproductive Medicine (ASRM). Revised ASRM classification for endometriosis: 1996. *Fertil Steril.* 1997;67:820.

Antonelli A. Urinary tract endometriosis. *Urologia.* 2012;79(3):167–170.

Arruda MS, Petta CA, Abrão MS, Benetti-Pinto CL. Time elapsed from onset of symptoms to diagnosis of endometriosis in a cohort study of Brazilian women. *Hum Reprod.* 2003;18(4):756–759.

Bassi MA, Podgaec S, Dias Jr JA, D'Amico Filho N, Petta CA, Abrao MS. Quality of life after segmental resection of the rectosigmoid by laparoscopy in patients with deep infiltrating endometriosis with bowel involvement. *J Minim Invasive Gynecol.* 2011;18(6):730–733.

Bazot M, Lafont C, Rouzier R, Roseau G, Thomassin-Naggara I, Darai E. Diagnostic accuracy of physical examination, transvaginal sonography, rectal endoscopic sonography, and magnetic resonance imaging to diagnose deep infiltrating endometriosis. *Fertil Steril.* 2009;92(6):1825–1833.

Bourdel N, Roma H, Mage G et al. Surgery for the management of ovarian endometriomas: From the physiopathology to the pre, peri and postoperative treatment. *Gynecol Obstet Fertil.* 2011;39(12):709–721.

Ceccaroni M, Clarizia R, Bruni F et al. Nerve-sparing laparoscopic eradication of deep endometriosis with segmental rectal and parametrial resection: The Negrar method. A single-center, prospective, clinical trial. *Surg Endosc.* 2012;26:2029–2045.

Chamie LP, Blasbalg R, Goncalves MO, Carvalho FM, Abrao MS, Oliveira IS. Accuracy of magnetic resonance imaging for diagnosis and preoperative assessment of deeply infiltrating endometriosis. *Int J Gynaecol Obstet.* 2009;106(3):198–201.

Chapron C, Chiodo I, Leconte M et al. Severe ureteral endometriosis: The intrinsic type is not so rare after complete surgical exeresis of deep endometriotic lesions. *Fertil Steril.* 2010;93(7):2115–2120.

Cornillie FJ, Oosterlynck D, Lauweryns JM, Koninckx PR. Deeply infiltrating pelvic endometriosis: Histology and clinical significance. *Fertil Steril.* 1990;53(6):978–983.

Darai E, Bazot M, Rouzier R, Coutant C, Ballester M. Colorectal endometriosis and fertility. *Gynecol Obstet Fertil.* 2008;36:1214–1217.

Darai E, Thomassin I, Barranger E et al. Feasibility and clinical outcome of laparoscopic colorectal resection for endometriosis. *Am J Obstet Gynecol.* 2005;192:394–400.

Davalos ML, De Cicco C, D'Hoore A, De Decker B, Koninckx PR. Outcome after rectum or sigmoid resection: A review for gynecologists. *J Minim Invasive Gynecol.* 2007;14:33–38.

De Ceglie A, Bilardi C, Bianchi S et al. Acute small bowel obstruction caused by endometriosis: A case report and review of the literature. *World J Gastroenterol.* 2008;14(21):3430–3434.

De Cicco C, Schonman R, Craessaerts M et al. Laparoscopic management of ureteral lesions in gynecology. *Fertil Steril.* 2009;92(4):1424–1427.

Dubree HJ, Senagore AJ, Delaney CP et al. Laparoscopic resection of deep pelvic endometriosis with rectosigmoid involvement. *J Am Coll Surg.* 2002;195(6):754–758.

Fanfani F, Fagotti A, Gagliardi ML et al. Discoid or segmental rectosigmoid resection for deep infiltrating endometriosis: A case-control study. *Fertil Steril.* 2010;94(2):444–449.

Fedele L, Bianchi S, Zanconato G, Berlanda N, Borruto F, Frontino G. Tailoring radicality in demolitive surgery for deeply infiltrating endometriosis. *Am J Obstet Gynecol.* 2005;193:114–117.

Fourquet J, Gao X, Zavala D et al. Patients' report on how endometriosis affects health, work, and daily life. *Fertil Steril.* 2010;93:2424–2428.

Frenna V, Santos L, Ohana E et al. Laparoscopic management of ureteral endometriosis: Our experience. *J Minim Invasive Gynecol.* 2007;14:169–171.

Giudice LC, Kao LC. Endometriosis. *Lancet.* 2004;364:1789–1799.

Gonçalves MO, Dias Jr JA, Podgaec S, Averbach M, Abrao MS. Transvaginal ultrasound for diagnosis of deeply infiltrating endometriosis. *Int J Gynaecol Obstet.* 2009;104(2):156–160.

Goncalves MO, Dias Jr JA, Podgaec S, Rossini L, Abrao MS. How transvaginal ultrasonography can help in the indication of surgical treatment of rectal endometriosis. *J Minim Invasive Gynecol.* 2008;15(6):36(s).

Goncalves MO, Podgaec S, Dias Jr JA, Gonzalez M, Abrão MS. Transvaginal ultrasonography with bowel preparation is able to predict the number of lesions and rectosigmoid layers affected in cases of deep endometriosis, defining surgical strategy. *Hum Reprod.* 2010;25(3):665–671.

Goncalves MO, Podgaec S, Dias Jr JA, Mattos LA, Abrao MS. Transvaginal ultrasonography with bowel preparation is a useful tool for predicting the surgical staging of endometriosis. *J Minim Invasive Gynecol.* 2011;18(6):61(s).

Guerriero S, Ajossa S, Gerada M et al. Diagnostic value of transvaginal "tenderness-guided" ultrasonography for the prediction of location of deep endometriosis. *Hum Reprod.* 2008;23(11):2452–2457.

Gustofson RL, Kim N, Liu S, Stratton P. Endometriosis and the appendix: A case series and comprehensive review of the literature. *Fertil Steril.* 2006;86(2):298–303.

Hart RJ, Hickey M, Maouris P, Buckett W. Excisional surgery versus ablative surgery for ovarian endometriomata. *Cochrane Database Syst Rev.* 2013;(5):CD004992.

Kennedy S, Bergqvist A, Chapron C et al. On behalf of the ESHRE Special Interest Group for Endometriosis and Endometrium Guideline Development Group. ESHRE guidelines for the diagnosis and treatment of endometriosis. *Hum Reprod.* 2005;20(10):2698–2704.

Koninckx PR, Meuleman C, Demeyere S, Lesaffre E, Cornillie FJ. Suggestive evidence that pelvic endometriosis is a progressive disease, whereas deeply infiltrating endometriosis is associated with pelvic pain. *Fertil Steril.* 1991;55:759–765.

Kovoor E, Nassif J, Miranda-Mendoza I, Wattiez A. Endometriosis of bladder: Outcomes after laparoscopic surgery. *J Minim Invasive Gynecol.* 2010;17(5):600–604.

Landi S, Ceccaroni M, Perutelli A et al. Laparoscopic nerve-sparing complete excision of deep endometriosis: Is it feasible? *Hum Reprod.* 2006;21(3):774–781.

Maggard MA, O'Connell JB, Ko CY. Updated population-based review of carcinoid tumors. *Ann Surg.* 2004;240(1):117–122.

Manassero F, Mogorovich A, Fiorini G et al. Ureteral reimplantation with psoas bladder hitch in adults: A contemporary series with long term follow-up. *Sci World J.* 2012;2012:379316.

Mencaglia L, Minelli L, Wattiez A. *Manual of Gynecological Laparoscopic Surgery.* Tuttlingen: Verlag Endo Press; 2008:48–55.

Mereu L, Gagliardi ML, Clarizia R et al. Laparoscopic management of ureteral endometriosis in case of moderate-severe hydroureteronephrosis. *Fertil Steril.* 2010;93(1):46–51.

Minelli L, Barbieri F, Fiaccavento A et al. Complete laparoscopic removal of endometriosis for the management of pain symptomatology. *J Am Assoc Gynecol Laparosc.* 2003;10(S):11.

Minelli L, Fanfani F, Fagotti A et al. Laparoscopic colorectal resection for bowel endometriosis: Feasibility, complications and clinical outcome. *Arch Surg.* 2009;144:234–239.

Mohr C, Nezhat FR, Nezhat CH, Seidman DS, Nezhat CR. Fertility consideration in laparoscopic treatment of infiltrative bowel endometriosis. *J Soc Laparosc Surg.* 2005;9:16–24.

Nezhat C, Pennington E, Nezhat F, Silfen SL. Laparoscopically assisted anterior rectal wall resection and reanastomosis for deeply infiltrating endometriosis of the rectum. *Surg Laparosc Endosc.* 1991;1:106–108.

Nezhat F, Nezhat C, Pennington E, Ambroze Q. Laparoscopic segmental resection for infiltrating endometriosis of the rectosigmoid colon: A preliminary report. *Surg Laparosc Endosc.* 1992;2:212–216.

Nisolle M, Donnez J. Peritoneal endometriosis, ovarian endometriosis, and adenomyotic nodules of the rectovaginal septum are three different entities. *Fertil Steril.* 1997;68(4):585–596.

Orbuch IK, Reich H, Orbuch M, Orbuch L. Laparoscopic treatment of recurrent small bowel obstruction secondary to ileal endometriosis. *J Minim Invasive Gynecol.* 2007;14(1):113–115.

Pastor-Navarro H, Gimenez-Bachs JM, Donate-Moreno MJ et al. Update on the diagnosis and treatment of bladder endometriosis. *Int Urogynecol J Pelvic Floor Dysfunct.* 2007;18:949–954.

Pearce CL, Templeman C, Rossing MA et al. Association between endometriosis and risk of histological subtypes of ovarian cancer: A pooled analysis of case-control studies. *Lancet Oncol.* 2012;13(4):385–394.

Podgaec S, Abrao MS, Dias Jr JA, Rizzo LV, de Oliveira RM, Baracat EC. Endometriosis: An inflammatory disease with a Th2 immune response component. *Hum Reprod.* 2007;22(5):1373–1379.

Radosa MP, Bernardi TS, Georgiev I, Diebolder H, Camara O, Runnebaum IB. Coagulation versus excision of primary superficial endometriosis: A 2-year follow-up. *Eur J Obstet Gynecol Reprod Biol.* 2010;150(2):195–198.

Remorgida V, Ragni N, Ferrero S, Anserini P, Torelli P, Fulcheri E. How complete is full thickness disc resection of bowel endometriotic lesions? A prospective surgical and histological study. *Hum Reprod.* 2005;20:2317–2320.

Roy C, Balzan C, Thoma V et al. Efficiency of MR imaging to orientate surgical treatment of posterior deep pelvic endometriosis. *Abdom Imaging.* 2009;34(2):251–259.

Senagore AJ, Duepree HJ, Delaney CP et al. Results of standardized technique and postoperative care plan for laparoscopic sigmoid colectomy: A 30-month experience. *Dis Colon Rectum.* 2003;46(4):503–509.

Simoens S, Hummelshoj L, D'Hooghe T. Endometriosis: Cost estimates and methodological perspective. *Hum Reprod Update.* 2007;13(4):395–404.

Vercellini P, Chapron C, De Giorgi O, Consonni D, Frontino G, Crosignami PG. Coagulation or excision of ovarian endometriomas? *Am J Obstet Gynecol.* 2003;188:606–610.

Vercellini P, Meschia M, De Giorgi O et al. Bladder detrusor endometriosis: Clinical and pathogenic implications. *J Urol.* 1996;155(1):84–86.

Woods RJ, Heriot AG, Chen FC. Anterior rectal wall excision for endometriosis using the circular stapler. *ANZ J Surg.* 2003;73:647–648.

Chapter 16

VAGINAL HYSTERECTOMY AND ADNEXECTOMY TECHNIQUE

Johnny Yi and Rosanne Kho

The vaginal route is the preferred approach for benign hysterectomy. In one Cochrane review of surgical approaches to hysterectomy involving over 4495 women in 34 randomized controlled trials, vaginal hysterectomy resulted in fewer complications, shorter hospital stay, and faster recovery and return to normal activity. It also provided the best cosmetic result with its single and concealed incision.

Despite strong evidence for greater advantage of the vaginal approach, there has not been an increase in the number of hysterectomies performed vaginally. In the United States, the rate has declined in 15 years from 24% in 1990 to 22% in 2005 and may even continue to be declining. In fact, less than 5% of gynecologic surgeons in the United States perform more than 10 vaginal surgeries in a year and a greater proportion, (>80%) perform less than five vaginal surgeries in a year.

The main stumbling blocks for many surgeons in choosing the vaginal route include challenges with exposure, entry into the anterior cul-de-sac, hemostasis, avoidance of ureteral and bladder injury, and removal of the large uterus. In addition to these intrinsic challenges, a contributing factor to the declining rates of vaginal hysterectomies may be the rising adoption of laparoscopic and robotic approaches to hysterectomy. While minimally invasive approaches to hysterectomy have increased overall, rates of vaginal hysterectomy have remained stable or slightly decreased. With more stringent work-hour restrictions, exposure and training during residency are limited further. Moreover, training continues to decline with the gradual attrition of mentors with expertise in vaginal surgery.

We describe the fundamental steps used to perform vaginal hysterectomy, highlighting different techniques and instrumentation that can help overcome common technical challenges. The incorporation of advanced energy-based surgical devices can facilitate both vaginal hysterectomy and adnexectomy.

PATIENT POSITIONING

Once adequate general anesthesia is obtained, the patient is placed in a high lithotomy position in candy cane stirrups. To avoid nerve injuries, the patient's hips should be flexed no greater than 90° to protect the femoral nerve.

Care is taken to avoid any contact of the patient's lower extremities with the metal stirrup. Overabduction and external overrotation of the hips should be avoided. In addition, adequate padding should be applied to the heels, legs, and hips. The patient's hips are carefully brought down to the end of the bed, allowing support of the sacrum, without interfering between a self-retaining retractor and the surgical bed. The bladder is drained with the red rubber catheter, and the Foley catheter is not kept in place during the procedure.

OBTAINING EXPOSURE

The use of a self-retaining retractor, such as the Magrina-Bookwalter vaginal retractor system (Symmetry Surgical, Tennessee), provides consistent and reliable exposure without requiring two surgical assistants at the bedside (Figure 16.1). Similar to the abdominal self-retaining retractor system, the post is attached to the rail of the operating table, and the ring is designed to fit the contour of the patient's perineum while in a high lithotomy position. Blades of multiple lengths are latched onto the retractor ring and placed in the four quadrants to maximize room for surgery. The arm is attached to the post on the bed and then to the ring at the 8 o'clock position. The ring is placed flush against the perineum with the bend in the ring at the level of the posterior fourchette. The posterior blade is attached first in order to allow the lateral blades to be positioned below the bend in the ring. The lateral blades are placed carefully and parallel to the vaginal sulcus to avoid undue pressure and sulcal lacerations. The small anterior blade is held manually behind the ring by the assistant until after the anterior cul-de-sac is entered.

PREEMPTIVE ANALGESIA AND FIRST INCISION

The cervix is grasped with the single-tooth or Jacobs tenaculum at 12 and 6 o'clock, the uterus is pulled downward, and the border of the bladder and the anterior cervix is inspected (Figure 16.2). Prior to vaginal incision, 20 mL of 0.5% bupivacaine with 1:200,000 of epinephrine is injected into the uterosacral ligaments bilaterally for preemptive local analgesia. Dilute vasopressin solution

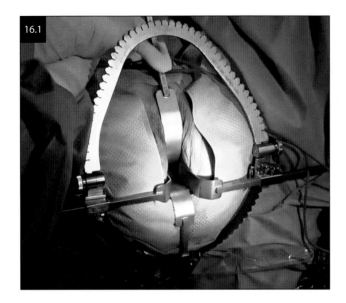

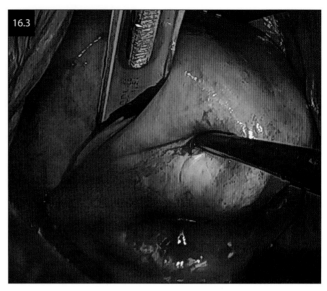

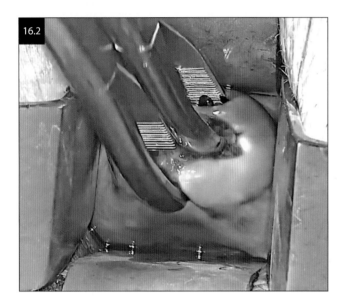

are transected. Dorsal traction of the posterior vaginal wall with ventral traction of the cervix allows safe exposure to the posterior cul-de-sac. The posterior peritoneum is grasped with forceps and tented downward, and Mayo scissors are used to incise the posterior peritoneum after the posterior epithelium is dissected off of the cervix. Scissors are placed parallel to the plane of the cervix to avoid inadvertent rectal injury (Figure 16.4). The operator should visually confirm the peritoneal entry before extending the incision laterally. A long self-retaining

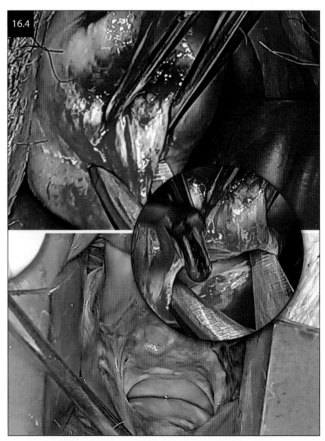

is then circumferentially injected under the vaginal epithelium. A scalpel is used to make a circumferential incision at the cervicovaginal junction. This circumferential incision should be at least 3–4 mm deep. Operators very often make a mistake of not making the incision deep enough (Figure 16.3). A careful approach is needed in patients with cystocele not to injure the bladder. The anterior vaginal epithelium is sharply dissected off the cervix until the vesicouterine space is reached. With the index finger, the bladder is pushed superiorly and also laterally in order to avoid bladder and ureteral injury with subsequent placement of the clamps. Entry into the anterior cul-de-sac is then delayed until adequate descensus of the uterus is obtained. Attention is now directed to entry into the posterior cul-de-sac.

POSTERIOR DISSECTION AND ENTRY

Posterior entry is often easier and also allows for better descensus of the uterus once the uterosacral ligaments posterior blade is positioned into the abdominal cavity and attached to the ring to provide exposure. If you do not have the Bookwalter retractor, a long weighted speculum can be used for this part of the procedure.

VESSEL-SEALING DEVICE

The uterosacral ligaments are clearly visualized and palpated. The operator should get in the habit of confirming the structures by palpating the ligaments with the index finger. A bipolar vessel-sealing device is used to seal and transect the uterosacral ligaments bilaterally (Figure 16.5). The device is placed across the ligament and rotated around the ligament so that the tips of the blade stay within the circular incision that was cut around the cervix. This allows gradual descensus of the uterus for better exposure for anterior entry. The use of vessel-sealing devices in vaginal hysterectomy helps overcome the limitation of tight vaginal access and has been proven to be feasible and safe. A number of bipolar vessel-sealing clamps are now available including the PK (Olympus), Ligasure Impact (Covidien), Super Jaw (Ethicon), and Altrus (Conmed). These devices can be particularly helpful in cases with a narrowed introitus and larger uterus. The choice of device is surgeon-dependent, and each requires a learning curve for safe and effective application.

ANTERIOR DISSECTION AND ENTRY

Once the uterosacral ligaments are transected, the cardinal ligaments can also be sealed and divided serially and gradually with the vessel-sealing device to gain further uterine descensus. It is important to keep the clamps lateral and inferior to the 3 and 9 o'clock positions in order to avoid injury to the bladder and the ureters. With better descensus, entry into the anterior cul-de-sac can be attempted with dorsal traction applied to the cervix with the Jacobs tenacula. The posterior

blade of the Bookwalter retractor is removed to achieve better exposure with a more pronounced angulation of the lower uterine segment. With ventral traction on the anterior vaginal wall, the bladder is separated from the anterior cervix using sharp dissection with the Mayo curved scissors. The vesicouterine fold is identified as a crescent-shaped peritoneal fold that can be lifted and divided for entry. Palpation of this peritoneal fold can aid and confirm the smooth texture of the thin peritoneum. Fine-toothed forceps and Metzenbaum scissors are preferred to allow precise incision. The vesical fold should be grasped and elevated with fine-toothed forceps, and the tissue should be cut with Metzenbaum scissors underneath the forceps. The scissor tips are pointed downward, aimed parallel to the plane of the cervix to reveal the avascular vesicouterine peritoneum (Figure 16.6). Understanding the anatomy and perceiving the different tissues are critical to mastering entry into the anterior cul-de-sac. Cutting into the cervix will feel tough against the tips of the Metzenbaum scissors, while cutting into the softer striated detrusor muscle will manifest with excessive bleeding. In cases where scarring between the bladder and uterus is encountered in patients having undergone multiple previous cesarean sections, sharp dissection is best performed lateral to the midline, away from centrally dense adhesions. This step should only be performed when there is adequate exposure of the tissue planes. The cardinal ligaments can also be further sealed and transected prior to anterior entry if it will allow better visualization and safer entry into the anterior cul-de-sac.

Upon entering the anterior cul-de-sac, the smooth serosa of the uterine corpus along with bowel should be visualized prior to proceeding with the hysterectomy. The anterior tenaculum blade is then placed in the abdomen to protect the bladder (Figure 16.7). Safe entrances to the posterior and anterior cul-de-sac are the crucial and probably the most difficult steps of vaginal hysterectomy.

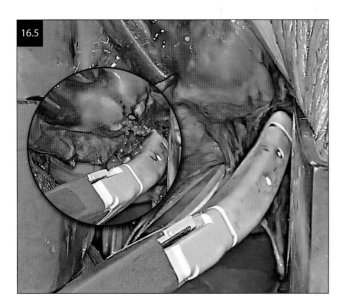

16.5

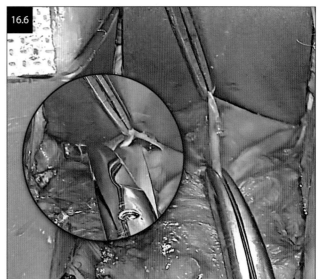

16.6

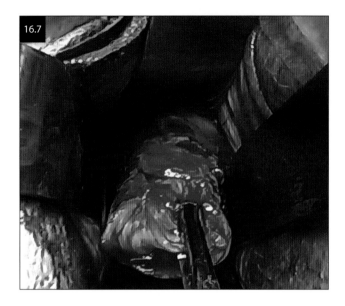

SECURING VASCULAR PEDICLES

Achieving hemostasis in vaginal procedures is challenging where there is limited space in placing a suture around the clamp and in securing knots with fingers deep within the vaginal canal. However, the suture placement and knot tying can be achieved with adequate exposure by skilled assistants. The vessel-sealing devices are used to seal the uterine blood supply to overcome this technical difficulty. Gentle traction is placed on the cervix while the vessel-sealing device is pushed up against the pedicle,

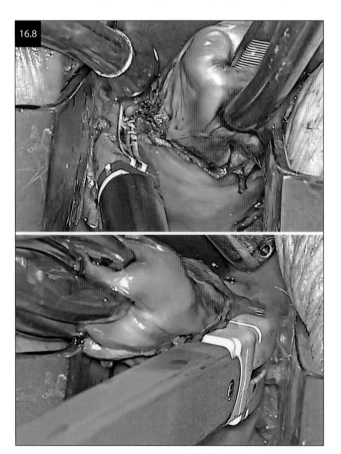

taking care to avoid leaning against any adjacent tissues or retractor blades to avoid thermal injury to the vaginal wall. A suction device can be used to quickly dissipate the hot steam that can be generated from the bipolar vessel-sealing device. The vascular pedicles are coagulated and transected on the left and right sides (Figure 16.8).

Once the uterosacral ligaments and cardinal ligaments are sealed and transected using the advanced bipolar device, the uterine vessels are secured under direct visualization. The vessel-sealing device is then advanced in a stepwise fashion beyond the level of the uterine vessels into the broad ligament. Once the vessels are secure, morcellation can be safely performed to decompress the uterus, and gain access to the utero-ovarian pedicles. The uteroovarian pedicle contains the uteroovarian ligament, round ligament, and fallopian tube.

To isolate the uteroovarian ligaments, the surgeon places a finger around the cornua of the uterus and follows with an open Heaney clamp (Figure 16.9). Each uteroovarian pedicle is clamped in its entirety, and the cornua are cut with Mayo scissors (Figure 16.10). Once clamped, each uteroovarian pedicle is suture ligated by passing a suture through the middle of the pedicle and tying around it. This pedicle can be doubly ligated if it is bulky.

REMOVAL OF FALLOPIAN TUBES AND OVARIES

Upon completion of the hysterectomy, the final pedicle is secured using an absorbable multifilamented suture as described above. This allows traction of the uteroovarian pedicle in preparation for salpingo-oophorectomy using the round ligament technique. First, identification of the tubes and ovaries is paramount. Two long Allis clamps are used to grasp the ovary and identify the fimbriated end of the fallopian tube. Once both ovary and tube are grasped, the round ligament is identified. Using a monopolar electrosurgical pencil with an extended tip, the round ligament is carefully transected, isolating the infundibulopelvic (IP) ligament. A modified Heaney

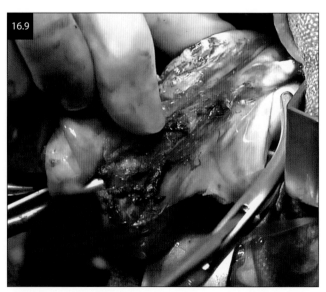

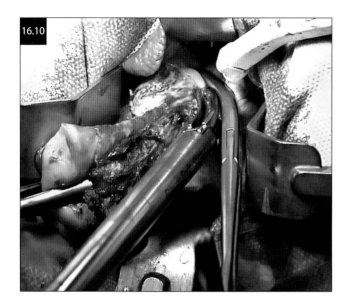

clamp that has been elongated and curved, also referred to as the ovarian clamp, is used to clamp the IP ligament (Figure 16.11). The tube and ovary are cut with scissors and inspected to ensure complete removal. A suture is used to secure the pedicle. This can be doubly tied at the surgeon's preference. Hemostasis is evaluated using a sponge stick to retract to the contralateral side.

Once hysterectomy is completed, a peritoneal suture is placed to ensure hemostasis and help prevent postoperative seroma or hematoma formation. The peritoneum

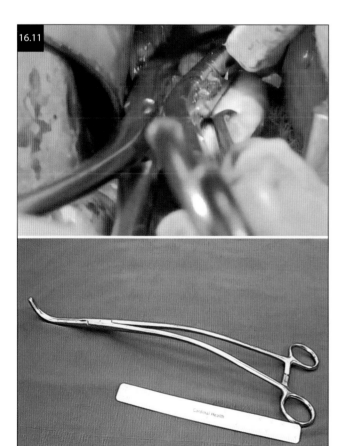

is brought to the vaginal cuff using a 2-0 Vicryl suture in a running locked fashion from the uterosacral pedicle to the cardinal pedicle bilaterally.

MODIFIED MCCALL CULDOPLASTY

McCall culdoplasty was first described in the literature by Dr. Milton McCall as an apical support suture for the treatment of pelvic organ prolapse. We perform our modification to the traditional McCall culdoplasty for apical support at the time of every vaginal hysterectomy. Our modification includes three McCall sutures: one suture placed in the midline—plicating bilateral uterosacral ligaments—and two ipsilateral sutures—lifting each vaginal lateral fornix to the ipsilateral uterosacral ligament.

A 1-polyglactin suture is used to take a full-thickness bite of the midline of the posterior vaginal wall and peritoneum. The posterior blade of the Bookwalter is used to retract the rectum to the contralateral side, and the posterior vaginal fornix is grasped with toothed forceps to delineate the uterosacral ligament. An intermediate length Deaver retractor is then placed at the 3 o'clock position to protect the ureter, which would be coursing in the 2–3 o'clock aspect of the pelvis. With traction of the vagina at the uterosacral ligament, the proximal uterosacral ligament is clearly visualized. The deep suture is placed 1–2 centimeters below the level of the ischial spine. The contralateral uterosacral ligament is similarly delineated and purchased. The midline McCall suture is then brought out through the posterior vaginal wall lateral to the entry stitch (Figure 16.12).

In a similar fashion, an ipsilateral McCall stitch incorporates the left vaginal fornix immediately below the 3 o'clock position. The uterosacral ligament is delineated with the retractors and purchased. The same stitch is then brought through the vaginal cuff near the entry site (Figure 16.13). A similar procedure is performed on the contralateral side with the entry stitch at the right posterior cuff placed immediately inferior to the 9 o'clock position. Due to an increased risk of ureteral compromise with high uterosacral sutures, cystoscopy is routinely performed following placement of these sutures. This can be performed after the vaginal cuff is closed in an interrupted fashion with 2-0 polyglactin suture. Once the vaginal cuff is closed, the McCall culdoplasty sutures are tied down, taking care to cinch and plicate down to the uterosacral ligaments. These sutures can be tagged with a clamp until cystoscopy confirms ureteral patency.

OVERCOMING CHALLENGES IN VAGINAL HYSTERECTOMY

Simple vaginal hysterectomy and adnexectomy can be performed using the techniques above. More challenging cases such as with the nonprolapsed and nulliparous patient, patients with multiple previous cesarean sections, and patients with large fibroid uteri can also be

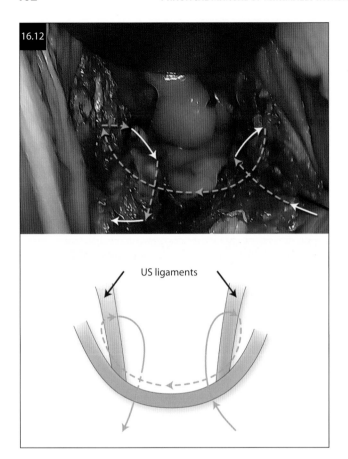

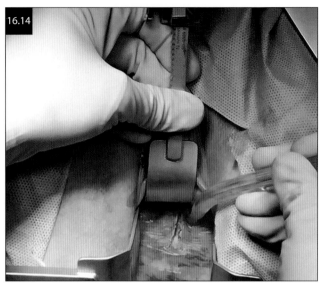

approached vaginally. We present additional techniques to approach these more challenging cases.

NARROW INTROITUS

In cases where the introital opening is limited (i.e., ≤2.5 cm), such as in nulliparous or menopausal women, a superficial 2–3 cm longitudinal incision is performed with the monopolar pencil in the midline and distal portion of the posterior vaginal wall (Figure 16.14). This provides additional width to allow placement of the

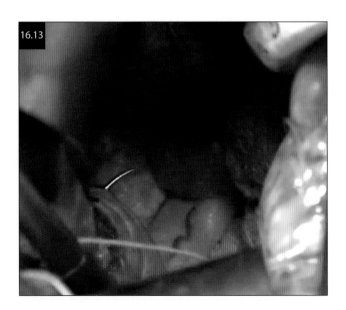

lateral and posterior self-retracting blades. This incision is 2–3 mm deep and is simply closed with absorbable suture in a continuous fashion at the end of the case.

INSUFFICIENT VISUALIZATION

Optimizing visualization is key to successfully performing a difficult vaginal hysterectomy. Additional light sources from a surgical headlight or flexible light source (such as the cystoscopy light) held with a Babcock clamp, or a lighted suction irrigator tip (such as Vital Vue, Covidien, Massachusetts) are extremely helpful when visualizing structures deep within the vagina (Figures 16.15 and 16.16). Providing the ability to accurately display every step of a vaginal hysterectomy in an ergonomic and high-quality manner, the VITOM 25 System from Karl Storz consists of an exoscope with integrated illumination along with a full HD camera with display and documentation system. It can be set conveniently in front of the vagina at a distance from 25 up to 60 cm from the surgical site, being held by a mechanical or pneumatic holding device. It provides a commendable depth of field, magnification, contrast, and color reproduction for full HD display (Figure 16.17).

Elongated Deaver retractors or Breisky-Navratil retractors (Figure 16.18) can improve visualization and retraction of the bowel to allow adequate visualization of the pelvic sidewalls. Standard retractors can be modified to increase the length of the blade to facilitate deep retraction, which is often necessary during pelvic reconstructive surgery or salpingo-oophorectomy. A long vaginal pack or moistened laparotomy sponge is also placed following hysterectomy to retract loops of bowel out of the operating field.

DIFFICULT PERITONEAL ENTRY

An inability to enter into either or both cul-de-sacs should not preclude continuation with the vaginal approach. Securing the uterine arteries can still be accomplished

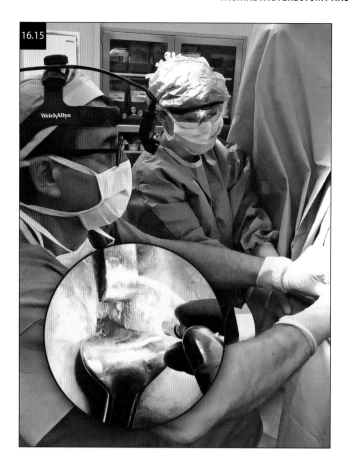

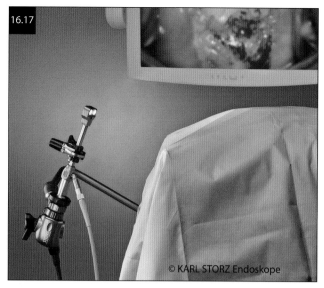

extraperitoneally until better descensus of the uterus is obtained. If posterior entry is difficult, a finger can be placed in the rectum to better palpate the rectovaginal space.

With anterior dissection, we prefer not to routinely drain the bladder with an indwelling catheter at the beginning of vaginal hysterectomy. This allows some fullness of the bladder and better visualization of the vesicouterine fold. If the bladder is entered, this also allows immediate recognition of the injury with the release of urine upon entry.

REMOVING THE LARGE UTERUS

Morcellation can be initiated after the uterine arteries have been sealed and divided on each side. Orientation of the uterus must be maintained by placing the Jacobs tenaculum at 3 and 9 o'clock positions on the cervix. Bivalve the cervix starting at the level of the lower uterine segment. If the anterior cul-de-sac has not yet been entered, bivalve to a centimeter below the vesicouterine peritoneal fold and start morcellation within the uterus (Figure 16.19).

Morcellation is performed with a double-toothed tenaculum placed on the myometrium, and a wedge excision is accomplished with a 10-blade. With the uterus bivalved to the level of the lower uterine segment, the endometrium can be excised entirely and sent to pathology. Serial wedges are performed to decompress the uterus. Entry into the anterior cul-de-sac can now be performed easily with better uterine descensus and visualization of the peritoneal fold. Avoid forceful traction

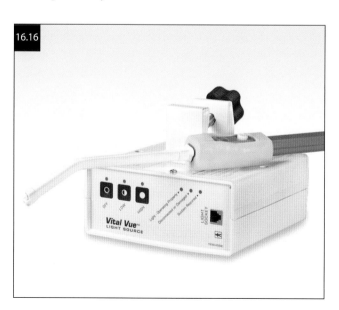

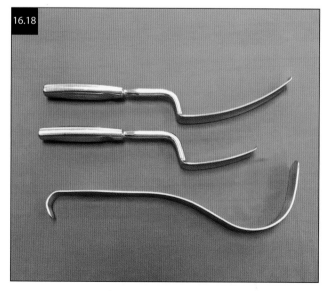

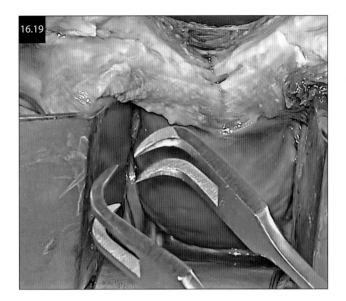

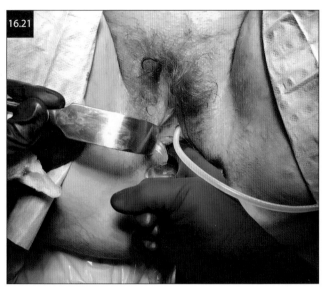

on the cervix during morcellation, which can cause the remaining vascular pedicles to avulse. Depending on the size of the uterus, morcellation can require a significant amount of time but can be performed safely and without risk of leaving pieces of myometrium in the abdominal cavity, as with laparoscopic morcellation (Figure 16.20). Morcellation can be continued to the level of the fundus and cornua, when the uteroovarian, round ligament, and fallopian tube can be safely secured. A sudden and slight increase in bleeding is often encountered when morcellation is near the fundus.

AVOIDING BLADDER AND URETERAL INJURY

Once the vesicouterine space is entered, bladder pillars are gently pushed superiorly and laterally with the index finger to avoid injury during placement of the vessel-sealing clamp. It is imperative that the surgeon is aware of the location of the ureters, which may be displaced and in close proximity to the cervicovaginal junction, especially in cases with uterovaginal prolapse. The ureters can be palpated with the index finger at 2 and 10 o'clock (for the left and right ureter, respectively) against a curved Deaver placed outside the peritoneal cavity on the lateral vaginal wall (Figures 16.21 and 16.22). Intraoperative cystoscopy at the end of the procedure should always be performed to diagnose inadvertent bladder and ureteral injury.

CYSTOSCOPY

Cystoscopic examination of the bladder and ureteral orifices ensures no bladder or ureteral compromise at the time of hysterectomy. Further, pelvic reconstructive surgeries can increase the risk of bladder and ureteral compromise, and routine cystoscopy should be performed in such cases. Close to the culmination of the procedure, 1 ampule of indigo carmine is given intravenously. A 70° rigid cystoscope is advanced and the bladder is

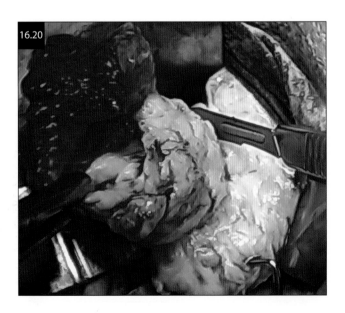

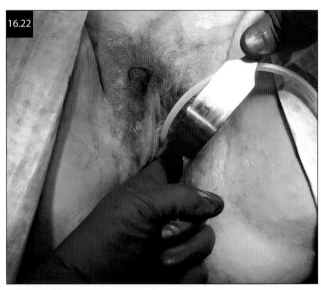

filled with 200–300 mL of saline. Then 360° evaluation of the bladder is performed to evaluate for any bladder injury. Normal and abnormal bladder anatomy should be documented. Ureteral efflux of the indigo carmine dye is clearly visualized at the ureteral orifices.

CONCLUSION

Vaginal hysterectomy should be incorporated in the surgical armamentarium of minimally invasive surgeons given its safe and cost-effective advantages. The technique described in this chapter has reviewed the step-by-step approach to vaginal hysterectomy, bilateral salpingo-oopherectomy, and McCall culdoplasty. As a surgeon improves his or her comfort level with vaginal hysterectomy, more complex and difficult cases can also be performed vaginally. Having knowledge of and familiarity with the anatomy and tools that are used, achieving adequate surgical exposure, and honing the surgical technique will allow the surgeon to perform the procedure safely and efficiently.

SUGGESTED READING

Aarts JW, Nieboer TE, Johnson N et al. Surgical approach to hysterectomy for benign gynaecological disease. *Cochrane Database Syst Rev*. 2015;(8):CD003677.

Brown J. Safe and sound: Vaginal hysterectomy with uncontained manual morcellation to effect uterine removal. *JMIG*. 2017;24(4):511.

Ding Z, Wable M, Rane A. Use of Ligasure bipolar diathermy system in vaginal hysterectomy. *J Obstet Gynaecol*. 2005;25(1):49–51.

Farquhar CM, Steiner CA. Hysterectomy rates in the United States 1990–1997. *Obstet Gynecol*. 2002;99(2):229–234.

Hefni MA, Bhaumik J, El-Toukhy T et al. Safety and efficacy of using the LigaSure vessel sealing system for securing the pedicles in vaginal hysterectomy: Randomised controlled trial. *BJOG*. 2005;112(3):329–333.

Jacoby VL, Autry M, Jacobson G et al. Nationwide use of laparoscopic hysterectomy compared with abdominal and vaginal approaches. *Obstet Gynecol*. 2009;114(5):1041–1048.

Levy B, Emery L. Randomized trial of suture versus electrosurgical bipolar vessel sealing in vaginal hysterectomy. *Obstet Gynecol*. 2003;102(1):147–151.

Long JB, Eiland RJ, Hentz JG et al. Randomized trial of preemptive local analgesia in vaginal surgery. *Int Urogynecol J Pelvic Floor Dysfunct*. 2009;20(1):5–10.

McCall M. Posterior culdeplasty; surgical correction of enterocele during vaginal hysterectomy; a preliminary report. *Obstet Gynecol*. 1957;10(6):595–602.

Mistrangelo E, Febo G, Ferrero B et al. Safety and efficacy of vaginal hysterectomy in the large uterus with the LigaSure bipolar diathermy system. *Am J Obstet Gynecol*. 2008;199(5):475.e1–475.e5.

Rogo-Gupta LJ, Lewin SN, Kim JH et al. The effect of surgeon volume on outcomes and resource use for vaginal hysterectomy. *Obstet Gynecol*. 2010;116(6):1341–1347.

Silva-Filho AL, Rodrigues AM, Vale de Castro Monteiro M et al. Randomized study of bipolar vessel sealing system versus conventional suture ligature for vaginal hysterectomy. *Eur J Obstet Gynecol Reprod Biol*. 2009;146(2):200–203.

Chapter 17

LAPAROSCOPIC-ASSISTED VAGINAL HYSTERECTOMY

Johan van der Wat

INTRODUCTION

To be a successful vaginal surgeon requires a certain mental attitude which is that of a pioneering spirit, an innovative mind, and persevering character.

The surgeon must be an astute clinician of sound judgment to make rational decisions based on the clinical evidence to provide the patient with the optimal surgical intervention to cure or ameliorate her condition. He or she must be capable of performing a variety of procedures that may include laparotomy when necessary. No vaginal hysterectomy is the same as another, and every procedure is individualized to suit the clinical situation and deal with the surgical realities as presented.

This chapter describes key clinical, anatomic, and surgical aspects of laparoscopic-assisted vaginal hysterectomy (LAVH) to enlighten and empower prospective surgeons who wish to incorporate this technique into his or her armamentarium.

DEFINITION

There are numerous definitions for LAVH. The simple definition is: LAVH is the procedure in which the laparoscopic approach is used to secure the upper uterine pedicles, whereas the uterine ligaments and vessels are typically secured transvaginally, enabling the uterus to be removed through the vagina after which the vaginal cuff is sutured vaginally. The two most technically challenging portions of a total laparoscopic hysterectomy are colpotomy and cuff closure; combining a laparoscopic with a vaginal approach can enable surgeons to perform a technically challenging hysterectomy by laparoscopy despite their lack of expertise in laparoscopic or vaginal surgery.

For the purpose of this chapter, the operational assumption is that the primary intent of LAVH is to remove the uterus vaginally and to use the laparoscope and other laparoscopic instruments only when ancillary pathology significantly interferes with this primary goal. Problematic pathology may include uterine fibroids, endometriosis, adnexal pathology, pelvic adhesions, and adenomyosis.

PATIENT SELECTION

Given appropriate training, most hysterectomies for benign gynecology can be performed vaginally. It is thus logical to initially consider all cases for hysterectomy as possible candidates for the vaginal approach. Preoperative history taking and clinical evaluation will give a good indication as to the probability of successfully removing the uterus vaginally. Abdominal palpation and a thorough vaginal examination with cervical traction can provide important information regarding the size, shape, mobility, descent, and vaginal space that may be available at the time of the surgical procedure. The best and final assessment, however, is in the operating room under anesthesia. This will give enhanced information about size, mobility, available parauterine space, and uterine descent. A shallow fornix along with a short cervix displaced cranially as well as concomitant adnexal and pouch of Douglas pathology, such as endometriotic nodules, will point to a difficult vaginal hysterectomy that could be facilitated using adjunctive laparoscopy. In certain cases, a minilaparotomy or even a conventional abdominal hysterectomy may be the most appropriate and prudent approach based on the extent of associated pelvic pathology.

The following situations should be considered as relative contraindications for vaginal hysterectomy:

- Uterine immobility in all directions (i.e., side to side as well as downward), commonly described as a "frozen pelvis." An enlarged and impacted uterus without descent may require laparoscopic assistance or even laparotomy.
- A history of any abdominal or pelvic surgery suspect for severe pelvic adhesions: In this circumstance, a laparoscopic assessment can be employed to assess the feasibility of a vaginal procedure. In certain cases, concomitant laparoscopic surgery can be proactively used to perform adhesiolysis or resection of endometriosis to help ensure the success of a vaginal procedure.

Absolute contraindications include the following conditions that must be ascertained and well characterized prior to attempting vaginal surgery:

- Inability to visualize the cervix after a full-length vaginal speculum has been introduced into the vagina. The cervix is the key organ and the starting point for the vaginal hysterectomy, and it must be accessible.
- Invasive cancer of the cervix, myometrium (sarcoma), and endometrium.
- Large adnexal mass suspicious for malignancy.

SIZE

An enlarged uterus, usually caused by fibroids, should be methodically assessed, including the use of specialized imaging techniques such as pelvic ultrasound and magnetic resonance imaging. For example, a large fundal fibroid that is not accessible to vaginal morcellation may be more effectively dealt with using other means, such as a total laparoscopic hysterectomy or by laparotomy. However, in experienced hands it is not uncommon to remove uteri up to 2 kg. As a general rule of thumb, uteri of 24w size and above may be very difficult to extirpate, especially if a narrow vagina and limited descent are also present. These types of cases could then be considered good candidates for LAVH, laparoscopic hysterectomy, or even abdominal hysterectomy using a self-retaining retractor. In case of a larger fibroid uterus, volume reduction can be considered depending on the size and location of fibroids. Various techniques are employed to achieve volume reduction, including bisecting, wedge morcellation, and coring. Transvaginal myomectomy can also be very effective to reduce uterine bulk. It is essential to ligate the uterine arteries prior to performing volume reduction in order to avoid excessive hemorrhage.

NULLIPARITY

The current literature does not support the notion that uterine descensus is a prerequisite for a successful vaginal hysterectomy. Nulliparity should be considered an associated factor rather than a justification to preclude vaginal hysterectomy. In a nulliparous female, the cervix can often be gradually pulled down with ease under anesthesia. This degree of "physiological" descent is often sufficient to commence surgery, secure the supporting ligaments, and ligate the uterine arteries, all key prerequisites needed to complete the operation vaginally.

PREVIOUS CESAREAN SECTION

Previous cesarean section has historically been considered a contraindication for vaginal hysterectomy. The challenge is opening the vesicouterine space along the cesarean section scar. This plane can be obliterated by dense fibrotic adhesions formed between the bladder base and the lower uterine segment. A partially filled bladder with saline or methylene blue can help demarcate the lower limit of the bladder in difficult cases.

For experienced vaginal surgeons, laparoscopic assistance to enter the vesicouterine space may not be beneficial as vaginal dissection is more direct and less likely to cause bladder injury. However, for the inexperienced vaginal surgeon, laparoscopic dissection can greatly help in identifying and entering this obliterated anatomic space.

ANATOMIC CONSIDERATIONS

The following anatomic structures have to be understood and surgically dissected in order to accomplish a safe and efficient LAVH:

1. Vaginal wall, pubocervical fascia, and cervix.
2. Pelvic floor ligaments that are condensations of the pelvic endopelvic fascia at the base of the broad ligaments. They suspend the uterine-cervical complex in the pelvis. There are four such ligaments: two uterosacral and two transverse cervical ligaments (Cardinal or Mackenrod). The uterosacral ligaments connect the cervix to the sacrum and suspend the cervix and vaginal fornices to the level of ischial spines. The transverse cervical ligaments connect the cervix to the pelvic side walls by attaching to the obturator fascia of the obturator internus muscle.
3. *Peritoneal surfaces and folds*: The uterovesicle peritoneal fold covers the dome of the bladder and extends backward over the upper cervix and anterior uterine wall.
   The posterior peritoneal fold extends from the posterior uterine surface over the pouch of Douglas onto the rectum.
4. *Major blood vessels*: The uterine arteries lie close to the lateral aspect of the cervix at the upper end of the transverse cervical ligaments.
   The ovarian arteries, which also supply the body of the uterus, extend downward from the aorta.
5. *Ureter*: The ureter lies in close proximity and just lateral to the uterine artery at the uterocervical junction, close to the point where the uterine arteries are secured during surgery. It is thus imperative to stay close to the cervix to avoid injury to the ureter.
6. *Adnexae*: These extend laterally from the fundus of the uterus through the cranial margin of the broad ligament and comprise the fallopian tubes, ovaries, and blood vessels.

TECHNICAL CONSIDERATIONS

INSTRUMENTS

No two sets of instruments are alike, as individual surgeons have their own preferences and sets are assembled to suit their individual needs. Two separate instrument tables are useful.

One instrument table should be for laparoscopic instruments and should include trocars, laparoscopic graspers, energy source, laparoscopic scissors, and suction irrigators (see Chapters 3 and 6).

The other table should include the vaginal tray.

A small table is also placed in front of and across the lap of the surgeon.

Retractors should include a weighted speculum and retractors of different sizes. These are needed to be inserted beneath the bladder into the peritoneal cavity as well as into the pouch of Douglas to facilitate dissection and mobilization in these areas. Hemostatic and pedicle clamps, whether curved or straight, must have longitudinal serrations to prevent slipping. It is also important that these clamps be sturdy, as some pedicles are thick and fibrous. Smaller hemostatic clamps are essential to control bleeders and to attach holding sutures to the drapes for identification. Two multi-toothed, curved tenacula are required to pull on the cervix. Lahey clamps are useful to deliver the corpus of the uterus through the posterior fornix. Both curved and straight needle holders are necessary to deliver suture material to the clamped pedicles. Good visualization is mandatory, so a headlight/spotlight can be useful.

It is wise to have suction connected to suck up blood collecting in the vagina and pouch of Douglas. This will allow for better judgment of blood loss.

SUTURE MATERIAL

Chromic catgut suture is preferred for the vascular pedicles as they tend to form a nonslip bite after the first throw. This is in contrast with Vicryl, which does not have this capability, resulting in loss of tension in critical situations where absolute knot control is demanded. Vicryl sutures are ideal for ligaments and vaginal closure, because they are not very vascular and can benefit from a longer resorption period.

VESSEL SEALING DEVICES

Advanced bipolar vessel sealing devices are helpful for completion of the laparoscopic portion of the procedure; however, this part of surgery can safely be performed using a combination of bipolar and monopolar electrosurgery.

Electrosurgical vessel-sealing devices for the vaginal part of the procedure have been recommended by many companies to secure vessels and ligaments during vaginal hysterectomy. After using these instruments for some time, some surgeons have abandoned them in favor of the time-tested clamp, cut, and tie routine for the following reasons:

- Poor management of the uterosacral/transcervical ligament complex, as anatomic detail is lost due to the fulguration and retraction of the ligament when current is applied.
- Hemorrhage: As the uterus is pulled down, most pedicles are on stretch. Applying the current under these circumstances can cause premature separation and traction of tissue and vessels before

sealing is complete, potentially leading to extensive hemorrhage.
- Cost: These devices are disposable and expensive, which can hugely impact on the total cost of the procedure, which is otherwise a low-cost procedure.

PRESURGICAL ROUTINE

1. The patient should be placed in the lithotomy position using adjustable leg support systems, as the legs may have to be adjusted during surgery to facilitate the procedure (Figure 17.1). The leg support systems should be well padded to prevent pressure and nerve injury. Straight leg holders and stirrups are considered hazardous as they can cause injury to the nerves on the dorsum of the feet. The patient should be positioned that the buttocks are 8–10 cm over the edge of the operating room table to allow for the weighted speculum to hang free.

2. The abdomen, pelvis, perineum, and vagina should be thoroughly cleansed, ideally with a clear disinfecting solution as brown or other colored solutions may stain the natural tissue and make it difficult to distinguish between natural tissue and dissecting planes.

3. *Drapes*: Drapes should cover the abdomen, legs, and perineum. They should be fixed with tape or clips as they tend to be dislodged during surgery.

4. *Empty the bladder*: It is not necessary to place an indwelling catheter for the duration of this surgery.

5. Perform an examination under anesthesia to confirm preoperative clinical findings. It is important to reevaluate size, mobility, and especially, cervical descent. The uterosacral ligaments must be identified and palpated digitally to identify pathology like endometriosis infiltration, which can hamper entry into the pouch of Douglas. The adnexa should be palpated to identify potential pathology.

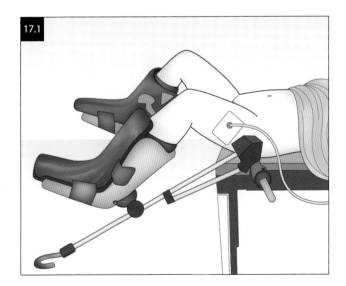

17.1

6. A reusable device such as the Hulka manipulator is introduced into the cervix to manipulate the uterus for the laparoscopic part of the procedure.

The procedure is started by establishing a pneumoperitoneum and introducing a 5 or 10 mm umbilical trocar for placement of the laparoscope. Two to three 5 mm ancillary ports are placed under vision for the introduction of various laparoscopic instruments (Figure 17.2). The abdominal cavity is inspected and any adhesions removed to restore normal anatomy. The laparoscope offers significant advantage for inspection of the pelvic anatomy for adhesions or endometriotic lesions, while providing safe methods to secure the upper uterine pedicles. If adhesions are present, laparoscopic adhesiolysis should be performed and normal anatomy restored before hysterectomy is started (see Chapter 9 for adhesiolysis). Upon identification of the course of the ureters, the upper pedicles can be coagulated and transected as described in Chapters 11, 18, and 19.

Depending on the surgeon's laparoscopic versus vaginal approach skills, the laparoscopic portion of the procedure can be terminated at different stages of surgery. If the surgeon feels more comfortable with the vaginal approach, the laparoscopic portion of the procedure can be terminated after inspection of the abdominal cavity and elimination of significant adhesions or after transection of the round ligaments, development of the broad ligament bilaterally, and mobilization of the vesicouterine fold. If the surgeon is experienced with the laparoscopic approach, the uterine arteries can be coagulated and transected laparoscopically under direct vision, whereas the colpotomy and cuff closure can then be carried out using the vaginal approach.

VAGINAL SURGICAL PROCEDURE (12 STEPS TO SUCCESS)

In this section, all of the steps used to perform vaginal hysterectomy will be presented without regard to laparoscopy. The vaginal part of the LAVH procedure will be truncated depending on how many steps are otherwise performed laparoscopically.

1. The weighted vaginal speculum is inserted into the vagina with the blade lodging behind the cervix.
2. If there are large labia minora present, it is necessary to suture them laterally to the vulval skin beyond the labia majora.
3. Empty the bladder with a sterile urinary catheter.
4. Secure the cervix with the curved multitoothed vulsellum both on the anterior and posterior cervical lips. When surgery is performed on the anterior cervix, the traction is downward, whereas it should be upward when working behind the cervix in the posterior fornix.
5. Infiltrate the cervix circumferentially with a hemostatic solution. This will promote hemostasis and open tissue planes. Posteriorly, also infiltrate the uterosacral ligaments (Figure 17.3).
6. *Cervical incision*: Using a scalpel, a circumferential incision is made around the cervix. The incision should be no more than a finger's breadth around the surface of the cervix (Figure 17.4). It is important not to make the incision high on the cervix as the bladder may be entered. If there is uncertainty as to the whereabouts of the margins of the bladder, a metal catheter can be inserted into the bladder and its cervical margins probed and identified. The incision should be through the mucosa and connective tissue until the white fibrous layer of the cervix is reached.
7. *Entering the utero-vesical space*: The bladder is carefully separated from the cervix using a blunt-tipped scissors and digital dissection using the tip of the index finger until the peritoneal reflection of the utero-vesical space is reached. The reflection can be identified as a thin white reflection line transversing the upper cervical surface.

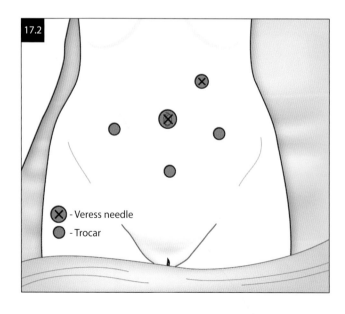

17.2

⊗ - Veress needle

● - Trocar

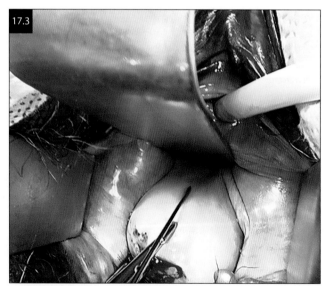

17.3

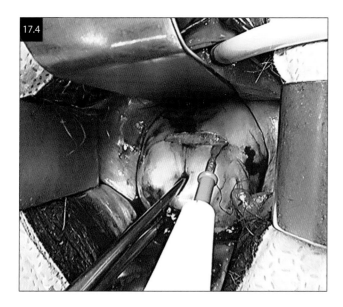

Before opening this peritoneal reflexion, it is wise to digitally spread open and free up the vesicouterine space. The peritoneum is now opened by holding it with a toothed dissecting forceps and cutting through with a scissors (Figure 17.5). Now spread the space open digitally until a retractor can easily be inserted into the space.

Danger points: The bladder can be entered if care is not taken. Use the curved scissors only if the curve points toward the cervix. If the bladder is

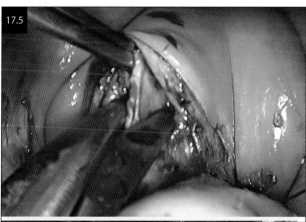

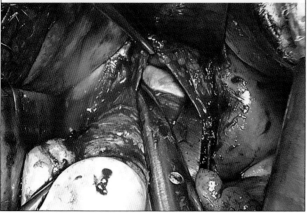

entered, it should be closed in two layers. It is not a reason to abandon the procedure.

Special situation: Cesarean section (C/S) is not considered a contraindication to vaginal hysterectomy. As more and more patients undergo C/S, the "previous C/S" scenario will become a regular presentation and may actually outnumber the "no C/S" cases. It is thus important to deal with the situation. C/S causes the normal tissue planes to be obliterated and replaced with dense fibrous tissue connecting the bladder to the C/S scar. With retraction of the scar tissue, the bladder may be "pulled" into a C/S scar. This can sometimes be observed in the presurgical ultrasound and should be an indication of a "difficult" dissection. However, in most cases, the dissection proceeds without a hitch, especially if small, careful bites with the scissors are taken to get through the fibrous tissue. Sometimes it is very difficult to complete this dissection through to the peritoneal cavity. Do not despair, it is not important at this stage to enter the anterior peritoneal space. As the uterine ligaments are separated from their cervical connections, there will be descent and the C/S scar will be presented to the surgeon "on a plate," so to speak. The vesicouterine space, however, will have to be entered at some point to complete the operation. This sometimes may become possible only when the uterine arteries are clamped and cut, allowing for further uterine descent.

The use of a laparoscopic approach may facilitate dissection of a severely scarred C/S scar. Capitalizing on the magnification and illumination of laparoscopy, normally recognized anatomic landmarks such as the pubocervical fascia can be used to guide the dissection in a lateral-to-medial fashion until the bladder is sufficiently mobilized for safe colpotomy.

8. *Entering the posterior peritoneal space (pouch of Douglas)*: Procedure: The cervix is elevated by pulling the vulsellum, grasping the cervix anteriorly. A digital examination of the uterosacral ligaments and the space between them is made. Nodularity should indicate pathology such as endometriosis, and it will be wise to do a laparoscopic assessment before proceeding with the surgery. The incised vaginal mucosa is now grabbed with a toothed forceps and pulled down. The rectovaginal space is dissected open with a scissors, and the peritoneum is opened by a sharp incision (Figure 17.6). The incision is extended laterally by using digital and sharp dissection. A good tip is to suture the peritoneum to the posterior vaginal wall to prevent oozing. At this point, it is appropriate to insert a retractor into the pouch of Douglas and inspect the peritoneal cavity. If intestine or omentum come into the operating field, the position of the patient can be adjusted to a steeper Trendelenburg position.

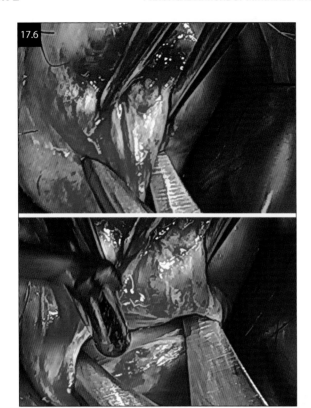

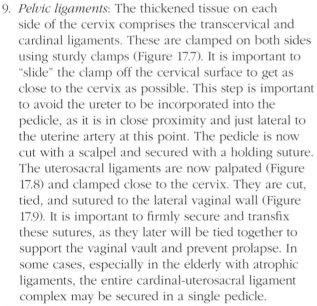

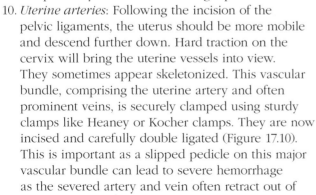

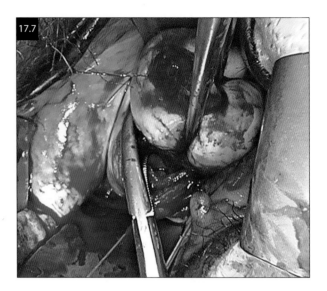

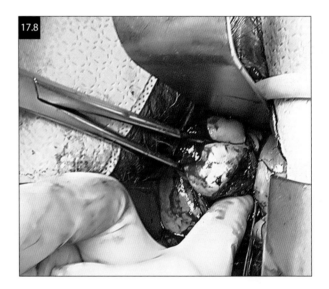

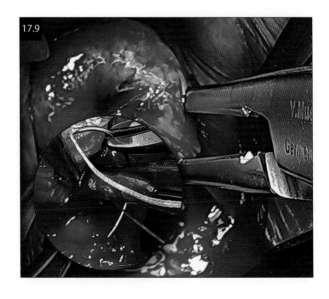

9. *Pelvic ligaments*: The thickened tissue on each side of the cervix comprises the transcervical and cardinal ligaments. These are clamped on both sides using sturdy clamps (Figure 17.7). It is important to "slide" the clamp off the cervical surface to get as close to the cervix as possible. This step is important to avoid the ureter to be incorporated into the pedicle, as it is in close proximity and just lateral to the uterine artery at this point. The pedicle is now cut with a scalpel and secured with a holding suture. The uterosacral ligaments are now palpated (Figure 17.8) and clamped close to the cervix. They are cut, tied, and sutured to the lateral vaginal wall (Figure 17.9). It is important to firmly secure and transfix these sutures, as they later will be tied together to support the vaginal vault and prevent prolapse. In some cases, especially in the elderly with atrophic ligaments, the entire cardinal-uterosacral ligament complex may be secured in a single pedicle.

10. *Uterine arteries*: Following the incision of the pelvic ligaments, the uterus should be more mobile and descend further down. Hard traction on the cervix will bring the uterine vessels into view. They sometimes appear skeletonized. This vascular bundle, comprising the uterine artery and often prominent veins, is securely clamped using sturdy clamps like Heaney or Kocher clamps. They are now incised and carefully double ligated (Figure 17.10). This is important as a slipped pedicle on this major vascular bundle can lead to severe hemorrhage as the severed artery and vein often retract out of

the field of view. These pedicles are not held by a holding suture.

Following the securing of the uterine vessels, a reevaluation of the surgical approach is done. The size of the uterus will determine if morcellation should be attempted or whether the fundus can be delivered through the pouch of Douglas or anterior UV space. A point of comfort is now reached in the knowledge that the major blood vessels to the uterus are now secured and that it is unusual to expect major or catastrophic hemorrhage as the surgery progresses. To illustrate this point, "bloodless" morcellation is often possible as blood supply to fibroids and other pathology are drastically reduced. If morcellation is required, it should be undertaken at this stage after the uterine vessels have been firmly secured. Depending on the pathology, enucleation of fibroids bivalving or coring may be necessary. The fundus can now be delivered through the posterior cul-de-sac (somersaulted) by traction on the fundus with a vulsellum or towel clamp. To facilitate this, it often helps to amputate the cervix. The ovarian ligament, round ligaments, and fallopian tubes are thus presented into the vagina to be secured. At this point, the final area of laparoscopic dissection is reached, and the uterus is freed and delivered vaginally. After the uterus has been removed from the pelvis, it is important to inspect the pelvis through the vaginal incision and to deal with any active bleeders. All the pedicles should be inspected including the major pedicles held by the holding sutures. At this point, if indicated, a McCall culdoplasty may be performed to elevate the vaginal vault. The vaginal incision is now closed in layers starting with the peritoneum.

11. *Closing the vaginal vault*: Ideally, a purse-string suture should now be placed in the peritoneum as it exteriorizes all the pedicles when tied. This suture is started posteriorly in the middle of the posterior vaginal wall, advancing through the right uterosacral

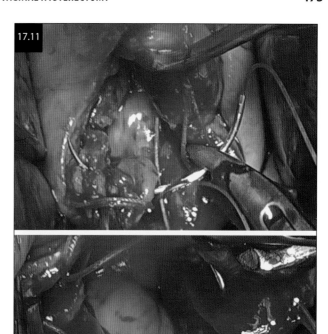

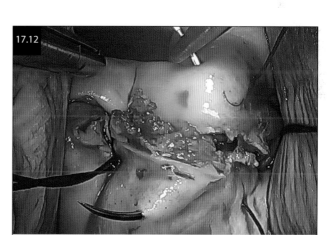

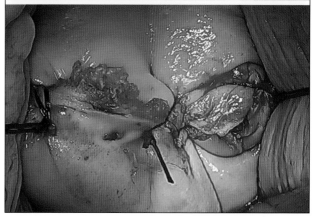

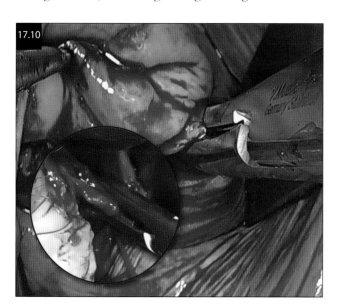

ligament complex up the right sidewall through the right round ligament complex. Then a few bites are taken through the bladder peritoneum before advancing the suture in a similar fashion down the left side to the original starting point.

Utmost care should be taken not to puncture the uterine artery when the purse-string suture is placed. The suture is now slowly and carefully pulled together and tied (Figure 17.11). At this stage, the holding sutures on US and cervical ligaments should be tied together. The holding sutures to the round ligaments/adnexal pedicle should be cut and not tied, as tying will bring the ovaries to the vaginal vault and cause dyspareunia. The vaginal wall is now closed using a Vicryl suture. The jury is still out on whether a horizontal or a vertical closure is best. Whatever is decided upon, make sure that good bites incorporating the full vaginal wall are taken (Figure 17.12).

12. An indwelling bladder catheter should now be placed, and the vagina may be packed with a long vaginal pack. Some surgeons perform a cystoscopy to inspect the integrity of the bladder and to ensure that the ureters have not been compromised.

SUGGESTED READING

King CR, Giles D. Total laparoscopic hysterectomy and laparoscopic-assisted vaginal hysterectomy. *Obstet Gynecol Clin North Am*. 2016;43(3):463–478.

Roy KK, Goyal M, Singla S, Sharma JB, Malhotra N, Kumar S. A prospective randomised study of total laparoscopic hysterectomy, laparoscopically assisted vaginal hysterectomy and non-descent vaginal hysterectomy for the treatment of benign diseases of the uterus. *Arch Gynecol Obstet*. 2011;284(4):907–912.

Sesti F, Cosi V, Calonzi F et al. Randomized comparison of total laparoscopic, laparoscopically assisted vaginal and vaginal hysterectomies for myomatous uteri. *Arch Gynecol Obstet*. 2014;290(3):485–491.

Shin JW, Lee HH, Lee SP, Park CY. Total laparoscopic hysterectomy and laparoscopy-assisted vaginal hysterectomy. *JSLS*. 2011;15(2):218–221.

Song T, Kim TJ, Kang H et al. A review of the technique and complications from 2,012 cases of laparoscopically assisted vaginal hysterectomy at a single institution. *Aust N Z J Obstet Gynaecol*. 2011;51(3):239–243.

CHAPTER 18

LAPAROSCOPIC SUPRACERVICAL HYSTERECTOMY

Jason Abbott

BACKGROUND

Surgical procedures, like so many other areas of our rapidly changing lives, respond to the rise and fall of fashion—and hysterectomy is a prime example of this. For the last century, whether to retain or remove the cervix at the time of hysterectomy has come and gone out of fashion, and the available scientific, rather than fashionable, evidence tells us that either is a reasonable option. Since the first description of laparoscopic supracervical hysterectomy (LSH) in 1991, this technique has had strong proponents and remains an excellent variant of hysterectomy. It is important to note both the technical aspects and the provision of a truly informed consent when discussing LSH with a woman. The LSH may be performed with a multiport, single-port (SILS), or robotic-assisted laparoscopic approach. Intraoperative technical considerations correspond to the level of cervical amputation and extraction of the corpus. Informed consent must include the possibility of ongoing intermittent vaginal bleeding, the need for continued cervical surveillance, the risk for reoperation for cervical prolapse, and the risk for various complications and outcomes that are now specifically known for LSH.

SELECTING THE WOMAN UNSUITABLE FOR A LSH

The indication for hysterectomy is an important consideration as to whether an LSH should be considered as an option. There are relatively few contraindications to LSH; however, gynecological malignancy should prompt cervical removal for most women—including the now heightened concern for leiomyosarcoma should this be known or suspected preoperatively. The heightened risk, albeit low, for recurrent disease after a history of cervical dysplasia should be frankly considered. LSH may be of limited value for women with chronic pelvic pain associated with collisional dyspareunia, as symptoms may persist if the cervix is not removed. The presence of pathology is also an important consideration, because retrocervical or paravaginal endometriosis, adenomyosis, or other cul-de-sac pathology in a woman with pelvic pain may lead to continued symptoms if the pelvic disease along with the cervix is not excised. Unless

the cervix will be retained as a surgical buttress for a concurrently performed sacrocervicopexy or other suspensory procedure in women with partial or complete uterovaginal prolapse, the risk for postoperative cervical prolapse should preclude LSH. Since amenorrhea cannot be guaranteed whenever the cervix is retained (see below for further discussion), LSH is contraindicated in women seeking eradication of their menstrual bleeding. For all other women, the choice of LSH is generally without contraindication and often requested after a balanced discussion about risks and benefits with her gynecological surgeon.

TECHNICAL CONSIDERATIONS

Whether employing conventional or robotically assisted laparoscopy, the technical approach for LSH is the same as for laparoscopic hysterectomy up to securing the uterine vessels (see Chapter 19).

There are three fundamental surgical steps during LSH:

1. Occlusion and transection of the uterine arteries
2. Transection of the uterine corpus
3. Tissue extraction of the uterine corpus

KEY STEPS TO REDUCE RISK DURING LSH

- The relationship between the uterine artery and the ureter, cervix, and uterine corpus should be noted (Figure 18.1).
- Since cervical preservation does not necessarily protect the ureter, it should be identified before any sidewall dissection and when securing the uterine vessels.
- The course of the ureter should be identified at the level of the pelvic brim before performing adnexectomy (Figure 18.2).
- The location of myoma(s) may have considerable impact on the capacity to complete the hysterectomy using a supracervical approach.
- With pathology that distorts the lower uterine segment, the uterine artery may be secured either via an anterior or posterior approach through the broad ligament and then secured either medial or lateral to the ureter (Figure 18.3).

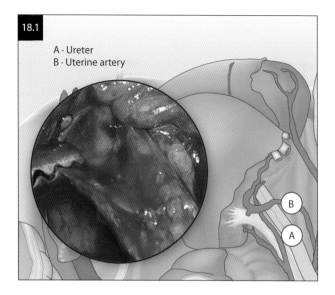

A · Ureter
B · Uterine artery

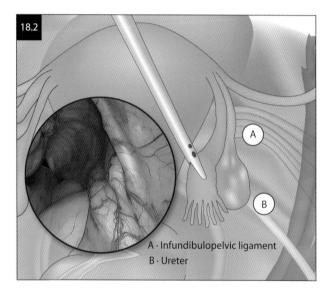

A · Infundibulopelvic ligament
B · Ureter

- The release of the posterior leaf of the broad ligament to allow the ureter to move inferiorly and laterally away from the cervix is required and will give further protection to the ureter (Figure 18.4).

- A large cervical myoma that requires removal of a substantial portion of the cervix may justify total hysterectomy as a better surgical alternative.

- In women having undergone cesarean delivery, the bladder may have been surgically advanced above the level of the internal os. Rather than employing blunt dissection, sharp dissection using mechanical scissors alone or with an energy-based surgical device combined with traction and countertraction may help reduce the risk for inadvertent bladder injury. Moreover, clarifying the pubocervical fascia anterior to the uterine vessels can be a dependable method to help identify the best surgical plane to initiate separation of the bladder from the lower uterine corpus.

- For the bladder that is adherent to the uterine body, the central component is typically the most affected. Backfilling through a Foley catheter may aid in determining its boundaries. Grasping the bladder with an atraumatic grasper to elevate anteriorly can help determine the proper dissection plane between it and the underlying pubocervical fascia (Figure 18.5). In this circumstance, a lateral approach to the bladder while noting the vascular bladder pillars during traction–countertraction along with sharp dissection may be another method to help reduce incidental cystotomy. A cervical colpotomy cup or tube can aid by placing upward traction on the tissue and provide additional landmarks to help mobilize the bladder downward along the lower corpus to the level of the internal os.

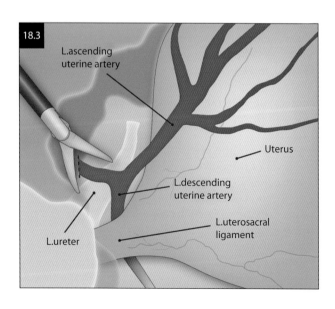

L.ascending
uterine artery

Uterus

L.descending
uterine artery

L.uterosacral
ligament

L.ureter

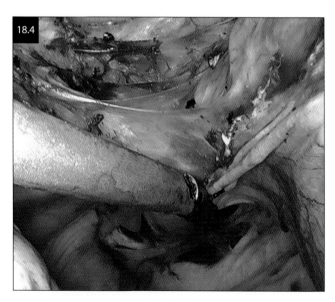

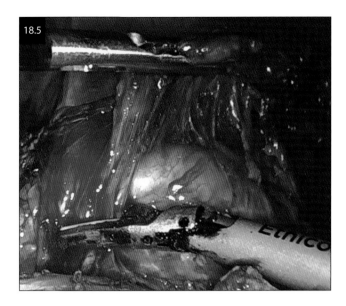

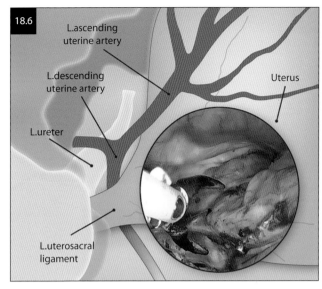

- Where pathology includes the bladder or there is concern about the integrity of the lower urinary tract, using a cystoscopic, oral or intravenous contrast agent will aid in the demonstration of any immediate damage. However, it may not prevent a delayed complication such as thermal injury from an energy source.

UTERINE AMPUTATION

After completing the procedure down to the level of the uterine vessels, it is important to consider where the uterus will be transected. To do this effectively, the following practical points should be considered:

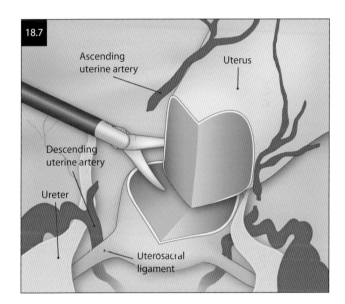

- Skeletonize the uterine vessels free of endopelvic tissue so that each vascular bundle may be clearly identified along the respective sides of the lower uterine corpus.
- Once the uterine arteries are secured by an energy source or suturing, there is no further need for vascular control of the uterus (Figure 18.6).
- Should there be bleeding from a uterine artery pedicle, the source of bleeding is more evident as it may be clearly visualized at the lower uterine corpus.
- If a uterine manipulator is being used, it is then generally removed at this time.
- If the uterine manipulator is left in place, the propensity for electrosurgical arcing with metal or liquefaction of plastic by ultrasonic energy must be considered during amputation.
- The uterus should be transected at or below the level of the internal os, ideally by fashioning a conical defect in reverse. As a general rule, always go with the goal to leave the cervix no more than 2 cm in length (Figure 18.7).
- The level of the internal os can always be interpolated by visualizing the nexus of the uterosacral ligaments with the posterior cervix.

- Transection of the cervix may be performed with "cold" instruments or with ultrasonic or electrosurgical instruments.
- There are specific electrosurgical loop devices that have been developed for amputation, decreasing the procedural time for fundal amputation by up to 80% (Figure 18.8).

PROCEDURES ON THE CERVIX TO REDUCE THE CHANCE OF BLEEDING

Despite a variety of methods to ablate or alter the endocervix, the simple fact remains that when the cervix is retained, there is always a chance of intermittent postoperative vaginal bleeding/spotting with a wide reported range of up to 37%. If bleeding occurs, the volume of vaginal loss is typically small and with minimal clinical

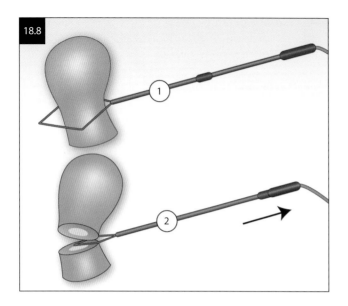

impact. The most important aspect of this outcome is that women should be preoperatively warned of this possibility following LSH. If the cervical epithelium is ablated using an energy source (bipolar or monopolar instrument, harmonics, or laser) (Figure 18.9), it is important that the energy be confined to the cervix to prevent advertent burning of the underlying vaginal epithelium. If using a monopolar or bipolar instrument, the cervix may be first palpated vaginally to determine when the instrument is through the endocervical canal, which is then retracted up into the canal before applying energy.

There is only one randomized controlled trial that has studied the impact of any adjunctive technique to the cervix in order to reduce postop intermittent vaginal bleeding. In this study, 140 women were randomized to LSH and reverse conization using a laparoscopic loop electrode ($n = 70$) or LSH without conization ($n = 70$). At 12 months postoperatively, there were no differences in vaginal bleeding rates, with 33% of women reporting vaginal bleeding without conization compared to 37%

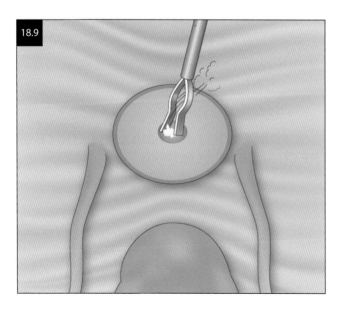

with conization. While the procedure of reverse cervical conization is a simple technical approach with a short procedure time (mean duration 61.9 seconds, SD 24.7%, 95% CI: 51–72.9) and no reported complications, it does not seem to reduce the chance of bleeding. Surgeons have also tried to predict the occurrence of post-LSH bleeding by taking endocervical biopsies of the cervical stump following amputation; this too is inaccurate, with no correlation between the histological findings of these biopsies and the clinical outcomes. In a large, retrospective series of 400 women treated by combination proprietary loop amputation device followed by electrosurgical coagulation of the cervical canal, only 2% of women reported intermittent postoperative vaginal bleeding.

THE CERVICAL STUMP

After the uterine corpus has been removed from the cervix and any additional cervical procedures are performed, the cervix may be focally coagulated with bipolar electrosurgery along the stump, peritoneal edges, or medial aspects of the uterine artery pedicles for any residual bleeding. Some surgeons elect to close the cervix with sutures based on custom and habit. The following technical considerations should be considered when suturing the cervical stump:

- Use an absorbable suture—either monofilament or braided.
- Ensure that the suture bites through the cervix posteriorly and anteriorly by the same margin to reduce the risk of bleeding from a missed cervical edge.
- Incorporate the canal into the suture line.
- For the bulky cervix, consider a two-layer closure with an imbricating initial suture to incorporate and invert the canal and a second layer to close the peritoneum posteriorly to the anterior cervical fascia and reduce any dead space within the cervix.
- If there is any prolapse, this should be addressed, since detachment of the pubocervical fascia, fascia of Denonvilliers, or laxity of the uterosacral ligaments may lead to prolapse even with the cervix retained.
- The cervix may be used as a central anchor point for any fascial defect with primary suture repair being a reasonable and low-risk approach.

REMOVAL OF THE UTERINE CORPUS

It is essential to remove the uterine corpus once it is transected from the cervix, and this may be achieved by a variety of surgical approaches. A more detailed account may be found in Chapter 14, which deals with tissue extraction. A posterior colpotomy has been described, as is simple mechanical morcellation with a scalpel or similar instrument through an enlarged abdominal port incision. This may be performed within a containment bag for reduction of any spilled material; however, the efficacy of containment to reduce malignant intraperitoneal seeding is not scientifically validated at this time. The introduction of electromechanical morcellators has substantially simplified tissue extraction at LSH with both reusable and single-use devices available. The tissue fragments may be removed through the morcellator body itself, through one of the existing abdominal ports, a posterior colpotomy, or by a transcervical uterine morcellator. Power morcellation within a containment bag is also described; however, this approach is no more validated than for mechanical morcellation performed in this manner, and risks must be weighed against benefit. There are no data to demonstrate superiority of any power morcellation approaches, and instrument and approach will depend on surgeon preference and availability. What is apparent is that all tissue fragments should be removed since retention may lead to substantial clinical sequelae (see discussion later in this chapter).

Safety and efficacy during electromechanical morcellation require strategic thinking and strict adherence to principles of best practice. Moreover, morcellation ideally requires a skilled assistant who is able to progressively feed tissue to the instrument while promoting safety from accidental visceral or vascular insult. Whereas morcellation is possible from any port site of sufficient diameter, it is commonly performed either transumbilically or suprapubically (Figure 18.10), since the distribution of parietal nerves perforating the rectus fascia results in less discomfort at the umbilical and midline suprapubic sites. Given that all current power morcellation devices are larger than 10 mm in diameter, any site lateral to the rectus sheath should be closed under direct laparoscopic vision, ideally with a fascial closure device to reduce the risk for postoperative hernia formation. Generally speaking, power morcellation may be safely and effectively performed using the following recommendations:

- Always keep the exposed blade clearly in view during morcellation.

- Maintain the depth of insertion by withdrawing tissue rather than advancing the morcellator (Figure 18.11).
- To facilitate more complete removal of tissue at primary extraction, the assistant should feed tissue into the morcellator.
- Using lateral port sites, align the shaft of the instrument as parallel as possible to the abdominal wall.
- Unless softened by degeneration, larger specimens are promoted by unpeeling rather than coring (Figure 18.12).

For *in situ* morcellation due to large leiomyomas, the following principles should be followed:

- Never morcellate leiomyomas prior to obliterating uterine blood supply.
- Perform hysterotomy parallel to the base of each leiomyoma.
- Always apply steady upward traction away from uterine corpus with a tenacious forceps.

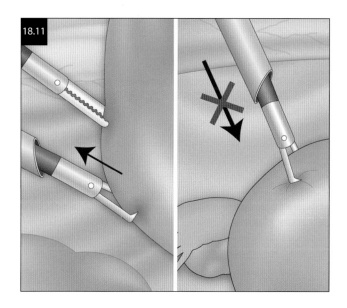

18.11

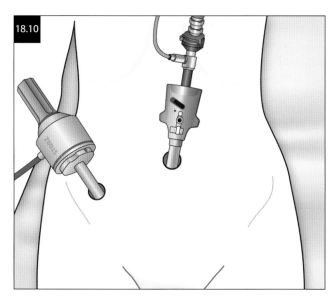

18.10

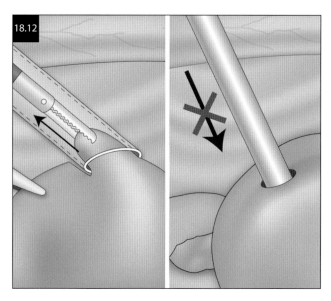

18.12

- Try to specifically target the interface between the myoma and uterus.
- Avoid this technique for low lateral or submucous leiomyomas.

More recently, the U.S. Food and Drug Administration has permitted the marketing of a new tissue containment system consisting of a containment bag and tubelike plunger for use with certain laparoscopic power morcellators to isolate uterine tissue that is not suspected to contain cancer. However, it has not been proven to reduce the risk of spreading cancer during these procedures. This device is intended for a limited patient population, with women who have been appropriately informed of the risks and are premenopausal and without uterine fibroids.

OUTCOMES FOLLOWING LSH

There are few clinical studies to compare the outcomes of LSH with other types of hysterectomy. One randomized controlled trial (RCT) reports no difference in blood loss or operative time for 71 women undergoing LSH compared with 70 undergoing total laparoscopic hysterectomy (TLH). From other data, there are no differences in complication rates or blood transfusions, with some studies reporting a statistical reduction in blood loss when LSH is undertaken and variable operative times that range from 47 to 181 minutes.

In a separate randomized study, 31 women randomized to LSH and 32 women to LAVH were followed for 6 months postoperatively with no difference reported in sexual function, pain, and psychological outcomes between the two techniques. Data from nonrandomized studies have suggested that LSH has less impact on sexual function compared with TLH with less vaginal pain, shortening and altered mucus production. It is likely that women undergoing LSH may return to vaginal intercourse sooner following surgery than women having TLH.

Theoretical advantages to bowel, bladder, and sexual function by performing LSH have not been borne out by studies, and these should not be claims made to women when considering this approach to hysterectomy.

GYNECOLOGICAL MALIGNANCY

A guideline produced by the American College of Obstetricians and Gynecologists recommends that for women with known or suspected gynecologic malignancy, current or recent cervical dysplasia, or endometrial hyperplasia, LSH should not be considered. This includes the risk of leiomyosarcoma, although it is recognized that this is difficult to diagnose preoperatively. In women who have had a LSH, the risk of cervical cancer remains very low at 0.1%–1.9%. A future risk of cervical cancer should not be a deterrent for women having a LSH with appropriate counseling, understanding that postoperative cervical surveillance remains essential.

For a woman who has undergone a LSH, there remains a risk of endometrial malignancy that is similarly increased if she takes unopposed estrogen. The rationale for hormone replacement therapy in a woman who has retained her cervix must be individualized, since there are no long-term data to support or refute any specific practice regarding potential benefit from including a progestin as part of her postmenopausal hormone replacement therapy.

COMPLICATIONS FOLLOWING LSH

It is important to note that nearly all complications that occur for laparoscopic hysterectomy are also reported for the LSH. There are few comparative studies, with only one RCT reported that shows no difference in complication rates, although the small number of just 141 women in total makes it unlikely that the study is sufficiently powered to detect a difference for many complications. Complication rates for LSH reported from other nonrandomized data range from 0% to 19%, with comparative retrospective data reporting comparable complication rates of laparoscopic total (1.59%) and supracervical hysterectomy (1.36%). Specific complications following LSH include a bladder injury risk in 0.25%–0.75% of cases, ureteral injuries in 0.19% of cases, and bowel injury in 0.2%–0.5% of cases. Together, these data suggest that LSH is no safer than other modes of hysterectomy, and this should not be suggested as a benefit of LSH.

MORCELLATION-ASSOCIATED COMPLICATIONS

Since retrieval of the uterine corpus is an integral component of the LSH, complications related to morcellation must be considered. Initial reports suggesting iatrogenic endometriosis may occur following morcellation do not appear to be more prevalent when compared to women who have other types of hysterectomy, where this pathology is also noted.

For women having LSH where myomas are the indication, and possibly for women without this initial pathology, there are rare reports of peritoneal leiomyomatosis demonstrated after morcellation. The true incidence is unknown, because a denominator for this practice is unavailable. It seems prudent clinical practice to remove all visible fragments of myometrium and myoma if morcellation is undertaken, and there are case reports of serious complications from retained tissue that include sepsis, subphrenic abscess, and bowel obstruction.

Should leiomyosarcoma be present at the time of morcellation following LSH, the malignancy is technically upstaged. It is unknown if dissemination is more likely to occur in this instance or the true impact on survival for this particularly aggressive form of malignancy.

PELVIC ORGAN PROLAPSE

It seems logical that keeping the pubocervical ring intact should decrease the rate of subsequent pelvic organ prolapse following LSH; however, there are no data to support this notion. Fascial defects may be present below the level of the cervical ring (such as uterosacral detachment, or fenestrations in the fascia of Denonvilliers) that may still result in pelvic organ prolapse if they are not specifically repaired at the time of the LSH. For women whose primary indication for surgery is prolapse, recurrence is more likely no matter what the approach of hysterectomy. Following LSH, there are case reports of cervical prolapse that was not present in the preoperative assessment. In summary, there is no evidence that LSH will protect against the future risk of pelvic organ prolapse.

SUGGESTED READING

American Association of Gynecologic Laparoscopists. AAGL practice report: Practice guidelines for laparoscopic subtotal/supracervical hysterectomy (LSH). *J Minim Invasive Gynecol.* 2014;21(1):9–16.

American College of Obstetricians and Gynecologists. ACOG Committee Opinion No. 388 November 2007: supracervical hysterectomy. *Obstet Gynecol.* [Practice Guideline]. 2007;110(5):1215–1217.

Berner E, Qvigstad E, Langebrekke A, Lieng M. Laparoscopic supracervical hysterectomy performed with and without excision of the endocervix: A randomized controlled trial. *J Minim Invasive Gynecol.* 2013;20(3):368–375.

Berner E, Qvigstad E, Myrvold AK, Lieng M. Pain reduction after total laparoscopic hysterectomy and laparoscopic supracervical hysterectomy among women with dysmenorrhoea: A randomised controlled trial. *BJOG.* 2015;122(8):1102–1111.

Bojahr B, De Wilde RL, Tchartchian G. Malignancy rate of 10,731 uteri morcellated during laparoscopic supracervical hysterectomy (LASH). *Arch Gynecol Obstet.* 2015;292(3):665–672.

Dequesne J, Schmidt N, Frydman R. A new electrosurgical loop technique for laparoscopic supracervical hysterectomy. *Gynaecol Endosc.* 1998;7(1):29–32.

Erian J, Hassan M, Pachydakis A, Chandakas S, Wissa I, Hill N. Efficacy of laparoscopic subtotal hysterectomy in the management of menorrhagia: 400 consecutive cases. *Obstet Gynecol Surv.* 2008;63(8):501–502.

Espen B, Qvigstad E, Langebrekke A, Lieng M. Laparoscopic supracervical hysterectomy performed with and without excision of the endocervix: A randomized controlled trial. *J Minim Invasive Gynecol.* 2013;20(3):368–375.

Flory N, Bissonnette F, Amsel RT, Binik YM. The psychosocial outcomes of total and subtotal hysterectomy: A randomized controlled trial. *J Sex Med.* 2006;3(3):483–491.

Lieng M, Berner E, Busund B. Risk of morcellation of uterine leiomyosarcomas in laparoscopic supracervical hysterectomy and laparoscopic myomectomy, a retrospective trial including 4791 women. *J Minim Invasive Gynecol.* 2015;22(3):410–414.

Lieng M, Qvigstad E, Istre O, Langebrekke A, Ballard K. Long-term outcomes following laparoscopic supracervical hysterectomy. *BJOG.* 2008;115(13):1605–1610.

Morelli M, Noia R, Chiodo D et al. Laparoscopic supracervical hysterectomy versus laparoscopic total hysterectomy: A prospective randomized study. Isterectomia sopracervicale laparoscopica versus isterectomia totale laparoscopica: Studio prospettico randomizzato. *Minerva Ginecol.* 2007;59(1):1–10.

Nesbitt-Hawes EM, Maley PE, Won HR et al. Laparoscopic subtotal hysterectomy: Evidence and techniques. *J Minim Invasive Gynecol.* 2013;20(4):424–434.

Ordulu Z, Dal Cin P, Chong WWS et al. Disseminated peritoneal leiomyomatosis after laparoscopic supracervical hysterectomy with characteristic molecular cytogenetic findings of uterine leiomyoma. *Genes Chromosomes Cancer.* 2010;49(12):1152–1160.

Schuster MW, Wheeler TL, 2nd, Richter HE. Endometriosis after laparoscopic supracervical hysterectomy with uterine morcellation: A case control study. *J Minim Invasive Gynecol.* 2012;19(2):183–187.

CHAPTER 19

TOTAL LAPAROSCOPIC HYSTERECTOMY

Nicole M. Donnellan and Ted Lee

BACKGROUND

Approximately 600,000 hysterectomies are performed in the United States each year, making it the second most common major operation that women undergo. Nearly one-third of all women in the United States will have a hysterectomy by the time they turn 60 years of age, with the most common indication being symptomatic fibroids. Historically performed through an abdominal approach, improvements in technology and training have led to a steady increase in the number of hysterectomies performed laparoscopically. The first laparoscopic hysterectomy was performed by Dr. Harry Reich in 1988, and since that time nearly 15% of all hysterectomies for benign disease in the United States are performed in this minimally invasive manner.

Professional societies advocate for the use of minimally invasive techniques for hysterectomy when safe and appropriate owing to the decreased morbidity compared to an abdominal approach. The American Congress of Obstetricians and Gynecologists states that "vaginal hysterectomy is the approach of choice whenever feasible," and that "laparoscopic hysterectomy is an alternative to abdominal hysterectomy for those patients in whom a vaginal hysterectomy is not indicated or feasible." Advantages of laparoscopic hysterectomy over the traditional abdominal approach are numerous and include improved intraoperative visualization of anatomy, shorter postoperative hospital stays, decreased postoperative pain, and improved cosmesis with smaller incisions. Drawbacks include the steep learning curve in mastering laparoscopic suturing and advanced dissections, as well as the associated costs of disposable instruments.

The decision to perform a hysterectomy through a laparoscopic approach is made when enlarged, distorted anatomy precludes the vaginal approach or preoperative concern for pathology necessitates a thorough examination of the pelvis. Relative indications include the need to evaluate pelvic pain, perform adhesiolysis, excise endometriosis, perform adnexal surgery, manage extremely large uteri distorted by fibroids, and perform lymphadenectomy when concerned about malignancy. There are very few contraindications to laparoscopy. Absolute contraindications include medical comorbidities that preclude general anesthesia and patient positioning as well as known malignancy when morcellation of the specimen is necessitated for retrieval. A contraindication is insufficient surgical training and experience.

A total laparoscopic hysterectomy (TLH) is performed entirely through a laparoscopic approach, including colpotomy and cuff closure.

INTRAOPERATIVE CONSIDERATIONS

OPERATING ROOM SETUP AND EQUIPMENT

Prior to entering the operating room, it is imperative to check that all necessary equipment for safe and efficient completion of the case is present and functioning. One should ensure that basic laparoscopic equipment, including camera and light source, are functioning, power sources for monopolar and bipolar instruments are connected, and an ample source of CO_2 gas is available. Further, the operating room table should be positioned such that it permits placement of tower and/or television screens that optimize surgeon ergonomics (Figure 19.1). When only one screen is available, placement should be between the patient's legs at surgeon eye level. If two screens are available, placement should be just lateral to each lower extremity, with the surgeon utilizing the contralateral screen to prevent neck strain.

The surgeon should also confirm the presence of necessary laparoscopic instruments, including atraumatic graspers, electrosurgical monopolar and bipolar instruments, a suction irrigator, needle holder and grasper, ports, and a uterine manipulator. Both 5 and 10 mm 0° laparoscopes should be available. Access to 30° and 45° laparoscopes is also recommended to assist in cases of large fibroids and distorted anatomy. Placement of laparoscopes in heated sterile water to 120°F prior to the start of the surgery greatly assists in fog prevention. Depending on the nature of the case, a morcellator, cystoscopy equipment, clip appliers, and vaginal/rectal probes should also be accessible.

PATIENT POSITIONING

Upon entry into the operating room, the patient should have sequential compressive devices placed and activated. Following induction of general anesthesia, an orogastric tube is placed to decompress the stomach. Once tubes and IVs are secured, the patient should be positioned by the surgical team in low lithotomy utilizing Allen stirrups

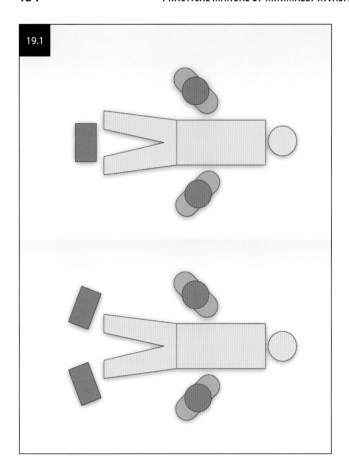

of the Allen stirrups aids in the ability to transition to high lithotomy in a sterile fashion. This position may be required for placement of the uterine manipulator and other vaginal instruments as well as for performing cystoscopy.

Patient arms are tucked on both sides in a neutral position using foam padding to prevent injury to the ulnar nerve (Figure 19.3). Tucking the arms creates a more ergonomic field for the surgeon and helps prevent brachial plexus injury. Any protruding IV tubing should be padded with 4×4 gauze pads prior to tucking the arms to minimize undue pressure at these sites. Bean bags or gel pads can be utilized to prevent patients from sliding during steep Trendelenburg position. A grounding dispersive electrode is placed on a lower extremity for monopolar instrumentation.

The abdomen is then prepped, followed by the perineum and vagina. A sterile drape with access to the vagina should be used. After placement of the Foley catheter, a uterine manipulator is placed. A manipulator with articulating ability is preferred for optimal assistance during the case (Figure 19.4). There are a number of manipulators on the market such as Pelosi (Cooper Surgical), RUMI (Cooper Surgical), V-Care (Covidien), and Clermon Ferrand (Karl Storz Endoscopy). Further, a manipulator with a colpotomizer cup is recommended for a total laparoscopic hysterectomy.

(Figure 19.2). The heel should be placed flush with the base of the stirrup, avoiding pressure on the common peroneal nerve, which runs parallel to the lateral head of the fibula making it prone to pressure injury. The lower extremities should be positioned with an approximately 45° flexion at the knee, and maintenance of this degree of flexion should be checked repeatedly throughout the case, as even slight patient migration may lead to leg straightening. While the laparoscopic portion of the case is performed with the patient in low lithotomy, the use

LAPAROSCOPIC ENTRY

Regardless of mode of entry, knowledge of the anatomy of the anterior abdominal wall is paramount for safe placement of laparoscopic trocars. Extra caution must be taken in thin patients, as the great vessels will be within centimeters of the umbilicus. Further, patients should *not* be placed in the Trendelenburg position during Veress needle and umbilical trocar placement, as this rotates the angle of the sacrum and great vessels anterior, making these structures more prone to injury at time of entry.

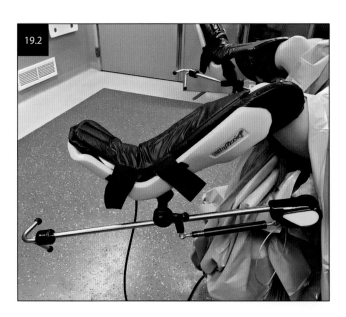

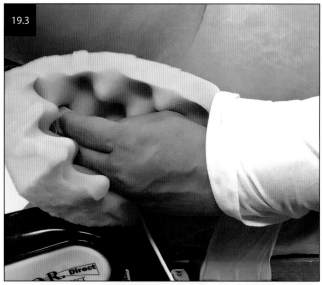

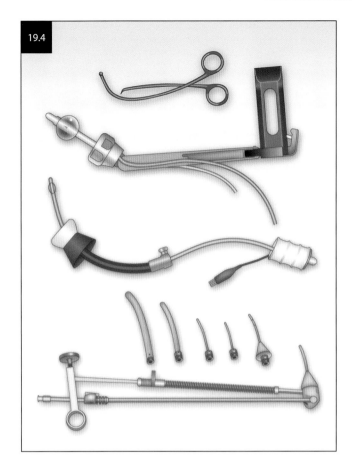

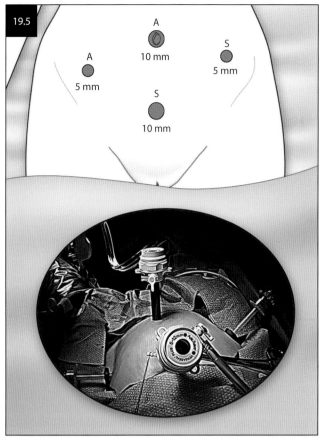

Following confirmation of access into the peritoneal cavity, pneumoperitoneum with CO_2 25 mm Hg should be obtained. After examining the area immediately below the location of entry to confirm no inadvertent injury, the patient is placed in Trendelenburg position. This position allows for optimal visualization of the pelvis, making use of gravity to displace the bowel from the posterior cul-de-sac. Accessory trocars are then placed under direct visualization. Lateral ports should be placed lateral to the inferior epigastric vessels, but medial and superior to the anterior superior iliac spine. The epigastric vessels can often be visualized laparoscopically lateral to the medial umbilical ligament, which is seen as a prominent peritoneal fold on either side of midline. A suprapubic port should be placed above the upper margin of the bladder, located approximately one-third of the distance between the pubic symphysis and the umbilicus (Figure 19.5).

FUNDAMENTAL STEPS OF A TOTAL LAPAROSCOPIC HYSTERECTOMY

Following placement of the uterine manipulator, Foley catheter, and trocars, the surgeon should work with the anesthesia team to ensure maximum Trendelenburg positioning. There are surgeons who do not advocate use of the uterine manipulator, but in our opinion, the uterine manipulator enables better uterine manipulation, and the addition of the colpotomy cup facilitates easier and safer colpotomy, especially for novice surgeons. It is imperative to take time at the start of the case to optimize visualization of the pelvis in order to facilitate a safe and efficient surgical procedure. If the bowel still limits adequate visualization after achieving Trendelenburg, the colon can be further mobilized cephalad by lysing the pericolic reflection of the rectosigmoid colon to the pelvic brim. If visualization is still unsatisfactory, the bowel can be deflected laterally by placing a suture through several epiploica and suspending the suture up through the left lower quadrant port. An effort should be made to identify the ureter at the pelvic brim and to follow it all the way down toward uterosacral ligaments. This can be achieved in the majority of patients.

It is important to keep in mind that normal anatomy should be restored first, which means taking down all adhesions of the omentum, bowel, and ovaries before starting the hysterectomy. The easy side should be done first to make sure that at least one uterine artery is coagulated, minimizing blood supply to the uterus.

A 10 mm 0° laparoscope can be used to complete most hysterectomies, and a 10 mm 30° laparoscope can be utilized when dealing with large fibroids and distorted anatomy. The right-handed surgeon stands on the patient's left side, operating through the left lower quadrant and suprapubic ports. The assistant drives the camera through the umbilical port and uses the right lower quadrant port for passage of surgical instruments. Prior to commencing the surgery, one should identify the ureter transperitoneally at the pelvic brim and trace its

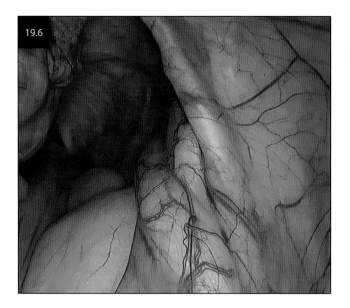

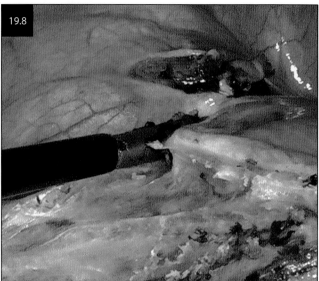

course into the pelvis. The path of the ureters should be constantly confirmed throughout the case (Figure 19.6).

The following steps outline a fundamental approach to a total laparoscopic hysterectomy. Variations to the sequence of these steps are often needed to overcome difficult pathology.

Step 1: Transecting the round ligament
Although some surgeons prefer to start the hysterectomy at the upper pedicles, we prefer to start by identifying the round ligament. The round ligament is grasped and tented upward. To avoid bleeding, the round ligament should be coagulated and transected laterally, making use of an avascular portion of the broad ligament (Figure 19.7).

Step 2: Developing the bladder flap
Using the manipulator, the uterus is placed in a retroverted position. The assistant can improve visualization of the anterior cul-de-sac with gentle downward traction on the uterine corpus. The anterior leaf of the

broad ligament is grasped at the laterally transected portion of the round ligament (Figure 19.8). Upward traction at this location permits CO_2 gas to dissect under the peritoneum and assists in increasing the distance between the peritoneum and underlying structures. A peritoneal incision is then made in the anterior leaf of the broad ligament, aiming toward the level of the colpotomizer cup. Once reaching the level of the cup, the incision is then curved upward to the contralateral round ligament.

Once the peritoneal incision is completed, the bladder is mobilized off the cervix and vagina. Bladder tissue is gently elevated to provide adequate countertraction (Figure 19.9). Identification of the endopelvic fascia confirms the correct vesicouterine plane. Using the colpotomizer cup as a landmark, blunt and sharp dissection is performed to ensure all bladder fibers are dropped well below the cervicovaginal junction (Figure 19.10). Care should be taken to avoid lateral dissection in order to minimize bleeding from the uterine vessels.

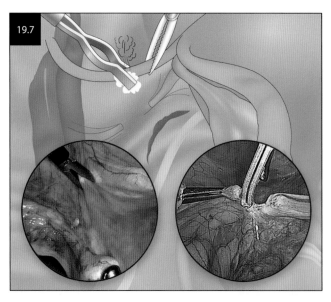

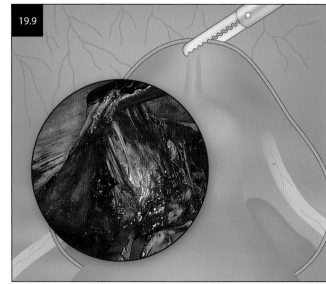

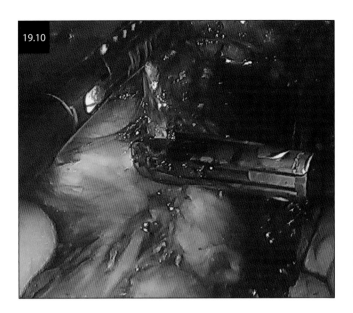

Step 3: Securing the upper pedicles

Optimal exposure to secure the upper pedicles is achieved by manipulating the uterus into a neutral, mid-position, with deviation to the contralateral side. Whether performing a salpingo-oophorectomy or conserving the ovaries, it is helpful to create a window in an avascular portion of the posterior leaf of the broad ligament. This window is made inferior to the vasculature of the upper pedicles but superior to the ureter (Figure 19.11). Creation of a window allows for isolation of the pedicle, which improves

hemostasis and ensures that the ureter is not included in the pedicle. If performing a salpingo-oophorectomy, the surgeon can secure the infundibulopelvic ligament at this point in time, and the ovary and fallopian tube are detached from the pelvic sidewall (Figure 19.12). If the ovaries are preserved, the uteroovarian ligament is coagulated and transected. When securing these upper pedicles, it is also important to avoid the cornual region of the uterus, as significant bleeding can occur (Figure 19.13). When preserving the ovaries, many surgeons prefer removal of the fallopian tubes during hysterectomy. The fallopian tubes are grasped and elevated, and the coagulation is performed along the mesosalpinx until the uterus is reached (Figure 19.14).

Step 4: Skeletonizing the uterine vessels

After anteverting the uterus with the manipulator, the assistant should gently grasp the round ligament stump to provide exposure to the posterior cul-de-sac (Figure 19.15). It is imperative that the assistant keeps the uterus

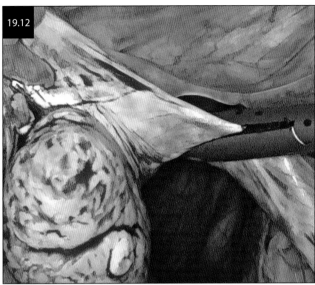

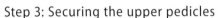

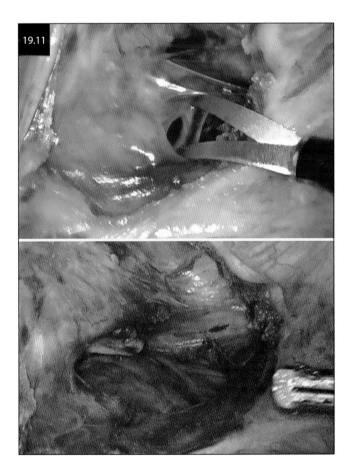

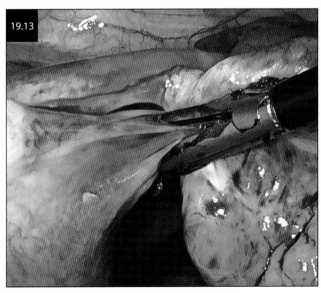

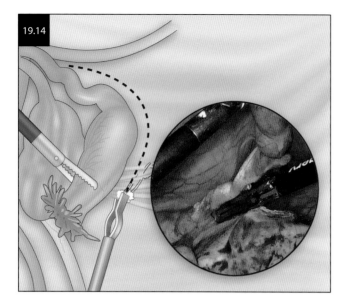

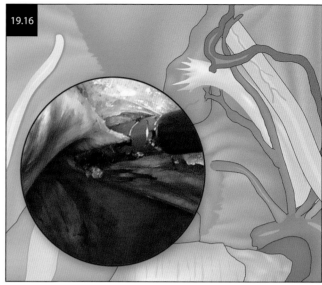

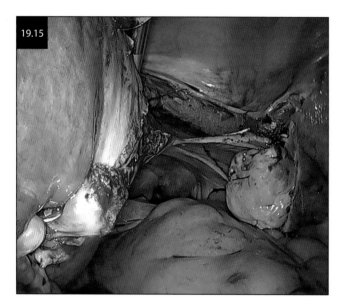

in appropriate anatomic location and does not "twist" the uterus to a more anterior or posterior location. Instructing the assistant to keep the round ligaments at 3 and 9 o'clock locations easily conveys this desired orientation.

The posterior leaf of the broad ligament is transected to the level of the ipsilateral uterosacral ligament, which is easily delineated by the superior margin of the colpotomizer cup (Figure 19.16). This dissection isolates the uterine artery at the level of the internal cervical os, ultimately allowing for the uterine artery to be secured in a more hemostatic manner without including the posterior peritoneum. In addition, by dropping the posterior leaf of the broad ligament, the ureter is also dropped, increasing its distance from the uterine artery pedicle.

Similar to the open approach, the uterine artery can then be further skeletonized. The areolar tissue surrounding the vessels is divided and retracted in a caudad direction.

Step 5: Securing the uterine vessels

Maintaining exposure as described above, the uterine vessels are coagulated at the level of the internal os with a bipolar instrument or advanced vessel-sealing device. Similar to the technique employed in open surgery with a Heaney clamp, it is critical to bounce off the cervix to ensure that all medial branches of the uterine artery are secured. If the uterine vessel is large, an atraumatic grasper can first be used to compress or "format" the pedicle such that the vessel-sealing device can be applied to the entire pedicle (Figure 19.17).

The colpotomizer cup serves as a landmark to delineate the level of the internal os. The ascending branch of the uterine artery should be coagulated superior to this location. Applying energy or sutures to any location lateral and inferior may place the ureter at risk of injury. To further minimize risk of injury to the ureter, the uterine manipulator should be under constant upward (cephalic) pressure to increase the distance between the ureter and uterine artery.

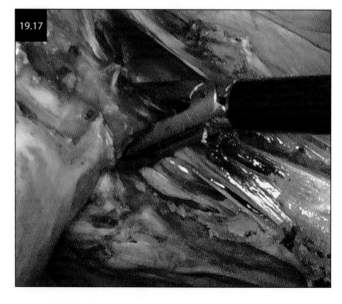

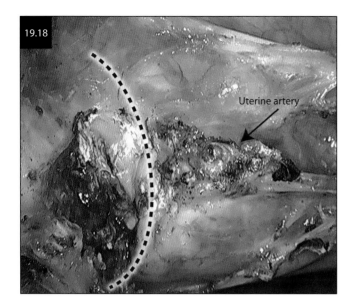

The uterine artery pedicle should then be further dissected and lateralized by coagulating and transecting the tissue medial to the artery. This dissection drops the uterine artery pedicle just lateral and inferior off of the colpotomizer cup (Figure 19.18). This ensures that the endopelvic fascia is cleared of any major vasculature when making the colpotomy.

Step 6: Creating the colpotomy

The creation of a colpotomy is greatly facilitated by the use of a colpotomizer cup. Every effort should be made to preserve the uterosacral ligament insertion to the paracervical ring to prevent further vaginal prolapse.

The colpotomy can be initiated anteriorly or in a posterior location above the uterosacral ligaments (Figure 19.19). Colpotomy can be performed using ultrasonic energy, monopolar scissors, or a monopolar hook electrode. When using monopolar energy, a pure cutting current at 50 watt setting should be employed. Continued repositioning of the uterine manipulator optimizes visualization for safe completion of the colpotomy (Figure 19.20). The assistant can provide countertraction on the uterus to delineate the edge of the cup when encountering thicker tissue. The cutting electrode should be exchanged between the lower ports to optimize angles and exposure for a safe transection.

Once the colpotomy is completed, the uterine specimen can be delivered through the vagina. If the specimen is too large, it can be morcellated (either manually through a vaginal approach or mechanically through an abdominal approach).

Step 7: Closing the vaginal cuff

A glove containing a Kerlix sponge is placed in the vagina, knot end first, to maintain pneumoperitoneum. There are several ways to close the vaginal cuff, and techniques are surgeon dependent. The cuff can be closed with interrupted figure-of-8 extracorporeal suturing or continuous intracorporeal running stitch. Some

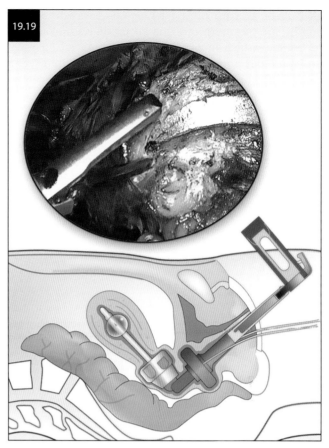

surgeons advocate vertical cuff closure for achieving longer vaginal length. The choice of suture is almost always absorbable or delayed absorbable suture with CT-1 or GS-21 needle. Regardless of what technique is used, care must be taken to incorporate the uterosacral ligaments into the vaginal cuff if the ligaments were detached during the colpotomy procedure.

The authors prefer to suture bilateral vaginal angles using a monofilament delayed absorbable suture (such

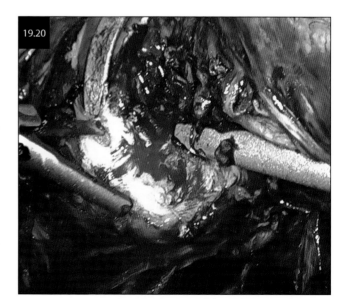

as PDS or Maxon) on a CT-1 or GS-21 needle. These angles are secured utilizing a modified Richardson technique, which incorporates the uterosacral ligament and provides improved hemostasis. The sutures can be brought up as "stay" sutures through the bilateral lower quadrant ports. This technique elevates the cuff and better delineates anatomy, making closure easier (Figure 19.21).

The vaginal cuff is then closed in a transverse fashion using interrupted, figure-of-8, continuous running or barbed suture techniques (Figure 19.22). Sutures can be tied down in an intra- or extracorporeal fashion or secured utilizing a Lapra-Ty device. Regardless of method, sutures should be placed approximately 1 cm apart. Depth of each throw should be approximately 1 cm, ensuring that adequate bites of endopelvic fascia are obtained, and vaginal mucosa is reapproximated.

VARIATIONS IN TOTAL LAPAROSCOPIC HYSTERECTOMY: OVERCOMING DIFFICULT ANATOMY

While a step-wise, systematic approach to a total laparoscopic hysterectomy is advocated, surgeons may encounter pathology that requires alternative approaches to overcome difficult anatomy.

Alternative entry via a left upper quadrant approach

Morbidly obese patients, patients with suspected adhesions, prior abdominal surgeries or abdominal wall hernia repairs, or large bulky pathology extending above the pelvic brim are at increased risk of visceral injury when entry is performed at the umbilicus. Such patients are best served with entry in the left upper quadrant at Palmer point. This location, below the left costal margin in the midclavicular line, provides a means of avoiding midline pathology. Surgeons, however, must be aware of the underlying structures at this location, which include the stomach, spleen, left lobe of the liver, pancreas, and transverse colon (see Chapter 5).

Alternative trocar placement

Enlarged fibroid uteri or unexpected dense pelvic adhesions can make visualization at the umbilicus difficult. In such cases, after achieving entry at the umbilicus, placement of a midline supraumbilical port approximately 5–10 cm above the umbilicus can greatly improve visualization (Figure 19.23). This alternative trocar can serve as an optical port providing a more distant, "global" view of the pelvis. In cases of extremely large uteri, lateral trocars should remain in the same location. The surgeon can use the umbilical port in place of a suprapubic port. With this alternative port placement, midline trocars are simply shifted upward, but operative techniques and approaches are akin to traditional placement. If instrument length limits safe operating in the case of a deep pelvis, a traditional suprapubic port can be placed to complete the procedure.

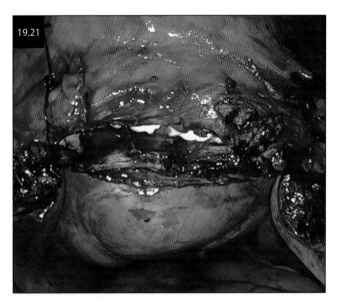

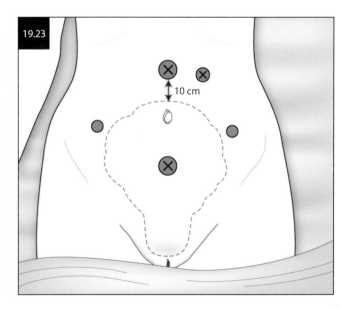

Even with placement of alternative trocars, visualization may still be suboptimal with large, bulky uteri. Further, manipulation of a large uterus is often extremely limited with a uterine manipulator. A suction irrigator placed through the suprapubic port can be used to manipulate the uterus to the contralateral side and greatly improves exposure. The same can be done by using a 5 mm single-tooth laparoscopic grasper or myoma screw to gently retract the uterus (Figure 19.24). Furthermore, the use of 30° and 45° angled laparoscopes can also assist in optimizing visualization.

Securing the uterine artery at the origin

Access to the ascending branch of the uterine artery may be limited by pathology. Large bulky fibroids or extensive fibrosis from endometriosis or prior surgeries can make the traditional approach to coagulation and transection of the ascending uterine artery unsafe or even impossible. In such situations, ligation of the uterine artery at its origin off the internal iliac artery facilitates safe completion of the hysterectomy.

Knowledge of the retroperitoneal anatomy, including the gynecologic pararectal space and the paravesical space, is paramount to performing this dissection. These two spaces can be depicted as triangles that share a common base represented by the uterine artery. The lateral border of the paravesical space is represented by the median umbilical ligament (obliterated umbilical artery that represents the terminal branch of the internal iliac), and the bladder represents the medial border. The gynecologic pararectal space is defined by the internal iliac laterally and the ureter medially.

The origin of the uterine artery can reliably be located by two approaches. The first approach utilizes the identification of the median umbilical ligament as it courses off of the anterior abdominal wall. Gentle upward and lateral traction of this ligament facilitates dissection deep into the retroperitoneal space. Dissecting along the median umbilical ligament, with good countertraction by the assistant, allows for easy identification of the uterine at its origin (Figure 19.25). A second approach starts with entry into the retroperitoneum at the pelvic brim. The ureter is identified as it courses over the brim along the posterior leaf of the broad ligament. Blunt dissection of the areolar tissue medial to the ureter assists in developing the gynecologic pararectal space. Continuing this blunt dissection in a caudad direction, the uterine artery is identified as it crosses over the ureter (Figure 19.26). Careful dissection laterally ultimately allows for identification of the uterine artery at the origin off the internal iliac artery.

Alternative techniques for developing the bladder flap

Dense adhesions owing to prior cesarean sections can make a traditional approach to the development of the bladder flap difficult. Thick fibrotic tissue alters surgical planes, and identification of the vesicouterine plane can be challenging. In such situations, limits of the bladder can be delineated by backfilling the bladder using irrigation fluid. Further, a uterine sound can be passed transurethrally and gently advanced to demarcate the superior border of the bladder.

Even when anatomy is well delineated, dense adhesions can greatly increase the risk of cystotomy with a traditional midline and superior approach to bladder flap development. At the time of cesarean section, bladder flap dissection occurs in a medial location,

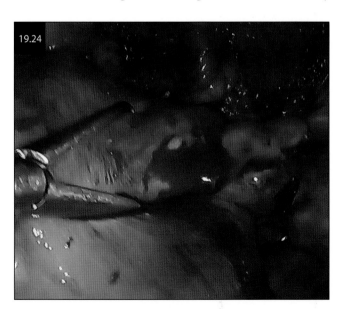

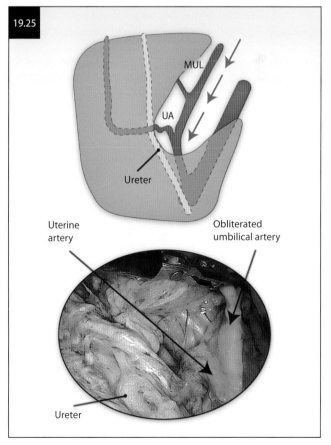

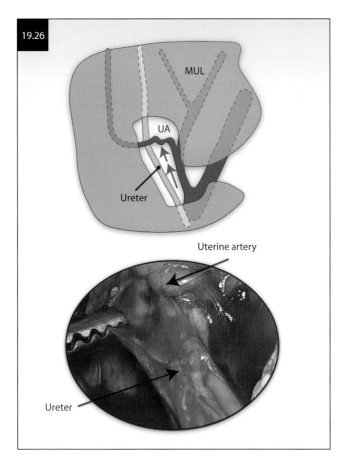

19.26

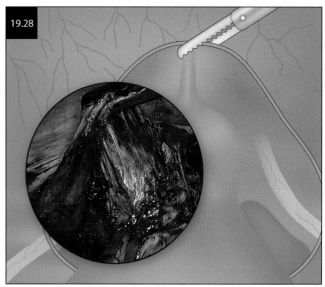

19.28

from a lateral location toward a medial location. An additional trick is to grasp the bladder with the laparoscopic grasper and place it on stretch, which will allow us to identify the plane between scarred bladder and the uterus (Figure 19.28).

Alternative technique for creating the colpotomy

In cases of enlarged uteri, visualization deep in the pelvis may be greatly impaired, making the traditional approach to colpotomy creation difficult and unsafe. In such situations, use of a 30° laparoscope can be helpful or in such cases the uterine corpus can be amputated at the level of the internal os (similar to the supracervical approach) with monopolar energy on a pure cutting current. A uterine manipulator with an obturator (and not a colpotomizer cup) best facilitates this technique. The assistant can gently elevate the cervix by passing an instrument posteriorly, to maximize distance between the cervix and underlying structures in the cul-de-sac. When the cervix is transected through to the canal and the obturator is visualized, the manipulator is removed. At this point, the assistant can grasp the lower uterine segment and reflect it back to optimize exposure to complete amputation of the posterior cervix. Following amputation, a colpotomizer cup is placed, and the colpotomy can be performed as described above to remove the remainder of the cervix.

In patients with previous conizations, flushed cervices, or small nulliparous cervices, anatomy often precludes placement of manipulators with a colpotomizer cup. A sponge stick or Scheiden vaginal retractors can be inserted vaginally to delineate the vesicovaginal junction in order to perform the colpotomy (Figure 19.29). Alternatively, a blue suction bulb on a sponge stick (used in labor and delivery for a baby's nasal suction) can be inserted vaginally. The blue bulb delineates the vagina clearly and serves as a guide to safely perform a colpotomy (Figure 19.30).

and resultant adhesions often favor a midline, superior location near the hysterotomy site. Initiating a dissection lower and more lateral to this location assists in identifying virgin endopelvic fascia underneath the bladder, which may be tethered up high to the lower uterine segment (Figure 19.27). Once endopelvic fascia is identified, the bladder can be more easily identified and isolated off of the lower uterine segment. The best way to free the bladder is to start the dissection

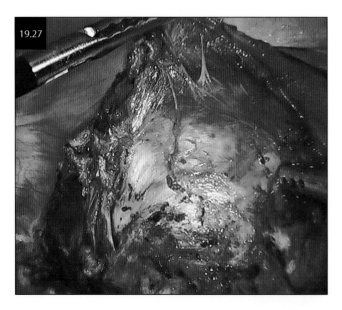

19.27

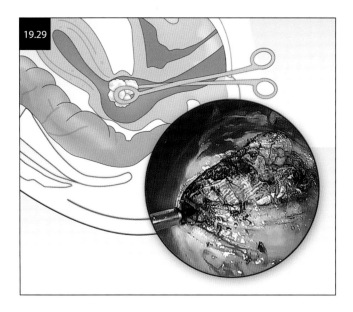

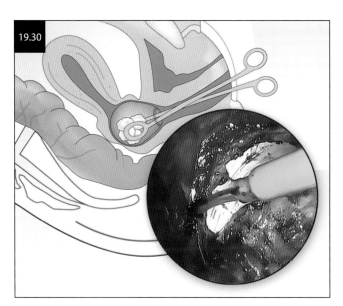

SUGGESTED READING

AAGL. AAGL position statement: Route of hysterectomy to treat benign disease. *J Minim Invasive Gynecol.* 2011;18(1):1–5.

ACOG. ACOG Committee Opinion No. 444: Choosing the route of hysterectomy for benign disease. *Obstet Gynecol.* 2009;114(5):1156–1158.

Cohen S, Einarsson J. Total and supracervical hysterectomy. *Obstet Gynecol Clin North Am.* 2011;38:651–661.

Johnson N, Barlow D, Lethaby A, Tavender E, Curr E, Garry R. Surgical approach to hysterectomy for benign gynecological disease. *Cochrane Database Syst Rev.* 2006;19(2):CD003677.

King C, Giles D. Total laparoscopic hysterectomy and laparoscopic-assisted vaginal hysterectomy. *Obstet Gynecol Clin North Am.* 2016;43:463–478.

Rahn DD, Phelan JN, Roshanravan SM, White AB, Corton MM. Anterior abdominal wall nerve and vessel anatomy: Clinical implications for gynecologic surgery. *Am J Obstet Gynecol.* 2010;202(3):e1–e5.

Reich H, DeCaprio J, McGlynn F. Laparoscopic hysterectomy. *J Gynecol Surg.* 1989;5:213–216.

Sandberg E, Twinjstra A, Driesse S, Jansen F. Total laparoscopic hysterectomy versus vaginal hysterectomy: A systematic review and meta-analysis. *J Minim Invasive Gynecol.* 2017;24:206–217.

Uccella S, Cromi A, Serati M, Casarin J, Sturla D, Ghezzi F. Laparoscopic hysterectomy in case of uteri weighting >1 kilogram: A series of 71 cases and review of the literature. *J Minim Invasive Gynecol.* 2014;21:460–465.

Xu Y, Wang Q, Wang F. Previous cesarean section and risk of urinary tract injury during laparoscopic hysterectomy: A meta-analysis. *Int Urogynecol J.* 2015;26:1269–1275.

CHAPTER 20

RETROPERITONEAL DISSECTION OF THE PELVIC SIDEWALL

Grace M. Janik

LAPAROSCOPIC SURGICAL ANATOMY

Anatomy is a constant, but its appearance varies based on how it is visualized and approached. Laparoscopy offers some distinct advantages in identifying anatomy during retroperitoneal dissection of the pelvic sidewall and cul-de-sac, areas that are particularly difficult to visualize while performing a laparotomy. During laparoscopy, the continuous illumination and magnification enable detailed identification and microdissection of tissue planes and vital structures. Visualization is further enhanced by the pneumoperitoneum, which reduces bleeding during dissection and improves avascular dissection. The disadvantages of laparoscopy are the fixed visual angles and the conversion of a three-dimensional pelvis to a two-dimensional image. While these limitations may prolong the learning curve of laparoscopy, they do not negate its significant advantages in retroperitoneal dissection.

Surgical anatomy emphasizes the clinically relevant aspects of anatomy that are essential for safe, efficient surgery. Knowledge of the anatomy of the pelvic brim and the three levels of the pelvic sidewall is required for retroperitoneal dissection (see Chapter 2). Special emphasis should be placed on the ureter, as it is the most frequently injured structure in gynecological surgery. A firm understanding of the ureter's path through the pelvis to the bladder is critical, especially its relationship to the pelvic vasculature. The ureter enters the pelvic cavity at the pelvic brim by crossing anterior to the bifurcation of the common iliac artery and just below the ovarian vessels of the infundibulopelvic ligament. The right ureter usually crosses over the external iliac, whereas the left ureter tends to run more medial and crosses over the common iliac. The anatomy at the pelvic brim pushes the ureter anteriorly with minimal connective tissue between the ureter and peritoneum, making this the most consistent location for identification of the ureter, particularly with severe pelvic disease or obesity (Figure 20.1). The ureter then courses in the medial leaf of the broad ligament toward the bladder, entering the cardinal ligament approximately 2 cm medial to the ischial spine and 2 cm lateral to the uterosacral ligament. The hypogastric artery and upper uterine artery run parallel, lateral, and deep to the ureter until the uterine artery crosses over the ureter at the base of the broad ligament. Figure 20.2 shows this relationship on the patient's left side. The ureter will then enter the ureteric tunnel in the vesicocervical ligament, bending abruptly anteriorly and medially for the final 1–2 cm of the ureter called the "knee."

While the anatomic relationship between the ureter and the pelvic vessels is the cornerstone of pelvic sidewall dissection, it is important to remember that there is a significant rate of urinary and vascular anomalies in the retroperitoneum: 1.6% and 13.6%, respectively. Dissection of avascular tissue planes should proceed bluntly with careful exposure of structures encountered to avoid injury of vascular and renal anomalies.

SURGICAL TECHNIQUE

There are two main approaches for retroperitoneal resection of the pelvic sidewall: the medial approach and the lateral approach. The lateral approach is most commonly used in gynecologic oncology for lymph node dissection (see Chapter 31). It can also be useful in benign surgery when the primary objective is isolating the uterine artery for laparoscopic uterine artery occlusion or hysterectomy. The medial approach is most useful for the majority of benign gynecologic pathologies, as the peritoneum of the ovarian fossa is commonly involved in the disease process (i.e., adnexal adhesions and endometriosis). The medial approach is also advantageous because below the pelvic brim, the main blood flow to the ureter is lateral. Both approaches require a responsive uterine manipulator to be able to achieve extreme anteversion. We prefer a RUMI manipulator by Cooper Surgical. Lateral port placement of the secondary trocars is optimal to achieve a useful angle to the pelvis and maximize the stability of the surgeon who uses two lateral ports on one side. The lower ports are placed 1–2 cm superior and lateral to the anterior superior iliac spine. The upper port is placed at the same level, lateral at the periumbilical level (Figure 20.3).

THE MEDIAL APPROACH

1. *Restore normal anatomic relationships*: The approach to a grossly distorted pelvis begins with the restoration of normal anatomic relationships of organs

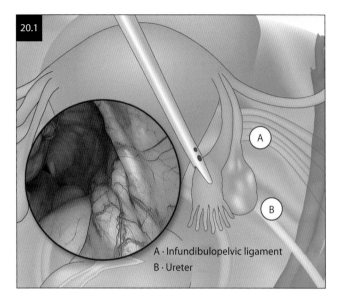

A · Infundibulopelvic ligament
B · Ureter

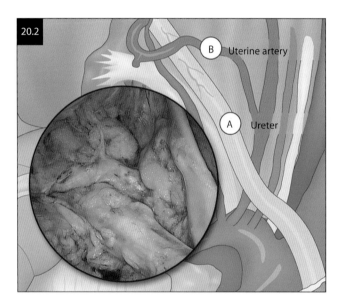

B Uterine artery

A Ureter

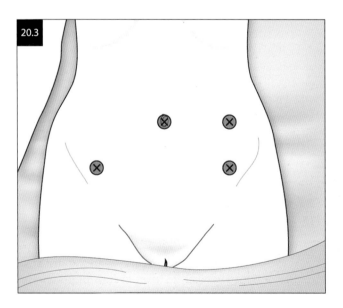

adherent to the pelvis, such as omentum and bowel. This is accomplished by blunt and sharp dissections depending on the density of the adhesions. Adhesiolysis of dense adhesions to the cul-de-sac and sidewall should not be addressed at this time.

2. *Identification of the ureter*: The ureter must be identified before surgery in the ovarian fossa or cul-de-sac is initiated. Identification of the ureter along the pelvic sidewall can be attempted, but if unsuccessful, attention should be directed to the pelvic brim where consistent identification is possible as the ureter crosses over the bifurcation of the common iliac artery (see Figure 20.1). Identification can be confirmed by grasping the suspected location of the ureter with an atraumatic grasper to stimulate peristalsis. The left ureter may require mobilization of the sigmoid mesentery from the abdominal sidewall to gain access to the pelvic brim (Figure 20.4).

3. *Ureterolysis*: Once the ureter is identified, it can be traced caudally until the pathology begins or the ureter is no longer visible. Just before this point, the peritoneum directly over the ureter is grasped and excised (Figure 20.5). CO_2 gas will quickly enter the retroperitoneal space, aiding in further dissection. The frequent peristalsis of the ureter within the loose retroperitoneal connective tissue creates a pseudosheath around the ureter. Ureterolysis can be continued down to the level of the uterine artery

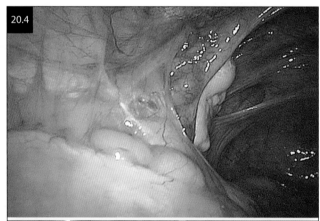

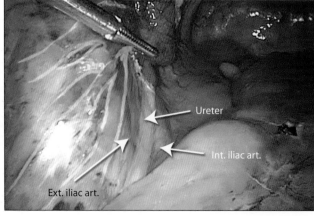

Ureter

Int. iliac art.

Ext. iliac art.

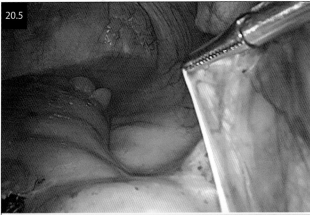

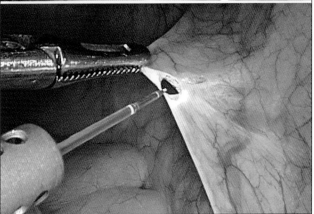

even deep fibrotic endometriosis that is responsible for hydroureter (Figure 20.7).

4. *Pathology-directed dissection*: After the ureters have been isolated, many operations can proceed without any further retroperitoneal dissection, such as hysterectomy, lysis of adnexal adhesions, oophorectomy, and peritoneal resection of endometriosis, provided that the pathology does not extend past the first layer of the pelvis. In some cases it may become necessary to extend the dissection to isolate the internal iliac artery and uterine artery. Following peritoneal resection in the ovarian fossa, the areolar spaces around the vessels can be easily dissected using blunt dissection, isolating the vessels from the pathology (see Figure 20.2). Inadvertent injury to the vessels is rare, but if it occurs, it is important to grasp the vessel with an atraumatic grasper to control the bleeding, and then confirm the location of the previously dissected ureter before coagulating or ligating the vessel.

5. *Extending the pelvic sidewall dissection to uterosacral ligaments and rectovaginal space*: If there is disease invading the uterosacral ligaments or cul-de-sac, the rectovaginal space can be opened after ureterolysis. The lateral pararectal space is between the ureter and the uterosacral ligament. It is relatively avascular with the hypogastric nerve running through it; resection in this area can proceed after the hypogastric nerve is identified. Mild bleeding may be encountered at the posterior lateral aspect of the uterosacral ligament, which is easily managed with bipolar cautery. The medial pararectal space is the area between the uterosacral ligament and rectum. Care must be taken when operating in this area because of the mesenteric vessels present in the perirectal fat. Dissection in this area can be aided by a rectal probe or a ring forceps in the rectum. The rectovaginal space is the large cavernous potential space between the rectum and posterior

by placing a grasper along the medial aspect of the ureter in the pseudosheath and dividing the overlying peritoneum (Figure 20.6). As the ureter approaches the uterine artery, the ureter will start to travel more posteriorly in relationship to the peritoneum. The depth of the pathology determines how close the dissection needs to be to the ureter. It is possible to dissect through the deepest layers of pseudosheath using a micrograsper to perform ureterolysis directly along the adventitia, liberating

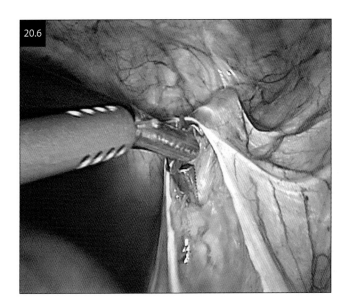

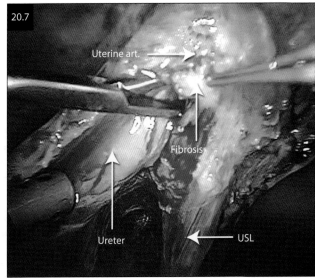

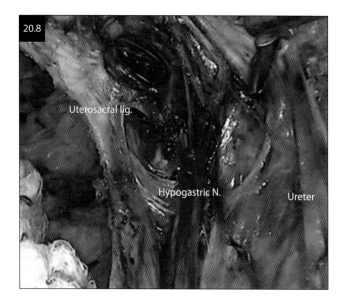

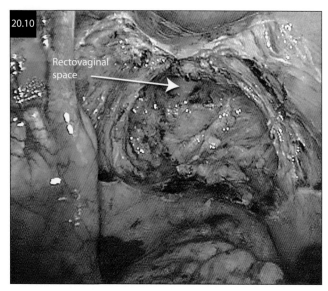

vagina. The ability to open this space is essential for pelvic reconstructive surgery and management of cul-de-sac endometriosis. The best place to enter the rectovaginal space is in the perirectal fat just medial to the attachment of the uterosacral ligament. If the ligament has not been transected, the peritoneum is incised. A blunt grasper is placed in the perirectal fat just medial to the uterosacral ligament, using blunt dissection parallel to the vagina opening the rectovaginal space (Figure 20.8). The space is expanded further by extending the lateral perirectal entry spaces medially using blunt dissection and dividing the medial peritoneum until the space is fully developed (Figure 20.9). The dissection can be accomplished by placing the gauze in the abdominal cavity through a 10 mm trocar and performing a blunt dissection with the gauze (Figure 20.10). Once the space is open, further surgery can proceed, such

as pelvic reconstruction or resection of endometriosis from the rectum or vagina.

LATERAL APPROACH

The lateral approach for pelvic sidewall dissection is described in detail for pelvic lymphadenectomy (see Chapter 31). Summary of the key steps in the lateral approach for benign disease are as follows:

1. *Peritoneal incision at the pelvic sidewall triangle*: The uterus is placed on contralateral traction exposing the triangle of the lateral broad ligament, created by the round ligament, the external iliac, and the infundibulopelvic ligament. An incision is made from the base of the triangle (the round ligament) to the apex (the junction of the external iliac and infundibulopelvic ligament) (Figure 20.11). It is

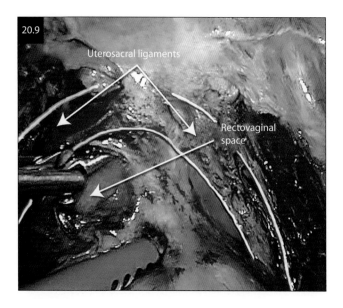

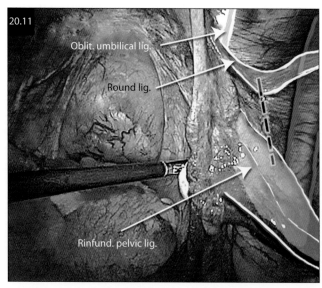

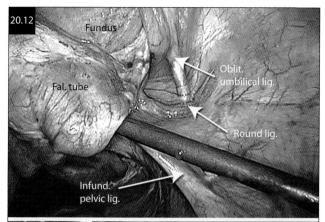

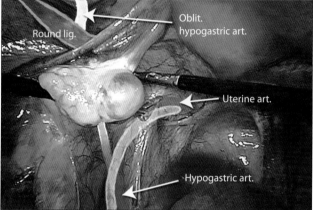

pelvic anatomy. The peritoneum can be severely thickened and fibrotic, making visualization and palpation of vital structures problematic. Fortunately, even in the most severe cases, dissection down to normal connective tissue planes and liberation of vital structures from fibrotic endometriosis are possible by following the steps for the medial approach to retroperitoneal dissection.

Peritoneal resection of endometriosis is a surgical approach for treatment of endometriosis, where all peritoneum with endometriosis is completely resected down to disease-free connective tissue. New peritoneum, free of endometriosis, will generate in 2–3 days with minimal *de novo* adhesion formation (Figure 20.13). Even though peritoneal resection of endometriosis can be surgically challenging, results for both pain control and fertility are encouraging. Long-term pain studies show over 80% of patients are pain free or have their pain controlled. Fertility rates as high as 68% have been reported for severe endometriosis. Even in cases of extensive cul-de-sac endometriosis requiring bowel resection, a 48% pregnancy rate can be achieved.

The surgical steps in peritoneal resection of endometriosis begin with a careful inspection of the pelvis to identify all areas of peritoneal endometriosis before the peritoneum is distorted by surgical ecchymosis. Close magnification and irrigation help identify more subtle lesions. Peritoneal windows are usually indicative of endometriosis, especially at the base of the pocket, which can extend deep into the pelvic sidewall. After all areas

important that the incision be extended sufficiently cephalad to enable adequate medial mobilization of the infundibulopelvic ligament and ureter.

2. *Dissection of paravesical space and identification of the ureter*: Using blunt dissection, the avascular paravesical space is dissected. The infundibulopelvic ligament and ureter are retracted medially. The attachment of the ureter to the medial leaf of the broad ligament is left intact, and the ureter is identified laterally. The identification may need to begin at the apex where the ureter crosses the common iliac artery. Care must be taken to minimize dissection lateral to the obliterated hypogastric artery as the external iliac vein is medial to the external iliac artery.

3. *Identification of the uterine artery*: Locating the uterine artery can be accomplished by identifying the obliterated hypogastric artery on the anterior abdominal wall (Figure 20.12) and tracing it retrograde to the uterine artery. The uterine artery can be ligated before it crosses the ureter. Pulling on the obliterated umbilical ligament can aid in identification.

ENDOMETRIOSIS

In no other gynecologic disease is adherence to a surgical anatomic approach more vital than in severe endometriosis. The cul-de-sac and ovary are the most frequently involved areas of endometriosis. Deep fibrotic endometriosis can cause dense adhesions, grossly distorting

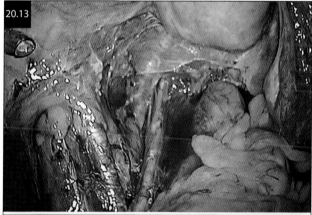

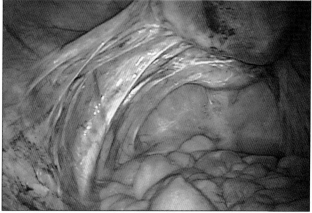

of endometriosis have been mapped out, the steps for the medial approach to retroperitoneal resection of the sidewall are initiated. Once the vital structures are isolated, *en bloc* resection is performed by circumscribing the peritoneum around the lesions, leaving a disease-free margin (Figure 20.14). The circumscribed peritoneum is then dissected from the underlying connective tissue. This technique is the same for both superficial and deep lesions. Endometriosis may invade so deeply that dissection may need to be extended to the third layer of the pelvis, isolating the obturator nerve and vasculature (Figure 20.15). In extreme circumstances, deep infiltrating endometriosis can be invasive to the bowel, bladder, vagina, or ureter, requiring resection and repair of these organs.

RETROPERITONEAL OVARY

Pelvic sidewall dissection is central to both the prevention and treatment of retroperitoneal ovaries. The

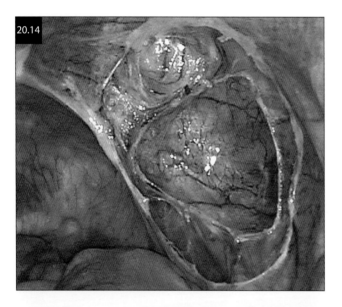

retroperitoneal ovary has two subcategories: residual ovarian syndrome and ovarian remnant syndrome. In residual ovarian syndrome, the ovary becomes encapsulated by adhesions secondary to previous surgery or pathologic process, such as endometriosis or pelvic inflammatory disease. Ovarian remnant syndrome is ovarian tissue persistent after oophorectomy. The main etiology is incomplete removal of the ovary, usually at the infundibulopelvic ligament or residual cortex adherent to the pelvic sidewall. Other proposed mechanisms are seeding during oophorectomy with fragment reattachment, or accessory ovaries. Predisposing factors to ovarian remnant syndrome are ovarian enlargement, periovarian adhesions, multiple previous surgeries, and most importantly, a history of endometriosis present in over 50% of cases. Adequate retroperitoneal dissection of the sidewall during these cases may reduce the incidence of ovarian remnant syndrome. Treatment of ovarian remnant can be difficult due to adhesions and distorted anatomy. Retroperitoneal dissection with identification of landmarks and vital structures enables location and removal of residual ovarian tissue (Figure 20.16). The recurrence of ovarian remnant has been reported as 8%–20%, but many of these cases were by laparotomy. The largest laparoscopic series by Nezhat reported an 8% recurrence rate. Complication rates in the literature range from 3% to 33%, with 5.8% reported in Nezhat's laparoscopic series.

COMPLICATIONS

The prime objective of retroperitoneal dissection of the pelvic sidewall is to reduce complications during difficult surgery with complex pathology. Even with a thorough understanding of surgical anatomy and meticulous dissection technique, the surgeon must be prepared to encounter surgical complications. It is important to control bleeding with pressure and evaluate the surrounding anatomy before coagulating the vessel. Preplanning

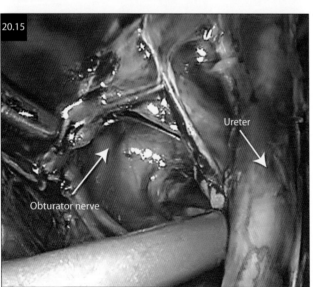

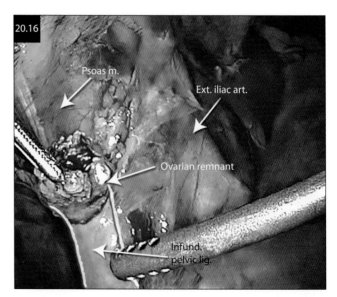

consultations with urology, general, and vascular surgeons can be helpful in formulating a detailed management plan for repair of injuries even before they occur. Many complications can be safely managed laparoscopically if suturing skills are solid and the same standards as open surgery are maintained.

SUGGESTED READING

Benedetti-Panici P, Maneschi F, Scambia G, Greggi S, Mancuso S et al. Anatomic abnormalities of the retroperitoneum encountered during aortic and pelvic lymphadenectomy. *Am J Obstet Gynecol* 1994;170(1 pt 1):111–116.

Koh CH, Janik GM. The surgical management of deep rectovaginal endometriosis. *Curr Opin Obstet Gynecol*. 2002;14(4):357–364.

Nezhat C, Kearney S, Malik S, Nezhat C, Nezhat F. Laparoscopic management of ovarian remnant. *Fertil Steril*. 2005;83(4):973–978.

Rogers RM, Pasic R. Pelvic retroperitoneal dissection: A hands-on primer. *J Minim Invasive Gynecol*. 2017;24(4):546–551.

CHAPTER 21
LOWER URINARY TRACT ENDOSCOPY

Sam H. Hessami and David Shin

INTRODUCTION

Gynecologists have not been traditionally trained in performing endoscopy of the lower urinary tract. Cystourethroscopy, when compared to hysteroscopy and laparoscopy, is one of the simpler procedures to teach and to learn. Medically speaking, given the close proximity of the genital organs to the urinary tracts, it is necessary for gynecologists to ensure the intactness of the urinary system after complicated pelvic procedures. Although the benefits of the routine use of cystoscopy after certain gynecologic procedures such as a vaginal hysterectomy have been debated, there is no question that with advances in pelvic reconstructive surgery and the use of synthetic and nonsynthetic grafts, it is incumbent on every surgeon to ensure intactness of the urinary tract. Failure to identify iatrogenic injuries intraoperatively will have life-changing and catastrophic sequelae for the patient. More complex vaginal procedures, such as those for advanced pelvic organ prolapse, where the ureters are at greatest risk for injury, also dictate routine cystoscopic evaluation at the end of the procedure.

The surgeon must be familiar with the different equipment and choose the best for the application, since there are multitudes of endoscopes and lenses currently available on the market. In this chapter, we focus on diagnostic cystoscopy only.

EQUIPMENT

ROD-LENS ENDOSCOPES

There are two types of endoscopes available on the market: rod-lens versus fiberoptic. Rod-lens endoscopes, familiar to all laparoscopists, are also known as rigid scopes. They are stiff, rod-shaped instruments with cylindrical lenses, where the angles of deflection range from 0° to 120° (0°, 30°, 70°, 90°, and 120°), depending on the specific use. A common property of all angled scopes is that the angle of view is always opposite to the light post (Figure 21.1). The rigid cystoscope must be attached to a bridge and then passed through a sheath before it can be inserted (Figure 21.2). The bridge will allow the attachment of the telescope to the sheath as well as the passage of instruments through its working channels, in case of operative cystoscopy. The sheath is used for atraumatic passage of the telescope into the urethra and then the bladder. The rigid endoscopes measure 4 mm in diameter, and the cystoscopic sheath ranges from 17Fr to 25Fr (Figure 21.3). In general, a 17Fr sheath is all that is required for diagnostic cystoscopy. Keep in mind that an adult female urethra measures 4 mm in diameter, and thus a 17Fr sheath is easily tolerated by patients even in an office setting with minimal use of a topical anesthetic gel (1 mm = 3 Fr). Larger-caliber sheaths are needed to allow for passage of instruments in cases of operative cystoscopy. It is important to understand the differences and benefits of different objective lenses. The 0° lens is used for urethroscopy. Even though a 30° lens also can be used for this purpose, it is not the lens of choice. A 30° lens is most suitable for abdominal teleoscopy, allowing for the visualization of both ureteral orifices. It is also used for transurethral inspection of the bladder and ureteral orifices. For diagnostic purposes, a 70° lens is preferred, as it allows for inspection of the ureteral orifices as well as bladder side walls and dome with minimal need for rotation and movement of the endoscope, thus resulting in conservation of movement and better tolerance by patients in an outpatient setting with topical use of anesthesia. Rigid scopes are sturdy, resulting in excellent longevity. They are the easiest to operate, and are more readily available when compared to flexible scopes. Their obvious limitation is their stiffness and lack of flexibility, which result in their inability to inspect the anterior bladder neck.

FLEXIBLE ENDOSCOPES

The flexible endoscopes contain fiberoptic bundles, which with the advancement in technology, can now offer excellent images but are still fragile. Their flexibility allows for a more comprehensive inspection of the bladder. A specific mechanical property of these devices, secondary deflection, allows for it to be retroflexed so that the bladder neck and the trigone can be easily inspected (Figure 21.4). The smallest size flexible cystoscope comes in 16Fr, which is easily tolerated by patients and smaller than the 17Fr rigid cystoscope sheath, the smallest diameter adult sheath. Flexible cystoscopes do not require a bridge or a sheath. Technically speaking, flexible cystoscopes are harder to master and also require careful handling due to their fragile nature.

CYSTOSCOPIC TECHNIQUE

The endoscopic inspection of the lower urinary tract must be systematic, beginning with the urethra. Prior to the procedure, the patient is prepped with an antiseptic

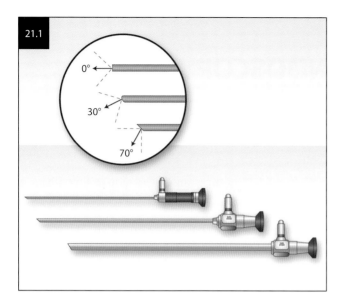

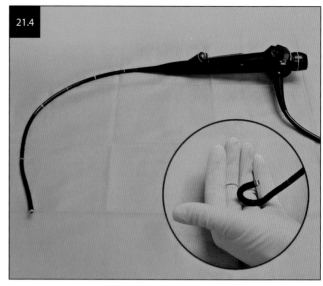

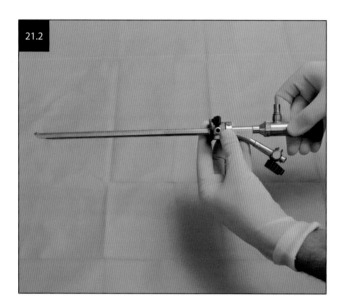

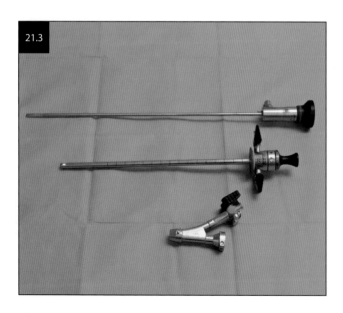

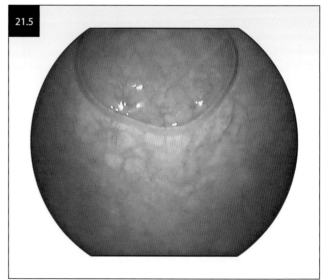

solution. The bladder is drained, as concentrated urine will interfere with the clarity of the image. About 5–10 cc of xylocaine jelly (Urojet 2%) are then injected transurethrally, while the cystoscope is being assembled. Sterile water and normal saline can both be used as irrigation for a diagnostic cystoscopy. If electrocautery is planned, solutions containing electrolytes must be avoided. When using a rigid scope, first attach the bridge to the scope. Then pass the cystoscope, with the bridge attached, through the sheath. The light stump and the deflection on the sheath should be pointing upward to 12 o'clock. In order to conserve movements, the light handle should be used to manipulate the cystoscope as opposed to the actual rotation of the cystoscope. The water tubing is then connected next to the bridge. The water tubing does not need to be primed. This is to allow for the passage of air into the bladder, and for identification of the bladder dome by visualization of the air bubble (Figure 21.5). This will also confirm the integrity of the bladder, as the bubble will escape from a perforated bladder. The laparoscopic camera should be held in an upward position with the nondominant hand, and the cystoscope can be directed by holding and rotating the light cable in the dominant hand. The bladder should be filled with 200 cc of sterile water to allow for adequate distention of the bladder walls. Keep in mind that overinflating the bladder will make it difficult to see the ureteral orifices, while underinflation will leave mucosal folds intact, resulting in inadequate inspection.

Upon insertion of a well-lubricated cystoscope, the urethra is inspected first. This should be done while the distending medium is flowing, thus allowing for the urethra to remain open. Upon entry into the bladder, and after adequate volume is instilled, a systematic inspection is performed.

After inserting the cystoscope, the light cord assists in orienting the lens as the operator inspects the trigone, the ureteric orifices, and the bladder walls. The cystoscope lens is always directed opposite from the light cord insertion (as shown in Figure 21.1).

First the bladder floor is inspected. This is where the interureteric ridge, just inside the bladder neck and along the trigone, is identified. A few centimeters lateral to the center of this ridge, the ureteral orifices are located. The ureteric orifices are located below the urethra and cannot be easily visualized with the 0° scope. Therefore, the operator should use a 30° or 70° scope to visualize the orifices. In order to visualize the patient's right orifice, the camera should be raised and moved toward the patient's left leg, pointing the tip of the cystoscope down toward the patient's right orifice. The camera should always be kept in the upright position. The light cord should be rotated 45° clockwise, pointing the 70° lens toward the patient's right side until the orifice is found (Figure 21.6). In order to visualize the left orifice, the camera should be held in the upright position and moved toward the patient's right leg, changing the axes of the scope, and pointing the tip of the cystoscope toward the left orifice. The light cord should be

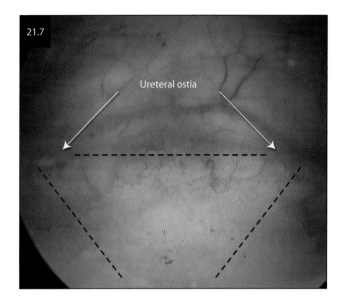

rotated counterclockwise until the left orifice is visualized. Laterally, on either side of the ureteral orifices, short ridges can also be identified, representing the most distal segment of ureters running intramurally through the bladder wall. The imaginary lines connecting the urethral opening to the two ureteral orifices, and the interureteral ridge form the three borders of the triangle of the trigone (Figure 21.7). The trigone is the most dependent and, therefore, the least forgiving part of the bladder in case of injuries. Injuries to this region are at high risk to fistulize despite adequate repair.

Indigo carmine may be administered intravenously approximately 2–3 minutes prior to performing a cystoscopy. Indigo carmine allows for the clear visualization of both ureteric orifices, as it causes the urine to turn blue, thus making for a very visible efflux of blue-colored urine (Figure 21.8).

After visualization of both ureteral ostia, the lateral walls and the bladder dome are inspected next. The camera is kept steady in the upright position; the light

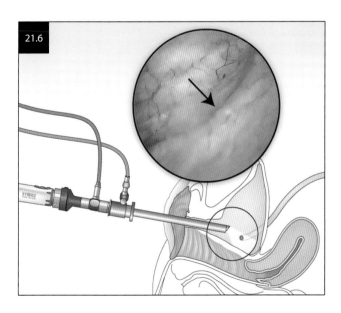

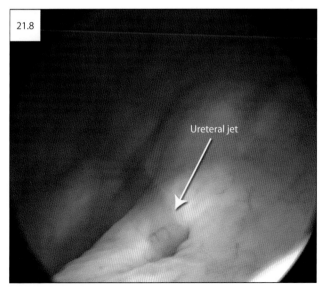

cable is rotated downward, pointing the tip of the cystoscope toward the bladder dome; and the rest of the bladder is inspected.

The anterior bladder wall is inspected last. This can be accomplished with a 90° or 120° telescope only.

Alternatively, a flexible cystoscope can be used. Flexible cystoscopes are handled slightly different. The tip of the scope is deflected up and down to inspect the entire bladder cavity. In general, as with rigid scopes, the trigone and the ureteral orifices are inspected first, followed by bladder walls, and then the dome of the bladder. The collection of air bubbles here serves as a consistent landmark, and also ensures intactness of the bladder. The secondary deflection property of flexible cystoscopes will allow it to retroflex and thus be capable of inspecting the bladder neck and the anterior wall, something that is not easily accomplished with rigid scopes. Flexible cystoscopes also have a working channel allowing for passage of instruments for tissue sampling and coagulation.

POOR MAN'S CYSTOSCOPY

Quick evaluation of the bladder integrity and ureteral patency can be accomplished by retrograde filling the bladder with 150 cc of sterile water through the Foley catheter and inserting a 30° 5 mm laparoscope through the urethra. This technique is mostly used after performing laparoscopic hysterectomy to inspect the bladder integrity and the presence of ureteral jets.

A 60 cc syringe is used to inject the sterile water through the port on the three-way Foley catheter after the tubing is clamped to prevent the water escaping to the Foley bag. If you are using the regular Foley catheter, the bladder can be retrograde filled through the Foley catheter. The Foley catheter is then removed, the 30° 5 mm laparoscope is inserted into the urethra, and the bladder is inspected (Figure 21.9). When using sterile water, rather than saline, for distention, ureteral jets can

be easily seen through the 30° laparoscope, obviating the need for any intravenous contrast.

URETERAL STENT

INDICATION

Ureteral stents are commonly placed to relieve obstruction within the urinary tract, whether for extrinsic compression on the ureter due to malignancy or internal blockage within the ureter due to stones. Ureter stents are also placed if suspected injury to the ureter has occurred during pelvic surgery. In gynecology, similar to colorectal cases, stents can also be placed in selected cases in order to make ureteral identification easier and thus avoid injury. Cases in which prophylaxis stent placement could be beneficial include suspected severe endometriosis and laparoscopic or robotic vault suspension procedures. Ureteral stents are also placed if suspected injury to the ureter has occurred during surgery. In these cases, intraoperative urology consultation should be obtained.

TECHNIQUE

A 22Fr or 23Fr rigid cystoscope is inserted through the urethra and advanced into the bladder to allow better visualization of the bladder and to provide a larger working channel to pass instruments. As previously noted, a 30° lens is used to visualize the trigone and ureteral orifices. Attention is then turned toward the ureteral orifice where the suspected injury may have occurred. An 8Fr cone-tipped catheter (Figure 21.10) is introduced through a working channel on the cystoscope and advanced within the cystoscope sheath until the cone tip is visualized. The cone tip is then advanced generally up to and into the ureter orifice causing temporary occlusion. Using a 10 cc syringe connected to the 8Fr cone-tipped catheter, a 50–50 mixture of Renografin contrast and normal

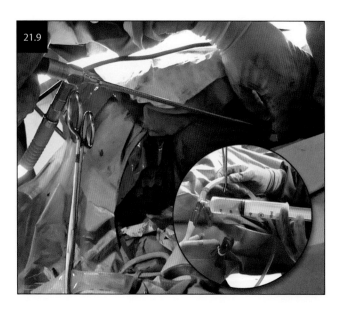

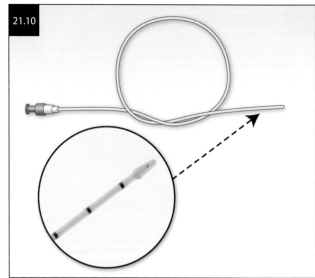

saline is injected into the catheter to perform the retrograde pyelogram. Under direct radiographic visualization, the dye should be seen to freely flow up the ureter and into the kidney without extravasation or blockage.

If extravasation of contrast is seen anywhere along the ureter, then one has to suspect that patency of the ureter has been compromised. At this point, a ureter stent should be placed to promote healing and prevent further damage to the ureter. Therefore, the 8Fr cone-tipped catheter is removed. A 0.035 in (2.7Fr) straight-tipped, stainless steel, polytetrafluoroethylene-coated guidewire (Cook Standard PFTE coated #635413) (Figure 21.11) is introduced through a working channel on the cystoscope and advanced within the cystoscope sheath until it is visualized. Once the tip of the guidewire is seen, it is placed into the opening of the ureteral orifice and passed up the ureter into the kidney. The tip placement is confirmed under fluoroscopy (i.e., a C-arm). The surgeon should encounter minimal resistance as the guidewire is advanced up the ureter. Placement of the wire is then confirmed by radiology. This confirmation is very important to ensure that the guidewire is within the urinary tract and did not migrate into the retroperitoneum.

After confirmation of placement, the surgeon has to choose the appropriate ureteral stent (Figure 21.12). The most common stent placed has both proximal and distal coils (double J or pigtail), which decreases the probability of migration out of the kidney or bladder. The length of the stent (the distance between the two pigtails) varies between 8 cm and 32 cm. The length choice by the surgeon will be dependent on the patient's height. For example, the typical stent placed is a ureteral catheter with a 6Fr diameter and 24 cm length (6 × 24 double-J stent), because it adequately drains urine in a person ranging in height from 5′5″ to 5′10″. Because of its versatility, the 6 × 24 double-J stent (Microvasive Polaris, Bardex Double Pigtail Soft Stent) is a popular choice for temporary internal stent placement. For persons less than 5′5″ in height, a shorter 6 × 22 double-J stent is a

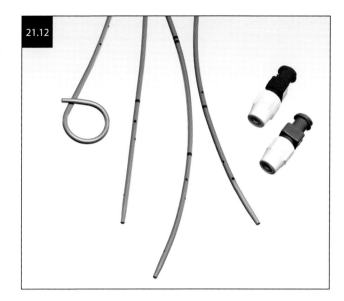

more appropriate choice. For persons more than 5′10″ in height, a longer 6 × 26 double-J stent is necessary to provide adequate urinary drainage.

Once the proper choice of ureteral stent is made, it is placed over the guidewire, and a second "pusher" catheter (included with the stent kit) is used to advance the ureter under direct visualization. Typically, five bars or one fat bar is an indication that the end of the stent is approaching. When the distal end of the stent is visualized in the bladder, the surgeon must also confirm by radiology that the proximal coil of the stent is within the pelvis of the kidney. Once the stent has been confirmed in the proper position, the guidewire is removed. Then, the cystoscope is carefully retreated out of the bladder and urethra while leaving the stent in place for a minimum of 6 weeks.

If during the injection of contrast media, the dye flow abruptly stops in the lower or midureter within the pelvis, then one has to strongly suspect obstruction of the ureter by hemostatic clips or suture. An attempt to place an

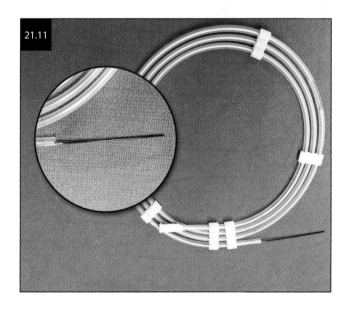

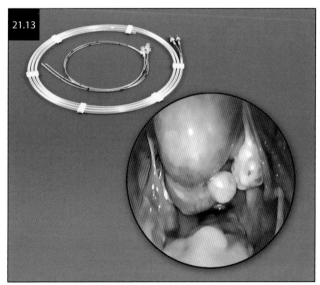

ureteral stent as described can be performed but should not be aggressively pursued if the guidewire does not easily advance up the ureter. At this point, open surgical exploration to repair any ureteral occlusion or injury should be performed. If the patient is clinically unstable, another option is to place a percutaneous nephrostomy tube to drain the urine directly away from the kidney.

URETERAL CATHETERIZATION

In cases where the ureters are at high risk for injury, the identification of the ureters can be facilitated by the preoperative insertion of ureteral catheters or lighted ureteral stents (LUSs) (Stryker Endoscopy, Santa Clara, California). Sigmoid resection or abdominal vault suspension procedures (sacrocolpopexy or high uterosacral vault suspension) are good examples, where a ureteral catheter can help in ureteral identification and ureterolysis. Lighted stents can facilitate localization of the ureters during laparoscopic surgery (Figure 21.13).

The technique for ureteral catheterization is almost identical to stenting. We generally use 6Fr olive tip ureteral catheters for this purpose. The catheter is passed through a 24Fr sheath attached to a 30° scope. Similar to stents, the olive tip catheter has 5 cm markings, demarcated by solid bars. For the purpose of ureteral catheterization,

the catheter is pushed up to 20–25 cm, depending on the height of the patient. The catheter is then connected to and held in place by passing it through a three-way connector and the Foley catheter, allowing for drainage of the kidney. The ureteral catheter is promptly removed at the end of the operative procedure.

CONCLUSION

Diagnostic cystoscopy is a relatively simple procedure. It should be mastered by all gynecologists who perform difficult pelvic cases or pelvic reconstructive cases as the lower urogenital system is at increased risk for injury. The procedure must be done in a systematic and organized manner, inspecting directly the bladder and urethra and indirectly the ureters by observing efflux of urine from ureteral orifices. This additional 5-minute procedure can save a patient and her surgeon a lifetime of headache and sorrow.

SUGGESTED READING

O'Hanlan KA. Cystoscopy with a 5-mm laparoscope and suction irrigator. *JMIG*. 2007;14:260–263.

Rosenberg BH, Averch TD. Ancillary instrumentation for ureteroscopy. *Urol Clin North Am*. 2004;31(1):49–59.

CHAPTER 22

LAPAROSCOPIC PARAVAGINAL REPAIR AND BURCH URETHROPEXY

J. Stephen Rich, C.Y. Liu, and Adam R. Duke

INTRODUCTION

Anterior vaginal compartment support defects are common and often result in symptomatic organ prolapse and urinary incontinence. The management of these defects varies according to several factors: the location and severity of the anatomical defect(s), the patient's physical status and symptomatology, the patient's desire for surgical correction, and the patient's expectations.

This chapter discusses two surgical techniques used to repair specific anterior support defects: the laparoscopic paravaginal repair and the laparoscopic Burch procedure. It is generally agreed that a paravaginal repair should be reserved for the treatment of a lateral defect cystocele and should not be used alone as the primary treatment for stress urinary incontinence. Consequently, the laparoscopic Burch colposuspension is often performed concomitantly for the treatment of genuine stress urinary incontinence.

DISSECTION OF THE SPACE OF RETZIUS

Surgery in the space of Retzius is complicated by limited space for suture placement and the proximity of neurovascular and urologic structures that are easily damaged. It must be emphasized that these types of operations require a surgeon experienced in sound retropubic anatomy and advanced operative laparoscopy with proficient laparoscopic suture and knot-tying techniques. A well-organized and experienced laparoscopic surgical team will yield the most efficient and best results in laparoscopic repair of anterior vaginal compartment defects.

There is considerable variability in operator preference regarding trocar placement, operating room setup, suture materials, and surgical instruments. We describe laparoscopic techniques for operating in the space of Retzius that we have found to be most useful.

The patient is placed in the modified dorsolithotomy position using padded support stirrups (e.g., the Allen Yellofin stirrups). It is important to avoid injury to the patient by using surgical stirrups that are safe and secure and do not allow excessive abduction, rotation, or flexion.

The surgical technologist is positioned between the stirrups, and the surgical assistant is positioned on the side of the patient opposite the surgeon.

An 18 Fr urethral catheter with a 30 cc bulb is inserted, and the bulb is inflated with 15–20 cc of sterile water. The bladder is drained prior to trocar insertion in order to avoid bladder injury. Gentle traction is placed on the catheter during the procedure, and the large catheter and bulb will aid identification of the urethra and bladder neck.

A 10 mm trocar port is inserted transumbilically, and two pairs of ancillary 5 mm trocar ports are inserted under direct visualization, using transillumination to avoid injury to the deep inferior epigastric vessels: one pair two fingerbreadths above the symphysis pubis and medial to the deep inferior epigastric vessels and the second pair about two fingerbreadths below the umbilicus and lateral to the abdominal rectus muscles (Figure 22.1).

The space of Retzius is entered by making a transverse incision approximately 2–3 cm above the symphysis pubis on the anterior peritoneum (Figure 22.2). The anterior peritoneum and loose areola tissues are then dissected away from the anterior abdominal wall until the symphysis pubis and the adjacent proximal part of Cooper ligaments are clearly identified (Figure 22.3). Approximately 200–300 cc of Ringer lactate solution is instilled into the bladder of the obese patient whose symphysis pubis is difficult to identify laparoscopically; this helps identify the dome of the bladder and, thus, avoid bladder injury on entering the space of Retzius. The bladder is drained as soon as the space of Retzius is safely entered.

The incision on the anterior abdominal peritoneum is extended bilaterally following the curvatures of Cooper ligament, taking care to stop short of the aberrant obturator vessels as they course from the external iliac vessels over the ligament. Sharp dissection with bipolar coagulation for hemostasis is utilized to open the space of Retzius. Special care must be paid to clearly identify all the important anatomic landmarks to avoid injuring them during the procedure. The important vessels located anterior to Cooper ligaments include aberrant obturator vessels, deep inferior epigastric vessels, and external iliac vessels, which are very close to the superior iliac crest (Figure 22.4). The structures posterior to Cooper ligaments are the obturator neurovascular bundles, arcus tendineus fascia of levator ani, arcus tendineus fascia of pelvis (ATFP), ischial spine, and coccygeal muscle. The

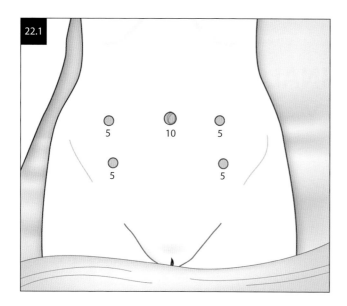

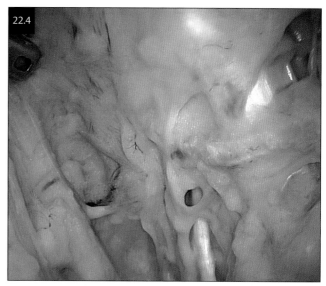

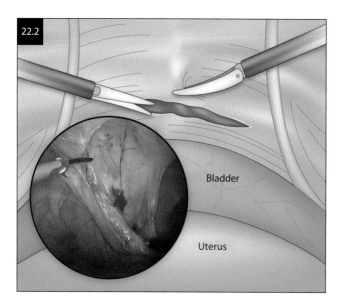

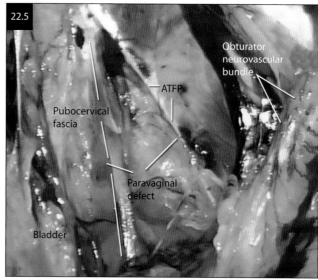

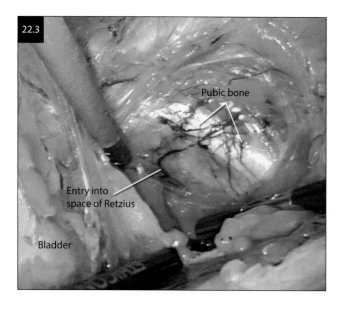

structures around the symphysis pubis, urethra, and bladder neck are the pubovesical muscles, posterior clitoral vessel, and paraurethral vascular plexus (Figure 22.5).

LAPAROSCOPIC PARAVAGINAL REPAIR

There are basically three different types of anterior vaginal defects:

1. *Lateral defect.* This is the detachment of pubocervical fascia from the pelvic sidewall at the level of arcus tendineus fascia of pelvis (ATFP, white line). This paravaginal defect accounts for 80%–85% of anterior compartment defects.
2. *Central defect.* This is the detachment of pubocervical fascia from the pericervical ring at the level of the cervix or vaginal apex. This is the condition of anterior enterocele, and it accounts for 10%–15% of anterior compartment defects.

3. *Midline defect.* This is where the pubocervical fascia breaks at the midline, usually as a result of previous anterior colporrhaphy. This paravaginal defect accounts for less than 5% of anterior vaginal defects (Figure 22.6).

The paravaginal defect was first described by White in 1909. In 1976, Cullen Richardson performed fresh cadaveric dissections and further defined the surgical anatomy and treatment of paravaginal defects. Subsequently, three types of paravaginal defects have been identified: (A) separation of the pubocervical fascia from the ATFP, (B) a midline disruption of the ATFP, and (C) complete avulsion of the ATFP from the obturator internus muscle (Figure 22.7).

TECHNIQUE

Following careful dissection of the space of Retzius and clear identification of all the important anatomic landmarks, the entire paravaginal space between the ischial spines and symphysis pubis are thus well exposed and the types of the paravaginal defects defined.

The strength of ATFP needs to be tested before repair of type A and B paravaginal defects. If the ATFP is not sturdy enough, then Cooper ligaments should be used to anchor the paravaginal suture. The type C paravaginal defect will have to be repaired by using Cooper ligament.

The surgeon inserts two fingers vaginally to aide in identification of the paravaginal defects and the margin of the pubocervical fascia. The surgical assistant retracts the bladder medially, and the surgeon's vaginal fingers are used to tent the pubocervical fascia lateral to the bladder; this further exposes the paravaginal defect.

The ischial spine is identified, and the first figure-of-8 sutures of 2-0 Prolene on a CT-2 needle are placed at approximately 1–1.5 cm caudad to the ischial spine between the pubocervical fascia and ATFP (Figure 22.8) and then four to five additional sutures are placed 1–2 cm

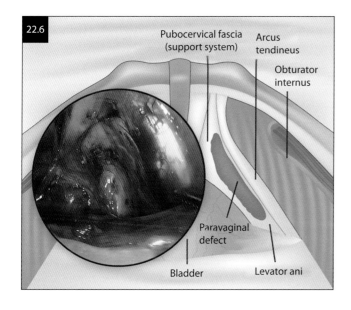

Figure 22.6. Pubocervical fascia (support system) — Arcus tendineus — Obturator internus — Paravaginal defect — Bladder — Levator ani

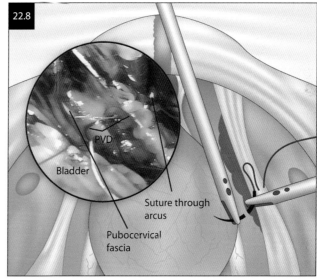

Figure 22.8. PVD — Bladder — Suture through arcus — Pubocervical fascia

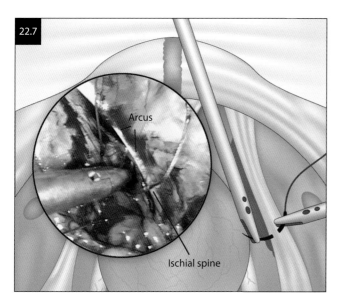

Figure 22.7. Arcus — Ischial spine

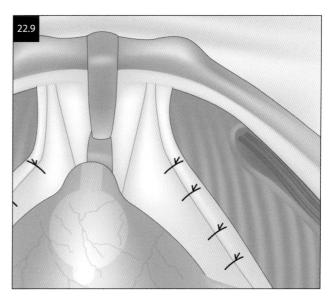

Figure 22.9.

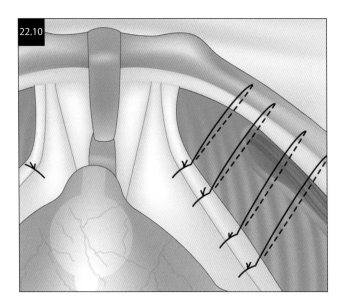

22.10

intervals toward the symphysis pubis (Figure 22.9). If the ATFP is weakened or avulsed from the obturator internus muscles, it is advisable to include Cooper ligament on the ipsilateral side in the repair of the defects (Figure 22.10). We routinely use a CV-0 GORE-TEX suture when Cooper ligament is included in the repair and the suture ligature includes the pubocervical fascia medially, the avulsed ATFP and obturator internus laterally, and Cooper ligament anteriorly. An extracorporeal knot-tying technique is used with an open knot pusher. Special care must be paid to avoid injury to the aberrant obturator vessels and external iliac vessels in placing the first sutures through Cooper ligament, which is close to the level of ischial spines.

LAPAROSCOPIC PARAVAGINAL REPAIR: RESULTS

The data regarding the laparoscopic approach to paravaginal defects are sparse and sometimes difficult to evaluate as paravaginal repairs are often done in combination with other procedures for pelvic organ prolapse. Recent studies are also scant because of the widespread adoption of the tension-free vaginal tape (TVT) approach in favor of the more technically challenging procedures in the space of Retzius.

Pulliam et al., in an observational study of 125 women who underwent a laparoscopic paravaginal repair, observed objective failure rates of 14.5% (95% CI [8.8%–22.4%]) in the anterior compartment using a preoperative and postoperative pelvic organ prolapse quantification (POP-Q) system. The mean length of follow-up was 335 days. The authors concluded, "laparoscopic paravaginal repair is an effective and safe means of repairing the displacement cystocele."

Behnia-Willison et al. longitudinally assessed 212 women with the POP-Q system prior to and following laparoscopic paravaginal repair. In patients with DeLancey level I defect ($N = 42$), the paravaginal repair was combined with a uterosacral hysteropexy or colpopexy. In patients with a concomitant posterior fascial defect ($N = 47$), the paravaginal repair was performed concurrently with a supralevator repair. Major complications were reported in nine women (4.2%) and 61 minor complications were noted. POP-Q assessment on follow-up at a mean of 14.2 months gave a prolapse cure of the laparoscopic repair of 76% (95% CI 70.7%–82.1%). Twenty-three women had a residual central defect, and 18 of these underwent a subsequent graft-reinforced anterior colporrhaphy, which increased cure rates to 84% (95% CI 79.6%–89.3%).

LAPAROSCOPIC MODIFIED BURCH URETHROPEXY

Genuine stress urinary incontinence (GSUI) is often due to a lack of periurethral support resulting in a hypermobile bladder neck. Since Marshall et al. first described in 1949 the vesicourethral suspension (Marshall-Marchetti-Krantz procedure) for urinary incontinence, numerous adaptations and permutations of the original procedure have evolved. The Tanagho Modification of the Burch colposuspension, utilizing a bridge of suture rather than approximating the pubocervical fascia and Cooper ligament, was originally performed abdominally in 1976. In 1993, Drs. Liu and Paek first reported on the laparoscopic modified Burch colposuspension, and since then the laparoscopic technique has been employed with comparable results to the open procedure.

TECHNIQUE

Following dissection of the space of Retzius, the surgeon inserts his or her second and third fingers vaginally to aid in the dissection of the pubocervical fascia just distal to the urethrovesical junction and lateral to the urethra (Figure 22.11). It is important to avoid aggressive dissection of the urethra, the bladder neck, the dorsal clitoral vein, and the obturator neurovascular bundle laterally.

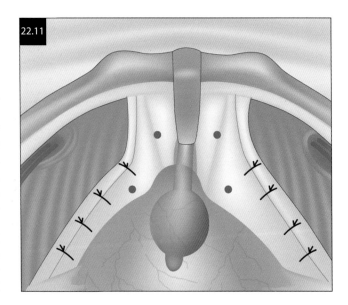

22.11

Significant bleeding can occur, and devascularization of the urethra is an undesirable consequence of overzealous dissection in these areas. The areolar and adipose tissue should be dissected off of Cooper ligament. The obturator neurovascular bundle should be visualized throughout the procedure and kept out of harm's way. A minimal amount of traction should be placed on the Foley catheter, and the vesicle's neck should be clearly identified by transvaginal palpation and abdominally under direct visualization (Figure 22.12). The pubocervical fascia is tented with the surgeon's vaginal index finger to aide in suture placement. A two-stitch approach is used, and the sutures should be placed and tied ipsilaterally. The first set of sutures of CV-0 GORE-TEX suture (polytetrafluoroethylene) is placed full thickness in the pubocervical fascia 1–2 cm distal to the mid-urethra bilaterally (Figure 22.13). The sutures should be placed 1–2 cm lateral to the urethra, and a double-bite technique through the pubocervical fascia is used, taking care to avoid locking the suture. A second set of sutures is placed at the urethrovesical junction using a similar technique. The sutures should be placed on tension prior to trying to make certain that a good purchase of the pubocervical fascia has been achieved. The sutures should be tied beginning distally and working proximally. Care should be taken to make certain that the sutures do not penetrate the vaginal mucosa. The CV-0 GORE-TEX sutures are passed through Cooper ligament at appropriate levels and the sutures secured beginning distally and working proximally. The vaginal fingers are used to assist in knot tying by elevating the pubocervical fascia. The knots are tied extracorporeally. Minimal tension on the midurethral sutures and avoidance of undue tension on the urethrovesical junction is mandatory to avoid postoperative voiding difficulty (Figure 22.14). A cystoscopy should be done to make certain that the bladder has not been injured and that the ureters have not been compromised. An ampule (5 mL) of indigo carmine dye should be given IV with 10 mg of Lasix, and good efflux of the dye from each ureteral orifice should be visualized cystoscopically.

LAPAROSCOPIC-MODIFIED BURCH RESULTS

A significant difference in failure rate was noted in the number of paraurethral sutures used to complete the colpopexy. Persson and Wolner-Hanssen reported a difference of 83% success rate using two single-bite sutures versus a 58% success rate using a single double-bite suturing technique ($p = 0.001$).

Analysis of the data directly comparing laparoscopic to open modified Burch colpopexy is complicated by differences in surgical technique, inconsistency in the definitions and criteria for "successful" outcomes, and variability in surgical skills and experience. The Medical Research Colposuspension Trial done in the United Kingdom reported objective data (1-hour pad test) demonstrating an 80% cure rate when the procedure was performed laparoscopically and a 70% cure rate when the procedure was done openly. The subjective cure rate

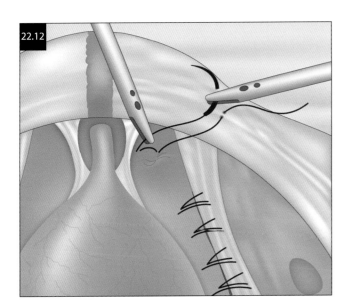

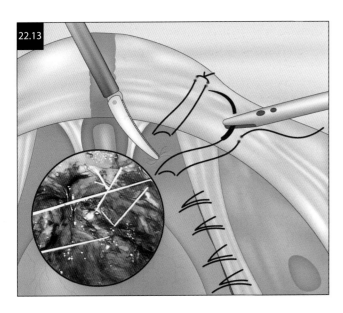

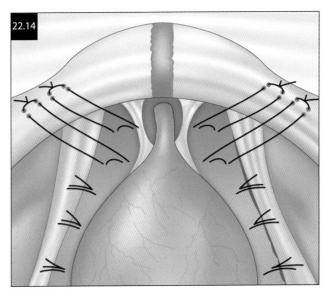

(perfectly happy/pleased) was noted to be 55% in this study.

Cheon et al. published results of 80 patients randomized to 43 in the open technique arm and 47 in the laparoscopic technique arm. At 1 year, they reported no difference in subjective or objective patient outcomes if done openly or laparoscopically. Importantly, the authors found no significant difference in the rate of complications, including *de novo* detrusor instability, urinary obstruction, enterocele, or dyspareunia.

Fatthy et al., in a study comparing open to laparoscopic-modified colpopexy, noted the following: (1) a 17 minute longer operating time in the laparoscopic group, (2) less blood loss (approximately 200 cc), (3) markedly reduced hospital stay, and (4) faster return to normal activities and work.

Notably, a 2009 Cochrane analysis identified 10 randomized or quasi-randomized trials that involved the comparison of laparoscopic with open colposuspension. The trials demonstrated a subjective (women's impression) cure rate that was favorable and similar for both techniques. In short- and medium-term follow-up, there was some evidence of better objective results for open colposuspension compared to the laparoscopic technique. Trends were shown toward fewer perioperative complications, less postoperative pain, and shorter hospital stay for laparoscopic compared with open colposuspension.

SPACE OF RETZIUS: SURGICAL COMPLICATIONS

Early studies regarding laparoscopic retropubic procedures for SUI and pelvic organ prolapse showed variable complication rates, perhaps due to the relative newness of the procedure and the lack of a uniform approach at the time.

In 2000, Speights et al. reported data from 171 patients that showed a 2.3% rate of bladder injury with laparoscopic colposuspension. Dwyer et al. presented data from 178 patients with a complication rate of 3.4%, which included three bladder sutures and three ureteral obstructions.

Scant data are available regarding *de novo* detrusor instability, but a 1995 meta-analysis by Jarvis showed a 9.6% mean incidence.

Complications encountered during a paravaginal repair are similar to those found in a laparoscopic colposuspension; however, since the paravaginal repair only corrects lateral sulcus defect, secondary midline, apical, and posterior prolapse requiring additional surgery have been reported. Increased risk of apical prolapse enterocele and posterior compartment prolapse following a modified Burch procedure are considered by many authors to be secondary to an alteration of the anterior vaginal axis.

Technological advances, as well as improved surgical experience in advanced laparoscopic techniques, have diminished the risk of laparoscopic retropubic surgery for stress urinary incontinence and pelvic organ prolapse. The most frequently reported complications of the modified Burch procedure and paravaginal repair are injury to the lower urinary tract and bleeding. Other reported complications include misplaced sutures in the bladder or urethra, urethral injury or obstruction, voiding dysfunction, and infection.

The importance of intraoperative or early recognition and repair of an injury cannot be overemphasized. Prior to completion of any procedure in the space of Retzius, routine confirmation of the integrity of the urinary tract should be accomplished.

The most common urinary tract injury is unintentional cystotomy, which frequently can be repaired laparoscopically using a layered closure of 3-0 absorbable suture, such as Vicryl (polyglactin).

The most common site of ureteral obstruction during a modified Burch procedure is in proximity to the urethrovesicle junction or vesicle neck, and the most common ureteral obstruction site during a paravaginal repair is the result of the plication suture placed in closest proximity to the ischial spine. When the surgery is complex, or there is any likelihood of ureteral injury, 5 mL of indigo carmine dye and 10–20 mg Lasix should be given intravenously, and a cystoscopy should be performed using a 70° lens. Good efflux of the dye should be noted from each ureteral orifice within 15 minutes of IV administration. If obvious effusion of the dye is not noted, a 4Fr or 5Fr whistle-tip catheter should be placed in retrograde fashion with laparoscopic observation during the advancement of the catheter. If resistance to passage of the catheter is encountered, or free drainage of urine is not noted, and the site of obstruction is not evident, a retrograde pyelogram should be accomplished by infusing the dye through the catheter. The site of the obstruction will be noted, and the offending suture should then be removed. If injury to the ureter is noted or suspected, a double-J ureteral catheter should be inserted under endoscopic guidance to stint the ureter and provide free urinary drainage.

The pelvic floor is highly vascularized, and brisk bleeding can occur during suture placement. While operating in the space of Retzius, care must be taken to avoid injury to the paraurethral vascular plexus during a Burch procedure, or injury to the pudendal vessels and obturator vessels, including the aberrant obturator vein, during a paravaginal repair. When bleeding occurs during the placement of the plication sutures during a paravaginal repair, cessation of bleeding usually occurs when the figure-of-8 sutures are secured during a paravaginal repair.

LAPAROSCOPIC BURCH PROCEDURE VERSUS TVT

Proponents of the laparoscopic Burch procedure for correction of stress urinary incontinence cite a proven history of success for the Burch procedure. But since Ulmsten et al. first described their tension-free midurethral sling procedure in the mid-1990s, this technique has garnered widespread popularity. The main reasons are thought to be that it is a technically easier surgery, with shorter operative times and a faster recovery time.

Early prospective, randomized trials between laparoscopic Burch and TVT found no significant difference in efficacy between the procedures with regard to SUI on urodynamic testing. However, Paraiso et al., in a 2004 randomized trial, compared the laparoscopic Burch colposuspension (36 patients) versus the TVT (36 patients) using multichannel urodynamic studies and Urogenital Distress Inventory and Incontinence Impact Questionnaire scores. At 1 year, 32 patients in the laparoscopic Burch arm of the study demonstrated an 18.8% incidence of urodynamic stress incontinence compared to 3.2% of patients in the TVT arm of the study ($p = .056$). This study demonstrated that the TVT had significantly better cure rates objectively and subjectively.

Reported complications of midurethral slings include hemorrhage, bladder perforation, vaginal erosion, fistula formation, obturator nerve injury, periostitis, voiding difficulties, graft rejection, urge incontinence, and overactive bladder.

In 2008, Ridgeway et al. looked at long-term follow-up data from the patients in Paraiso's original study. No significant difference was noted long term between the laparoscopic Burch and TVT arms of the trial, with 58% of subjects compared with 48% of subjects reporting any urinary incontinence in their respective groups 4–8 years following surgery (Relative Risk (RR):1.19; 95% CI: 0.71–2). The median follow-up duration was 65 months.

Paraiso's 2004 study noted overall complication rates were not different between the two arms, though the study did mention that complications in the TVT arm tended to be more serious. A 2007 Swedish study under Ankardal constructed a health-care cost model and found that the TVT procedure generated a lower direct cost than both open and laparoscopic colposuspension.

Although the U.S. Food and Drug Administration (FDA) has specifically exempted TVT from its 2011 communiqué regarding mesh safety, patient concerns over the perceived dangers of transvaginal mesh may lead to a return to the more "traditional" paravaginal repair and laparoscopic Burch procedure.

CONCLUSIONS

The treatments for pelvic organ prolapse and stress urinary incontinence have evolved over the years, and various surgical approaches to treatment have been developed. Currently, the midurethral sling procedures, especially the TVT and the transobturator tape, have in many institutions largely replaced the traditional paravaginal repair and the modified Burch procedure. Since no one procedure is optimal for all patients, it seems prudent that the traditional procedures should remain in the armamentarium of the advanced gynecologic surgeon.

SUGGESTED READING

Ankardal M, Järbrink K, Milsom I, Heiwall B, Lausten-Thomsen N, Ellström-Engh M. Comparison of health care costs for open Burch colposuspension, laparoscopic colposuspension and tension-free vaginal tape in the treatment of female urinary incontinence. *Neurourol Urodyn.* 2007;26(6):761–766.

Behnia-Willison F, Seman EI, Cook JR, O'Shea RT, Keirse MJ. Laparoscopic paravaginal repair of anterior compartment prolapse. *J Minim Invasive Gynecol.* 2007;14(4):475–480.

Chapple CR, Zimmerin PE, Brubaker L, Smith ARB, BØ K. *Multidisciplinary Management of Female Pelvic Floor Disorders.* Elsevier; 2006.

Cheon WC, Mak JH, Liu JY. Prospective randomized controlled trial comparing laparoscopic and open colposuspension. *Hong Kong Med J.* 2003;9:10–14.

Dean N, Ellis G, Herbison GP, Wilson D. Laparoscopic colposuspension for urinary incontinence in women. *Cochrane Database Syst Rev.* 2010;(3):CD002239.

Dwyer PL, Carey MP, Rosamilia A. Suture injury to the urinary tract in urethral suspension procedures for stress incontinence. *Int Urogynecol J Pelvic Floor Dysfunct.* 1999;10(1):15–21.

Fatthy H, El Hao M, Samaha I, Abdallah K. Modified Burch colposuspension: Laparoscopy versus laparotomy. *J Am Assoc Gynecol Laparosc.* 2001;8:99–106.

FDA and CDRH. Urogynecologic Surgical Mesh: Update on the Safety and Effectiveness of Transvaginal Placement for Pelvic Organ Prolapse. 2011: Available at https://www.fda.gov/downloads/medicaldevices/safety/alertsandnotices/ucm262760.pdf.

Jarvis GJ. Surgery for genuine stress incontinence. *Baillieres Best Pract Res Clin Obstet Gynaecol.* 2000;14(2):315–334.

Kitchener HC, Dunn G, Lawton V et al. Laparoscopic versus open colposuspension—Results of a prospective randomized controlled trial. *BJOG.* 2006;113:1007–1013.

Liu CY. *Laparoscopic Ureteral Injury. Prevention and Management of Laparoscopic Surgical Complications.* Chap 28, Society of Laproendoscopic Surgeons http://laparoscopy.blogs.com/prevention_management/chapter_28_ureteral_surgery/.

Liu CY. Laparoscopic treatment of genuine urinary stress incontinence. *Clin Obstet Gynecol.* 1994;8:789–798.

Liu CY, Paek W. Laparoscopic retropubic colposuspension (Burch procedure). *J Am Assoc Gynecol Laparosc.* 1993;1:31–35.

Lucas M. Traditional surgery and other historical procedures for stress urinary incontinence. In: Cardozo L, Straskin D. eds. *Textbook of Female Urology and Urogynecology,* 3rd ed. Boca Raton, FL: CRC Press; 2016:661–662.

Marshall VF, Marchetti AA, Kratnz KE. The correction of stress incontinence by simple vesicourethral suspension. *Surg Gynecol Obstet.* 1949;88:509–578.

Paraiso MF, Walters MD, Karram MM, Barber MD. Laparoscopic Burch colposuspension versus tension-free vaginal tape: A randomized trial. *Obstet Gynecol.* 2004;104(6):1249–1258.

Persson J, Wolner-Hanssen P. Laparoscopic Burch colposuspension for stress urinary incontinence: A randomized comparison of one or two sutures on each side of the urethra. *Obstet Gynecol.* 2000;95:151–155.

Pulliam S, Chelmow D, Weld A, Rosenblatt P. Laparoscopic Paravaginal Repair: A Case Series, 2005.

Richardson AC, Lyon JB, Williams NL. Treatment of stress urinary incontinence due to paravaginal fascial defect. *Obstet Gynecol.* 1981;57:357–362.

Ridgeway B, Walters MD, Paraiso MF et al. Early experience with mesh excision for adverse outcomes after transvaginal mesh placement using prolapse kits. *Am J Obstet Gynecol.* 2008;199(6):703.e1-e7.

Scotti RJ, Garely AD, Greston WM et al. Paravaginal repair of lateral vaginal wall defects by fixation to the ischial periosteum and obturator membrane. *Am J Obstet Gynecol.* 1998;179:1436–1445.

Shull BL, Baden WF. A six-year experience with paravaginal defect repair for stress urinary incontinence. *Am J Obstet Gynecol.* 1989;160:1432–1440.

Speights SE, Moore RD, Miklos JR. Frequency of lower urinary tract injury at laparoscopic Burch and paravaginal repair. *J Am Assoc Gynecol Laparosc.* 2000;7(4):515–518.

Tanagho EA. Colpocystourethropexy: The way we do it. *J Urol.* 1976;116:751–753.

Ulmsten U, Henriksson L, Johnson P, Varhos G. An ambulatory surgical procedure under local anesthesia for treatment of female urinary incontinence. *Int Urogynecol J Pelvic Floor Dysfunct.* 1996;7(2):81–85; discussion 85.

Vashisht A, Cutner A. Laparoscopic colposuspension. In: Cardozo L, Straskin D. eds. *Textbook of Female Urology and Urogynecology,* 3rd ed. Boca Raton, FL: CRC Press; 2016:909–928.

White GR. Cystocele, a radical cure by suturing lateral sulci of vagina to white line of pelvic fascia. *J Am Med Assoc.* 1909;53:1707–1711.

CHAPTER 23

MIDURETHRAL SLING PROCEDURES FOR STRESS URINARY INCONTINENCE

J. Ryan Stewart

HISTORY

Up to 35% of women are affected by stress urinary incontinence (SUI), and approximately 1 in 1000 women will undergo surgical treatment for SUI symptoms in her lifetime. Treatment options consist of lifestyle modifications, pessary use, and surgery. Traditional surgical treatments included open, and more recently laparoscopic, retropubic urethropexy (aka retropubic colposuspension) procedures such as the Marshall-Marchetti-Krantz (MMK) and Burch procedures, needle suspension procedures, and Kelly plication. In 1990 Ulmsten and Petros introduced their "Integral Theory" and used this theory to develop the first vaginal approach for the treatment of SUI, which Ulmsten and colleagues described in 1996. Since the initial description of this technique in 50 patients, millions of women have undergone these midurethral sling (MUS) procedures for the treatment of SUI and it has become the procedure of choice for patients refractory to conservative treatments. Modifications of this technique to decrease morbidity and operative time have continued to develop during the 20 years since first being reported.

PATHOPHYSIOLOGY

In the normal female, the urethra is supported by a combination of the endopelvic fascia and the anterior vaginal wall—structures that connect laterally to the arcus tendineus fascia pelvis and the levator ani muscles. This suburethral support is static and provides a stopping point for the intraabdominal forces that are transferred to the bladder and urethra during laugh, cough, and sneeze. This static support absorbs increases in intraabdominal pressure, resulting in coaptation of the urethra, thus maintaining continence. When damage to these "ligamentous" connections occurs, the static support is dissipated, and the forces are spread over a larger area decreasing the extent of coaptation and leading to urinary incontinence (Figures 23.1 and 23.2).

APPROACHES

The mechanism by which the MUS provides a high rate of success (85%–95%) directly relates to the recreation of the suburethral vaginal hammock, providing support as intraabdominal pressure is applied with a laugh, cough, sneeze, etc. The original description of the procedure required the blind passage of trocars from the vagina up through the retropubic space (bottom-up) (Figure 23.3). The first commercially available product for this approach was the Gynecare TVT. Although no longer commercially available, trocar-based retropubic procedures are often referred to as a "TVT." Variations of this surgery have evolved in an attempt to further decrease operative time and morbidity (Figure 23.4, Table 23.1).

The decision regarding choice of approach is highly individualized and guided by patient history, physician experience, comorbidities, informed consent, and physical exam.

> AT A MINIMUM, ALL PATIENTS SHOULD FIRST UNDERGO THE FOLLOWING EVALUATIONS PRIOR TO SLING PLACEMENT: (1) HISTORY, (2) PHYSICAL EXAMINATION, (3) DEMONSTRATION OF URETHRAL MOBILITY (Q-TIP TEST), (4) SUPINE OR STANDING COUGH STRESS TEST TO DEMONSTRATE SUI, (5) URINALYSIS, AND (6) MEASUREMENT OF POSTVOID RESIDUAL URINE VOLUME.

In a multicenter, randomized equivalence trial, Richter and colleagues evaluated subjective and objective treatment success in patients receiving either a retropubic or transobturator sling. They found that, using objective outcomes, the two approaches met criteria for equivalence. Evaluations of subjective outcomes did not show the same equivalence with success rates of 62.2% and 55.8% between the retropubic and transobturator groups, respectively. Analysis of complications showed a difference between the two approaches in terms of voiding dysfunction (retropubic 2.7%, transobturator 0%) and neurologic symptoms (retropubic 4%, transobturator 9.4%). Regardless of approach, there was no difference in quality of life, satisfaction, or postoperative urge incontinence.

Because of this, many physicians who are skilled in both retropubic and transobturator sling placement prefer retropubic slings for patients with a higher risk of failure or postoperative pain complaints. Alternatively, retropubic slings are often avoided in patients at high risk for voiding dysfunction or irritative voiding symptoms.

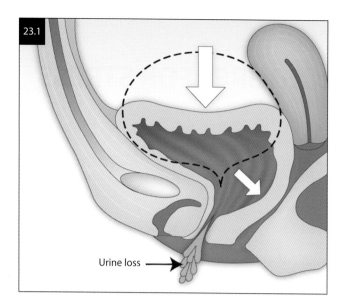

23.1

Urine loss

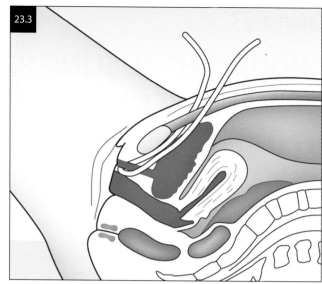

23.3

Clearly, the risk of bladder perforation is higher with retropubic slings. As such, an ability to perform routine cystoscopy is a prerequisite to this approach.

A robust systematic review and meta-analysis by Abdel-Fattah and colleagues, performed in 2011 and repeated in 2014, evaluated single-incision ("mini") slings compared to traditional (i.e., retropubic and transobturator) slings and found no significant difference in subjective or objective outcomes combined with less pain, faster recovery, and faster return to work. The authors go on to advise caution in the interpretation of their results due to the short-term nature of the data and trends toward improved outcomes with traditional slings and higher rates of reoperation with mini-slings.

The choice of approach is complex and often comes down to the individual surgeon's interpretation of the data and a thorough discussion of risks and benefits with the patient. Factors such as patient habitus, pure stress versus mixed incontinence, intrinsic sphincter deficiency, and the presence of chronic pain syndromes often play a role in the decision-making process. A review of this literature is beyond the scope of this text.

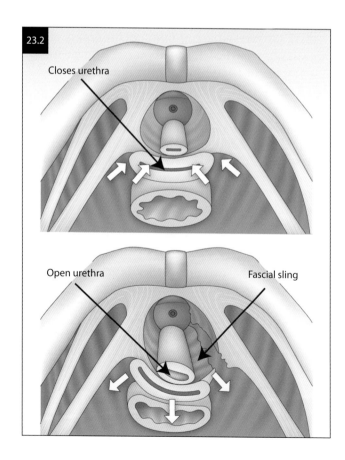

23.2

Closes urethra

Open urethra

Fascial sling

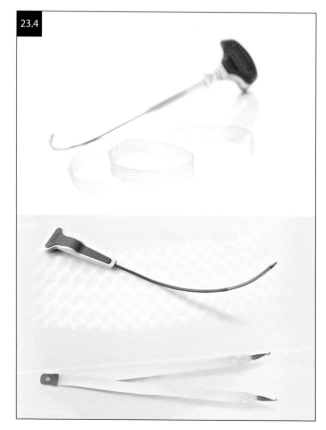

23.4

TABLE 23.1

MIDURETHRAL SLING MATERIALS AND KITS AVAILABLE AT THE TIME OF PUBLICATION

APPROACH	PASSAGE	TRADE NAME	MANUFACTURER	COMMENTS
RETROPUBIC	BOTTOM-UP	ADVANTAGE	BOSTON SCIENTIFIC	
RETROPUBIC	BOTTOM-UP	ADVANTAGE FIT	BOSTON SCIENTIFIC	SAME AS ADVANTAGE SYSTEM, BUT WITH TIGHTER TROCAR CURVE AND SMALLER-GAUGE TROCAR
RETROPUBIC	BOTTOM-UP	DESARA TV	CALDERA MEDICAL	
RETROPUBIC	BOTTOM-UP OR TOP-DOWN	DESARA	CALDERA MEDICAL	
RETROPUBIC	BOTTOM-UP OR TOP-DOWN	SUPRIS	COLOPLAST	
RETROPUBIC	TOP-DOWN	LYNX	BOSTON SCIENTIFIC	
TRANSOBTURATOR	INSIDE-OUT	DESARA, DESARA SL	CALDERA MEDICAL	DESARA SL IS 12 CM IN LENGTH
TRANSOBTURATOR	OUTSIDE-IN	ARIS	COLOPLAST	
		DESARA, DESARA SL	CALDERA MEDICAL	
		OBTRYX	BOSTON SCIENTIFIC	
SINGLE INCISION	NA	ALTIS	COLOPLAST	
		SOLYX	BOSTON SCIENTIFIC	

SOURCE: FROM AMID PK. CLASSIFICATION OF BIOMATERIALS AND THEIR RELATED COMPLICATIONS IN ABDOMINAL WALL HERNIA SURGERY. *HERNIA* [INTERNET]. 1997 MAY;1(1):15–21, WITH PERMISSION.
ALL MESH IS AMID TYPE I (MACROPOROUS, MONOFILAMENT) POLYPROPYLENE.

PROCEDURES

PREOPERATIVE

The decision for method of anesthesia should involve discussion between patient, surgeon, and anesthesiologist preference. These procedures have been performed successfully under local, regional, and general anesthesia. Some studies suggest higher rates of postoperative voiding dysfunction with general anesthesia. Many physicians perform the procedure using local anesthesia with monitored anesthesia care (MAC). The area along the path of the sling insertion is liberally infiltrated with local anesthetic from above and from below (Figure 23.5). The patient should receive antibiotic prophylaxis prior to incision. Medication and dose protocols vary somewhat by institution and have been set forth in the ACOG Practice Bulletin 104. Recent documentation of a sterile urine should be confirmed. Sequential compression devices for deep vein thrombosis (DVT) prophylaxis should be considered unless contraindicated.

RETROPUBIC

DESCRIPTION OF PROCEDURE (BOTTOM-UP APPROACH)

Intraoperative

After adequate anesthesia is obtained and the patient prepped and draped in supine lithotomy, a Foley catheter

is placed. The suprapubic exit sites are identified and marked with a pen 2 cm lateral to the midline at the superior edge of the pubic bone. A weighted speculum or right-angle retractor is then placed into the posterior vagina in an effort to view the anterior vaginal wall and urethra. Allis clamps are then placed 1.5 cm proximal and distal to the midurethra, which can be identified by palpation of the urethrovesical junction (demarcated by

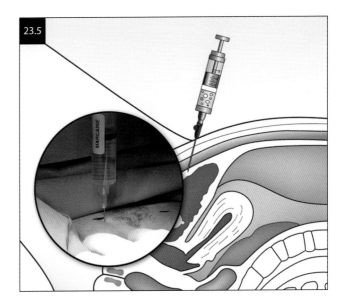

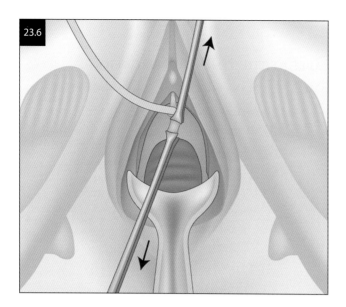

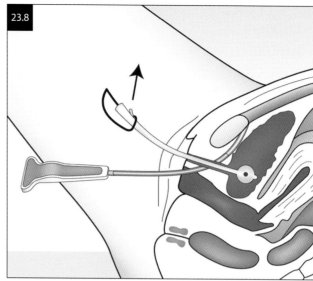

the Foley balloon) and the urethral meatus. These Allis clamps provide a point of countertraction for the following injection and dissection (Figure 23.6).

Injection of a dilute vasopressin solution (20 units in 100 mL saline) under the vaginal epithelium is useful to minimize bleeding and to hydrodissect the epithelium from the underlying urethra. This injection is continued laterally to the level of the ischiopubic ramus. A 1.5 cm full-thickness incision is then made over the midurethra. The epithelial edges are then grasped with Allis Adair clamps, and the epithelium is dissected away from the underlying urethra. The future sites of trocar placement are then dissected laterally with Metzenbaum scissors (Figure 23.7). Special attention should be paid to maintain full thickness as the dissection is carried superiorly and anteriorly toward the ischiopubic ramus. The endopelvic fascia should not be penetrated in this step.

Local anesthetic and/or vasopressin is then injected into the retropubic space by passing a spinal needle

from the previously marked exit sites to behind the pubic bone. A Foley catheter guide can then be placed and used to deflect the bladder contralateral to the side of trocar passage. The tip of the trocar is then placed in the previously created tunnel with the surgeon's dominant hand. Fingers of the nondominant hand are placed in the vagina palpating the inferior pubic ramus and are used to guide the tip of the trocar to the back of the pubic bone (Figure 23.8). As soon as the tip is posterior to the pubic bone, the dominant hand is dropped, and the curve of the trocar is used to pass the needle along the back of the pubic bone through the retropubic space. During passage of the trocar, special attention should be paid to aim the tip of the needle to the patient's ipsilateral shoulder. This is accomplished by keeping the eyes along the long axis of the trocar and keeping the handle parallel to the floor. Resistance is felt just before the hand is dropped (as the trocar passes through the endopelvic fascia) and near the end of the

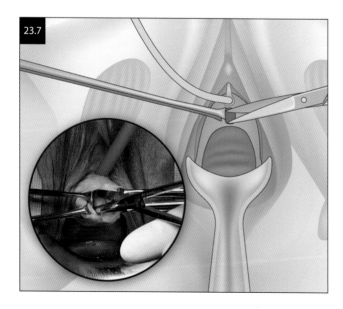

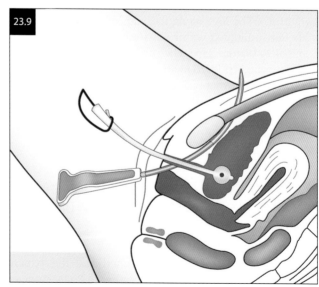

trocar passage (as the trocar passes through the rectus sheath and skin) (Figure 23.9). The trocar is then withdrawn, and the sheath of the mesh is grasped with a large clamp to prevent migration of the sheath while the opposite side is placed.

The bladder is then deflected to the opposite side and the exact procedure is repeated. With the sheath still in place, cystoscopy should be performed. During cystoscopy, the bladder should be filled until completely distended. The bladder should be examined in a clock-like and systematic fashion. Movement of the large clamps previously placed on the sheath should show that the sheaths are freely movable in the space of Retzius. There should be no evidence of tenting or perforation. If these signs are detected, the sheath should be removed and replaced, and the cystoscopy should be repeated. Likewise, after cystoscopy confirms no injury, the urethra should be systematically inspected for damage from dissection.

After confirmation that the sling is appropriately placed, the large clamps can be pulled toward the ceiling in order to tension the mesh. A large clamp or Metzenbaum scissors should be placed between the mesh and the urethra while the sling is drawn anteriorly. The sling should lie flat without folding or twisting. With gentle countertension on the Metzenbaum scissors, the sheath is removed from the mesh (Figure 23.10). The scissors should be able to be inserted and removed into this space without difficulty. If the procedure is being performed under MAC, the patient is asked to cough vigorously at this point—only small amounts of urine leakage (if any) should be seen. Alternatively, some physicians perform a Crede maneuver to provide feedback when tightening.

Copious irrigation of the vaginal wound is then performed, and the vaginal incision is closed with a 2-0 absorbable suture. Care should be taken to ensure a full-thickness closure. The suprapubic mesh is trimmed flush with the anterior abdominal wall. The skin should be elevated so the mesh lies within the subcutaneous fat. The incisions are then closed with a single suture, skin glue, or adhesive strips.

Postoperative care

The patient is taken to the recovery room where the Foley catheter is removed. Given the approximately 30% incidence of temporary postoperative urinary retention, a trial of voiding after catheter removal is recommended. If the patient is unable to adequately empty her bladder, she is discharged with a Foley catheter in place for 2–4 days until a repeat voiding trial can be performed. Alternatively, patients can be taught to perform intermittent self-catheterization prior to discharge.

TRANSOBTURATOR

DESCRIPTION OF PROCEDURE (OUTSIDE-IN APPROACH)

As with the retropubic sling, the transobturator approach can be done under MAC, regional, or general anesthesia. After adequate anesthesia is obtained and the patient is prepped and draped in supine lithotomy, a Foley catheter is placed. The "pinch test" is performed in which the surgeon palpates the inferior edge of the ischiopubic ramus and the obturator foramen (Figure 23.11). The exit sites in the groin are then marked with a sterile pen at the location where a horizontal line drawn from the clitoris intersects with the lateral edge of the labia majora, bilaterally (Figure 23.12). A weighted speculum or right-angle retractor is then placed in the posterior vagina in an effort to view the anterior vaginal wall and urethra. Allis clamps are then placed 1.5 cm proximal and distal to the midurethra, which can be identified by palpation of the urethrovesical junction (demarcated by the Foley balloon) and the urethral meatus. These Allis clamps provide a point of countertraction for the following injection and dissection.

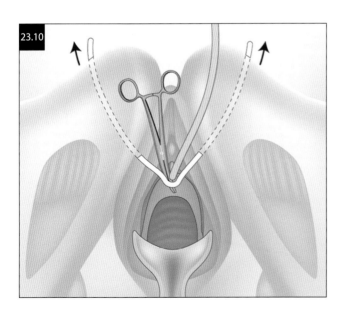

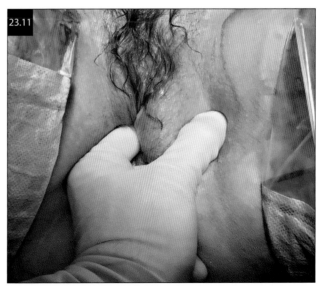

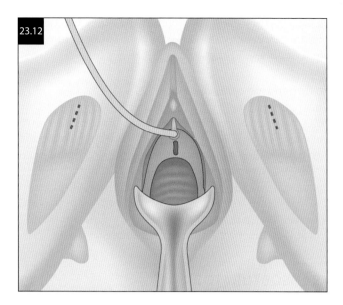

23.12

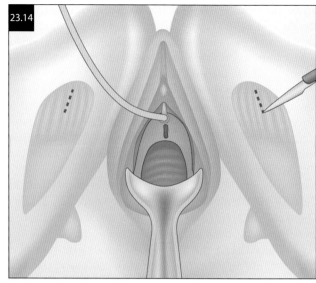

23.14

Injection of a dilute vasopressin solution (20 units in 100 mL saline) under the vaginal epithelium is useful to minimize bleeding and to hydrodissect the epithelium from the underlying urethra. This injection is continued laterally to the level of the ischiopubic ramus. A 1.5 cm full-thickness incision is then made over the midurethra. The epithelial edges are then grasped with Allis Adair clamps, and the epithelium is dissected away from the underlying urethra (Figure 23.13). The future sites of trocar placement are then dissected laterally with Metzenbaum scissors. Special attention should be paid to maintain full thickness as the dissection is carried superiorly and anteriorly toward the ischiopubic ramus. Many surgeons will repeat the "pinch test" at this point with one finger in the dissection, palpating the obturator internus muscle internally and visualizing the path of sling placement. Local anesthetic is then injected at the marked groin sites following the future path of the sling to the obturator internus muscle. Then 5 mm stab incisions are made at the marked entry points (Figure 23.14).

Note: There are two primary types of introducers used for transobturator sling placement: curved and helical (Figure 23.15). The primary difference between the introducers is the orientation of the handle during passage; the choice of introducer is a matter of physician preference. The passage of the helical trocar using an "outside-in" approach is described in the following text. Regardless of the approach, the surgeon should be familiar with, and follow, the manufacturer's recommendations for each system.

With the dissection complete, the tip of the introducer is placed into the stab incision lateral to the labium majora. The handle of the introducer is grasped with one hand, while the index finger of the opposite hand is placed in the vaginal dissection on the ipsilateral site (Figure 23.16). This step essentially recreates the "pinch test" using the introducer and the surgeon's finger. While this contact between finger and instrument is maintained, the introducer is rotated to pass the tip medially as the finger is withdrawn. With this motion, the introducer is

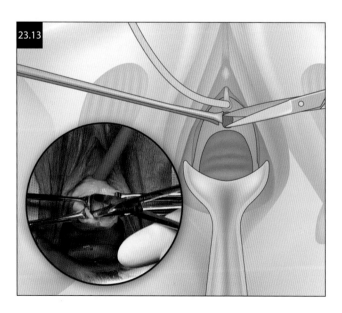

23.13

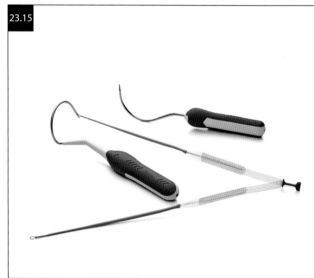

23.15

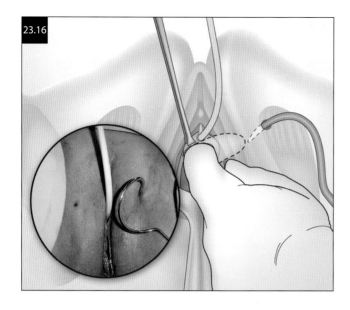

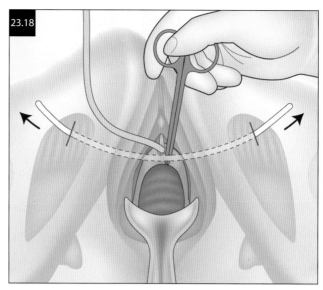

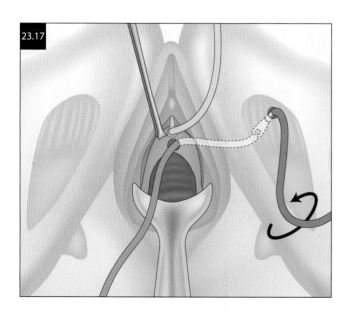

sequentially passed through the following structures: 1, skin; 2, subcutaneous tissue; 3, gracilis; 4, adductor brevis tendon; 5, obturator externus muscle; 6, obturator membrane; 7, obturator internus muscle; 8, endopelvic fascia; and finally 9, the vaginal dissection "tunnel."

When the tip of the introducer is seen, the sling is attached and the movement of the introducer is reversed, pulling the sling laterally out through the vaginal tunnel, obturator muscles, and skin (Figure 23.17). The same procedure is repeated on the opposite side. As with the retropubic sling, routine cystourethroscopy after placement of transobturator slings should be performed before removal of the sling's sheath.

After confirmation that the sling is appropriately placed, the mesh can be tensioned. A large clamp or Metzenbaum scissors should be placed between the mesh and the urethra while the sling is drawn anteriorly. The sling should lie flat without folding or twisting. With gentle countertension on the Metzenbaum scissors, the sheath is removed from the mesh. The scissors should be

able to be inserted and removed into this space without difficulty (Figure 23.18). If the procedure is being performed under MAC, the patient is asked to cough vigorously at this point—only small amounts of urine leakage (if any) should be seen. Alternatively, some physicians perform a Crede maneuver to provide feedback when tightening.

Copious irrigation of the vaginal wound is then performed, and the vaginal incision is closed with a 2-0 absorbable suture. Care should be taken to ensure a full-thickness closure. The mesh is trimmed flush with the skin of the groin. The skin should be elevated so the mesh lies within the subcutaneous fat. The incisions are then closed with a single suture, skin glue, or adhesive strips.

Postoperative care

The patient is taken to the recovery room where the Foley catheter is removed. Though the risk of postoperative voiding dysfunction is less with the transobturator than the retropubic approach, a trial of voiding after catheter removal should nevertheless be performed. If the patient is unable to adequately empty her bladder, she is discharged with a Foley catheter in place for 2–4 days until a repeat voiding trial can be performed. Alternatively, patients can be taught to perform intermittent self-catheterization prior to discharge.

SINGLE INCISION

DESCRIPTION OF PROCEDURE (INSERTION INTO OBTURATOR INTERNUS)

After adequate anesthesia is obtained and the patient is prepped and draped in supine lithotomy, a Foley catheter is placed. The "pinch test" is performed in which the surgeon palpates the inferior edge of the ischiopubic ramus and the obturator foramen. A weighted speculum or right-angle retractor is then placed in the posterior vagina in an effort to view the anterior vaginal wall and

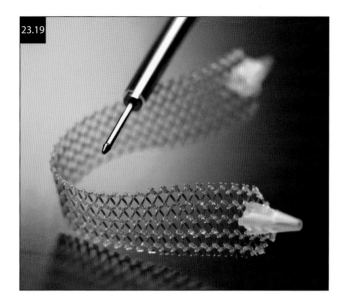

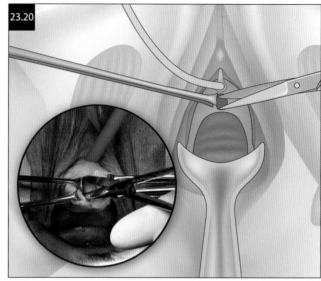

urethra. Allis clamps are then placed 1.5 cm proximal and distal to the midurethra, which can be identified by palpation of the urethrovesical junction (demarcated by the Foley balloon) and the urethral meatus. These Allis clamps provide a point of countertraction for the following injection and dissection.

The mini sling procedure does not require other entry sites, and the sling is anchored into the *endopelvic fascia* or into *the obturator internus muscle* (Figure 23.19).

Note: There are two placement types used for single-incision slings: (1) U-type, which anchors into the endopelvic fascia, and (2) H-type, which anchors to the obturator internus muscle. The placement of the H-type anchors is described in the following text. Regardless of the approach, the surgeon should be familiar with, and follow, the manufacturer's recommendations for each system.

Injection of a dilute vasopressin solution (20 units in 100 mL saline) under the vaginal epithelium is useful to minimize bleeding and to hydrodissect the epithelium from the underlying urethra. This injection is continued laterally to the level of the ischiopubic ramus. A 1.5 cm full-thickness incision is then made over the midurethra. The epithelial edges are then grasped with Allis Adair clamps, and the epithelium is dissected away from the underlying urethra. The future sites of sling placement are then dissected laterally with Metzenbaum scissors (Figure 23.20). Special attention should be paid to maintain full thickness as the dissection is carried superiorly and anteriorly toward the ischiopubic ramus. The endopelvic fascia should not be penetrated. The dissection should be large enough to accommodate the width of the chosen sling product so that the mesh will lie flat after placement.

The "pinch test" is then repeated to envision the future path of the trocar and anchor sites. The tip of the trocar is then placed in the previously created tunnel with the surgeon's dominant hand. Fingers of the nondominant hand are placed in the vagina palpating the inferior pubic ramus and are used to guide the tip of the trocar toward the inferior pubic ramus. The tip of the device will meet resistance at the endopelvic fascia, and a slight push into this layer will result in a "pop" as the fascia is penetrated. Continued rotation of the trocar results in contact with the obturator internus muscle and its overlying fascia. A second "pop" occurs as anchors are placed. Some devices employ the use of a removal suture in the event that the second anchor needs to be removed or replaced (Figure 23.21). Others have a "deployment mechanism" built into the device handle. In either case, proper placement and tensioning should be performed before removal of the trocar. Unlike its retropubic and transobturator predecessors, the single-incision slings require close approximation to the urethra. Many surgeons use a small clamp between the urethra and the sling to prevent overtensioning. Others tension by sight alone or by having the conscious patient perform a cough stress test. Cystoscopy can be performed at the surgeon's discretion. Copious irrigation of the vaginal wound is then performed and then it is closed with a 2-0 absorbable suture. Care should be taken to ensure a full-thickness closure.

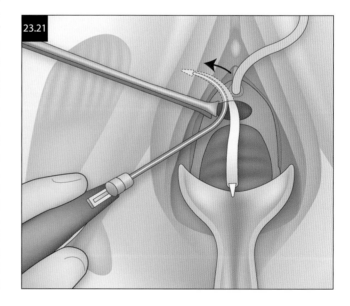

Postoperative

As mentioned for previous approaches, a postoperative voiding trial after catheter removal should be performed. If the patient is unable to adequately empty her bladder, she is discharged with a Foley catheter in place for 2–4 days until a repeat voiding trial can be performed. Alternatively, patients can be taught to perform intermittent self-catheterization prior to discharge.

CONCLUSION

Traditional (retropubic and transobturator), minimally invasive, midurethral slings are the most well-studied surgical procedure for stress urinary incontinence and have widely been accepted as the standard of care for this condition. Data from the Trial of Midurethral Slings (TOMUS) reported 1 year objective and subjective success rates of 78% and 62%, respectively. Additionally, Nilsson and colleagues reported on a prospective cohort of 90 women 17 years after their initial procedures, showing objective and subjective success rates of 90% and 87%, respectively, with only a single, small, and asymptomatic mesh erosion. In well-trained hands, the midurethral sling procedures are effective, safe, and durable.

ACKNOWLEDGMENT

Dr. Stewart would like to acknowledge contributions of Drs. Miklos and Moore for the work on this chapter in the previous edition of the book.

SUGGESTED READING

Abdel-Fattah M, Ford JA, Lim CP, Madhuvrata P. Single-incision mini-slings versus standard midurethral slings in surgical management of female stress urinary incontinence: A meta-analysis of effectiveness and complications. *Eur Urol.* 2011;60(3):468–480.

American College of Obstetricians and Gynecologists (ACOG). 104 Antibiotic Prophylaxis. *Obstet Gynecol [Internet].* 2009;114(106): 192–202.

American College of Obstetricians and Gynecologists (ACOG). Urinary incontinence in women. Practice Bulletin No. 155. *Obs Gynecol.* 2015;126:66–81.

Amid PK. Classification of biomaterials and their related complications in abdominal wall hernia surgery. *Hernia [Internet].* 1997;1(1):15–21.

DeLancey JO. Structural support of the urethra as it relates to stress urinary incontinence: The hammock hypothesis. *Am J Obstet Gynecol [Internet].* 1994;170(6):1713–1723.

Duckett JRA, Patil A, Papanikolaou NS. Predicting early voiding dysfunction after tension-free vaginal tape. *J Obstet Gynaecol [Internet].* 2008;28(1):89–92. Available from: http://www.ncbi.nlm.nih.gov/pubmed/18259908.

Jonsson Funk M, Levin PJ, Wu JM. Trends in the surgical management of stress urinary incontinence. *Obstet Gynecol [Internet].* 2012;119(4):845–851.

Koops SES, Bisseling TM, van Brummen HJ, Heintz APM, Vervest HAM. What determines a successful tension-free vaginal tape? A prospective multicenter cohort study: Results from The Netherlands TVT database. *Am J Obstet Gynecol [Internet].* 2006;194(1):65–74.

Mostafa A, Lim CP, Hopper L, Madhuvrata P, Abdel-Fattah M. Single-incision mini-slings versus standard midurethral slings in surgical management of female stress urinary incontinence: An updated systematic review and meta-analysis of effectiveness and complications. *Eur Urol [Internet]. European Association of Urology.* 2014;65(2):402–427.

Nilsson CG, Palva K, Aarnio R, Morcos E, Falconer C. Seventeen years' follow-up of the tension-free vaginal tape procedure for female stress urinary incontinence. *Int Urogynecol J Pelvic Floor Dysfunct.* 2013;24(8):1265–1269.

Petros PE, Ulmsten UI. An integral theory of female urinary incontinence. Experimental and clinical considerations. *Acta Obstet Gynecol Scand Suppl [Internet].* 1990;153:7–31.

Richter HE, Albo ME, Zyczynski HM et al. Retropubic versus transobturator midurethral slings for stress incontinence. *N Engl J Med [Internet].* 2010;362(22):2066–2076.

Ulmsten U, Henriksson L, Johnson P, Varhos G. An ambulatory surgical procedure under local anesthesia for treatment of female urinary incontinence. *Int Urogynecol J Pelvic Floor Dysfunct [Internet].* 1996;7(2):81–86.

CHAPTER 24

LAPAROSCOPIC SACROCOLPOPEXY AND CERVICOPEXY

Sean L. Francis and Ali Azadi

INTRODUCTION

Historical improvements on sacro- and cervicocolpopexy deemed it the "gold standard" of repair for the vaginal apex. Addison suggested distribution of mesh over as wide a portion of the vagina as possible using multiple sutures. Few changes have been made to this already effective technique; however, one of the most beneficial recent advancements has been the successful conversion to a minimally invasive surgical procedure due to technological advancements in imaging, monitors, and better laparoscopic instruments. Despite the success of early surgeon adopters, the steep learning curve has hindered many gynecologists from incorporating this technique into their armamentarium. Robotic technology, discussed elsewhere in the text, may prove to be the pivotal enablement to overcome the technical challenges.

ANATOMY

Knowledge of the pelvic anatomy is critical to perform this procedure. The course of the ureters should be carefully charted as they descend from the kidneys and follow the psoas muscle until they enter the pelvis at the pelvic brim. They do so by traversing the common iliac vessels just superior to the bifurcation of the external and internal iliac vessels (Figure 24.1). The ureter then travels to the bladder along the medial leaf of the broad ligament crossing beneath the uterine vessels. Also, it is essential to understand that within the pelvis the blood supply to the ureter is from vessels lateral to the ureter within the pelvis. This anatomy becomes quite relevant during dissection through the peritoneum over the sacrum and in closing the peritoneum.

The aortic bifurcation is above the sacral promontory. A series of cadavers and computed tomography (CT) scans were reviewed, and analysis revealed that the average distance from the sacral promontory to the bifurcation of the aorta is 5.3 cm. The left common iliac vein was demonstrated to be the closest large vascular structure to the promontory (Figure 24.2).

The middle sacral artery branches directly from the aorta. It should be avoided during dissection and suturing around the sacral promontory; however, it is reasonable to ligate this vessel using electrosurgery prior to placing any sacral sutures.

The presacral venous plexus is another potentially dangerous anatomic area that is occasionally encountered during this procedure. Injury to this avalvular vascular system, potentially masked by increased intraperitoneal pressure and resting out of the surgeon's field of view by Trendelenburg position, can result in hemorrhage requiring transfusion, and even mortality. This vascular plexus is composed of anastomoses between the lateral and median sacral veins from which blood courses into the pelvic fascia covering the body of the sacrum. Cadaveric studies of this anatomy have demonstrated that the best way to avoid this plexus is to suture within a 3×3 cm square above the third sacral foramen in the center of the promontory (Figure 24.3).

As retraction of the small intestine out of the pelvis and to the right toward the ileocecal junction will often improve visualization of the sacrum, it is important to understand the anatomy of the large and small intestines within the pelvis. Retraction of the sigmoid to the left will also facilitate dissection; however, one will occasionally encounter redundant bowel, diverticulosis, or significant adipose, which can make retraction difficult. If such circumstances arise, there are certain tips that might prove useful. Placement of a Keith needle with Monocryl suture first through the abdominal wall, then the epiploic fat and back through the abdominal wall is one solution. Providing an adequate number of ports to allow the assistant to hold the sigmoid is another option. Finally, specific laparoscopic instruments, such as a fan or the T'Lift, are made specifically for this problem (Figure 24.4). Finally, it is essential to know the core anatomy of pelvic floor support.

Delancey described three levels of pelvic support (Figure 24.5). Level 1 consists of the attachment of the vagina to the uterosacral ligaments and cardinal ligament complex, providing the highest level of support. It is believed that the sacral colpopexy mimics this support if performed appropriately. Level 2 consists of the lateral attachment of the upper vagina to the arcus tendineus fascia pelvis (white line). A paravaginal defect will be present if there is a defect at the Level 2 support. Level 3 support consists of the attachment of the vagina to the urogenital diaphragm and provides the lowest level of support.

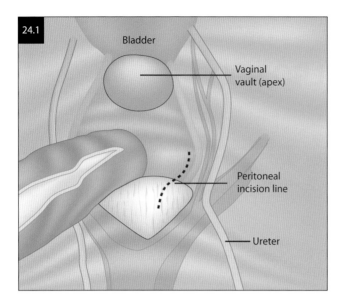

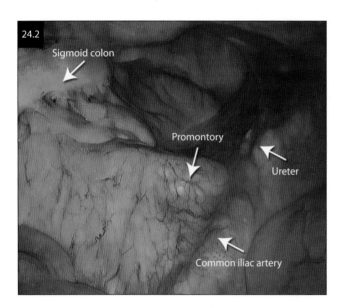

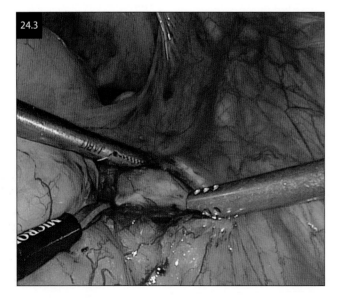

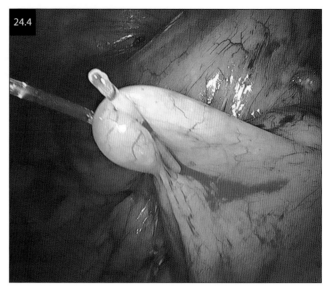

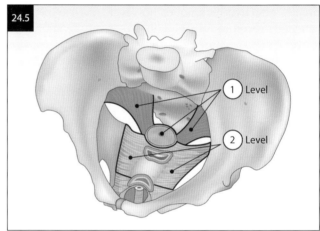

The degree of the prolapse can be assessed using different systems while the patient is awake and during straining. The POP-Q (pelvic organ prolapse quantification) and Baden-Walker grading systems are among the most commonly used. The POP-Q has the benefit of communicating the specific part of the vaginal anatomy that is prolapsed and of not relying on the surgeon's perspective regarding the organ behind the prolapsing part (Figure 24.6).

MESH/GRAFT

The graft used for sacral colpopexy has evolved in several ways from a single strap to two straps or a "Y"-shaped graft of polypropylene mesh. Alternative materials have been tried and studied, including fascia lata that is discussed later in this section.

Based on scientific publications demonstrating increased success rates, the standard practice among most female reconstructive surgeons is to use monofilament, large-pore, lightweight polypropylene mesh. Knitted mesh is preferred over woven for two reasons: The knitted product results in larger pore size, allowing macrophages to traverse the mesh, and allows for the establishment of the most ideal

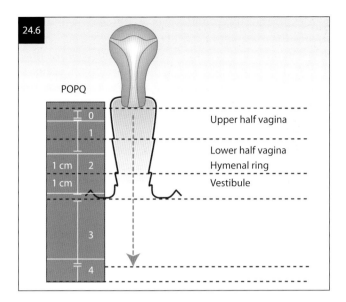

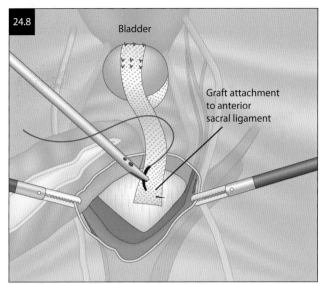

collagen type. Given this, companies that produce mesh have developed premanufactured Y-shaped grafts affording excellent strength, durability, and surgical adaptability with sufficient porosity for necessary tissue ingrowth.

If using the Y-mesh, the anterior arm is typically cut to approximately 4 cm and the posterior flap to approximately 8 cm depending on the extent of the dissection (Figure 24.7). Tensioning of the mesh is subjective; however, alleviating tension is crucial in avoiding erosions and failures. The vaginal probe is inserted into the vagina as far as possible while holding on to the sacral portion of the mesh. The probe is then left in a passive position by removing all force on the probe. The mesh is then released until there is no tension while making allowance for closing the peritoneum over the mesh. The mesh graft also may be tailored to fit the specific patient anatomy by cutting two independent rectangular-shaped sections of mesh from a larger piece. The caudal portions of the flaps are attached to anterior and posterior vaginal walls with cephalad portions attached to the sacrum (Figure 24.8). The tension on

the anterior and posterior vaginal wall therefore may be adjusted independently, providing an opportunity to correct the most prominent vaginal wall compartment defect. Some meshes have blue lines in the sacral and vaginal flaps, illustrating the bidirectional nature of the material. This aids in orientation and visibility and facilitates accurate suture placement. Biologic grafts may be used in patients with contraindication to mesh; however, their use for sacrocolpopexy may be technically challenging because they are opaque. In randomized controlled trials conducted at these authors' home institution, biologic grafts were shown to be inferior compared to synthetic materials 1 and 5 years following surgery.

The graft to the anterior portion of the vagina is first positioned with at least four interrupted, permanent, nonbraided sutures, and the posterior segment with at least eight sutures if possible (Figure 24.9). Recent data suggest delayed absorbable suture, such as PDS may be used for attaching the mesh to the vagina, however, permanent suture remains the preferred suture at the sacrum. This is

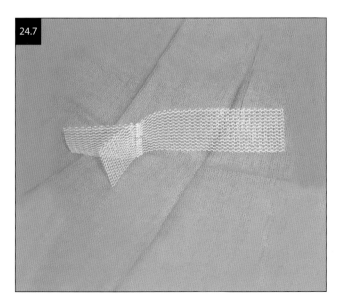

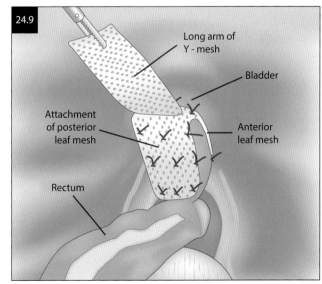

based on reported findings after open colpopexy and the strong contention that any significant deviation from the traditionally performed open technique changes the procedure and may therefore affect the outcome as reported after the introduction of the laparoscopic approach to performing the Burch colposuspension procedure. Similar suture selection is used to attach the sacral portion.

INFORMED CONSENT

Obtaining comprehensive informed consent is a critical and essential process. The patient should be apprised of all significant risks from the proposed surgery, including specific complications from implanted mesh materials, and contemporary alternatives to surgery including conservative nonsurgical therapies. In some cases, natural tissue repair without the use of mesh should be considered for surgical correction of primary prolapse.

In a public health notification released by the U.S. Food and Drug Administration (FDA) in 2008, and then updated in 2011, both practitioners and patients were warned about the complications of mesh. It was stated that mesh placed abdominally for pelvic organ prolapse repair appears to result in lower rates of mesh complications compared to comparable transvaginal surgery with mesh. The FDA recommended that when obtaining informed consent for these procedures, physicians should notify patients that implantation of surgical mesh is permanent, that some complications associated with the implanted mesh may require additional surgery, and that mesh may or may not correct the complication. They further recommended that patients be informed about the potential for serious complications and effects on quality of life, including pain during sexual intercourse, scarring, and narrowing of the vaginal wall in pelvic organ prolapse repair using surgical mesh. Furthermore, it is recommended that practitioners provide patients with a copy of the patient labeling from the surgical mesh manufacturer. Finally, the FDA recommends that health-care providers recognize that in most cases, pelvic organ prolapse may be treated successfully without mesh, thus avoiding the risk of mesh-related complications. Mesh surgery should be chosen only after weighing the risks and benefits of surgery with mesh versus all surgical and nonsurgical alternatives. Patients should be told and notified in writing that complete removal of mesh may not be possible and may not result in complete resolution of complications, including pain.

PROCEDURE

Laparoscopic sacrocolpopexy should be performed with consideration of the same surgical principles, techniques, and materials used in the abdominal approach.

POSITIONING

The patient should be placed in the dorsal lithotomy position with careful attention to avoid neurologic

injuries to the upper and lower extremities while optimizing the surgeon's visibility and access (see Chapter 38). The patient is placed in steep Trendelenburg position as this allows small bowel and redundant colon to move out of the pelvis. Some studies have suggested equal feasibility using less Trendelenburg in an attempt to minimize risk. The patient's arms should be tucked to the sides paying careful attention to the safety of the fingers. This maximizes the surgeon's ability to maneuver around the patient while providing the most ergonomic position. A Foley catheter is inserted into the bladder after the patient is prepped and draped but before trocars are placed to avoid perforation of the bladder upon trocar placement.

TROCAR PLACEMENT

Entry into the abdomen may be obtained by several different laparoscopic methods. Such options include the Veress needle, open technique, and visual access trocars. Visual access trocars and the open technique provide visualization of all layers successively during entry. All accessory trocars should be placed under direct visualization and with care to avoid injury to superficial and inferior epigastric vessels. The locations of trocars naturally vary according to each surgeon's preference. The goal is to provide adequate access to perform all of the required laparoscopic tasks. Figure 24.10 illustrates the port placement techniques used by the authors.

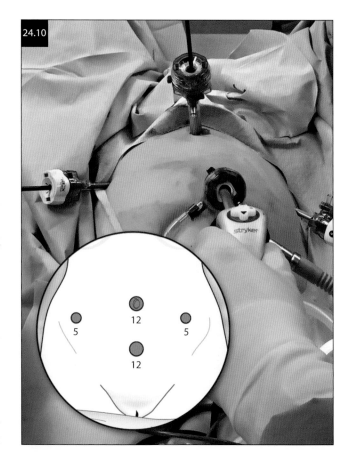

RESTORING ANATOMY

In the event that adhesions of the bowel to pelvic organs or abdominal/pelvic walls are encountered, lysis of adhesions should be performed in an attempt to restore normal anatomy. Key pelvic structures, especially the path of the ureters, should be identified. If a hysterectomy is to be coincidently performed, either a total laparoscopic (TLH) or supracervical hysterectomy (LSH) are sufficient (details of these surgeries are described in other chapters). Some surgeons prefer to perform vaginal hysterectomy or laparoscopic-assisted hysterectomy to avoid any thermal injury to the vaginal cuff, understanding there is a lack of evidence-based literature comparing supracervical hysterectomy to TLH for risk of erosion after sacral colpopexy; however, the available data lean toward supracervical hysterectomy resulting in a decreased rate of erosions. Moreover, one may consider closing the vaginal cuff in two layers, thereby imbricating the vaginal cuff when performing a TLH and sacrocolpopexy.

DISSECTION

Vesicovaginal and rectovaginal dissection

The vesicovaginal and the rectovaginal dissections are performed using a combination of sharp and blunt techniques. When performing the anterior dissection, the bladder is mobilized down and away from the vagina for 5–6 cm so that an adequate portion of vaginal length for suturing is exposed (Figure 24.11). The same is done posteriorly by mobilizing the rectovaginal septum to expose a vaginal length of 5–6 centimeters (Figure 24.12).

Placing a vaginal manipulator in the vagina provides elevation and countertraction, and facilitates dissection. Figure 24.13 shows some common instruments used as vaginal probes. A sponge stick may be used for similar manipulation of the vagina; however, one must be cautious as sutures penetrating the vagina may result in the sponge and/or sponge parts attaching to the lumen of the vagina. The peritoneum over the vagina should be

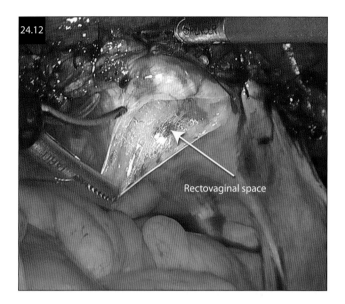

Rectovaginal space

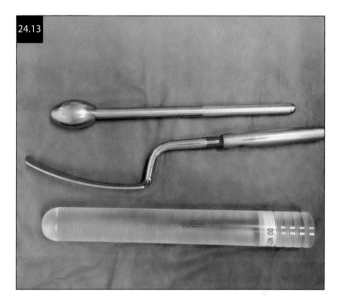

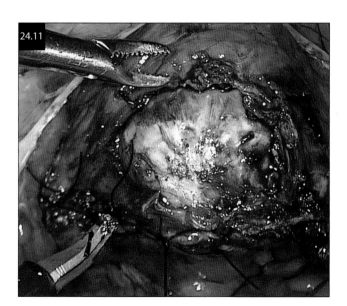

identified, lifted, and excised. Identifying the border of the bladder and rectum may be difficult in some cases; consequently, backfilling the bladder or placing an EEA sizer in the rectum may prove helpful in identifying these structures. The extent of dissection on the anterior and posterior walls depends on the quantity of prolapse and the location of the defect. If excessive perineal descent exists, the surgeon may consider attaching the most distal portion of the posterior mesh leaf to the perineum. Alternatively, a simple posterior repair may be accomplished if examination indicates this will be sufficient.

The sacral promontory

Excellent visualization is essential for this step of the procedure. Use of a 30° scope to obtain such visualization can be extremely helpful. After the sigmoid colon is retracted to the left, the right ureter should be visualized and the peritoneal incision made by elevating the peritoneum covering the sacral promontory medial to the right ureter (Figure 24.14). The assistant surgeon should

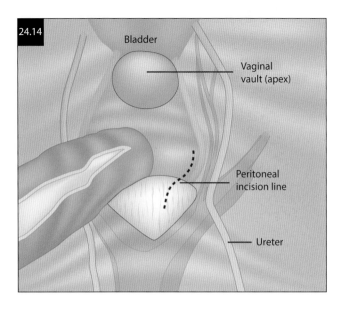

24.14

Bladder

Vaginal vault (apex)

Peritoneal incision line

Ureter

coagulate prior to suturing the mesh to the sacrum. The presacral venous plexus may bleed excessively if injured during the dissection and can be minimized by avoiding lower sacral dissection and by affixing the mesh to the upper portion of the sacral promontory. Placement on top of the promontory is not consistent with the original description or the physiologic axis of the vagina. Such placement is also believed to expose the posterior vagina to defects post surgery and may increase the possibility of bowel becoming entrapped under the mesh resulting in bowel obstruction. Due to the venous nature of bleeding in this type of injury, pressure should be applied to obtain hemostasis. Other methods may include bone wax, titanium thumb tacks, topical hemostatics, or a portion of rectus muscle applied to the bleeding sacrum and then deeply coagulated to stop bleeding. Conversion to laparotomy to attain hemostasis should not be considered a therapeutic failure.

grasp and elevate the peritoneum on the right side with the surgeon on the left. Using gentle traction, the area on top of the promontory should be cleared, and the presacral longitudinal ligament is then exposed (Figure 24.15). Due to the proximity of large vessels and the right ureter, all the structures must be visualized while identifying the right ureter through its entire course. The aortic bifurcation, right common iliac artery, and left common iliac vein are also in close proximity to the dissection. (Figure 24.2 shows the anatomy of the sacrum and the related structures.) The initial longitudinal incision over the peritoneum may be performed using laparoscopic scissors or with any form of energy-based cutting. Once the peritoneum is opened, the pneumoperitoneum naturally facilitates further mobilization and dissection of the retroperitoneal space. The presacral space is then dissected, and the retroperitoneal fat is cleaned off using a combination of blunt and sharp techniques to reach the anterior longitudinal ligament of the sacrum. The middle sacral vessels should be carefully identified to avoid or

The uterosacral ligaments

Once the presacral dissection is completed, the peritoneum medial to the pelvic side wall over the uterosacral ligaments should be opened from the sacral promontory to the cul-de-sac (Figure 24.16). It is important to remain in the space between the right ureter and the rectum. The right ureter should be in direct visualization throughout this step. Perirectal fat is a useful landmark to show proximity to the rectum. The assistant surgeon should elevate the right edge of the peritoneum, as the surgeon, while grasping the left edge, sharply performs the dissection. Placement of a vaginal elevator facilitates connecting this dissection to the rectovaginal space. A technique using tunneling beneath the peritoneum can also be utilized.

VAGINAL MESH ATTACHMENT

Once the appropriate dissection is completed, the mesh may be introduced through a port. The mesh is then

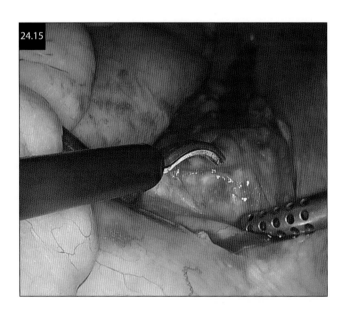

24.15

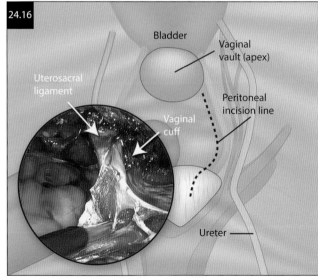

24.16

Bladder

Vaginal vault (apex)

Uterosacral ligament

Peritoneal incision line

Vaginal cuff

Ureter

attached to the anterior and posterior surfaces of the vagina using permanent interrupted sutures, such as Ethibond, GORE-TEX, or Prolene. Attachment using delayed absorbable sutures has also been described. More recently, knotless barbed sutures have been used to attach the mesh, thereby eliminating the need to tie sutures. Care must be taken to incorporate the vaginal fibromuscular tissue while avoiding penetration of the vaginal epithelium. The mesh is typically sutured first to the anterior vaginal wall by placing a low midline suture to fix the mesh to the lowest part of the anterior vaginal dissection. Tracting upward with a vaginal probe can help with this step of the procedure. The mesh is than fixated with five to six additional sutures. These sutures can be tied intracorporeally or extracorporeally (Figure 24.17). Surgeons outside the United States typically employ intracorporeal suturing to save sutures. Once the anterior mesh is secured, it is positioned on the posterior vaginal wall and then fixated with five to six sutures. Traction using a Breisky vaginal retractor can help expose the posterior vaginal wall to facilitate suturing. The assistant surgeon plays an important role in positioning the mesh during this step. Ultimately, the degree and type of the prolapse should direct the extent of vesicovaginal and rectovaginal dissection as well as placement of the mesh, such as attachment to the perineal body in cases of perineal descent noted during office examination or in those experiencing defecatory dysfunction.

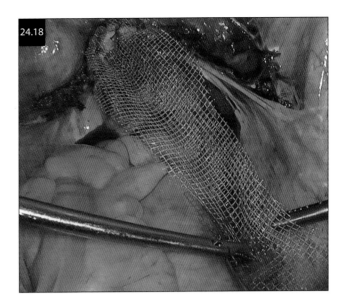

SACRAL MESH ATTACHMENT

The longer tail of the "Y" mesh is sutured to the anterior longitudinal ligament of the sacrum. The tension of the mesh is then carefully verified using vaginal examination (Figure 24.18). The mesh is ideally placed "tension free" given the inevitable shrinkage after implantation. Overtightening may cause pelvic pain, dyspareunia, and even failure. The mesh may be attached using a variety of techniques (Figure 24.19). Typically, two to four

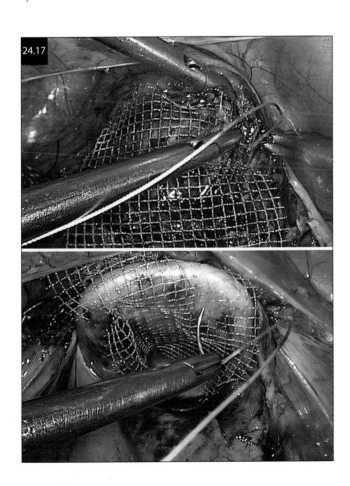

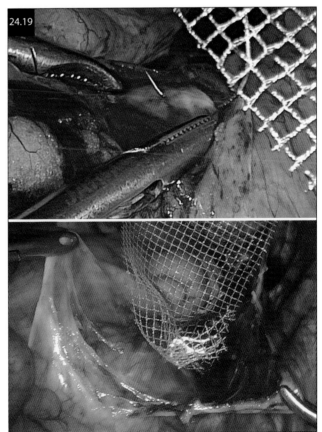

permanent sutures are utilized to secure the mesh to the anterior longitudinal ligament. Since penetrating too deeply may increase risk for discitis or osteomyelitis, the 60° drop of the sacral promontory must be considered when placing these sutures. Hemostasis should be assessed by lowering intraabdominal pressure prior to closing the peritoneal defect.

PERITONEUM CLOSURE

The peritoneum may be closed using a variety of methods, including interrupted or running sutures. It is important to ensure complete re-peritonealization (coverage of all the mesh by the peritoneum) to avoid contact with the bowel and possible erosion into the viscera (Figure 24.20). Moreover, bowel obstruction has been reported after sacrocolpopexy from bowel passing beneath an exposed bridge of mesh. This type of complication should also be prevented by proper closure of the peritoneum.

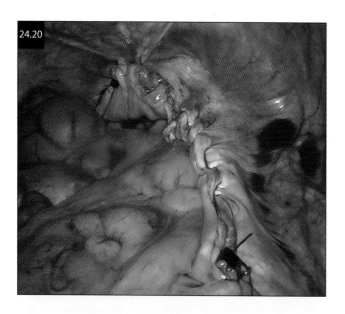

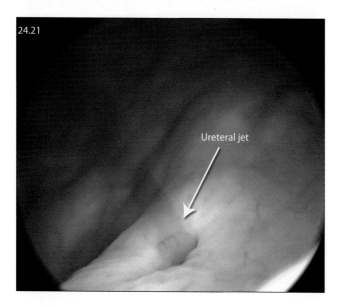

CYSTOSCOPY

Cystoscopy at the end of the case is essential to ensure the integrity of the bladder and patency of the ureters. One should additionally confirm that there is no suture or mesh penetrating the bladder. Indigo carmine may be given intravenously to aid in visualization of ureteral efflux (Figure 24.21). Trocars should be left in place until cystoscopy is completed. A 70° cystoscope using sterile water facilitates visualization of efflux from the ureters and allows the surgeon to examine difficult-to-reach parts of the bladder. Generally speaking, the potential for litigation is significantly reduced whenever a complication is revealed prior to leaving the operating room. Studies exist demonstrating a significant reduction in missed complications when cystoscopy is used after gynecological surgeries.

POTENTIAL COMPLICATIONS

The immediate complications of laparoscopic sacrocolpopexy include blood loss, hematoma, enterotomy, and injury to bladder and ureters. Due to its proximity to major vessels, life-threatening hemorrhage is a risk. Control of bleeding from the presacral venous plexus may be difficult, as these vessels can retract. Effective use of techniques described above during these circumstances may prove to be life saving.

Long-term complications may include bowel obstruction, infection, hernia formation, erosion or exposure of the mesh (about 5%), pelvic pain, and dyspareunia. Obesity, tobacco use, and concomitant hysterectomy are among risk factors for mesh erosion. Albeit rare, sacral osteomyelitis and discitis require removal of the mesh graft and long-term use of antibiotics.

LONG-TERM OUTCOME

The laparoscopic sacrocolpopexy provides excellent pelvic support with a low failure rate using a minimally invasive approach. Studies evaluating its anatomical success have shown that it is superior to vaginal approaches. A Cochrane database review showed better anatomical support, lower reoperation rate, and less dyspareunia in sacrocolpopexy compared to vaginal sacrospinous fixation. When counseling patients, these benefits should be considered and measured against potential complications, longer surgical times, and increased cost when compared to a vaginal approach. The reoperation rate for *de novo* stress urinary incontinence has been reported as high as 30%.

SUGGESTED READING

Benson JT, Lucente V, McClellan E. Vaginal versus abdominal reconstructive surgery for the treatment of pelvic support defects: A prospective randomized study with long-term outcome evaluation. *Am J Obstet Gynecol.* 1996;175(6):1418–1421; discussion 1421–1422.

Brubaker L, Nygaard I, Richter HE et al. Two-year outcomes after sacrocolpopexy with and without Burch to prevent stress urinary incontinence. *Obstet Gynecol.* 2008;112(1):49–55.

Carter JE, Winter M, Mendehlsohn S, Saye W, Richardson AC. Vaginal vault suspension and enterocele repair by Richardson-Saye laparoscopic technique: Description of training technique and results. *JSLS.* 2001;5(1):29–36.

Cundiff GW, Varner E, Visco AG et al. Pelvic Floor Disorders Network. Risk factors for mesh/suture erosion following sacral colpopexy. *Am J Obstet Gynecol.* 2008;199(6):688.e1–688.e5.

DeLancey JO. Anatomic aspects of vaginal eversion after hysterectomy. *Am J Obstet Gynecol.* 1992;166(6 Pt 1):1717–1724; discussion 1724-1728.

Jonsson Funk M, Edenfield AL, Pate V, Visco AG, Weidner AC, Wu JM. Trends in use of surgical mesh for pelvic organ prolapse. *Am J Obstet Gynecol.* 2013;208(1):79.e1–79.e7.

Miklos JR, Kohli N, Lucente V, Saye WB. Site-specific fascial defects in the diagnosis and surgical management of enterocele. *Am J Obstet Gynecol.* 1998;179(6 Pt 1):1418–1422; discussion 1822–1823.

Moore RD, Miklos JR. Laparoscopic sacral colpopexy. *Surg Technol Int.* 2008;17:195–202.

Nezhat CH, Nezhat F, Nezhat C. Laparoscopic sacral colpopexy for vaginal vault prolapse. *Obstet Gynecol.* 1994;84(5):885–888.

Paraiso MF, Jelovsek JE, Frick A, Chen CC, Barber MD. Laparoscopic compared with robotic sacrocolpopexy for vaginal prolapse: A randomized controlled trial. *Obstet Gynecol.* 2011;118(5):1005–1013.

Tan-Kim J, Menefee SA, Luber KM, Nager CW, Lukacz ES. Prevalence and risk factors for mesh erosion after laparoscopic-assisted sacrocolpopexy. *Int Urogynecol J.* 2011;22(2):205–212.

Tate SB, Blackwell L, Lorenz DJ, Steptoe MM, Culligan PJ. Randomized trial of fascia lata and polypropylene mesh for abdominal sacrocolpopexy: 5-year follow-up. *Int Urogynecol J.* 2011;22(2):137–143.

U.S. Food and Drug Administration (FDA). FDA Safety Communication: Update on serious complications associated with transvaginal placement of surgical mesh for pelvic organ prolapse. (2011-07-13) [2012-05-02]. http://www.fda.gov/MedicalDevices/Safety/AlertsandNotices/ucm262435.htm (2011).

Walters MD, Ridgeway BM. Surgical treatment of vaginal apex prolapse. *Obstet Gynecol.* 2013;121(2 Pt 1):354–374.

Warner WB, Vora S, Hurtado EA, Welgoss JA, Horbach NS, von Pechmann WS. Effect of operative technique on mesh exposure in laparoscopic sacrocolpopexy. *Female Pelvic Med Reconstr Surg.* 2012;18(2):113–117.

Wattiez A, Canis M, Mage G, Pouly JL, Bruhat MA. Promontofixation for the treatment of prolapse. *Urol Clin North Am.* 2001;28(1):151–157.

CHAPTER 25

LAPAROSCOPIC UTEROSACRAL LIGAMENT SUSPENSION

Elizabeth Babin and Timothy B. McKinney

INTRODUCTION

The surgeon is challenged daily to weigh his or her evaluation of an individual patient to the body of current evidence in order to propose effective treatment plans. Laparoscopic uterosacral ligament suspension is one effective minimally invasive surgical option for repair of DeLancey level 1 support defects of the *posthysterectomized* cervix or vaginal vault as well as for the *in situ* uterus. The uterosacral ligament complex can be utilized in the treatment of existing defects as well as for prophylaxis of iatrogenic defects created during hysterectomy. This complex of endopelvic fascia was first purported to be a successful option for surgical repair of prolapse in 1927 by Dr. Miller. The 2013 Cochrane database review suggests that sacrocolpopexy has superior outcomes to uterosacral colpopexy as well as other vault suspension procedures; however, many women and surgeons are migrating back to native tissue repair and trying to avoid biologic or synthetic mesh and their potential complications. The uterosacral ligament suspension is the native tissue equivalent to the mesh-augmented sacrocolpopexy. The cardinal-uterosacral ligament complex supports the upper vertical axis of the vagina, holding the pelvic viscera horizontally on the levator plate. The skeletal matrix of the endopelvic fascia that comprise the uterosacral ligament starts on the sacrum at the lateral aspect of S2, S3, and S4, extending down to fuse on the levator ani muscles and posterior cervicovaginal ring (Figure 25.1). Avulsions of these attachments lead to herniation or prolapse of the uterus or vaginal vault through the urogenital levator hiatus. The goal of uterosacral ligament suspension is to reattach these natural ligamentous avulsions in order to pulley the uterus or vaginal vault back up to its original level at the ischial spine. The uterosacral ligament also allows for the most anatomic repair when compared to other vault suspension methods, such as sacrospinous ligament fixation or iliococcygeal fixation, in that the uterosacral ligament will restore the vagina to its original axis of orientation for sexual function. The laparoscopic approach to this procedure allows direct visualization of the uterosacral ligament, the avulsed attachment of the ligament, and the closely approximated ureter and rectum. Several authors have demonstrated the feasibility of this procedure to be performed laparoscopically. Cadaver studies have demonstrated that sutures in the uterosacral ligament placed via a laparoscope have similar or slightly greater pull-out strength than those placed vaginally. The improved visualization and dissection available to the laparoscopic surgeon, with subsequent improved tissue capture, likely explain this trend. In addition, the laparoscopic approach facilitates concomitant laparoscopic procedures, such as paravaginal defect repair for the correction of anterior compartment defects. Low posterior defects tend to be more easily addressed as a concomitant repair through a combined vaginal-laparoscopic approach. High defects are very approachable via the laparoscopic route. An understanding of the uterosacral ligament complex in relation to the anatomy and biomechanics of pelvic support and a description of the laparoscopic uterosacral ligament suspension procedure are the focus of this chapter.

LITERATURE REVIEW

There is limited level 1 evidence related to uterosacral ligament suspension. To date, there is one prospective randomized controlled trial; however, several other non-randomized prospective studies and many retrospective case series and reviews suggest excellent anatomic and functional outcomes. One of the earliest reports of uterosacral ligament suspension being accomplished laparoscopically was from 1996 by Ostrzenski et al. In 2001, Karram et al., in a large retrospective study of high uterosacral vaginal vault suspension with fascial reconstruction, reported a 99% success rate over a 21.6 month follow-up time interval. Rardin et al. did a retrospective analysis of uterosacral suspension accomplished via laparoscopic versus transvaginal route at the time of vaginal hysterectomy. They reported similar outcomes with a trend toward fewer symptomatic failures (4.6% versus 12.5%) along with fewer ureteral and rectal injuries through the laparoscopic route versus the vaginal route. In 2010, Natale et al. performed a prospective randomized study comparing high levator myorrhaphy to uterosacral ligament suspension via the vaginal route. They defined success as stage 2 or better anatomical outcome and found a 96.6% cure rate for levator myorrhaphy and a 98.3% cure rate for uterosacral ligament suspension.

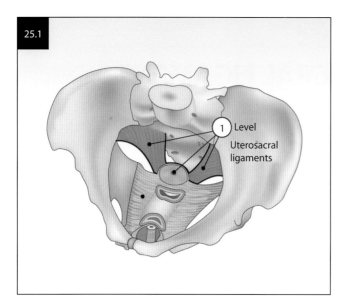

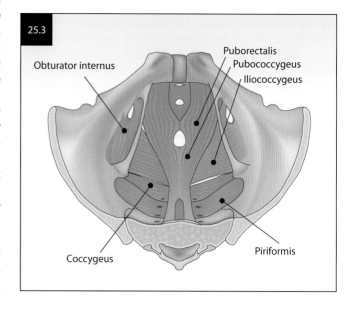

Marguiles et al. published a systematic review and meta-analysis of transvaginal uterosacral ligament suspension outcomes in 2010 that suggested 98% anatomical success and 82%–100% pooled analysis subjective symptom relief. As previously mentioned, the 2013 Cochrane database review of surgical management of women with pelvic organ prolapse noted that sacrocolpopexy has higher overall success than uterosacral suspension, but this must be weighed against the risk:benefit ratio of permanent synthetic mesh placement. Additionally, the vast majority of the uterosacral suspension studies included in the database review were of the vaginal route. Further studies of the laparoscopic outcomes of this procedure are needed; however, it appears to be a viable alternative to the mesh-augmented sacrocolpopexy.

ANATOMY AND BIOMECHANICS OF PELVIC SUPPORT

The various bulges encountered in the vagina (i.e., cystoceles, urethroceles, uterine prolapse, enteroceles, and rectoceles) all represent some failure of the pelvic floor to support one or more of the visceral structures resting on or contained within it. Isolated breaks in the rectovaginal septum cause rectoceles, as well as breaks between the rectovaginal septum and pubocervical fascia give rise to enterocele (Figure 25.2). The pelvic floor acts as a unit. It is divided into three layers of support from the inside out: the endopelvic fascial network, the striated levator ani muscles of the pelvic diaphragm, and the urogenital diaphragm and bony pelvis (Figures 25.3 and 25.4). The mechanism of failure is always from the inside out in pelvic organ prolapse. Therefore, in all major prolapses, there are isolated breaks in the innermost layer or endopelvic fascia. Surgically, these endopelvic fascial structures (i.e., the uterosacral ligament complex, pubocervical fascia, and rectovaginal fascia) each individually need to be addressed in all repair procedures to help ensure anatomical correction. The clinical identification

of these defects allows for appropriate repair. When contemplating the various supportive structures, it is helpful to consider the vagina as a flattened fibromuscular tube lined with vaginal epithelium. The top of the tube is the pubocervical fascia. The bottom is the rectovaginal fascia or septum (Figure 25.5). The top of the tube, as well as the uterus, are supported above the pelvic diaphragm by structures identified as the cardinal/uterosacral ligament complex. DeLancey described three levels of support for the pelvic viscera (Figure 25.6). The uterosacral ligaments

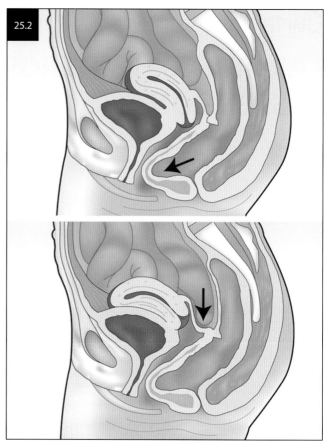

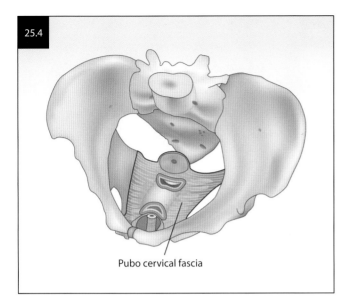

Pubo cervical fascia

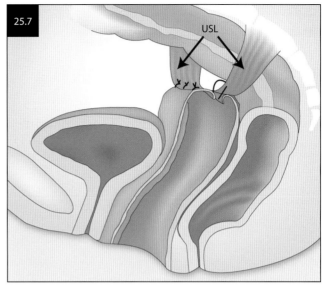

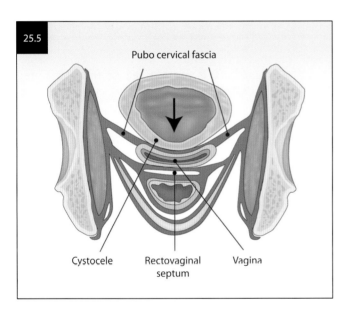

Pubo cervical fascia

Cystocele   Rectovaginal   Vagina
             septum

represent the level 1 support of endopelvic fascia. In the woman that is standing, the uterosacral ligaments suspend the pericervical ring and vagina (Figure 25.7). The midportion of the endopelvic fascia support, or level 2, attaches the vagina to the levator ani muscles from the ischial spines to the urogenital diaphragm. The anterior vaginal wall, pubocervical fascia, as well as the posterior vaginal wall, attach laterally at the same spot, the arcus tendineus ligament, and form a restraining layer that prevents the bladder and rectum from protruding into the vagina (Figure 25.8).

On the distal end of the tube, DeLancey level 3, there is a fusion with the urogenital diaphragm and perineal body (Figure 25.9). In the normally functioning pelvis, the levator ani muscles are always contracted, keeping the pelvic floor closed and allowing for minimal transmission of increased abdominal pressure on the endopelvic fascia. The endopelvic fascia network simply suspends the organs in their proper position above the levator ani muscles. This interaction between the pelvic floor

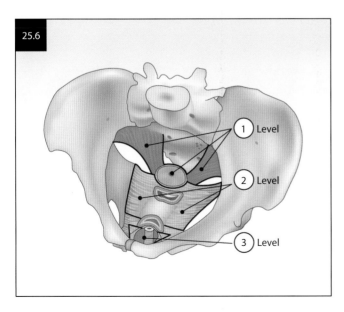

1 Level
2 Level
3 Level

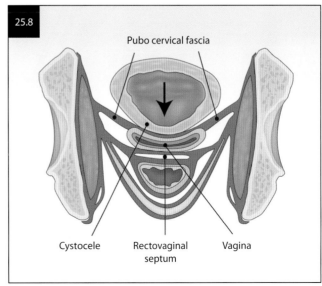

Pubo cervical fascia

Cystocele   Rectovaginal   Vagina
             septum

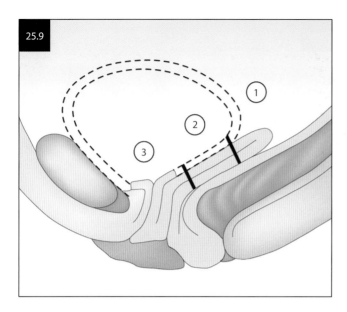

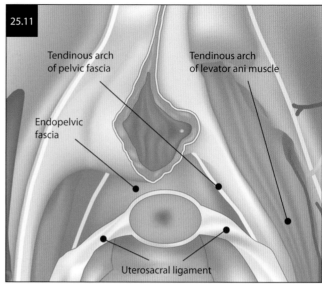

muscles and fascia is critical to proper pelvic floor support and function. If the pelvic floor muscles are damaged or relaxed for prolonged periods of time, increases in intraabdominal pressure and gravity can damage the underlying endopelvic fascia or expose weaknesses in the fascia. These defects in the endopelvic fascia in conjunction with poorly functioning levator ani muscles result in genital organ prolapse (Figure 25.10).

ENDOPELVIC FASCIA

The endopelvic fascia is the most important element responsible for maintenance of the normal anatomical relationship. It is a skeletal matrix made up of a meshwork of collagen, elastin, and smooth muscle (Figure 25.11). The endopelvic fascia serves two important purposes: first, to support the pelvic viscera in a proper orientation. In a standing female, the bladder, the upper two-thirds of the vagina, and the rectum lie in the horizontal axis; thus, the endopelvic fascia serves as support

(Figure 25.12). This mechanism is critical in preventing prolapse of organs through the urogenital levator hiatus. The mechanism by which this works to maintain organ position is that during times of intraabdominal pressure, a perpendicular force is exerted against the vagina and pelvic viscera. Simultaneously, the contracting levator ani plate elevates the pelvic floor, pinning organs and entrapping them in a flapper valve mechanism that prevents organ descent when standing. This mechanism is what we aim to reestablish during our surgical reconstruction. The second purpose of the endopelvic fascia is to envelop and support blood vessels, visceral nerves, and lymphatics as they course through the pelvis. The first support axis, DeLancey's level 1, represents the upper vertical axis and is delineated by the cardinal-uterosacral ligament complex holding the pelvic viscera horizontally over the levator plate. The uterosacral ligament does not contain any of the major blood supply or ureters. This structure represents a complex of endopelvic fascia beginning on the sacrum at the lateral aspect of S2, S3,

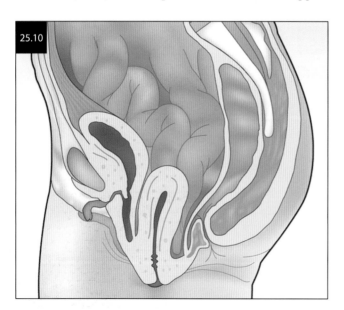

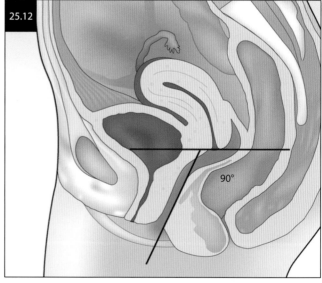

and S4 and extending to fuse with the vagina and the levator ani muscles below (see Figure 25.1). Clinically, they cannot be seen or palpated unless tension is applied to their distal margins. Therein lies the problem with their identification and utilization in the repair of significant uterine and vaginal vault prolapse where the attachment has been ruptured. Richardson et al. demonstrated that the pelvic connective tissue is more likely to be damaged by rupture than by stretching. Carter et al. published on the Richardson-Say technique for laparoscopic identification and utilization of the uterosacral ligament in the repair of uterine or vaginal vault prolapse. The uterosacral ligaments provide bilateral attachment of the upper end of the vagina and uterus to prevent prolapse downward through the urogenital hiatus. The advantage to using these ligaments is that it allows free mobility of the attached vagina laterally and superiorly, which is essential in proper sexual function. These ligaments when properly tensioned suspend the vagina to the level of the ischial spine.

The second support axis or DeLancey's level 2 is a horizontal axis from the ischial spine to the posterior aspect of the pubic bone. The paravaginal or lateral supports of the bladder, upper two-thirds of the vagina, and rectum are derived from this axis. They are supported by the pubocervical fascia anteriorly, and the rectovaginal septum posteriorly, which are attached laterally to the arcus tendineus ligament or white line (see Figures 25.6 and 25.8). If defects are noted in this compartment, they should be repaired concurrently with the uterosacral ligament suspension (Figure 25.13).

The third support axis, DeLancey's level 3, is responsible for the almost vertical orientation of the urethra, lower third of the vagina, and anal canal (see Figure 25.9). It travels perpendicularly to the urogenital triangles. The lower third of the vagina passes through the levator hiatus, forming an almost 90° angle due to the puborectalis muscle posteriorly, and the pubocervical fascia hammock anteriorly. This allows for an almost 90° angle for the urethra to descend through and contributes greatly to the continence mechanism. Posterior level 3 defects are most effectively handled vaginally, as the angle of repair laparoscopically makes it more difficult to accomplish.

PERIOPERATIVE PREPARATION

Maximum vaginal estrogenization with at least 6 weeks of therapy is recommended prior to any repair. When examining relative risks and benefits, as recently reported, bowel preparation has been discouraged in gynecologic surgery; however, debulking the bowel for better visualization may be more important for advanced laparoscopic reconstructive surgery and is recommended by some authors.

Intraoperative technique

The intraoperative technique includes positioning, exam under anesthesia, vaginal portion of repair if indicated, and trocar placement.

The patient is first placed in a low semilithotomy position allowing the laparoscopic instruments to be rotated 360° around the abdomen after anesthetic induction. Kendal boots or a sequential compression device are placed to reduce blood clotting. Allen-type stirrups should be used to allow for safe positioning to avoid neurologic injury and allow for some adjustments of the position during surgery. An examination under anesthesia should be performed to reassess all site-specific defects that need to be addressed. A Foley catheter is placed into the bladder for dependent drainage. If a level 3 low transverse defect of the perineal body (i.e., distal rectovaginal septal area) were noted, it could be repaired first through a vaginal incision (Figure 25.14). The dissection of the rectovaginal septum free from the vaginal epithelium to the vaginal apex minimizes the work needing to be performed on the laparoscopic side, as the distal rectovaginal septum has a difficult angle to dissect safely without increased risk of rectal injury. The high defect of the posterior compartment

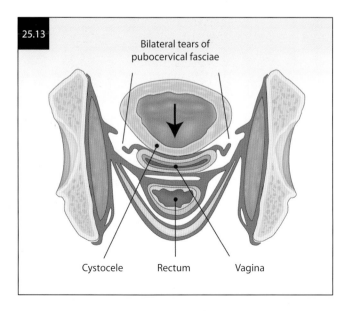

25.13

Bilateral tears of
pubocervical fasciae

Cystocele   Rectum   Vagina

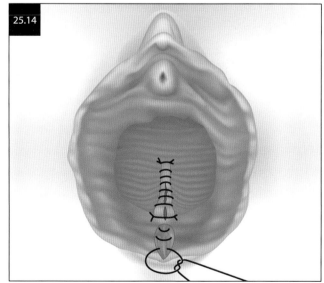

25.14

and enterocele can be further addressed during the laparoscopic portion of the procedure.

Laparoscopy

Begin with the camera port by making a vertical incision within the umbilicus and introducing a 5 mm or 10–12 mm trocar. Three ancillary ports are recommended: one just in a suprapubic hairline area (5 mm), and the other two just lateral to transversalis fascia and at about the level of McBurney point (1–12 and 1–5 mm) (Figure 25.15). The patient is then placed in a steep Trendelenburg position. Once the abdomen has been insufflated, trocars should be placed, an abdominal survey completed, and the bowel moved out of the pelvis by atraumatic instrumentation or T-lifts to decrease the risk of bowel perforation. Then the ureters should be clearly identified as they cross over the bifurcation of the common iliac vessels. The vaginal vault or cervical stump can be easily exposed by using either a vaginal blunt manipulator or an EEA rectal sizer. The procedure may also be completed with the uterus *in situ* or with a supracervical hysterectomy if a uterine manipulator, such as a Valchev/Pelosi manipulator, is in place. A critical step in the procedure is to clearly identify the uterosacral ligaments. Palpation of the anatomy vaginally will help locate the ureterosacral ligaments if they are difficult to identify and if needing any orientation during the surgical procedure. The anatomy in and around the ischial spine is predictably consistent. The pudendal nerve runs 1 cm below and lateral to the ischial spine. The inferior gluteal nerve/artery/vein bundle runs 1 cm medial and inferior to the sacrospinous ligament attached to the ischial spine. The ureter is 1 cm medial and superior. The obturator nerve runs 4–5 cm superior to the ischial spine. Finally, 2 cm cephalad run the uterine vessels with ureter giving way to our popular adage "water under the bridge." The uterosacral ligament runs 1 cm medial and at a 70° angle downward from the ischial spine. Once the anatomy is defined, begin with a ureterolysis at the level of the repair by making a linear releasing incision with laparoscopic

scissors or the harmonic scalpel just underneath the ureter at the level of the ligament's sacral insertion point. The peritoneal window is extended down the line of the ureter into the deep pelvis (Figure 25.16). A semitraumatic grasper can then be utilized to grab the uterosacral ligament structures including the peritoneal wall as well as all the tissue dissected free from the ureter downward toward the ischial spine area to ensure that the dissection is adequate for sustained support. The uterosacral ligament is then elevated toward the anterior abdominal wall while utilizing a closed grasper to pluck the tensed uterosacral ligaments (Figure 25.17). If this tissue stretches, you have not identified the ligament appropriately and should continue to grasp the tissue until finding the true ligament. In the authors' experience of well over 500 cases of laparoscopic vault suspension, the uterosacral ligaments were found in every patient, except one who had a radical hysterectomy. Next, the bladder should be mobilized off the vagina. If identification of the bladder flap is difficult, a three-way

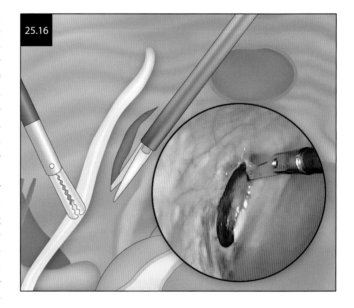

25.16

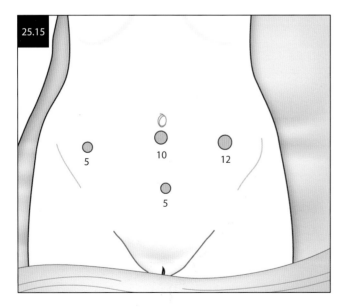

25.15

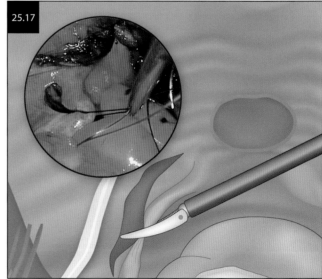

25.17

Foley catheter can be back-filled with 60–200 cc of saline to expand the bladder, helping denote the location of the vesical peritoneal fold. The bladder is mobilized all the way down to the pillars on either side, exposing the pubocervical fascia at this level (Figure 25.18). In patients with severe paravaginal defects, be aware that the ureter may have shifted medial into the plane of the vesicovaginal dissection, and suture placement may then compromise the ureter. In patients with mild to moderate degrees of clinically recognized post–total laparoscopic hysterectomy vault or post–laparoscopic supracervical hysterectomy cervix descensus as well as prophylaxis of procidencia, just the uterosacral ligament suspension can be performed. However, in patients with advanced descent, especially for post–total hysterectomy frank vault or post-supra cervical hysterectomy (SCH) frank cervical prolapse, an approach with reconstruction of the recto vaginal septum is recommended. In those cases, attention is then directed posterior to the vagina where the peritoneum is entered and dissection is conducted to identify the rectovaginal septum (Figure 25.19). This layer should be avascular and, therefore, should separate fairly easily. The dissection is carried out laterally until you reach the levator muscles and, if performed earlier in the procedure, until you reach the previously dissected plane vaginally. Once again, it is often helpful to perform a vaginal or rectal exam at this time to identify the ischial spine as well as any particular site-specific defects that may exist. Once the dissection is completed and identification of a site-specific defect is ensured, grab the actual rectovaginal septum and reapproximate it back to its normal support area. While holding it in the correct position, again perform a rectovaginal exam and identify whether this corrects the defect. With this accomplished, repair the rectovaginal septal defects. Place interrupted stitches from the arcus tendineus ligament to the rectovaginal septum building the rectovaginal septum back to the ischial spine if this has not been completed through the vaginal route (Figure 25.20). This needs to be performed bilaterally and can be tested again with a

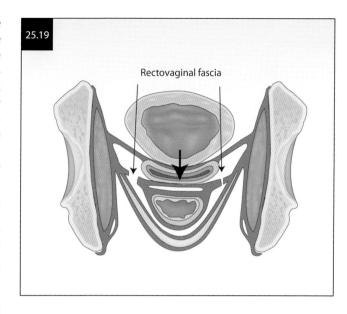

25.19

Rectovaginal fascia

rectal exam. Once the rectovaginal septum is intact, a permanent suture of the surgeon's choice—generally Prolene or GORE-TEX—is run through the uterosacral ligament, rectovaginal septum, and then back to the uterosacral ligament to be tied down securely. Repeat this on the other side so that an individual attachment of the rectovaginal septum into the uterosacral ligament at the level of the ischial spine and the top of the uterosacral ligament is formed. A second stitch is then placed through the uterosacral ligament 1 cm proximal to the previous suture continuing onto the pubocervical fascia anteriorly, rectovaginal septum posteriorly, and then back to the uterosacral ligament (Figure 25.21). It is generally recommended to perform the sutures bilaterally before tying them down. The sutures should be passed through separate ports to avoid entanglement, especially when tying knots. If needed, additional stitches may be placed through the pubocervical fascia and rectovaginal septum in the midline until the enterocele is covered. The sutures are then tied down securely, thus closing any of the enterocele defect as well

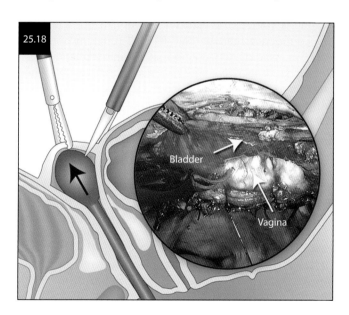

25.18

Bladder

Vagina

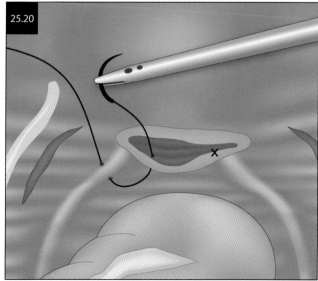

25.20

X

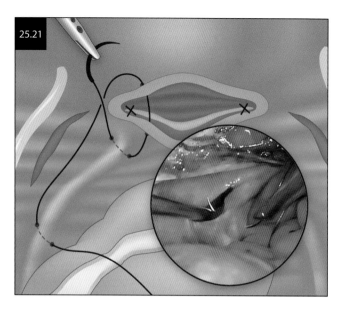

as creating the level 1 suspension (Figure 25.22). It is rare that any vaginal epithelium needs to be removed during the course of this technique, as most of the vaginal epithelium will remold itself into the exoskeleton of the vagina within 6 weeks. A large blunt-tip vaginal probe is then reinserted to expand the vaginal apex and check if all defects have been addressed. If there are any further defects, sequential stitches are placed to gain the proper support. It is best to avoid plicating the uterosacral ligaments in the midline as it closes down the cul-de-sac, which is designed to fill with stool. If this space is overly compromised, it could lead to pain, increased constipation, or increased risk of failure from the peristalsis pushing against the repair. Once the vault suspension is complete, sterile irrigation is performed. An underwater examination at low air pressure of 6 mm Hg should identify any active bleeding that will need to be controlled prior to closure. If there are any paravaginal defects, they are addressed via an incision made in the space of Retzius. The ischial spines and arcus tendineus are directly

visualized along with any remaining pubocervical fascial defects. These defects are then sequentially repaired with a monofilament permanent suture in an interrupted fashion as described in Chapter 22. If stress incontinence or potential stress incontinence has been identified on prior workup, an incontinence procedure can be accomplished prior to completion of the case as discussed in Chapter 23. Last, prior to closure, cystoscopy is performed to ensure that the ureters and bladder have not been compromised. The fascia of the large ports should be closed to avoid herniation via the surgeon's preferred method of closure. In the case of uterine preservation or supracervical hysterectomy, this entire procedure is performed as described above except that the sequential interrupted stitches are placed from the uterosacral ligament into the pericervical ring and cervical stroma at the level of uterosacral origin on the cervix.

POSTOPERATIVE CARE

The patient is transferred to recovery with a Foley catheter in place and advanced to oral analgesia as quickly as tolerated. In the past it was common practice to start these patients on patient-controlled analgesia (PCA) and to keep them in the hospital for 2–3 days. Over the last several years it has become common practice for patients to be admitted as 23 hour stays without PCA. Pain is now controlled via oral or breakthrough intravenous administration of analgesics. The patient's Foley catheter is usually removed as soon as the patient is ready to ambulate with a bladder trial. Just prior to removal of the Foley catheter, the bladder is filled with a known quantity of fluid, between 200 and 400 cc, until the patient feels an urgency to void. The catheter is removed and the patient instructed to void within a short interval of time, generally 30 min to 1 hour. This allows for a rapid and accurate measure of recovered voiding function after surgery and anesthesia. Knowing the volume of urine infused and volume voided allows by simple subtraction a postvoid residual urine to be calculated. If greater than 50% of the volume is voided, the catheter can be left out with relative confidence that the bladder will function normally; however, voiding dysfunction and urinary retention are common, especially when concomitant incontinence procedures are performed. The vast majority of patients are discharged within 23 hours and many on the same day as surgery either with or without a Foley leg bag depending on the results of the voiding trial. They are seen at follow-up 2 and 6 weeks post-op. They are sent home with prescriptions for narcotic analgesic for pain, stool softener to avoid constipation, and Pyridium if bladder spasms are reported. When the patient has recovered for a period of 12 weeks, biofeedback is recommended. Patients who undergo pelvic floor reconstruction should ideally be placed on some form of pelvic floor rehabilitation postoperatively to maximize the strength of the muscle support to reduce stress on the ligaments, much like the orthopedic surgeon would require after a knee

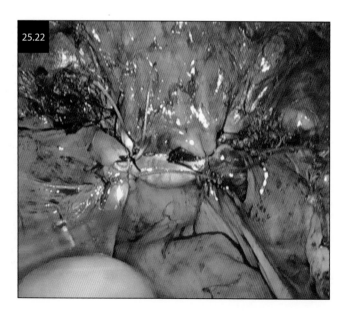

replacement. It is also important to encourage continued health of the vaginal mucosa during recovery. This can be readily accomplished through vaginal estrogenization, if not contraindicated.

SUGGESTED READING

Carter JE, Einter M, Mendehlsohn S et al. Vaginal vault suspension and enterocele repair by Richardson-Saye laparoscopic technique: Description of training technique and results. *J Soc Laparoendos Surg.* 2001;5:29–36.

Culligan PJ, Milklos JR, Murphy M et al. The tensile strength of uterosacral ligament sutures: A comparison of vaginal and laparoscopic techniques. *Obstet Gynecol.* 2003;101:500–503.

DeLancey JO. Anatomy and biomechanics of genital prolapse. *Clinical Obstet and Gynecol.* 1993;36(4):897–909.

Harris RL, Cundiff GL, Theofrastus JP et al. The value of intraoperative cystoscopy in urogynecologic and reconstructive pelvic surgery. *Am J Obstet Gynecol.* 1997;177:1367–1371.

Karram M, Goldwasser S, Kleeman S et al. High uterosacral vaginal vault suspension with fascial reconstruction for vaginal repair of enterocele and vaginal vault prolapse. *Am J Obstet Gynecol.* 2001;185(6):1339–1343.

Klauschie JL, Cornella JL. Surgical treatment of vaginal vault prolapse: A historic summary and review of outcomes. *Female Pelvic Med Reconstr Surg.* 2012;18(1):10–17.

Lin LL, Phelps JY, Liu CY. Laparoscopic vaginal vault suspension using uterosacral ligaments: A review of 133 cases. *J Minim Invasive Gynecol.* 2005;12:216–220.

Maher C, Feiner B, Baessler K et al. Surgical management of pelvic organ prolapse in women. *Cochrane Database Syst Rev.* 2013;(4):CD004014.

Marguiles Ru, Rogers M, Mogran DM. Outcomes of transvaginal uterosacral ligament suspension: Systematic review and metaanalysis. *Am J Obstet Gynecol.* 2010;202(2):124–134.

Miklos JR, Kohli N, Lucente V et al. Site-specific fascial defects in the diagnosis and surgical management of enterocele. *Am J Obstet Gynecol.* 1998;179:1418–1423.

Miller NE. A new method of correcting complete inversion of the vagina. *Surg Gynecol Obstet.* 1927;44:550–555.

Natale F, La Penna C, Padoa A et al. High levator myorrhaphy versus uterosacral ligament suspension for vaginal vault fixation: A prospective, randomized study. *Int Urogynecol J Pelvic Floor Dynsfunct.* 2010;21(5):515–522.

Ostrzenski A. Laparoscopic colposuspension for total vaginal prolapse. *Int J Gynecol Obstet.* 1996;55:147–152.

Rardin CR, Erekson EA, Sung VW et al. Uterosacral colpopexy at the time of vaginal hysterectomy: Comparison of laparoscopic and vaginal approaches. *J Reprod Med.* 2009;54(5):273–280.

Richardson AC, Lyon JB, Williams NL. New look at pelvic relaxation. *Am J Obstet Gynecol.* 1976;126:568–573.

Seman EI, Cook JR, O'Shea RT. Two-year experience with laparoscopic pelvic floor repair. *J Am Assoc Gynecol Laparosc.* 2003;10:38–45.

Won H, Maley P, Salim S. Surgical and patient outcomes using mechanical bowel preparation before laparoscopic gynecologic surgery: A randomized controlled trial. *Obstet Gynecol.* 2013;121(3):538–546.

Chapter 26

LAPAROSCOPY IN CHILDREN AND ADOLESCENT PATIENTS

Claire Templeman, S. Paige Hertweck, and Traci Ito

INTRODUCTION

In adults, laparoscopy is an established alternative to open surgery. However, until recently, concerns regarding proven benefit and adequate equipment have limited its use in pediatric patients. The advent of microendoscopic equipment has made pediatric endoscopy more practical, but there are some important technical differences between it and adult laparoscopy, which are the focus of this chapter.

INDICATIONS

There is now considerable experience with laparoscopy for appendectomy, cholecystectomy, splenectomy, exploration of nonpalpable testis, hernia repair, and trauma in children. Some relevant indications for gynecologists who treat young children and adolescents are listed in Table 26.1. Specific techniques for the management of ovarian masses and uterovaginal anomalies are detailed in Chapters 11 and 27.

When contemplating laparoscopy in a pediatric patient, an experienced anesthetic team is essential. Insufflation of the abdomen with carbon dioxide gas (CO_2) increases intraabdominal and intrathoracic pressure with the potential for ventilation and perfusion abnormalities. Correct insufflation pressure is critical in infants because they rely on diaphragmatic excursion for adequate ventilation. Overinsufflation may result in restricted diaphragmatic movement.

It has been demonstrated in animal models that intraabdominal pressures maintained between 0 and 10 mm Hg do not deleteriously affect ventilation or gas exchange. An insufflation pressure of 8 mm Hg with a flow rate of 0.5 L/min is appropriate for neonates or infants with pressures of 10–12 mm Hg appropriate for older children. Carbon dioxide insufflation may also result in hypercapnia and metabolic acidosis if the end tidal CO_2 and oxygen saturation are not monitored closely. A minute ventilatory rate that maintains the end tidal CO_2 in the range of 30–45 mm Hg is required, and in neonatal patients undergoing laparoscopy, this has been found to be 30%–40% more than that required at laparotomy. The use of humidified gas (37°C) is advisable, since it has also been shown to decrease the risk of hypothermia that

may occur in pediatric patients undergoing laparoscopy. Intravenous fluids such as lactated Ringer solution should be administered to maintain urine output at 1 mL/kg/h. Recent work suggests that the creation of a pneumoperitoneum in pediatric patients may adversely affect urine output during surgery. Anuria has been noted in infants less than 1 year of age and oliguria in about one-third of patients over 1 year of age. These phenomena appear to be completely reversible but highlight the inaccuracies of using urine output in the calculation of fluid administration requirements during laparoscopic surgery in infants.

PATIENT POSITIONING

In pediatric patients, the supine position is used almost exclusively since there is no need to instrument the uterus (Figure 26.1). If access to the vagina is required, proper use of padded stirrups that align the ipsilateral heal with the contralateral hip and shoulder are important. Stirrups that place the hips in hyperflexion are occasionally used in children because they give maximum access to the perineum; however, they place the patient at risk for femoral nerve damage, particularly if the case is lengthy.

Irrespective of age, tucking the child's arms by his or her side also allows the surgeon maximum flexibility while operating.

INSTRUMENTATION

There is now a range of instrumentation available that provides adequate optics for work in neonatal and pediatric patients, including 3–5 mm trocars for 2.7–4.5 mm instruments (Figure 26.2). It has been shown that the use of these smaller-caliber instruments in pediatric patients is associated with greater postoperative comfort. Traditional 10 mm laparoscopes can be used in adolescents if required.

Trocars are available as reusable metal, disposable plastic, and newer radially expanding models (Figure 26.3). The choice of trocar is important, since leakage from around these sites and compensatory rapid CO_2 insufflation into the abdomen may contribute to hypothermia, especially in neonates. A recent report suggests that the radially expanding trocars may be the most

TABLE 26.1

GYNECOLOGIC INDICATIONS FOR LAPAROSCOPY IN THE PEDIATRIC AND ADOLESCENT POPULATION

AGE GROUP	INDICATION
NEONATAL	COMPLEX, ENLARGING, OR SYMPTOMATIC OVARIAN MASS
	ABDOMINAL MASS OF UNCERTAIN ORIGIN
PREPUBERTAL	PERSISTENT OVARIAN CYST OR MASS
	PARATUBAL CYST
	OVARIAN TORSION
	OOPHOROPEXY
ADOLESCENT	PERSISTENT OVARIAN CYST OR MASS
	OVARIAN TORSION
	PARATUBAL CYST
	SUSPECTED ENDOMETRIOSIS
	UTEROVAGINAL ANOMALIES
	OOPHOROPEXY
	PELVIC INFLAMMATORY DISEASE

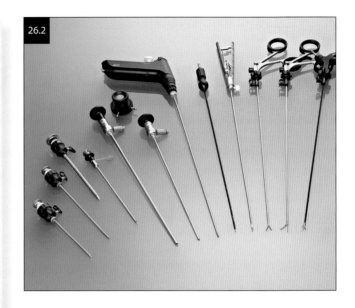

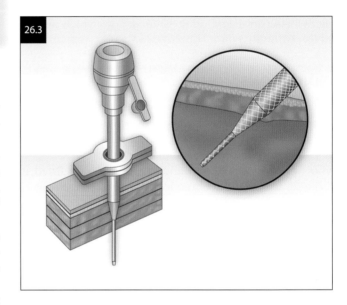

effective in very young patients, because they have a lower incidence of slippage from the abdominal wall.

Laparoscopes ranging from 2.7 to 10 mm in diameter with angles from 0° to 45° allow the surgeon a wide choice of views depending on the size of the patient. The newest cameras offer an autorotation feature maintaining an upright image irrespective of the angle of the camera. All these features are helpful when large masses or adhesions obscure the view within the abdomens of small infants.

In addition to conventional energy sources such as monopolar and bipolar cautery, the ultrasonically activated, harmonic scalpel can be a useful tool in pediatric laparoscopy (Figure 26.4). It uses mechanical energy, generated by a vibrating crystal in the handpiece, to cut

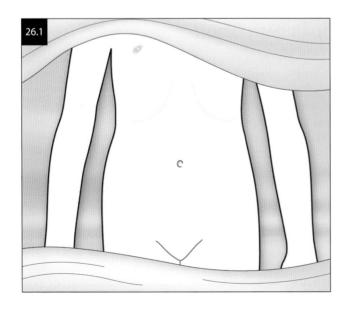

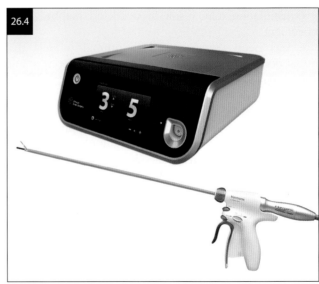

and coagulate without the transmission of energy to structures out of immediate view. This instrument has been used to coagulate gonadal and bowel vessels in very small infants, including neonates. The reported benefit of this dual-action instrument in pediatric patients is a decrease in operating time resulting in a shorter time under anesthesia.

PORT PLACEMENT AND ENTRANCE INTO THE ABDOMEN

Surgical complications in pediatric laparoscopy are often related to the introduction of the Veress needle or the first trocar. In a large review of 5400 laparoscopic surgeries performed in patients ranging in age from 0 to 20 years, the significant predictors of complications were operator experience and the method used to create a pneumoperitoneum. Specifically, the Veress needle was associated with a 2.6% major complication rate (viscus or major blood vessel injury) compared with 1.2% for the open technique. This difference continued even in experienced operators (>100 laparoscopic cases). This finding has led to the suggestion that the open technique is the method of choice for the creation of the pneumoperitoneum in pediatric patients; however, the Veress needle is used by many practitioners.

In neonates, the umbilical vessels may still be patent at the time of surgery; therefore, correct identification and ligation of the vessels are essential prior to abdominal entry. This can be done following skin incision at the umbilical site with the use of small claw retractors on the skin and fine hemostat clamps to dissect the superficial tissue. After the skin is incised (Figure 26.5), the fascia is identified and grasped with the clamp. Then, the next step is to identify the umbilical vessels, which are clamped and suture ligated after they are located. Abdominal entry is obtained using blunt dissection with the hemostat (Figure 26.6). We routinely achieve entry with open (Hasson) technique using WECK Vista

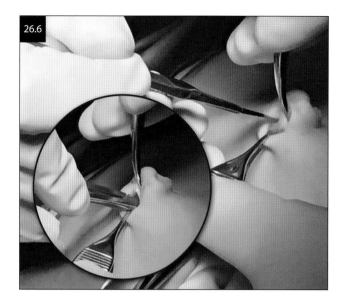

(Teleflex Medical, Westmeath, Ireland) 5 mm trocar with a short shaft. After the trocar is inserted into the abdominal cavity, the stitch is placed through the fascia and the conical plug of the trocar to keep the cannula in place (Figure 26.7).

Due to the intraabdominal location of the bladder, there is a reduced margin of safety in children in comparison with adolescents or adults. Preoperative emptying is therefore very important in avoiding secondary trocar injury, especially if suprapubic trocars are used.

Port placement on the abdomen depends on the operation contemplated and surgeon preference. However, in prepubertal patients with large ovarian masses, the placement of secondary trocars that are high, typically two fingers above the umbilicus, and lateral to the inferior epigastric artery may assist with access to the pathology (Figure 26.8). The primary trocar in a neonate is placed through the umbilicus, and the ancillary ports are placed superior and lateral to this in the midclavicular line (Figure 26.9).

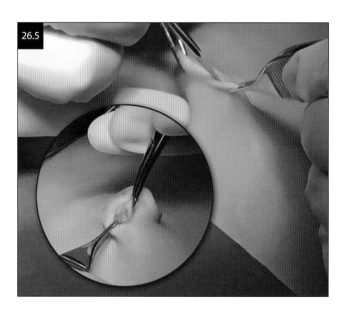

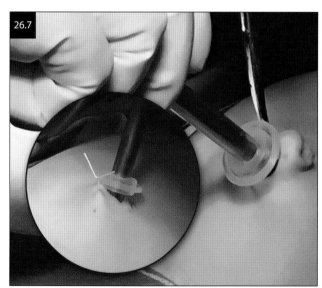

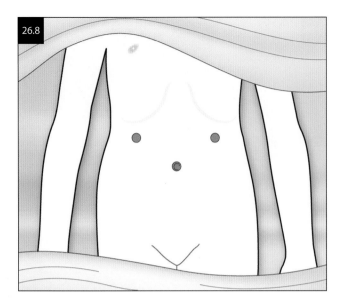

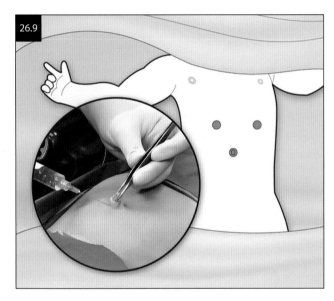

The fascia of all ports ≥5 mm in diameter should be closed in pediatric patients since there is a reported 2.7% incidence of port site hernia through open incisions. More recently, there have been reports of omental herniation through a 2-mm port site. Closure can be achieved with claw retractors at the site of incision, identification of the fascia with Kocher clamps, and closure with an 0 Vicryl suture on a UR5 needle.

OVARIAN MASSES

A young girl with a persistent or complex appearing ovarian mass is a typical indication for surgery in the pediatric population, and the likely ovarian pathology is dependent on patient age. The techniques for removing ovarian masses including cystectomy, oophorectomy, and the use of an endobag are the same in children as adults and are described in Chapter 11. In neonates, ovarian cysts are functional as the result of maternal gonadotrophin stimulation during the antenatal

period. Therefore, indications for surgery are complex in scenarios of enlarging or symptomatic masses where torsion is suspected or the diagnosis is in doubt. Since the incidence of ovarian malignancy in this age group approaches zero, laparoscopy is appropriate for operators experienced with neonatal surgery. In the prepubertal age group, approximately 11% of noninflammatory ovarian masses requiring surgery are malignant; therefore, careful investigation on an individual basis is essential. If preoperative assessment suggests malignancy, laparotomy and staging are indicated unless the surgeon is proficient with laparoscopic oncologic surgery.

Ovarian torsion occurring in the pediatric population is often associated with either a normal ovary or benign ovarian pathology. Laparoscopic management utilizing detorsion with or without cystectomy is becoming more common. Long-term follow-up of these children reveals folliculogenesis and resumption of normal size over time.

An additional scenario to consider is the management of fetal ovarian cysts, which have been discussed in the literature. These are likely the product of stimulation of the fetal ovary by placental chorionic gonadotropin causing follicular dysgenesis. They were first described by Valenti et al. in 1975, but the most recent reported incidence of neonatal cysts is around 34%. These can be simple or complex in nature. As hormonal stimulation decreases, the simple type often regresses spontaneously. However, if the cyst is greater than 5 cm in size, the potential complication of torsion exists. In addition to concerns for torsion, surgical management is necessary for large, uncomplicated cysts within the first few days after the fetus is delivered. This management is critical to this particular patient population to minimize ovarian tissue loss affecting future fertility.

CONCLUSION

In conclusion, laparoscopy, when performed by experienced practitioners, is a safe and practical approach to the surgical management of a variety of gynecologic problems in children.

SUGGESTED READING

Backman T, Arnbjornsson E, Kullendorff CM. Omentum herniation at a 2-mm trocar site. *J Laparoendosc Adv Surg Tech A*. 2005;15(1):87–88.

Celik A, Ergun O, Aldemir H et al. Long-term results of conservative management of adnexal torsion in children. *J Pediatr Surg*. 2005;40(4):704–708.

Esposito C, Ascione G, Garipoli V et al. Complications of pediatric laparoscopic surgery. *Surg Endo*. 1997;11(6):655–657.

Fujimoto T, Segawa O, Kobayashi H, Lane G, Miyano T. Endosurgery in children: Prospects and problems—An analysis of 88 cases. *Ped Endosurg Innov Tech*. 1997;1(3):189–195.

Fujimoto T, Segawa O, Lane GJ et al. Laparoscopic surgery in newborn infants. *Surg Endosc*. 1999;13:773–777.

Gomez Dammeier BH, Karanik E, Gluer S et al. Anuria during pneumoperitoneum in infants and children: A prospective study. *J Pediatr Surg*. 2005;40(9):1454–1458.

Peters CA. Complications in pediatric urological laparoscopy: Results of a survey. *J Urol*. 1996;155(3):1070–1073.

Pujar VC, Joshi SS, Pujar YV, Dhumale HA. Role of laparoscopy in the management of neonatal ovarian cysts. *J Neonatal Surg*. 2014;3(2):16.

Rubin SZ, Davis GM, Sehgal Y, Kaminski MJ. Does laparoscopy adversely affect gas exchange and pulmonary mechanics in the newborn? An experimental study. *J Laparoendo Surg*. 1996;6(Suppl 1):S69–S73.

Templeman CL, Fallat M, Blinshevsky A, Hertweck SP. Noninflammatory ovarian masses in girls and young women. *Obstet Gynecol*. 2000;96:229–233.

Templeman CL, Reynolds AJ, Hertweck SP, Nagaraj H. The laparoscopic management of neonatal ovarian cysts. *J Am Assoc Gyn Laparosc*. 2000;7:401–404.

Ure BM, Bax NM, van der Zee DC. Laparoscopy in infants and children: A prospective study on feasibility and the impact of routine surgery. *J Ped Surg*. 2000;35(8):1170–1173.

CHAPTER 27

ENDOSCOPIC DIAGNOSIS AND CORRECTION OF MALFORMATIONS OF FEMALE GENITALIA

Leila V. Adamyan, Katerine L. Yarotskaya, and Assia A. Stepanian

Congenital malformations of female genitalia comprise about 4% of all congenital anomalies. These malformations are associated with extragenital anomalies in about 74% of cases manifesting as skin marks and skeletal defects, as well as breast, heart, renal, and digestive system anomalies. Diagnoses of malformations of the uterus and/or vagina present significant difficulties that may confuse the character of the disease and cause incorrect and, sometimes, unwarranted or aggressive radical surgery in 24%–34% of patients. The high rate of diagnostic mistakes may be due to the absence of a universal classification of genital malformations. Suggested classifications do not reflect all clinical-anatomic features of malformations, which are essential for an optimal treatment strategy that will be beneficial for the patient's health, reproductive and sexual function, and general quality of life.

Presently, invasive diagnostic tools (ultrasonography, hysterosalpingography, magnetic resonance imaging [MRI], and spiral computer tomography [CT]) together with endoscopic techniques may permit the determination of the real character of a malformation of the uterus and/or vagina, and reveal concomitant extragenital anomalies of the urinary and digestive systems. Correct diagnosis will allow the rational management of anomalies. Based on the results of clinical examination and treatment of 855 patients, using modern imaging techniques, hysteroscopy and laparoscopy, L.V. Adamyan and coauthors (1993) introduced a classification of genital malformations and outlined a paradigm of examination, surgical treatment, and rehabilitation of patients with malformations. Updated in 2014, this morphofunctional classification included the experience in management of over 2000 women with various types of genital malformations. We primarily utilize reconstructive plastic surgery as an endoscopic approach for these types of complex pelvic anatomies (Table 27.1).

CLASS I: UTEROVAGINAL APLASIA (MRKH)

Aplasia of the vagina and uterus (Mayer–Rokitansky–Küster–Hauser syndrome) is a malformation characterized by congenital absence of the uterus (usually presented by two muscular rudiments, but other variants can also be encountered: asymmetric muscular mounds,

complete absence of rudiments, etc.) and vagina, normally functioning ovaries, female phenotype and karyotype (46, XX), and is often accompanied by other congenital anomalies including skeletal, urinary, and gastrointestinal (Figures 27.1 through 27.4). Figure 27.2 presents a laparoscopic view of aplasia of the uterus and vagina: absence of uterine rudiments. A laparoscopic view of aplasia of the uterus and vagina with symmetric uterine rudiments is shown in Figure 27.3, and a laparoscopic view of aplasia of the uterus and vagina with asymmetric uterine rudiments is presented in Figure 27.4.

The main clinical features of uterine and vaginal aplasia are the absence of menstruation and inability to have vaginal sexual intercourse. The uterine rudiments may be affected by adenomyosis, causing pelvic pain.

The diagnosis is based on the patient's complaints, physical examination, ultrasonographic data, and other methods of visualization (MRI and CT scan), which are necessary to determine if associated malformations (especially of the urinary system, which occurs in almost 40% of cases) are present.

Surgical correction, although not absolutely necessary, is required if normal sexual activity is anticipated. Gynecologists have long discussed the ethics involved in creating an artificial vagina. Most surgeons are in agreement that safe and reliable methods are needed to achieve the goal of a functional vagina. Different methods of colpoelongation appear to be minimally invasive but require considerable time and are not always effective.

Another approach to correct this malformation is based on techniques to create a canal between the urinary bladder and rectum. In this case, subsequent tamponade and dilatation with various prosthetic appliances and devices are required. Another possibility is creating a lining with skin flaps or segments of rectum, sigmoid, small intestine, or pelvic peritoneum. One-stage colpopoiesis from pelvic peritoneum results in immediate formation of neovagina with minimal risk in experienced hands. This method supplies a better quality of neovagina with rapid epithelization and sufficient capacity and depth. In 1993, L.V. Adamyan introduced a method of colpopoiesis incorporating pelvic peritoneum using laparoscopy in all the main steps of the operation, confirming diagnosis, identification, and opening of the peritoneum, and creation of a vaginal vault, which we

TABLE 27.1

CLASSIFICATION OF MALFORMATIONS OF UTERUS AND/OR VAGINA

CLASS I: UTEROVAGINAL APLASIA (MRKH)
  A. NONFUNCTIONAL UTERINE RUDIMENTS
  B. FUNCTIONAL RUDIMENTS

CLASS II: VAGINAL APLASIA
  A. HYMENAL ATRESIA
  B. PARTIAL VAGINAL APLASIA (ONE-THIRD OR TWO-THIRDS OF THE VAGINA)

CLASS III: CERVICOVAGINAL APLASIA
  A. COMPLETE VAGINAL AND CERVICAL APLASIA WITH FUNCTIONAL UTERUS
  B. CERVICAL APLASIA WITH FUNCTIONAL UTERUS

CLASS IV: UNICORNUATE UTERUS WITH
  A. COMMUNICATING FUNCTIONAL UTERINE HORN
  B. NONCOMMUNICATING FUNCTIONAL UTERINE HORN
  C. NONFUNCTIONAL UTERINE HORN
  D. WITHOUT RUDIMENTAL HORN

CLASS V: UTERUS DUPLEX
  A. SYMMETRIC FORM WITH DUPLICATION OF ONE-THIRD, TWO-THIRDS, OR ENTIRE LENGTH OF THE VAGINA
  B. ASYMMETRIC FORM—WITH APLASIA OF HEMIVAGINA

CLASS VI: BICORNUATE UTERUS
  A. COMPLETE FORM
  B. INCOMPLETE FORM
  C. ARCUATE UTERUS

CLASS VII: INTRAUTERINE SEPTUM
  A. INCOMPLETE SEPTUM
  B. COMPLETE SEPTUM (WITH VAGINAL DUPLICATION OR WITH NORMAL VAGINA)

CLASS VIII: ANOMALIES OF THE OVARIES AND/OR FALLOPIAN TUBES
  A. UNILATERAL OR BILATERAL ADNEXAL APLASIA
  B. GONADAL DYSGENESIS (OVARIAN HYPOPLASIA)

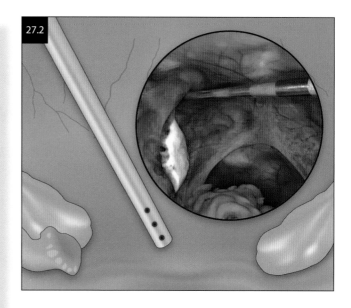

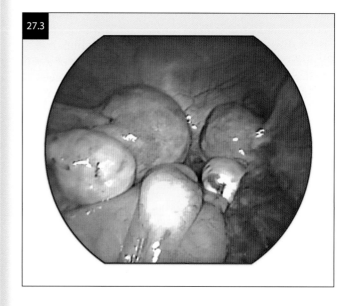

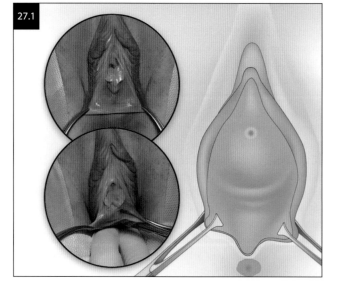

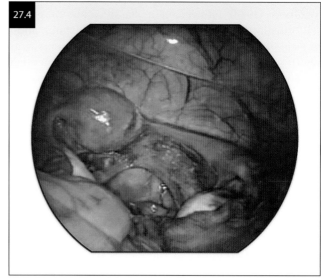

consider to be a method of choice for correction of this anomaly.

SURGICAL TECHNIQUE

Surgery is performed using a combined laparoscopic-perineal approach. The patient is placed in the lithotomy position with legs wide apart. Under general (endotracheal) anesthesia, diagnostic laparoscopy is carried out to specify the character of malformation and to evaluate the mobility of the peritoneum. The number and location of muscular rudiments and their status are noted. Enlarged uterine rudiments, causing pelvic pain and possibly affected by adenomyosis, should be removed laparoscopically with subsequent restoration of the peritoneum.

After laparoscopy, the perineal step is initiated: the skin is incised 3–3.5 cm transversally between the rectum and urinary bladder at the level of the lower border of the labia minora (Figure 27.5). By sharp and/or blunt dissection, in a strictly horizontal direction along the urinary bladder, the new canal is created (Figure 27.6). This step is the most difficult because of the risk of possible injury to the bladder and rectum. Rectal injury was observed in 1 out of over 350 patients who underwent colpopoiesis in our department. Most difficulties occur in the case of atypical (low) location of the urethra and when scarring is present at the site of the potential introitus. Scarring may be caused by repeated courses of colpoelongation, attempts at sexual intercourse, or perineal surgery, which may lead to formation of a false passage directed toward the rectum. The canal is formed up to the pelvic peritoneum.

The most crucial step of the operation—identification of the peritoneum—is performed using the laparoscope (Figure 27.7). The most mobile part of the peritoneum is between the bladder and the rectum and is often divided by the transverse fold between two muscular rudiments. It is identified, then marked with an atraumatic

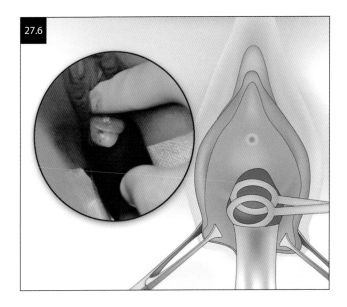

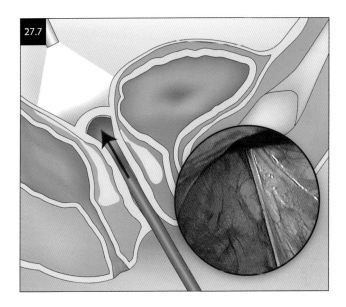

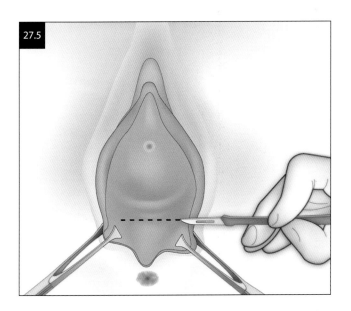

laparoscopic instrument (a manipulator or forceps), and is brought down into the created canal. The peritoneal fold is grasped in the canal by the forceps and transected either laparoscopically or from below (Figure 27.8). The edges of peritoneal incision are brought down and sutured to the edges of the skin incision with interrupted Vicryl stitches, forming the introitus (Figures 27.9 and 27.10). In case of previous scarring and excessive bleeding in the canal, fibrin glue made from the patient's blood may be applied for better attachment of the peritoneum to the canal walls. A moist sponge or vaginal probe is then placed at the introitus of the neovagina, to reestablish the pneumoperitoneum.

Formation of the neovaginal vault—the final step of the operation—is performed by laparoscopic placement of one purse-string or two semi-purse-string nonabsorbable sutures on a curved needle, incorporating the bladder peritoneum, muscular uterine rudiments, and peritoneum lining the pelvic sidewall and the serosa of

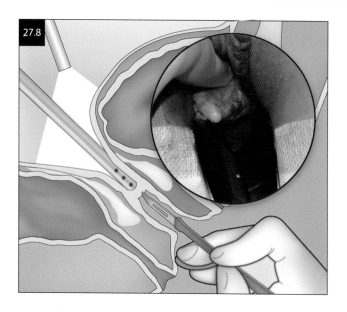

the sigmoid colon (Figure 27.11). The suture is tied with an extracorporeal knot. In case there is too much tension in the tissues, the vault can be formed by separate sutures, connecting the transverse peritoneal fold with muscular rudiments and peritoneum of the pelvic sidewall (Figure 27.12).

When muscular rudiments are absent (e.g., in patients with testicular feminization) and there is a shortage of peritoneum, the neovaginal vault can be formed using biologically compatible polymeric material (e.g., copolymer of glycolide and lactide [Vicryl mesh] or polyglycolic acid [Dexon mesh]). The mesh is sutured endoscopically to the anterior, posterior, and lateral aspects of the pelvic edge of the neovaginal tunnel to provide the barrier between the pelvic cavity and the neovagina.

In experienced hands, laparoscopically assisted colpopoiesis takes approximately 25–45 minutes, and the operation can be bloodless. Prophylactic antibiotics are recommended with continued therapy for 24–36 hours

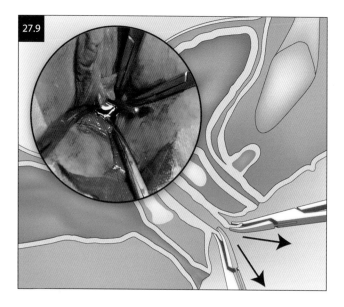

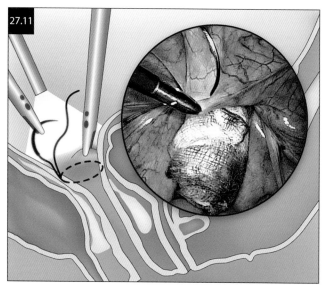

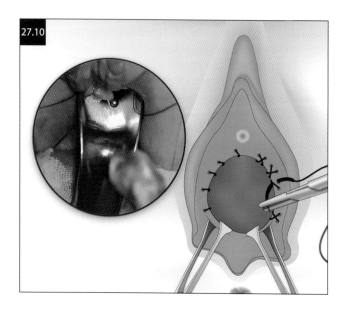

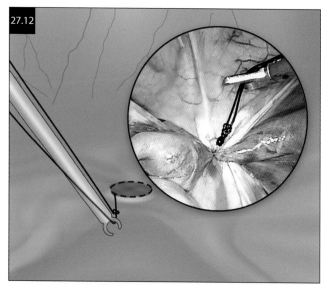

only if there is a high risk for infectious complications. A Foley catheter is placed into the bladder immediately after the operation to facilitate urination, which may be difficult in the early postoperative period due to a displacement of the urethral orifice by tension of the anterior neovaginal wall and vaginal packing. A gauze sponge moistened with an antiseptic solution and Vaseline is introduced into the neovagina for 1–2 days (Figure 27.13). The patients are allowed to sit and stand 5–6 hours after surgery. Gynecologic examination is performed on the fifth to seventh postoperative day to assess the reaction and patency of the tissues of the neovagina. The neovagina usually permits insertion of two fingers, and its length varies from 11 to 12.5 cm. The patient is asked to wear a sterile glove and to insert her index finger lubricated with K-Y Jelly into the neovagina. This manipulation is necessary to acquaint the patient with her new anatomy, and for maintenance of the neovaginal caliber until she starts regular sexual activity, which is allowed 2–4 weeks after this procedure. Most patients do not feel any discomfort during coitus and appear to be satisfied with their sexual activity, which significantly contributes to their psychological well-being.

The main features of the neovagina (the ability to perform a vaginal examination and to permit intercourse) are assessed. On examination, the border between the introitus and neovagina itself is absent; the vagina is about 11–12.5 cm long with sufficient caliber. The walls are moderately rugated, producing some mucus. Morphologic and electron-microscopic examination of the neovaginal wall reveals that 3 months after colpopoiesis, the neovaginal epithelium is similar to the stratified squamous epithelium of a normal vagina in all patients. This is most likely due to metaplasia.

In cases in which elasticity and extendibility of the peritoneum are limited, a laparoscopic-only approach to peritoneal colpopoiesis can be highly useful. In these cases care is applied to bring the epithelium of the vaginal dimple to the peritoneum with the use of

a rubber-coated manipulator of up to 5 cm in diameter (Figure 27.14). Traction of the manipulator is applied to the vaginal dimple toward the most mobile aspect of the pelvic peritoneum between the urethra and bladder anteriorly and the rectum posteriorly. Through such traction with the manipulator, the distance between neighboring organs increases and the urogenital diaphragm becomes better exposed.

Two control stitches are applied on the exposed prominent aspect of the peritoneum for the lateral control of the peritoneal incision. An incision over the peritoneum, preperitoneal adipose tissue, and urogenital diaphragm is sequentially made between these stitches until 1.5–2 cm of the manipulator is seen (Figure 27.15). Identification of the exact positions of the rectum and the bladder is needed at all times. The peritoneum is dissected off the underlying preperitoneal adipose tissue and urogenital diaphragm (Figure 27.16). Peritoneal edges are then fixed with the graspers and approximated with the skin of the vaginal dimple using interrupted

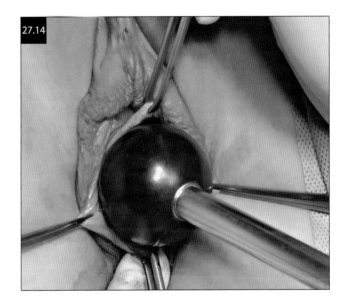

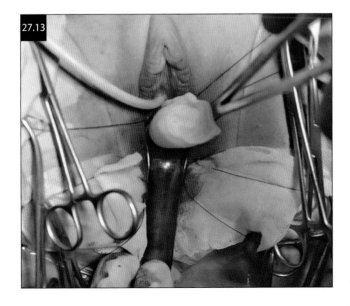

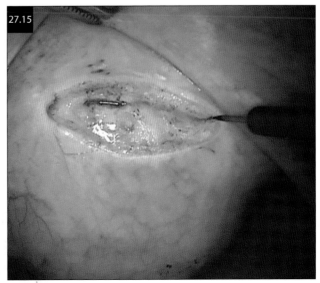

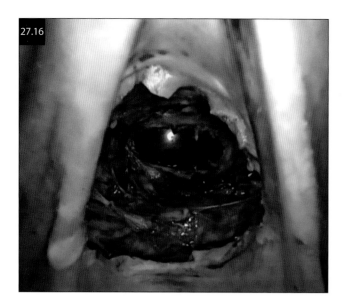

absorbable stitches (Figure 27.17). A Foley catheter is then placed. A tight gauze roll is placed vaginally beyond the perineo-peritoneal suture line. The apex of the vagina is formed in a fashion identical to the method described above.

Additional modifications include a laparovaginal approach in which the lateral peritoneal stitches are placed and then brought through the perineal opening to allow more efficacious and secure introduction of the pelvic peritoneum vaginally.

CLASS II: INCOMPLETE VAGINAL APLASIA

Incomplete vaginal aplasia presents itself as atresia of the hymenal ring or partial vaginal aplasia. Patients with both forms of vaginal aplasia present with absence of menstruation, presence of cyclic or persistent pelvic pain since menarche, and an inability to have vaginal sexual intercourse. In patients with partial vaginal aplasia hemato- and/or pyocolpos are found.

Laparoscopy in this malformation is recommended for evaluation of the status of the internal genitalia (the character of the malformation, damage caused by menstrual reflux) and for correction of pathology (pelvic irrigation, drainage of the hematosalpinx, adhesiolysis, endometriosis elimination, etc.). Conventional vaginoplasty is needed for correction of the partial vaginal aplasia when a functional uterus is present.

CLASS III: COMPLETE CERVICAL AND VAGINAL APLASIA

Patients with complete cervical and vaginal aplasia with functional normal or rudimentary uteri (Figures 27.18 and 27.19) present with symptoms similar to those of patients with incomplete vaginal aplasia.

Due to the more proximal level of obstruction, symptoms involving the uterus and pelvis are more often seen. In most of the patients, hemato- and/or pyometra, chronic

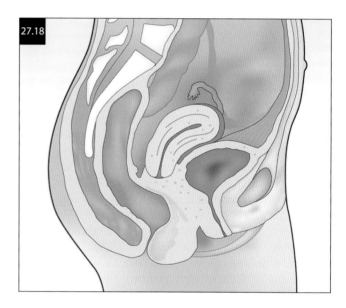

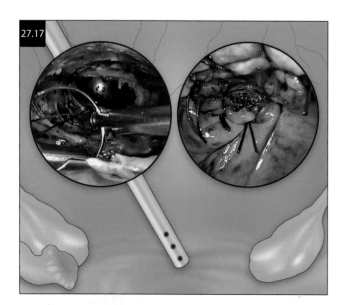

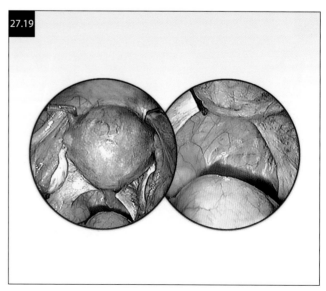

endometritis, and parametritis are found. Diagnosis is based on the patient's complaints, physical examination, laboratory analysis, ultrasonographic data, and other methods of visualization (MRI, SCT [spiral computed tomography]). Diagnostic difficulties may lead to unjustified surgery (in 24%–65% of cases).

Surgical correction is necessary and should be undertaken as soon as the diagnosis is established. One should remember that this malformation usually manifests itself in adolescence and may result in a distortion of the reproductive organs' anatomy. Definitive surgery is essential for the further reproductive health of these patients.

METHODS OF SURGICAL CORRECTION

In patients with complete aplasia of the vagina and a functional uterus, the first crucial aspect to be determined in order to choose the correct surgical modality is absence or presence of a cervical canal. For this purpose, we have introduced a method of retrograde hysteroscopy (by laparoscopic approach) by perforating the uterine fundus (Figure 27.20). The correction, which may be attempted to preserve a functional rudimentary uterus in patients with cervical and vaginal aplasia, is the creation of a tunnel between the uterus and neovagina, which can be performed as follows:

OPERATIVE TECHNIQUE

- Transverse incision of perineal skin between the urethra and lower border of labia minora
- Creation of a canal between the urinary bladder and rectum
- Simultaneous laparoscopy, pelvic revision, and final diagnosis
- Laparoscopic grasping and opening of peritoneum of rectouterine pouch
- Bringing down of the peritoneal incision edges and suturing to the introital skin

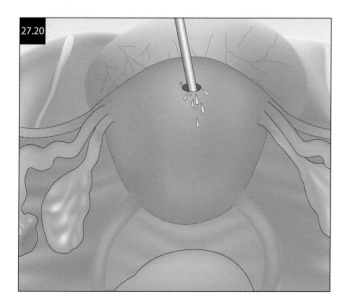

27.20

- Laparoscopic hysterotomy and retrograde hysteroscopy for identification of a site for further tunnel creation between the uterine cavity and neovagina
- Canalization of the uterine wall toward the created tunnel
- Fixation of the uterus at the tunnel, introduction of the dilator into the neocanal

If such correction appears impossible or ineffective, resulting in atresia of the previously created tunnel, the method of choice is total laparoscopic hysterectomy and laparoscopically assisted colpopoiesis from pelvic peritoneum. Total laparoscopic extirpation of a functional uterus in case of cervical and vaginal aplasia is performed according to our technique of laparoscopic hysterectomy applied for other uterine pathology, and includes the following steps:

- Coagulation and transection of round ligaments with simultaneous dissection of the plica vesical-utero fold, downward bladder dissection, and anterior dissection of uterine vessels.
- Fenestration of posterior leaves of broad ligaments and dissection to the uterosacral ligaments with their partial transection and simultaneous exposition of the uterine vessels.
- Ligation of ovarian ligaments and proximal uterine tubes.
- Suturing of ascendent uterine vessels.
- Transection of ovarian ligaments and uterine tubes (if technically advisable).
- Transection of uterine vessels and circular dissection of posterior aspect of the uterus from the pelvic fascia with transection of rudiments of cardinal and uterosacral ligaments. The specificity of this step of the operation is substantiated by abnormal development of the uterus (absence of cervix and normal cardinal and uterosacral ligaments).

Another peculiarity of this operation is the inability to use a uterine manipulator. Therefore, this requires the manipulation of the uterus with laparoscopic graspers or tenacula introduced through secondary laparoscopic ports. The uterus is removed from the abdominal cavity by electromechanical or contained morcellation. Colpopoiesis is performed according to the technique described above, with particular care of the peritoneum, which can be damaged by hysterectomy, adhesiolysis, and removal of endometriosis, and when forming the neovaginal vault.

CLASS IV: UNICORNUATE UTERUS

Unicornuate uterus is an anomaly caused by formation of only one paramesonephric duct, whereas the other has remained undeveloped. From an embryologic view, a unicornuate uterus is half of a normal uterus. The variants of the horn, or unicornuate uterus with a supplementary

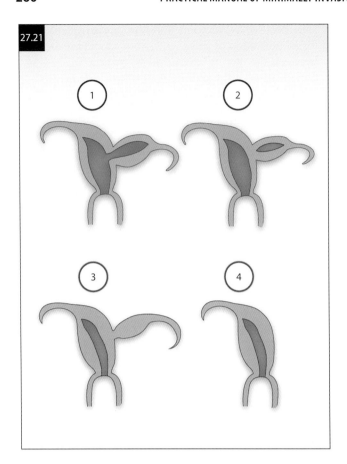

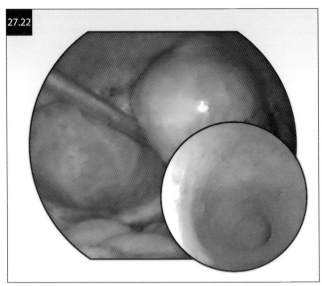

SURGICAL CORRECTION

Laparoscopic removal of the rudimentary horn is performed according to the hysterectomy technique:

- The horn is grasped, and round ligament, proximal tube, and ovarian ligament are coagulated and transected.
- Broad ligaments and uterovesical fold are dissected up to the level of junction between the principal and rudimentary horn, exposing uterine vessels supplying the rudimentary horn.
- The vessels are secured by extracorporeal suturing or bipolar coagulation (as the diameter of vessels is rather small).
- The rudimentary horn is transected by monopolar cutter or ultrasonic scalpel.
- Endosutures are placed at the uterine incision.
- The rudimentary horn is removed from the abdominal cavity by electric morcellation or through a colpotomy.

Our technique of resection of the rudimentary horn when incorporated in the uterine wall allows preservation of the uterine wall due to minimal resection of myometrium:

1. The wall is opened over the rudimentary horn cavity.
2. The cavity lining is ablated by CO_2 laser.
3. The uterine wall is restored by suturing.

These techniques are usually free from complications. Patients may stand and walk 2–3 hours after surgery. Pregnancy is allowed 2–3 months after operation, and a vaginal delivery may be performed.

CLASS V: UTERUS DUPLEX

Uterus duplex is characterized by the presence of two uteri and one or two vaginas (Figure 27.23). The

rudimentary horn, may be encountered (Figure 27.21). Sometimes the rudimentary horn is embedded in the wall of the main horn.

Unicornuate uterus without a supplementary horn usually does not cause any gynecologic or obstetric problems. On the contrary, patients with a supplementary noncommunicating (or obstructed) rudimentary horn with functioning endometrium complain of painful menses from menarche or of perimenstrual pain due to the formation of hematometra. One of the potential dangers in this malformation is the possibility of an ectopic pregnancy in the rudimentary horn, as well as a high rate (over 50%) of endometriosis. Thus, the removal of a rudimentary horn is substantiated by a range of indications.

Preliminary diagnosis is based on the patient's complaints, physical examination (pelvic mass), and information provided by imaging techniques—ultrasonography, MRI, or SCT. Definite diagnosis, however, is possible only during laparoscopy and hysteroscopy (Figure 27.22), which allow the differentiation of four variants of this malformation: (1) unicornuate uterus with supplementary rudimentary horn communicating with principal horn; (2) unicornuate uterus with supplementary noncommunicating horn (sometimes embedded in the wall of the main uterine horn); (3) unicornuate uterus with supplementary horn without endometrial cavity; and (4) unicornuate uterus without supplementary rudimentary horn.

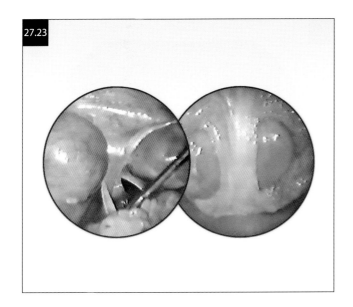

27.23

following variants of this malformation are differentiated: uterus duplex without obstruction to menstrual outflow; uterus and vagina duplex with partial vaginal aplasia; and uterus and vagina duplex where one uterus is nonfunctional.

Clinical manifestation depends on the malformation variant. The first variant (uterus duplex without obstruction to menstrual outflow) in most cases does not cause any problems and is often an occasional discovery, but, if not previously diagnosed, there may be difficulty in choosing the mode of delivery in a pregnant patient. Uterus and vagina duplex with partial aplasia of one hemivagina is accompanied by pelvic pain, caused by hematocolpos. Sometimes the diagnosis presents difficulties when one uterus is normally menstruating. Patients in whom one uterus is nonfunctional may appear infertile if intercourse involves the vagina of the nonfunctional uterus.

The patient's complaints, physical examination, ultrasonographic data, and other methods of visualization (MRI, SCT) contribute to the preliminary diagnosis, but only simultaneous hysteroscopy and laparoscopy provide the final differentiation between uterus duplex and other symmetric malformations (complete intrauterine septum and bicornuate uterus).

SURGICAL CORRECTION

Uterus duplex without obstruction to menstrual outflow itself does not necessitate surgical correction. In patients with uterine and vagina duplex with complete or partial aplasia of one of the hemivaginas, laparoscopy is used for final diagnosis, correction of associated gynecologic disease, and control after resection of the wall of the obstructed hemivagina which must provide a wide communication between the latter and the functional vagina. Laparoscopy with simultaneous correction of gynecologic disease during vaginoplasty in patients aged 12–15 years provides normal reproductive function.

CLASS VI: BICORNUATE UTERUS

Bicornuate uterus is a malformation where the upper part of the uterine body is divided into two horns. In some patients the bicornuate uterus is found during routine examinations or treatment for other gynecologic diseases. In some patients this malformation may be a cause of miscarriage, isthmic-cervical insufficiency, and abnormal labor.

None of the available diagnostic tools (ultrasonography, CT, MRI, HSG, hysteroscopy or laparoscopy alone) is adequate to provide 100% accuracy in differentiation between bicornuate and septate uterus. The hysteroscopic picture may look like that of an intrauterine septum. Laparoscopic examination performed together with hysteroscopy is crucial because the definitive diagnosis is possible only after visual evaluation of the external shape of corpus uteri (Figure 27.24).

SURGICAL CORRECTION

The only indication for surgical correction of this malformation is miscarriage. We use our own methods of combined laparoscopic-hysteroscopic metroplasty based on the principles of the conventional Strassman technique, comprising creation of a united cavity that includes:

1. Dissection of the uterine fundus in the frontal plane with opening of both hemicavities
2. Suturing of the uterine wound in the sagittal plane

In case of incomplete bicornuate uterus, and if simultaneous distension of both hemicavities is possible, the operation is started by hysteroscopy. Five percent mannitol or 5% glucose solution may be used as the distension media. The mucosal-muscular layer of the uterine wall is dissected using a resectoscopic hook electrode up to the serosa in the frontal plane, avoiding the tubal ostia. The depth of dissection is visually controlled hysteroscopically and laparoscopically by transillumination of the uterine wall (Figure 27.25). The hysteroscopic step is

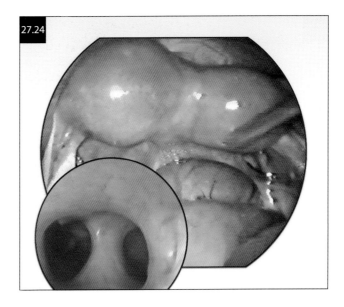

27.24

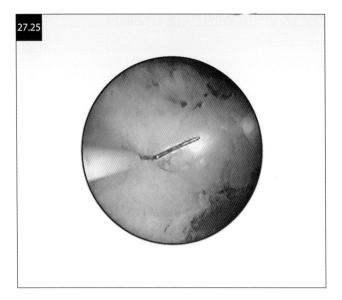

27.25

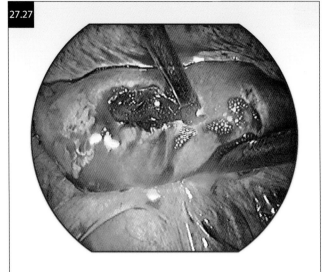

27.27

terminated by planned perforation of the uterus, which is necessary to determine the direction of the incision of the serosa. Further steps are performed laparoscopically (Figure 27.26).

Laparoscopy is performed through four punctures of the anterior abdominal wall. The uterine serosa is transected in the frontal plane by a monopolar or bipolar electrode, laser, or ultrasonic scalpel (Figure 27.27). Hemostasis is achieved by bipolar coagulation (Figure 27.28). Two layers (mucosal-muscular and muscular-serosal) of absorbable sutures are placed at the uterine wound in the sagittal direction (Figures 27.29 and 27.30). The ends of the first layer of sutures are withdrawn from the abdominal cavity through a central puncture outside the trocar sleeve and are left untied until the last suture is placed. The ligatures are then consecutively introduced into the trocar sleeve and tied extracorporeally. To avoid excessive tension and tissue sawing during knot-tying, both halves of the uterus are brought to the midline with the manipulators. The serosal-muscular suture may be

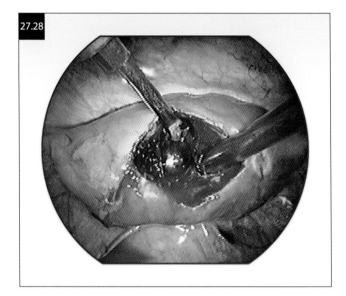

27.28

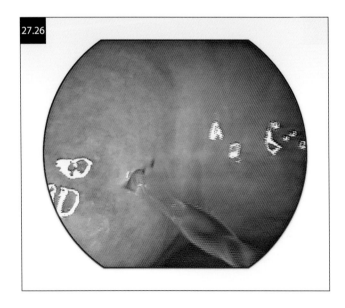

27.26

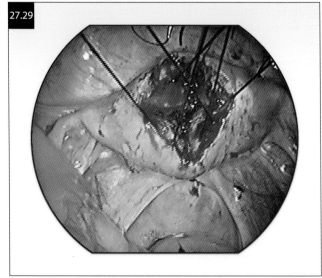

27.29

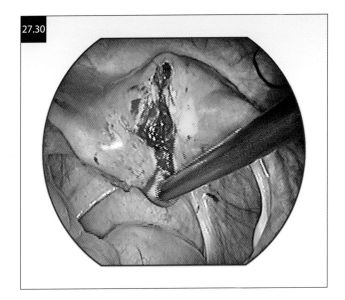

placed continuously. Second-look laparoscopy and hysteroscopy performed 3 months after endoscopic metroplasty have shown no evidence of adhesions either in the pelvis or in the uterine cavity. Satisfactory results of endoscopic metroplasty lead us to believe that minimally invasive approaches are more effective than conventional laparotomic techniques.

CLASS VII: INTRAUTERINE SEPTUM

Intrauterine septum is a symmetric malformation in which the uterine cavity is divided into two hemicavities by a longitudinal septum of varying length. The patients with intrauterine septum often suffer from reproductive failures (miscarriages). Final diagnosis is possible only under simultaneous hysteroscopy and laparoscopy. Laparoscopy shows united corpus uteri. Hysteroscopy is necessary to evaluate the volume of the uterine cavity and the length and thickness of the septum (Figure 27.31). Two variants of malformation exist:

1. Complete septum
2. Partial septum (not reaching internal ostium)

This intervention is incomparably less invasive than laparotomic metroplasty using the Jones or Tompkins techniques. Our method provides excellent anatomic effectiveness and is almost free from complications and disadvantages, such as formation of pelvic adhesions and the necessity of subsequent cesarean section.

Hysteroscopic resection is performed in the early follicular phase of the menstrual cycle (preferably immediately after menstruation) or after medical preparation of the endometrium (for reduction of its thickness, operative blood loss, and for better visualization) with 2 months of hormonal contraception or GnRH agonists, according to the following technique (Figure 27.32):

- The cervical canal is dilated up to 10.5–11.5 Hegar.
- A resectoscope is inserted into the uterine cavity; the intrauterine septum is consecutively transected in its middle part from the summit to the base with small movements of the hook electrode, and by monopolar pure cutting current of 100–130 W, until the uterine cavity assumes a normal triangular shape.
- Bleeding is controlled by a coagulating current of 40–60 W.

For distension, 5% glucose solution or other nonelectrolytes are used. The fluid (2–6 L, depending on the septum length and thickness) is delivered at a rate of 150–400 mL/min; average pressure in the cavity is maintained at 60–80 mm Hg. If the procedure duration exceeds 20 min, 20 mg of Lasix can be given intravenously for prevention of complications associated with possible fluid overload. Laparoscopic control during hysteroscopic resection of the intrauterine septum has been advised by some considering the risk of perforation of the uterus, and for the simultaneous evaluation and correction of associated pelvic disease.

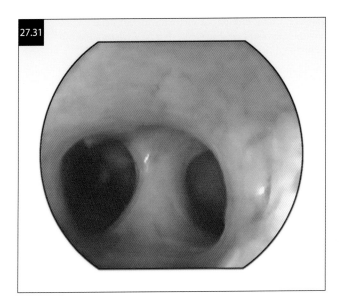

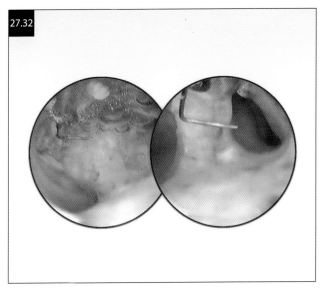

The patient is allowed to stand up 2 hours after surgery, and to leave the hospital on the same day. Contraception is recommended for 2–3 months. Reproductive function is restored in up to 64% of patients who have undergone this type of hysteroscopic resection, and the patients usually deliver vaginally, provided there are no obstetric indications for operative delivery.

CLASS VIII: ANOMALIES OF THE OVARIES AND/OR FALLOPIAN TUBES

Unilateral or bilateral aplasia of fallopian tubes or ovaries is included in this class. The absence of the ovarian tissue can be treated hormonally. In the event gonadal dysgenesis is present, biopsy of the ovarian tissue needs to be performed in order to establish its morphological diagnosis.

Not included in the updated version of the classification are combined anomalies, of which bladder extrophy is best known. Correction of these defects requires a highly specialized team in the correction of anomalies, including gynecologic surgeons, urologists, general, and general reconstructive surgeons. Parturition in patients after correction of bladder extrophy needs to be via cesarean section.

CONCLUSION

To conclude, laparoscopy and hysteroscopy not only help provide the definitive diagnosis of the full spectrum of malformations of the genitalia, but are the most rational methods to correct the majority of these gynecologic anomalies using minimally invasive operative approaches. In fact, endoscopic approaches are applicable and preferred for all classes of genital anomalies other than combined complex malformations.

SUGGESTED READING

Adamyan LV. Additional international perspectives: Colpopoiesis in vaginal and uterine aplasias. In: Nichols D, ed. *Gynecologic and Obstetric Surgery*. St. Louis, MO: Mosby; 1993:1167–1182.

Adamyan LV. Laparoscopic management of vaginal aplasia with or without functional noncommunicating uterus. In: Arregui ME, Fitzgibbons RJ Jr, Katkhouda N, McKernan JB, Reich H, eds. *Principles of Laparoscopic Surgery: Basic and Advanced Techniques*. Heidelberg: Springer; 1995:646–652.

Adamyan LV. Laparoscopic management of vaginal aplasia with or without functional noncommunicating rudimentary uterus. In: Arrequi ME, Fitzgibbons RJ, Katkhouda N, McKernan JB, Reich H, eds. *Principles of Laparoscopic Surgery*. New York, NY: Springer-Verlag; 1995:646.

Adamyan LV. Laparoscopy in surgical treatment of vaginal aplasia: Laparoscopy assisted colpopoiesis and perineal hysterectomy with colpopoiesis. *Int J Fertil*. 1996;41(1):40–45.

Adamyan LV. Therapeutic and endoscopic perspectives: Colpopoiesis in vaginal and uterine aplasias. In: Nichols D, ed. *Gynecologic, Obstetric and Related Surgery*. St. Louis, MO: Mosby; 1999:187–195.

Adamyan LV, Makyan ZN, Uvarova EV et al. Malformations of female genitalia: Classification and management issues. In: *Proceedings: XII International Congress with Endoscopic Course: "New Technologies for Diagnosis and Treatment of Gynecologic Disease,"* Moscow, 2009 June (rus/engl).

Adamyan LV, Stenyayeva NN, Makiyan ZN. Sexual function of women after surgical correction of the vaginal and uterine aplasia. In *Proceedings of XXVII Congress of*, Moscow, Russia, June 2014.

Adamyan LV, Stepanian AA. Neovagina creation with the use of the pelvic peritoneum. In: Grimbizis G, Campo R, Tarlatzis B, Gordts S, eds. *Female Genital Tract Congenital Malformations*. London: Springer; 2015.

Buttram VC, Jr. Mullerian anomalies and their management. *Fertil Steril*. 1983;40:159.

Frank RT. The formation of artificial vagina without operation. *Am J Obstet Gynecol*. 1938;35:1053–1055.

Jones HJ, Wheeless C. Salvage of the reproductive potential of women with anomalous development of the Mullerian ducts: 1868-1968-2068. *Am J Obstet Gynecol*. 1969;104:348–364.

Kulakov VI, Adamyan LV, Minbayev OA. Correction of genital malformations. In: Kulakov VI, Adamyan LV, Minbayev OA, eds. *Operative Gynecology—Surgical Energies*. Moscow: Medicine; 2000:691–694 (rus).

Monks P. Uterus didelphys associated with unilateral cervical atresia and renal agenesis. *Aust NZJ Obstet Gynaecol*. 1979;19:245–246.

CHAPTER 28

LAPAROENDOSCOPIC SINGLE-SITE (LESS) SURGERY

Patrick Yeung, Jr. and Brigid Holloran-Schwartz

INTRODUCTION

Laparoendoscopic single-site (LESS) surgery continues to be considered as a progression of a minimally invasive surgery for gynecologic procedures. This procedure has the benefit of consolidating the fascial defect to a single site at the umbilicus, and at the same time, avoiding lateral puncture wounds. In so doing, there is the potential that LESS surgery is an improved route for certain procedures, with the potential for improved cosmesis and decreased postoperative pain. Although technological innovation has permitted a surge in interest and demonstrated feasibility of this methodology, many challenges still exist for the widespread adoption of LESS. Acknowledging the present challenges with LESS, this chapter reviews the potential benefits, available instrumentation, and surgical principles of LESS surgery.

WHY PERFORM LESS?

Advances in surgical techniques and instrumentation now empower gynecologic surgeons to attain the maximal benefits of laparoscopy, while minimizing the incisional footprint on the abdominal wall. LESS surgery offers the advantages of fewer abdominal incisions and improved cosmesis, with the benefits of minimally invasive surgery (Figure 28.1). In 1991, Pelosi et al. reported on the first laparoscopic hysterectomy with bilateral salpingo-oophorectomy using a single umbilical puncture instead of multiple ports. This approach did not gain widespread acceptance until recently, due to the many inherent challenges of this procedure, and the lack of appropriate technology and instrumentation.

Traditional laparoscopic surgery is performed via multiple abdominal ports. The camera port is typically placed in the midline at the umbilicus, while lateral ports provide for triangulation of instruments at the level of the target organ or tissue. The placement of lateral ports can be a source of potential morbidity to muscles, nerves, and vessels in the abdominal wall. In fact, injury to the inferior epigastric vessels has been reported to be the most common complication in laparoscopic-assisted vaginal hysterectomy (LAVH). Lateral ports may also cause neuropathic pain if the iliohypogastric or ilioinguinal nerves are injured at the time of placement or during

suture closure of the fascial incision site. Moreover, incisional hernia is more apt to occur (for an equivalent size fascial defect) at a lateral port than at the umbilicus.

In LESS surgery, there is a single fascial defect and skin incision usually located at the umbilicus. Whereas the size of the fascial incision (about 2–2.5 cm) may be similar to the total fascial defect (when added together) of multiport laparoscopy, creating the fascial defect at a natural scar (the umbilicus) without the need for multiple lateral puncture sites can reduce some of the complications associated with multiport laparoscopy (described above), including postoperative pain. In addition, the larger umbilical fascial defect with the LESS approach potentially makes it the *preferred* approach for procedures that require removal of larger specimens through the abdominal wall, such as oophorectomy, ovarian cystectomy, hysterectomy, and myomectomy. A small wound retractor or laparoscopic bag placed through the umbilical fascial defect, combined with efficient manual morcellation techniques (such as the "paper roll" technique) (Figure 28.2), can facilitate efficient specimen removal for even larger tissue specimens.

For many surgeons and patients, the most convincing reason for opting for LESS surgery is the superior cosmesis. The entire skin incision can be hidden in the natural creases of the umbilicus to create a near scarless result. One study examining cosmetic preferences for abdominal incisions concluded that the lack of "visibility" of incisions in the mid-abdomen might be the most important factor for women's preferences, although there was difficulty in depicting real cosmetic results. While results may vary, of course, a truly "scar-less" result is in fact achievable (Figure 28.3). Even if there was no other comparative advantage for LESS surgery, cosmesis alone may be convincing enough to explore adopting or mastering this route of surgery.

WHY NOT DO LESS?

There are many challenges of LESS surgery including loss of instrument triangulation and reduced operative working space, resulting in instrument crowding and sword-fighting (instrument collisions). The introduction of the laparoscope and surgical instruments in a parallel approach, through the same incision, reduces both

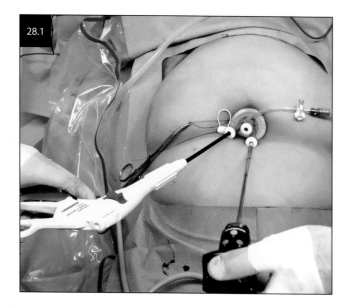

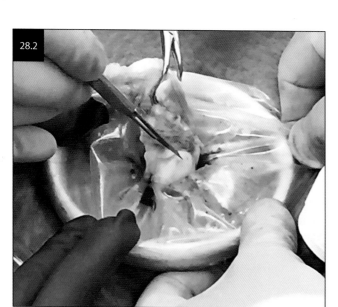

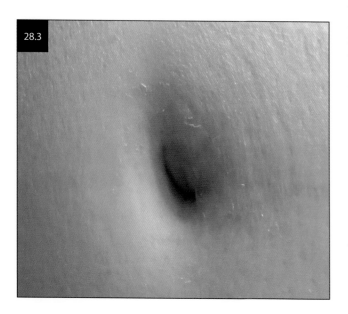

intraabdominal and external operative working space while reducing visualization and triangulation. Newer instruments including single-incision laparoscopic ports, articulating laparoscopic instruments, and automated suturing devices allow gynecologic surgeons to accommodate for some of these challenges. There is a steep learning curve for learning to use the LESS instrumentation and to get used to creating triangulation through a single fascial defect. LESS surgery is best viewed as a natural progression after the techniques of multiport laparoscopy have been mastered.

Concerns have been raised about potentially increased rates of umbilical hernia formation from the larger fascial defect. This question was addressed by Gunderson in 2012, who described a low hernia rate after LESS surgery for gynecologic procedures, especially in patients without comorbidities. This low rate may be attributed to the fact that the fascial defect was closed using a running delayed absorbable suture such as 0-PDS.

LESS PORTS: HOW TO MAKE ONE INTO THREE OR MORE

Technological innovation has greatly enabled the performance of LESS surgery. Initially, LESS surgery was performed through a single umbilical skin incision, with multiple ports placed through separate fascial incisions. Still, there are places where LESS surgery is performed using low-cost options including a simple wound retractor and a latex glove. However, several manufacturers have developed ports that accomplish the following: (1) make a single fascial incision able to accommodate multiple instruments, while (2) maintaining pneumoperitoneum and (3) allowing an escape valve to evacuate plume from the intraabdominal cavity. These ports provide flexibility of instruments that can be employed, while expanding their functionality.

The TriPort Access System from Olympus America (Center Valley, Pennsylvania) permits the placement of up to three laparoscopic instruments, while the QuadPort allows for up to four instruments. The TriPort can accommodate two 5 mm and one 12 mm instruments, and the QuadPort can accommodate one 5 mm, two 10 mm, and one 12 mm instruments (Figure 28.4). The TriPort may be the port of choice for the smallest fascial incision (about 18 mm) possible.

The SILS port from Covidien (Norwalk, Connecticut) is a single-piece, flexible port made from a sponge-like elastic polymer. It can accommodate three 5 mm instruments, or two 5 mm and one 5/12 mm port. These ports can be interchanged throughout the case. Once the incision has been made, a curved retractor (such as an "S" retractor) is often required and placed within the inferior aspect of the incision, to "shoe-horn" the port in place. The port can be removed and replaced throughout the case to facilitate specimen retrieval (Figure 28.5).

The AirSeal port from SurgiQuest (Orange, Connecticut) appears similar to any other rigid laparoscopic trocar but

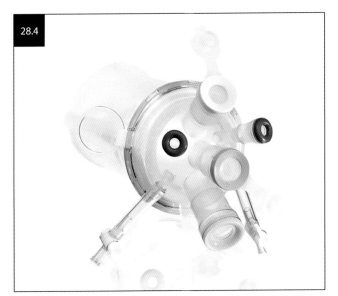

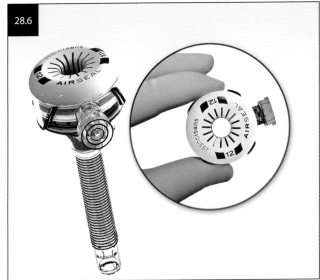

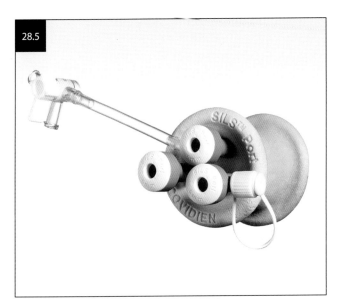

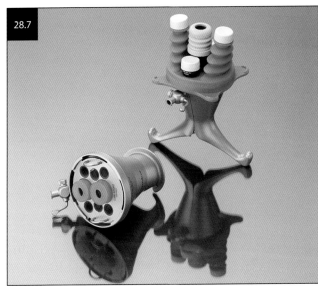

lacks an inner mechanical valve. Pneumoperitoneum is instead maintained by a pressure gradient (through the entire abdominal cavity) created within the housing of the trocar, with the pressure gradient within the port exceeding the pressure created by the pneumoperitoneum. The system uses a specialized air pump and tubing, and the circulating air is filtered to help to remove smoke. Oddly shaped or traditional instruments may be passed through the device unencumbered (Figure 28.6).

Karl Storz (Tutlingen, Germany) offers the S-PORTAL products, which include a variety of long, specially curved instruments along with reusable peritoneal access ports. The X-Cone consists of two metal halves that, once within the peritoneal cavity, are joined together by a silicone cap. Within the cap are three access channels that can accommodate instruments up to 12 mm in diameter (Figure 28.7). The ENDOCONE contains channels for six 5 mm instruments and two 12 mm instruments.

The GelPoint Advanced Access Platform single-incision system by Applied Medical (Rancho Santa Margarita, California) incorporates the company's Alexis wound retractor with the GelSeal cap. The GelSeal cap creates a PseudoAbdomen that floats above the fascial incision and provides for a very flexible fulcrum around which the cannulas can move entirely independent of one another. They come in two sizes, Gelpoint that fits on a 1.5–7 cm incision and is 10 cm in diameter, and Gelpoint Mini that fits a 1–3 cm incision and is 6 cm in diameter (Figures 28.8 and 28.9). This cap can be removed and replaced during the surgical procedure to facilitate specimen retrieval through the wound retractor, which can stay in place in the abdominal wall.

LESS INSTRUMENTATION: FACILITATING TRIANGULATION

Loss of triangulation, reduced operative working space, and instrument clashing are common challenges encountered during a LESS procedure, such as hysterectomy. Fortunately, there are various surgical devices and

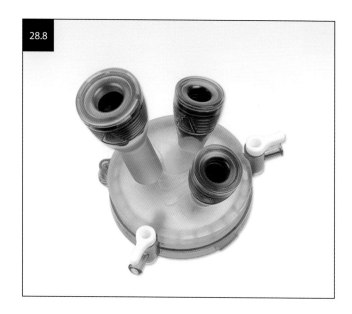

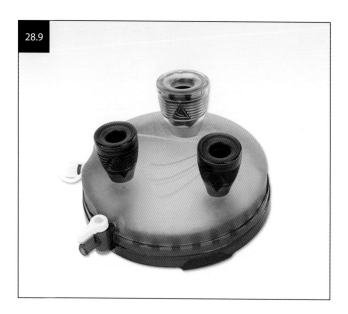

with KOH colpotomizer (Cooper Surgical, Trumbull, Connecticut), Pelosi uterine manipulator (Apple Medical Corporation, Marlborough, Massachusetts) and the VCare uterine manipulator (ConMed Corporation, Utica, New York) (see Chapter 3).

Each uterine manipulator has its own unique advantages and disadvantages. The RUMI Uterine Manipulator has a 140° range of uterine manipulation through a rotating handle, The VCare or the Delineator (by Cooper Surgical) uterine manipulators are disposable, single-use devices that have a long curved handle with a tip that conforms to the angle of the sacral curve, but has a fixed curve and does not ante- or retroflex across a joint. Both of these devices have a colpotomy cup that assists with lateral displacement of the ureters, anterior displacement of the bladder off the cervix, and delineation of the cervicovaginal junction. The Pelosi uterine manipulator is a reusable device that allows movement from 0° to 90° to maximize anteversion of the uterus, and a handle long enough to maximize uterine elevation.

ARTICULATING INSTRUMENTATION

The challenges encountered with loss of triangulation, reduced operative working space, and instrument collision can be partially mitigated with the use of articulating instrumentation. These instruments are invaluable in creating an internal type of triangulation that assists the surgeon with appropriate tissue manipulation. Since instruments are typically introduced through a single, multichannel port during a LESS hysterectomy procedure, it is essential that at least one instrument, but often preferably two, are able to articulate.

There are several articulating instruments that are currently commercially available for use in LESS hysterectomy procedures. The Covidien Roticulator is a rigid 5 mm laparoscopic instrument that provides up to an 80° articulating distal tip with 360° rotation at all articulation angles (Figure 28.10). This instrument is not a

instruments available to allow surgeons to help compensate for these challenges.

UTERINE MANIPULATION

In a traditional multiport total laparoscopic hysterectomy procedure, the uterus can be manipulated from above using a laparoscopic grasper through any auxiliary port. Uterine manipulation is more challenging during a LESS hysterectomy procedure due to the parallel nature of instrument insertion through a single-incision port, combined with the potential difficulties of instrument collision and reduced operative working space. An effective alternative method is the use of a uterine manipulator, which essentially acts as an auxiliary port. This enables the surgeon to fully manipulate the uterus without the instrument limitations imposed by the use of a single-incision port. Some of the more common uterine manipulators currently available include the RUMI uterine manipulator

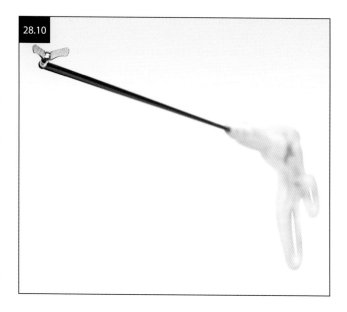

fully articulating instrument because it does not articulate in all directions or around the axis of the tip. The Roticulator instrument can be fixed in a specific articulation angle to allow triangulation to be recreated at the level of the tissue during a LESS procedure. However, there is a "crossover effect" since the instrument is going through the midline, meaning that retraction to the right in the surgical field corresponds to retraction of the instrument to the left outside the abdomen, and vice versa. Although this type of movement may be counterintuitive for a traditionally trained laparoscopic surgeon, it can become natural with practice. Covidien also makes a full line of true articulating instruments where the tip can bend (and lock in position) to any direction, and where the blades rotate around the axis of the tip. Other companies are also currently developing similar articulating instruments.

LESS LAPAROSCOPES

There are currently two flexible-tip laparoscopes that are in widespread use in LESS procedures (Figure 28.11). The Olympus EndoEYE is a 5 mm flexible endoscope, with a distally mounted CCD chip. The deflectable distal tip provides a 100° field of view in an all-in-one design with integrated light cable and camera system. The Stryker IDEAL EYES HD is a 10 mm articulating endoscope, with over 100° of flexion in all directions, that transmits both HD (1280 × 1024) and HDTV (720p) video signals for enhanced visualization. The handles of these laparoscopes allow the surgeon to change the surgical view without having to move the camera head, and allow for a locking mechanism to fix the view. Storz also has the ENDOCAMELEON "variable direction view" laparoscope, which has a prism at the end of a rigid 10 mm laparoscope that can be directed to views of 0°–120° as needed without having to move the camera head.

Systems

These flexible-tip, or variable direction view, laparoscopes are especially useful in LESS surgical procedures, since they allow the surgeon to create a surgical view with the camera head out of the way of other instrument handles. They do take some getting used to, since surgeons comfortable with traditional multiport laparoscopy have been conditioned to change the surgical view by moving the entire camera head. If flexible-tip laparoscopes are not available, then a 30° or 45° angled rigid laparoscope is preferred. The use of a rigid bariatric scope with a right-angle light connector also allows the surgeon to keep the camera out of the working space above the port.

The Stryker Wingman, a pneumatic-driven scope-holding system, can be used to stabilize any 5 mm or 10 mm laparoscope and camera. This allows the surgeon to fix the laparoscope in place, and frees up an extra hand, which may allow the surgeon to operate more efficiently (Figure 28.12). This is especially important in LESS surgery, when the gynecologic surgeon is required to not only position but also to articulate the instruments during the procedure. The Wingman is also very useful to stabilize the flexible-tip laparoscopic handle against the exterior anterior abdominal wall, so that the working space above the single-incision port is maximized, which improves efficient manipulation of the instruments. Since the flexible-tip laparoscopes have controls on the handle to deflect the tip in multiple directions, the laparoscope can remain in a single position throughout most of the surgical procedure, and visualization can be adjusted without moving the body of the laparoscope. The ViKY robotic laparoscope holder (Endocontrol Medical, La Tronche, France) can be used in a similar manner, but it offers the benefit of a robotic approach to laparoscopic manipulation through voice recognition or footswitch control. The FreeHand laparoscopic camera controller (Prosurgics, Cupertino, California) also gives the surgeon hands-free movement of

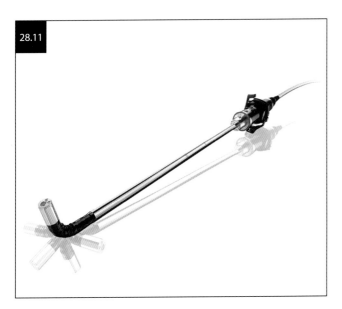

28.11

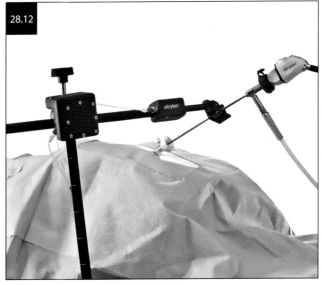

28.12

the laparoscope through a robotic platform that uses surgeon head movement and an activation controller. These laparoscope holders enable surgeons to perform LESS procedures as truly a single-operator procedure.

LESS TECHNIQUE: IT IS ALL IN THE SETUP

Gynecologic surgeons should not attempt to advance to LESS surgery until they are comfortable with multiport laparoscopy. There is a natural progression to minimize the number of port sites to a single port: (1) after one has mastered abdominal entry and trocar placement, (2) after one has the ability to view and understand key anatomy through a laparoscope, and (3) after one has comfortably learned to triangulate and operate with instruments through multiple ports. Whereas each of these steps needs to be modified or adapted when performing LESS surgery, confidence and skills with multiport laparoscopy provide the necessary foundation. In fact, if a situation arises where a LESS approach is limiting or inadequate, then a port (or several ports) should be added as necessary to complete the procedure. Multiport laparoscopy, then, is both the starting point and a possible backup plan for LESS surgery.

There are many techniques and preferences that surgeons commonly employ when performing a LESS surgery. This section, while not intending to be a comprehensive description of all techniques used, will describe several preferences or techniques of the authors. The topics to be discussed include (1) abdominal entry and port placement, (2) the use of "plane"-ing and retraction away from midline to avoid clashing of instrument handles, (3) aids in carrying out tissue manipulation, and (4) vaginal cuff closure.

An open Hasson technique is used for abdominal entry at the umbilicus. The skin incision is strictly independent of the fascial incision or entry point. The umbilicus can vary greatly in size, depth, and shape.

There are two basic skin incisions used for abdominal laparoscopic entry. One is the "Omega" incision, and the other is a linear incision directly through the center of the umbilicus (Figure 28.13). The "Omega" incision has two components—a "U"-shaped incision that follows the natural curve of the inferior aspect of the umbilical crater, and the arms of the "Omega" that extend from it. All of these components exist in perpendicular planes. The "U" is made at the base of the umbilical crater (visualized as a cylinder), while the arms rise up vertically along each side of this cylinder. Most importantly, this incision is made without incising skin outside the edge of the umbilical crater.

The linear incision tends to give a better cosmetic result and can be made in any orientation through the center of the umbilicus. Most commonly, this incision is made in a line axial to the body.

A variation of the linear incision is a "hockey stick" incision, where the linear incision is bent or redirected at the midline; this incision can be tailored to the natural

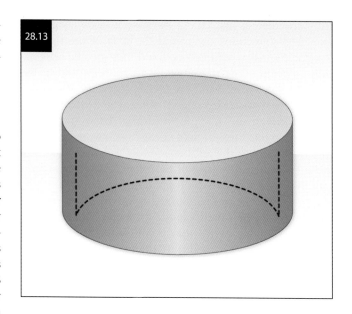

28.13

creases of the skin and umbilicus for the best cosmetic result (Figure 28.14). Regardless, the incision is still kept within the borders of the umbilical crater.

Regardless of the skin incision, the skin edges are retracted using Allis clamps. The fascial incision is independent of the skin incision. The fascia is usually entered in the same manner for all cases. At the last of where the umbilical stalk meets the fascia, there is a natural weakness that can be used as an advantage for entering the fascia. This point is identified at the base of the umbilical stalk, and is entered sharply with scissors or a scalpel, or bluntly using the tip of a curved hemostat (Figure 28.15). The fascial incision is extended using traction and countertraction, or sharply under direct visualization, usually in a horizontal fashion. The fascial edges are usually tagged for traction, and to assist with closure at the end of the procedure. The port is then placed according to the manufacturer's recommendations.

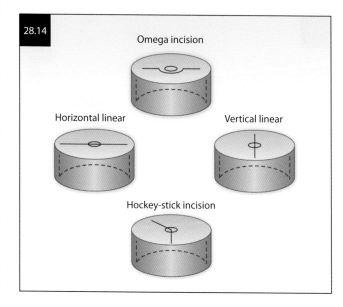

28.14   Omega incision

Horizontal linear   Vertical linear

Hockey-stick incision

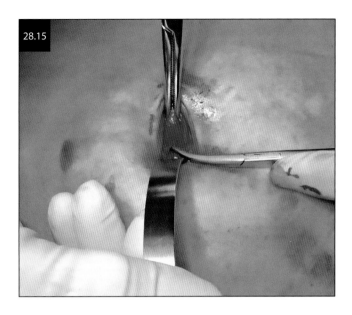

Instrument collisions can be minimized by using smaller-diameter laparoscopic instruments, those with smaller handles, and articulating instruments. This will help minimize the potential conflict of instrument handles above the abdominal wall. Retraction of an instrument handle, when possible, should also be configured such that the instrument handle is ideally retracted away from the midline. The concept of "plane"-ing also helps to prevent instrument handle clashing or collision (Figure 28.16). The space above the abdominal wall of the patient can be thought of as three planes, or three heights above the abdominal wall (lowest, middle, and highest slices). When using pistol grip handles, gripping sideways will enable movements, if necessary, over one another in different "planes."

The camera is usually positioned first in the lowest height or plane. The instrument providing traction is then positioned such that the instrument handle is being retracted away from the midline. If these two guidelines are followed, then the operating hand (usually the

energy device) has space in the center, and at the highest height, to move freely without clashing. A simpler way to think of it is to keep all instruments, but the energy device, away from the "bulls-eye" space directly in front of the umbilicus. Unlike multiport laparoscopy, it is best to minimize movement of the instrument handles above the abdominal wall, which usually involves setting up the camera and grasper first, and then focusing solely on the energy instrument so that only one instrument handle is moving at a time.

The steps of a LESS procedure are essentially the same as those for a traditional multiport procedure. Some key steps, or slight variations of steps that have been adopted while performing a LESS procedure, will be highlighted. Difficulty with appropriate tissue retraction can sometimes be encountered during a LESS procedure for many reasons. In patients with a previous cesarean section, or redundant bladder tissue, the Covidien Endo Mini-Retract 5 mm instrument can be used to retract the bladder flap and maximize visualization. A myoma screw is also useful for uterine manipulation throughout the procedure, especially for controlling the fundus of a large uterus, since the instrument can be placed, or replaced, at different positions within the uterus. If the procedure cannot be completed without assistance from additional auxillary ports, the Teleflex (Teleflex Inc., Wayne, Pennsylvania) MiniLap grasper can be used in place of a traditional 5 mm port, since the 2.3 mm diameter shaft will produce minimal pain and scarring (Figure 28.17). A surgeon may

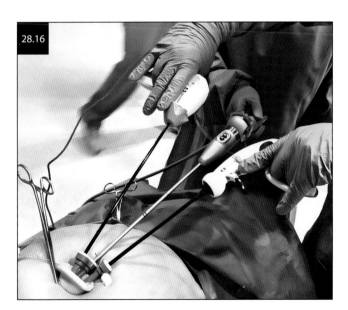

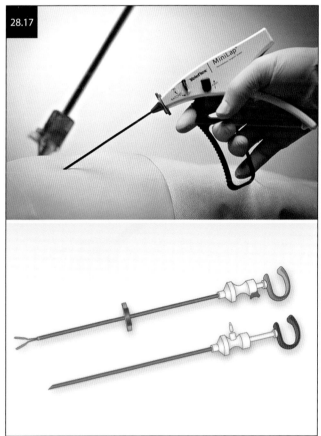

also elect to routinely place the Teleflex MiniLap grasper in the suprapubic location, at the start of every procedure, for added tissue manipulation and reassurance during the LESS hysterectomy procedure. Regardless, adding additional ports as needed during any LESS procedure is prudent surgical management.

Closure of the vaginal cuff can be accomplished utilizing a straight needle driver and an articulating grasper, or vice versa, though laparoscopic suturing during a LESS procedure is very challenging. Automated suturing devices such as the Endostitch, or the articulating SILS stitch, provide a controlled and efficient method for laparoscopic suturing during these procedures. These instruments allow a small, straight needle to be passed back and forth through the tissue, between the instrument jaws, in order to achieve effective suturing (Figures 28.18 and 28.19). A variety of suture types and lengths are available for vaginal cuff closure, although the authors typically use a 0 Polysorb suture with a 48 inch suture length. The vaginal cuff can be closed with either an interrupted, "figure-of-8" or running technique, per the surgeon's preference. The 48 inch suture also allows the surgeon to pull the suture out between tissue bites so that traction can be maintained extracorporeally.

LESS BASICS: GETTING STARTED

An accomplished laparoscopic surgeon can transition to LESS surgery quite easily for hysterectomy and

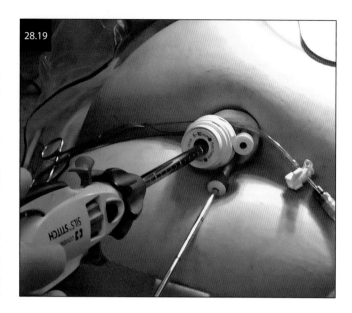

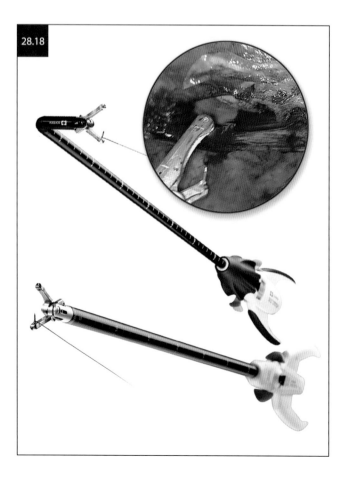

adnexectomy with a minimal learning curve following some basic principles. LESS is a technique that builds on the principles of traditional laparoscopic surgery; therefore, comfort and expertise with multiport laparoscopy are important. Two studies by experienced laparoscopists suggest that it may take between 10 and 20 cases to significantly decrease operative times and achieve proficiency using a single-incision approach. It is important to note that these studies did not show an increase in complications during the time that proficiency was achieved. If difficulty is encountered during a single-incision procedure, additional traditional ports can easily be added to complete the procedure, while still providing the benefits of laparoscopy.

This learning curve is based on subtle differences between single- and multiport laparoscopy. For example, creation of the single umbilical port site has been refined over the years to where one can literally create a "scarless" incision by following the natural folds of the umbilicus. Our preferred technique is to carefully inspect the natural folds of the umbilicus and mark out a 2 cm incision. The incision should always remain in the "basin" of the umbilicus following these natural folds in either a vertical or "hockey stick" configuration, depending on the individual patient's fold. The goal is that the incision does not extend outside of the umbilical crater. The center will always be at the exact base of the umbilicus, which is the shortest distance into the abdominal cavity where the skin, fascia, and peritoneum come together. This "stalk" of the umbilicus can be followed to its base. The fascia is grasped adjacent to the stalk while keeping the stalk itself intact, and entered sharply using an open, Hasson technique. We believe keeping the stalk intact can help recreate the natural appearance of the original umbilicus. The fascia is extended superiorly and inferiorly under direct visualization to 2 cm. This incision should accommodate most single ports and serves as an excellent site for specimen morcellation, as in laparoscopic supracervical hysterectomy, or removal of adnexal structures. We find this approach over the "omega" incision is superior in achieving a cosmetically preferred, "scarless," incision.

The choice of an endoscope is important to recreate an angled view of the operative field. Using a 30°–45° 5 mm, angled bariatric laparoscopic is useful. A standard laparoscope is 30 cm. A bariatric laparoscope is 45 cm, which allows displacement of the camera head farther away from the abdomen than the handles of the other instruments (by 15 cm). This configuration helps to prevent collision of the instruments. Further, a 90° light cord adaptor can be used to deflect the light cord backward, as opposed to upward, to again aid in avoiding collisions. Alternatively, and preferably, a flexible 5 mm laparoscope can be utilized to provide these offset views as well, though they are more expensive. A flexible laparoscope (e.g., EndoEye 5 by Olympus) allows one to change the surgical view by the use of levers, without moving the camera head. They also allow a greater degree of deflection (up to 85°) and are thin at 5 mm. A variable view laparoscope (e.g., EndoCAMeleon by Storz) offers angled views up to 120° but is bulkier at 10 mm.

When a bariatric or flexible laparoscope is not available, a standard-length laparoscope can be used with a 45 cm energy source (i.e., LigaSure, Covidien). This places the handle of the energy source 15 cm farther behind the camera head, as another way to avoid handle collisions.

It is best to start with more straightforward procedures such as removal of fallopian tubes, ovaries, or a simple hysterectomy. We do not advise ovarian cystectomy as a first procedure, as it can be more of a challenge given the need for traction, countertraction, and triangulation of instruments. Collision of the instrument handles is the primary frustration and obstacle for gynecologic surgeons who are comfortable with multiport laparoscopy.

For hysterectomy, starting with uteri that have reasonable access to the lateral attachments and uterine arteries is ideal. Manipulation of the uterus to expose these attachments can be accomplished with a uterine manipulator. If additional exposure is needed, as in the case of leiomyomas, a myoma screw is ideal to elevate and retract the uterus. The use of a myoma screw is preferred over an articulating grasper for superior, firm traction and the ability for a single uterine puncture to often expose both the anterior and posterior leaves of the broad ligament without readjustment. The primary energy source can then be inserted above or below the fixed myoma screw with minimal instrument clashing. Most hysterectomies can be completed without the use of any other instruments, articulating or nonarticulating, using the same technique as in multiport. Alternatively, an articulating grasper can be used to recreate the triangulation of traditional laparoscopy.

Removal of adnexal structures as in a bilateral sapling-oophorectomy (BSO) will often require assistance exposing the ovarian blood supply. The objective of reserving the midline space above the single port for the primary surgeon with the energy source should be maintained at all times. Therefore, if a grasper is needed to expose the ovarian vessels of the right ovary, for example, the assistant grasper should be placed in the trocar to the right of the primary energy source, allowing the assistant's handle to be displaced to the right, away from the midline, while avoiding crossing instrument handles on the outside of the patient. This maintains the midline area above the port for the primary surgeon's energy source without instrument clashing. The single incision site is again ideal for specimen removal.

LESS FUTURE: WHERE DO WE GO FROM HERE?

LESS surgery, though not new, has seen a surge in adoption due to technological innovation and newer instrumentation. Although the first LESS hysterectomy was done by Pelosi 20 years ago, LESS surgery is only beginning to realize its potential with the introduction of enabling technologies, including single-site robotics. The success and scope of LESS surgery will depend on technology, and the ability of industry to develop devices and instrumentation that enable surgeons to overcome the limitations of operating through a single site, and to operate in a natural and intuitive way.

Articulating laparoscopes and instruments will continue to play an increasingly important role in LESS gynecologic surgery. Recreation of the basic principles of triangulation is essential for effective and efficient performance of any laparoscopic procedure. Articulating laparoscopes allow for the same surgical view to be created from different angles, which provides the opportunity for more space outside the abdomen. Introduction of articulating energy devices will further reduce instrument collisions outside the abdomen. Innovative delivery systems in the future may also allow single or multiple instruments to be inserted through a single "stem" that then has the ability to separate, to deploy multiple arms, and to create triangulation at the level of the tissue.

Robotic surgical platforms, and other advanced technologies, have the potential to overcome reduced operative working space and the crossover effect of LESS surgery (where an instrument is controlling tissue from the opposite side). Still in its infancy, robotic platforms will continue to mature to become smaller, allow for more intuitive operation, and be more cost effective. Advanced technological development will provide a reduced learning curve for LESS surgery, yet will allow for operation through a single site with greater dexterity and precision. The potential of LESS surgery is limited only by technology, and widespread adoption should ultimately be driven by patient benefit.

SUGGESTED READING

AAGL Advancing Minimally Invasive Gynecology Worldwide. AAGL position statement: Route of hysterectomy to treat benign uterine disease. *J Minim Invasive Gynecol.* 2011;18:1–3.

Chen YJ, Wang PH, Ocampo EJ, Twu NF, Yen MS, Chao KC. Single-port compared with conventional laparoscopic-assisted vaginal hysterectomy: A randomized controlled trial. *Obstet Gynecol.* 2011;117:906–912.

Cho YJ, Kim ML, Lee SY, Lee HS, Kim JM, Joo KY. Laparoendoscopic single-site surgery (LESS) versus conventional laparoscopic surgery for adnexal preservation: A randomized controlled study. *Int J Womens Health.* 2012;4:85–91.

Escobar PF, Starks DC, Fader AN, Barber M, Rojas-Espalliat L. Single-port risk-reducing salpingo-oophorectomy with and without hysterectomy: Surgical outcomes and learning curve analysis. *Gynecol Oncol.* 2010;119:43–47.

Fader AN, Rojas-Espaillat L, Ibeanu O, Grumbine FC, Escobar PF. Laparoendoscopic single-site surgery (LESS) in gynecology: A multi-institutional evaluation. *Am J Obstet Gynecol.* 2010;203:501. e1–501.e6.

Fagotti A, Bottoni C, Vizzielli G, et al. Postoperative pain after conventional laparoscopy and laparoendoscopic single site surgery (LESS) for benign adnexal disease: A randomized trial. *Fertil Steril.* 2011;96:255–259.e2.

Fanfani F, Fagotti A, Gagliardi ML, et al. Minilaparoscopic versus single-port total hysterectomy: A randomized trial. *J Minim Invasive Gynecol.* 2013;20:192–197.

Garry R, Fountain J, Brown J, et al. EVALUATE hysterectomy trial: A multicentre randomised trial comparing abdominal, vaginal and laparoscopic methods of hysterectomy. *Health Technol Assess (Winchester, England).* 2004;8:1–154.

Gunderson CC, Knight J, Ybanez-Morano J, et al. The risk of umbilical hernia and other complications with laparoendoscopic single-site surgery. *J Minim Invasive Gynecol.* 2012;19:40–45.

Huang M, Musa F, Castillo C, Holcomb K. Postoperative bowel herniation in a 5-mm nonbladed trocar site. *JSLS.* 2010;14:289–291.

Hulka JF, Levy BS, Parker WH, Phillips JM. Laparoscopic-assisted vaginal hysterectomy: American Association of Gynecologic Laparoscopists' 1995 membership survey. *J Am Assoc Gynecol Laparosc.* 1997;4:167–171.

Johnson N, Barlow D, Lethaby A, Tavender E, Curr L, Garry R. Methods of hysterectomy: Systematic review and meta-analysis of randomised controlled trials. *BMJ.* 2005;330:1478.

Jung YW, Lee M, Yim GW, et al. A randomized prospective study of single-port and four-port approaches for hysterectomy in terms of postoperative pain. *Surg Endosc.* 2011;25(8):2462–2469.

Langebrekke A, Qvigstad E. Total laparoscopic hysterectomy with single-port access without vaginal surgery. *J Minim Invasive Gynecol.* 2009;16:609–611.

Li M, Han Y, Feng YC. Single-port laparoscopic hysterectomy versus conventional laparoscopic hysterectomy: A prospective randomized trial. *J Int Med Res.* 2012;40:701–708.

Murji A, Patel VI, Leyland N, Choi M. Single-incision laparoscopy in gynecologic surgery: A systematic review and meta-analysis. *Obstet Gynecol.* 2013;121:819–828.

Pelosi MA, Pelosi MA 3rd. Laparoscopic hysterectomy with bilateral salpingo-oophorectomy using a single umbilical puncture. *N J Med.* 1991;88:721–726.

Reich H, De Caprio J, McGlynn F. Laparoscopic hysterectomy. *J Gynecol Surg.* 1989;5:213–216.

Romanelli JR, Earle DB. Single-port laparoscopic surgery: An overview. *Surg Endosc.* 2009;23:1419–1427.

Sobolewski C, Yeung PP Jr, Hart S. Laparoendoscopic single-site surgery in gynecology. *Obstet Gynecol Clin North Am.* 2011;38:741–755.

Wheeless CR Jr. Elimination of second incision in laparoscopic sterilization. *Obstet Gynecol.* 1972;39:134–136.

Wong WS, Lee TC, Lim CE. Novel vaginal "paper roll" uterine morcellation technique for removal of large (>500 g) uterus. *J Minim Invasive Gynecol.* 2010;17:374–378.

Yamamoto M, Minikel L, Zaritsky E. Laparoscopic 5-mm trocar site herniation and literature review. *JSLS.* 2011;15:122–126.

Yeung PP Jr, Bolden CR, Westreich D, Sobolewski C. Patient preferences of cosmesis for abdominal incisions in gynecologic surgery. *J Minim Invasive Gynecol.* 2013;20:79–84.

Chapter 29

LAPAROSCOPIC BOWEL SURGERY

Jeff W. Allen and Benjamin D. Tanner

After mastering basic laparoscopic techniques such as tissue handling, intracorporeal suturing, and optical facility with 0° and 30° telescopes, operations that are more difficult can be performed using a minimal access approach. This includes many operations on the small and large bowel. This chapter reviews some advanced laparoscopic procedures such as colon resection and also some of the problems encountered during operations such as closure of an iatrogenic enterotomy.

COLON RESECTION

The laparoscopic approach to colon resection for benign disease is now preferred over the open operation in many circumstances. With malignant disease, concerns about issues of port site malignant recurrences, inadequate oncologic resections, and intraperitoneal tumor spread with pneumoperitoneum have all made laparoscopic colectomy controversial. A 2004 prospective, randomized study by Nelson et al. showed no differences in the overall or surgical wound rates of recurrence between laparoscopic and open colectomy for malignancy. The caveat in this study was that all surgeons who participated had performed at least 20 laparoscopic colon resections for benign disease prior to enrolling in the study, and the results were for only 3 years of follow-up. Benign diseases treated by laparoscopic partial colectomy include diverticular disease, some polyps, arterial venous malformations, endometriosis, benign strictures, and certain cases of colitis. Patients can significantly benefit from the laparoscopic approach to colon resection because there is a decrease in postoperative pain and wound infections. Most studies also demonstrate earlier return of bowel function, decreased hospital stay, along with improvements in pulmonary function and cosmesis.

SIGMOID COLECTOMY

For laparoscopic sigmoid colon resection, the patient is strategically positioned in Allen-type stirrups. Care is taken to adequately pad the legs in the stirrups to help prevent neuropraxia and neuropathy. The patient is placed in the Trendelenburg position, and the operating table is rolled so that the patient's left side is elevated. Some surgeons advocate a full lateral position with the use of beanbag support. The pneumoperitoneum is obtained with 5 mm working trocars placed in the left upper quadrant, left lower quadrant, and right lower quadrant (Figure 29.1). Since the extended incision of the left lower quadrant port is often the site for specimen extraction, this port can be 10 mm in size. A 10 mm camera port is placed below the umbilicus. A 30° laparoscope enables maximum viewing.

After port placement, the sigmoid colon is grasped using atraumatic bowel graspers or a Babcock, and retracted medially. The white line of Toldt is incised using scissors equipped with electrosurgery placed through the left lower quadrant port (Figure 29.2). Retroperitoneal structures including the ureter and left common iliac artery are identified. This dissection is continued cephalad to the splenic flexure. In some instances, the splenic flexure must be fully mobilized to ensure an adequate length of colon for a tension-free anastomosis.

After the colon is completely mobilized and the ureter identified, the major terminal portion of the inferior mesenteric artery is identified and ligated close to its origin. The vessel is most easily located by visualizing the arterial pulsations in the mesentery, while the colon is retracted toward the anterior abdominal wall. Ligation of this vessel includes creating a mesenteric window on either side of the artery and transecting it either with a linear laparoscopic stapler or large clips (Figure 29.3). In most patients, this vessel is too large for safe division with the harmonic scalpel.

Next, the remainder of the sigmoid colon mesentery is divided using the harmonic scalpel. It is important not to divide too far into the mesentery of the descending colon, because this can decrease the length of viable bowel available for anastomosis. After the mesentery has been divided, a linear laparoscopic stapler is fired across the distal sigmoid colon at the rectosigmoid junction below the area of pathology (Figure 29.4). It is important to identify the ureter prior to transecting the bowel.

The incision at either the left lower quadrant or the infraumbilical port site is extended, and the specimen with the attached proximal colon is delivered from the peritoneal cavity (Figure 29.5). The proximal end is transected with a firing of the laparoscopic stapler and opened. The anvil of an end-to-end (EEA) 25 mm stapler is placed in this colotomy and secured with a purse-string suture of 2-0 polypropylene (Figure 29.6). The 25 mm EEA is the size most suitable for this anastomosis, but other sizes can be used depending on the circumference of the descending colon. The descending colon

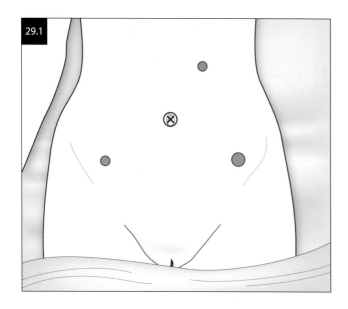

29.1

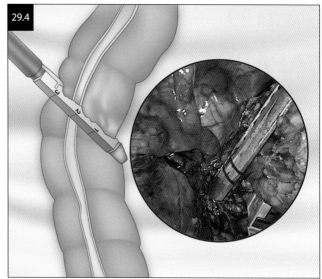

29.4

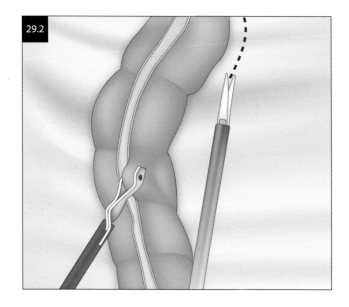

29.2

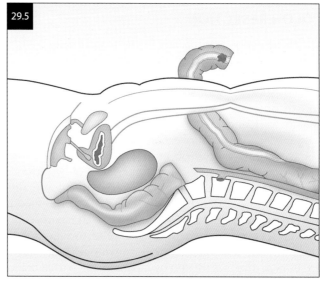

29.5

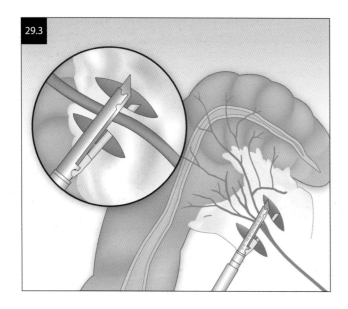

29.3

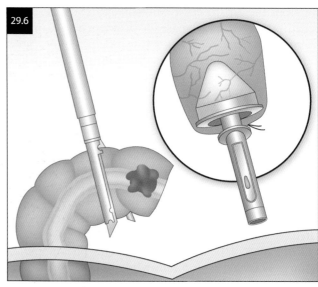

29.6

with anvil in place is then returned to the abdomen and the incision closed. It is important to make this closure airtight to reestablish a pneumoperitoneum. The EEA stapler is introduced per rectum, and the spike is deployed through the rectal stump. The proximal colon with anvil in place is stretched into the pelvis to the spike (Figure 29.7). If the anastomosis appears to be under tension, it is best to further mobilize the splenic flexure before performing the intracorporeal anastomosis in order to prevent a leak. The EEA stapler spike is then interfaced with its anvil, closed, and fired. The entire stapling apparatus is removed. It is important to test this anastomosis by clamping the colon proximal to the staple line with a noncrushing grasper, filling the pelvis with sterile saline or water, and then insufflating with air (Figure 29.8). A rigid sigmoidoscope can also be used to visualize the staple line and check for leakage. If a leak is noted, 2-0 silk sutures should be used to close the area by taking full-thickness bites using an intracorporeal suturing

technique. The pneumoperitoneum is decompressed, and the skin incisions are closed. The fascial defect at all port sites larger than 5 mm is customarily closed to prevent herniation.

RIGHT HEMICOLECTOMY

The patient is placed in a supine position on the operating room table. No stirrups are used, and the arms are tucked and padded in an adducted position at the patient's side. Rotating into the left lateral position then provides maximal exposure. Peritoneal access is obtained using an open Hasson technique via a 10 mm infraumbilical trocar. Working ports of 5 mm are placed into the right lower, the right upper, and the left lower quadrants, respectively (Figure 29.9). The table is rolled toward the patient's left side to increase visualization by allowing the small intestine to fall away from the right colon. The terminal ileum, appendix, and cecum are located, and the white line of Toldt is identified, and incised as previously described. This mobilization continues so that the cecum is freed from its retroperitoneal attachments (Figure 29.10). Often, this dissection is continued around the hepatic flexure as the harmonic scalpel is used to prevent bleeding. At this point, the ureter must be identified and protected along its entire path. Medial and inferior traction on the right and transverse colon is applied, and the duodenum is visualized and bluntly dissected away from the transverse mesocolon. Once the duodenum is completely freed, the pathologic process is identified, and a 5 cm distal margin is obtained. The transverse colon is transected using a linear 45 mm laparoscopic stapler. The mesentery is divided using the harmonic scalpel, and the laparoscopic stapler is used to divide the right colic artery (Figure 29.11). Alternatively, large clips may be used and the vessel divided with endoscopic shears. The specimen is delivered through a port site that has been extended. Either the infraumbilical or right lower quadrant incision may be used for this purpose. It is important to note that

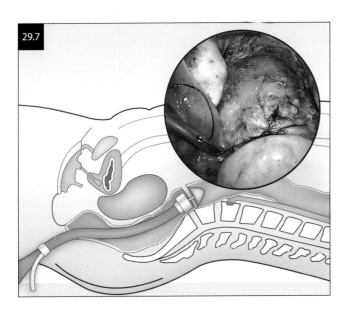
29.7

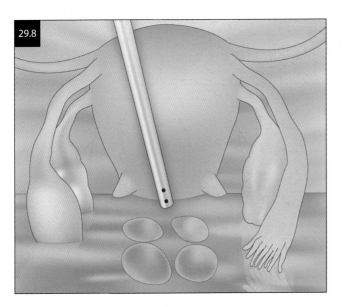
29.8

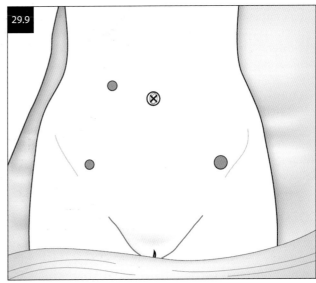
29.9

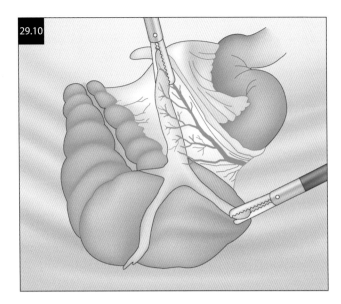

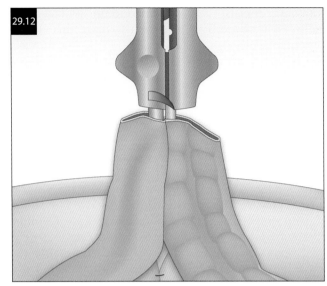

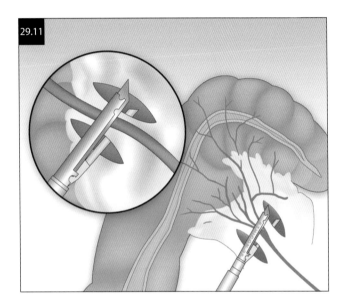

the ileum is still attached to the right colon and delivered out of the abdomen due to its lack of attachments. The ileum is then transected with a 45 mm linear stapler 5–10 cm proximal to the ileocecal valve. A hand-sewn end-to-end or side-to-side stapled anastomosis is performed extracorporeally (Figure 29.12). The mesenteric defect is closed with silk sutures, the ileocolic segment is returned to the abdomen, and the abdominal incisions are closed. Alternatively, this may be performed entirely intracorporeally with a side-to-side stapled anastomosis and closure of the common stoma with running 2-0 silk sutures tied intracorporeally. The specimen may then be delivered through an extended incision.

COLOSTOMY CREATION

Sigmoid or transverse colostomy is easily created using minimally invasive techniques. First, the pneumoperitoneum is obtained via an infraumbilical skin incision and working ports are then placed in the right upper and left lower quadrants. The large bowel is identified, and a sling is placed around it for easy manipulation (Figure 29.13). This is helpful because the colostomy site can be located based on how easily the colon reaches the skin site, as opposed to vice versa. After the colostomy site is identified, any necessary mobilization along the line of Toldt is undertaken as previously described. Once the loop can reach freely, an incision is made, and the colon is pulled through and matured in the usual fashion. A colostomy bar may replace the sling through the same aperture.

An end colostomy, with or without colon resection, entails identifying the site for the colostomy and dividing the colon and mesentery for proper length. The colon proximal to the colostomy is stretched to the site for the colostomy, a skin incision is made, and the colon is then delivered. The colostomy is matured in a standard fashion (Figure 29.14).

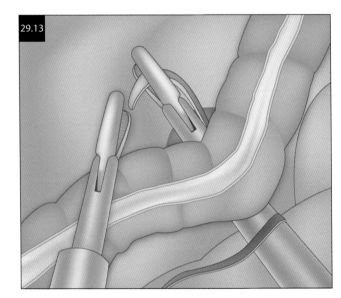

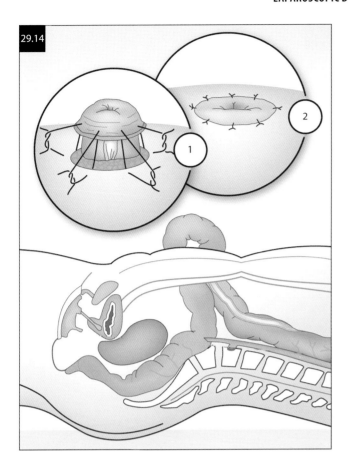

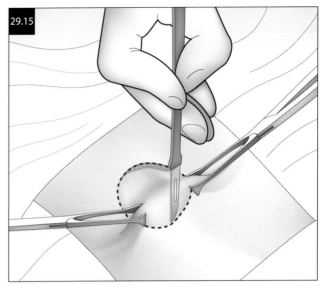

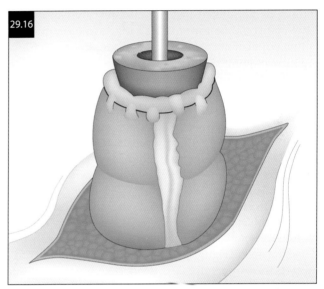

COLOSTOMY CLOSURE

The takedown of a colostomy is often a more morbid procedure than colostomy creation itself, because of the large adhesiolysis that is often required, along with the potential difficulty in identifying the distal colon for anastomosis.

Using the laparoscopic approach, the patient is carefully placed in the supine position and in stirrups. Care is taken to pad the legs to prevent neuropraxia and neuropathy. Port placement is based on previous incisions and the assumption that there will be less risk for significant adhesions to the bowel under unscarred skin. During the ensuing dissection, the peristomal area is cleared, and the colon that is proximal to the colostomy is mobilized. This often involves mobilizing the splenic flexure in the case of a descending colostomy.

Next, the colonic stump is identified. At this point, the pneumoperitoneum is released, and a peristomal incision is made with dissection of the colon off the fat and skin (Figure 29.15). The colostomy is then equipped with the anvil of a 25 mm EEA stapler secured with a pursestring suture of 2-0 polypropylene and replaced into the abdominal cavity (Figure 29.16). The colostomy incision is closed in an airtight fashion. The skin may be closed over drains or left open based on the preference of the surgeon. Next, the pneumoperitoneum is reestablished, and the colon with anvil is directed into the pelvis. The EEA stapler is passed per rectum following the curve of the sacrum. Once the EEA stapler is observed in the

rectal stump, the sharp spike is deployed, and the anvil and spike are interfaced. The stapler is fired after the appropriate pressure is obtained by closing the stapler (Figure 29.17). The anastomosis is checked as previously described.

APPENDECTOMY

The laparoscopic approach to appendectomy remains a controversial subject with regard to indications and cost. It is most beneficial for patients when the diagnosis is uncertain. This is often the case in obese patients, in those with history of inflammatory bowel disease, and particularly so in premenopausal women who present with adnexal pathology that may mimic appendicitis. A 1997 prospective study evaluated 161 premenopausal women with a diagnosis of acute appendicitis who underwent diagnostic laparoscopy. An appendectomy was performed in 55%, whereas 23% thought to have appendicitis actually had a gynecologic diagnosis. The

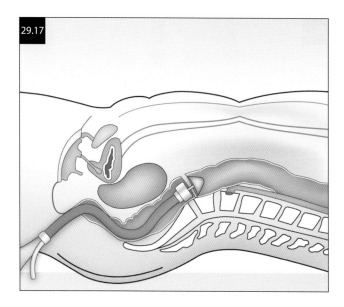

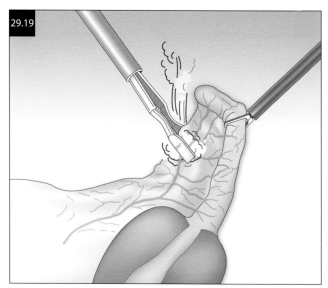

authors demonstrated that the false-negative appendectomy rate could be lowered with diagnostic laparoscopy in this population.

For maximum cosmesis, an infraumbilical incision is made for the camera port, and two lower 5 mm incisions are placed in the hairline (Figure 29.18). This technique involves creation of a pneumoperitoneum, establishing a diagnosis that confirms the need for appendectomy, and then isolating the appendix from its surrounding structures. Occasionally, the appendix is adherent to retroperitoneal structures by filmy adhesions, which must first be incised and mobilized.

After freeing the appendix, the mesoappendix is divided with clips and scissors, or alternatively with bipolar electrocautery (Figure 29.19), the harmonic scalpel, or a linear stapler (Figure 29.20). Once the appendix is free from its mesoappendix, it is divided with the linear stapler. This step may also be safely and cost-efficiently performed using a series of looped ligatures (Figure 29.21). The appendix is then delivered through the largest port.

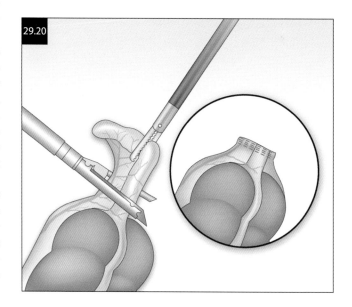

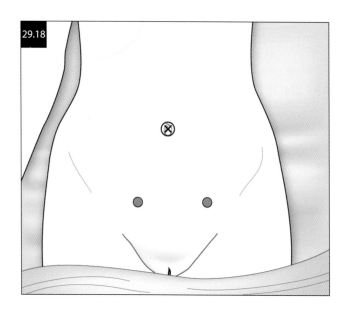

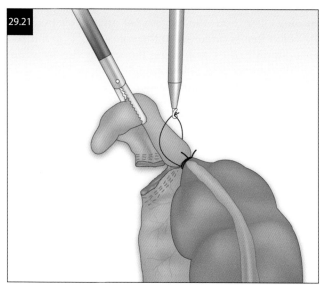

To minimize contamination at the port site, a specimen retrieval bag is used for extraction. Alternatively, to decrease costs, the thumb of a large powderless glove may be used. The operative field is inspected for bleeding, and the appendiceal stump is checked for security. The entire abdomen should undergo peritoneal lavage and aspiration to decrease the chance for abscess formation.

MECKEL RESECTION

An asymptomatic Meckel diverticulum is best treated without an operation. However, in cases when a symptomatic Meckel's is discovered or when an operation is performed for abdominal pain with no clear cause, a resection is indicated. Surgery to remove a Meckel diverticulum is either by a simple diverticulectomy or a small bowel resection with enteroenterostomy.

A diverticulectomy is performed most commonly in the laparoscopic realm with a laparoscopic linear stapler fired at the base of the diverticulum (Figure 29.22). This is performed after proper alignment and identification of the Meckel's. It is important not to excessively impinge on the lumen of the small bowel and equally important not to leave heterotopic mucosa behind.

In cases when the Meckel's is causing gastrointestinal hemorrhage, the diverticulum is large (>5 cm), or when an associated omphalomesenteric band is present, a small bowel resection is indicated. This can be accomplished with the use of just two ports including a 10 mm infraumbilical port for the camera and a 5 mm port to grasp and elevate the small bowel. The diverticulum is grasped and then removed from the abdomen through an extension of the 10 mm site. The resection and subsequent anastomosis are performed and then returned intraabdominally (Figure 29.23). This can also be performed intracorporeally, by firing a linear stapler across the bowel proximal and distal to the Meckel's and then fashioning a side-to-side stapled anastomosis. It is

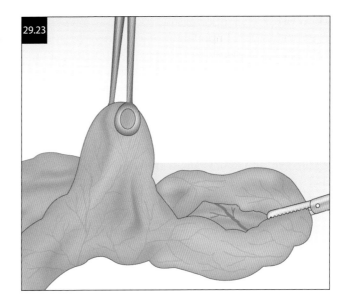

imperative to have generous margins, because the small bowel mucosa is likely to be the source of bleeding in the case of hemorrhage due to the proximal heterotrophic gastric acid-producing diverticulum. After firing a stapler proximal and distal to the Meckel's, the mesentery is transected either with a harmonic scalpel or with an additional load of the linear stapler. A side-to-side anastomosis is then fashioned using the stapler. The common stoma is then closed with a running intracorporeally tied suture as previously described. The specimen is then delivered through the largest port while housed in a protective bag.

INCIDENTAL ENTEROTOMY

Accidental bowel injury during gynecologic laparoscopic surgery can occur during trocar placement, adhesiolysis, resection of endometriotic implants, or by applying energy close to the bowel. If the injury is recognized intraoperatively, it can often be fixed laparoscopically.

As the skills of the laparoscopic surgeon increase, so does his or her ability to laparoscopically manage complications such as a bowel injury. A surgeon with the skill to perform intracorporeal suturing may safely repair an iatrogenic enterotomy given appropriate circumstances. Contraindications include heavy spillage, hypotension, inadequate exposure, or the belief that additional unrecognized enterotomies exist. In fact, there is sufficient evidence in the trauma literature to support primary repair for nondestructive colon wounds when the patient has no peritonitis, significant underlying disease, or evidence of shock. These same basic recommendations can be applied to bowel injury encountered during laparoscopic surgery.

STOMACH

Injury to the stomach can occur during Veress needle or trocar insertion in the left upper quadrant. This is more

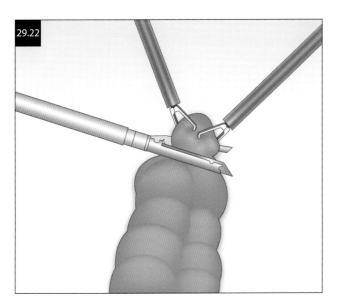

apt to occur after prior gastric surgery. To prevent this complication, it is important to decompress the stomach with either an orogastric or nasogastric tube prior to trocar placement in this area of the abdomen.

In the event of a single, 5 mm trocar injury to the stomach, repair is typically unnecessary. Nevertheless, a small stomach injury can be repaired using a single, full-layer closure with 2-0 or 3-0 Vicryl suture. However, if the injury is caused by a larger trocar, the defect should be repaired in all circumstances. Typically, a single figure-of-8 suture with 2-0 or 3-0 Vicryl can be used to close the injury. A second imbricating layer is then placed to strengthen the wound closure (Figure 29.24). Following repair, a nasogastric tube is left in place for 24–48 hours postoperatively.

SMALL BOWEL

Small bowel injury most commonly occurs when the bowel is immobile from adhesions during initial trocar placement. This is more apt to occur in patients having undergone previous abdominal surgery.

Serosal injury

Superficial injuries to the wall of the small bowel that do not involve the mucosa can be reapproximated using interrupted sutures of 2-0 or 3-0 Vicryl. An SH needle is preferred, and intracorporeal knot tying is used to decrease tension on the site. Imbricating sutures can then be placed through the serosa and muscularis layers to completely cover the injury (Figure 29.25).

Transmural injury

Simple lacerations to the small bowel that do not involve the mesentery can be closed transversely, using laparoscopic suturing techniques. Transverse closure is optimal as it avoids narrowing of the bowel lumen as the defect heals.

If irregular, the edges of the defect should first be trimmed. A simple, interrupted suture of 2-0 or 3-0 Vicryl is placed at each corner of the defect and then they are used to elongate the laceration transversely (Figure 29.26). Next, simple, interrupted sutures are placed approximately 2–3 mm apart to close the remainder of the injury. A finer needle, such as an SH, is preferentially used given the delicacy of the tissue. Each suture should incorporate 4–5 mm of serosa, including the edge of mucosa on each side of the laceration. Intracorporeal knot tying is used to avoid placing excessive tension on the tissue.

Depending on surgeon preference and the visual integrity of the repair, an additional layer of interrupted imbricating Vicryl sutures can be placed through the serosa and muscularis on each side of the repaired laceration to reinforce the closure (Figure 29.26). The site is then copiously irrigated with sterile saline and inspected for hemostasis and adequate repair.

Thermal injury

Thermal injuries to the small bowel may require a more extensive repair. Superficial injuries that do not involve a full thickness of the bowel wall can be oversewn using imbricating sutures of 2-0 or 3-0 Vicryl on an SH needle. Again, these sutures should be placed in a transverse orientation to avoid constriction of the bowel lumen (Figure 29.27). Given a single, full-thickness thermal injury, the edges of the affected tissue must be excised sharply to expose healthy, vascularized tissue. Repair

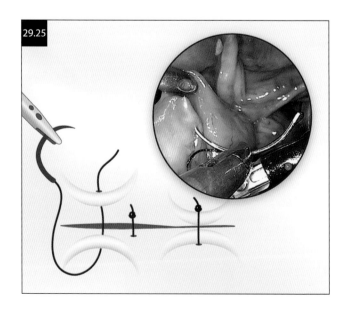

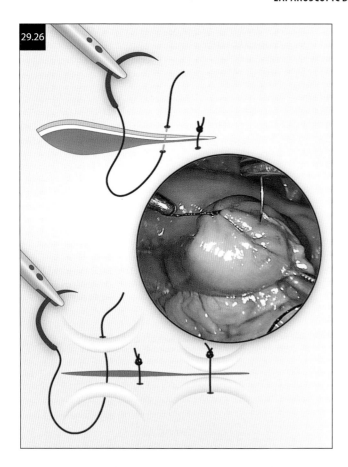

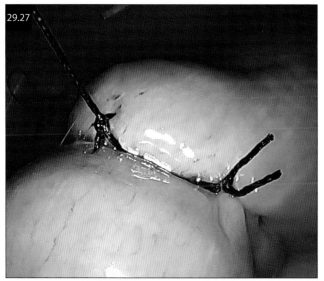

Injury can occur during adhesiolysis, deep pelvic dissections, or resection of extensive endometriosis.

When an injury is recognized, it is important to assess the extent of the injury, whether or not it is isolated, and whether there is intraperitoneal fecal contamination. If fecal contamination is minimal and the laceration does not compromise blood supply, repair can be managed by primary closure. Routine bowel prep is usually recommended in patients undergoing resection of endometriosis involving the bowel.

Serosal injury

Simple, superficial lacerations of the large bowel without involvement of the bowel mucosa can be closed transversely to minimize the potential risk of stricture of the bowel lumen. The choice of suture is a 3-0 or 2-0 absorbable suture material such as Vicryl or Monocryl on a SH needle. Simple stitches are placed through bowel serosa and muscularis in a transverse direction until the defect is closed (Figure 29.28).

Transmural injury

If there is a full-thickness injury to the large bowel, a 3-0 Vicryl suture on an SH needle is used for a through-and-through closure (Figure 29.29). Initial sutures are placed at each corner of the laceration and are used for gentle traction. The remaining interrupted sutures can then be placed to close the remainder of the injury. This is followed by a second, imbricating layer of 3-0 Vicryl suture, taking care to purchase only muscularis and serosa while being placed in an interrupted fashion (Figure 29.30). Again, intracorporeal knot tying is performed.

Some surgeons alternatively use a single-layer, transmural closure using 2-0 Vicryl on SH needle in an interrupted fashion.

The area is then copiously irrigated with saline solution. The repair should ideally be checked for integrity by insufflating air, or irrigating methylene blue, or povidone-iodine (Betadine) transrectally. Whenever there is

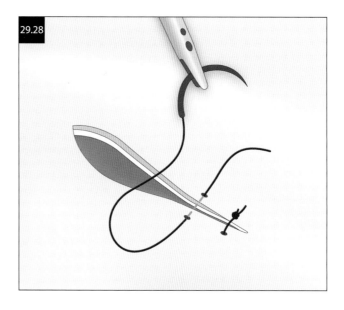

then proceeds in a similar fashion as outlined in the section on "Transmural injury."

Multiple thermal injuries or devascularization of a portion of the small bowel may require resection with reanastomosis. For these more complicated injuries, intraoperative consultation with a general or colorectal surgeon is highly recommended.

LARGE BOWEL AND COLON

The portion of the large bowel most commonly encountered in benign gynecologic surgery is the rectosigmoid.

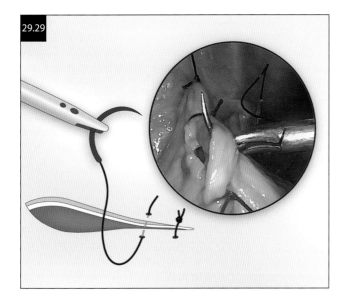

29.29

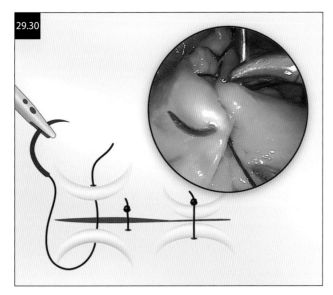

29.30

colon and rectum may be repaired as above and then diverted proximally with an end sigmoid colostomy.

When the gynecologic surgeon encounters any type of bowel injury, requesting an intraoperative consultation from General Surgery/Colorectal Surgery is appropriate. Though simple serosal injuries can be managed easily and safely without formal consultation, complicated or extensive injuries may require bowel resection and/or colostomy. Depending on one's expertise with managing bowel injuries, obtaining a prompt opinion from a specialist when faced with an unexpected complication is always prudent.

SUGGESTED READING

Berne JD, Velmahos BG, Chan LS, Asensio JA, Demetriades D. The high morbidity of colostomy closure after trauma: Further support for the primary repair of colon injuries. *Surgery.* 1998;123:157–164.

George SM, Fabian TC, Voeller GR, Kudsk KA, Mangiante EC, Britt LG. Primary repair of colon wounds: A prospective trial in nonselected patients. *Ann Surg.* 1989;209:728–734.

Gonzalez RP, Merlotti GJ, Holevar MR. Colostomy in penetrating colon injury. Is it necessary? *J Trauma.* 1996;41:271–275.

Jager RM. Laparoscopic right hemicolectomy in left lateral decubitus position. *Surg Laparosc Endosc.* 1994;4:348–352.

Laine S, Rantala A, Gullichsen R, et al. Laparoscopic appendectomy. Is it worthwhile? A prospective, randomized study in young women. *Surg Endosc.* 1997;11:95–97.

Muckleroy SK, Ratzer ER, Fenoglio ME. Laparoscopic colon surgery for benign disease: A comparison to open surgery. *JSLS.* 1999;3:33–37.

Nelson H, Sargent DJ, Wieand HS, et al. Clinical Outcomes of Surgical Therapy Study Group: A comparison of laparoscopically assisted and open colectomy for colon cancer. *N Engl J Med.* 2004;350(20):2050–2059.

Nezhat C, Nezhat F, Ambroze W, Pennington E. Laparoscopic repair of small bowel and colon. *Surg Endosc.* 1993;7:88–89.

Sasaki LS, Allaben RD, Golwala R, Mittal VK. Primary repair of colon injuries: A prospective randomized study. *J Trauma.* 1995;39:895–901.

The Clinical Outcomes of Surgical Therapy (COST) Study Group. A comparison of laparoscopically assisted and open colectomy for colon cancer. *N Engl J Med.* 2004;350:2050–2059.

any question about the best course of management, the need for better surgical exposure, or the ability of the surgeon to repair the injury, consultation with a general surgeon and/or conversion to an open procedure are indicated.

If viability is in question or when there has not been previous bowel preparation, injuries to the distal sigmoid

Chapter 30

LAPAROSCOPIC RADICAL HYSTERECTOMY

Masaaki Andou, Keiko Ebisawa, Yoshiaki Ota, and Tomonori Hada

Laparoscopic radical hysterectomy has become the mainstay of minimally invasive treatment for early stage cervical carcinoma. The total laparoscopic approach offers a panoramic view of the operative field, and the magnification elucidates pelvic anatomical structures. Laparoscopy also has the advantage of facilitating access to the deep pelvis, making it possible to perform complicated procedures in this very difficult to access zone. Laparoscopic procedures demand unique knowledge not required in the case of open surgery. Knowledge of anatomy in the laparoscopic environment, surgical skills such as instrument manipulation, and the ability to interpret images from the laparoscope must be mastered. To attain this level of knowledge, dry-box training with laparoscopic instruments and in-depth study of pelvic anatomy are essential.

During this procedure, all steps are performed laparoscopically aside from the preparatory step of creating a vaginal cuff to prevent the scattering of tumor cells. The essential goals of this surgery are to perform a safe, complete procedure meeting oncologic requirements that offer the patient the advantages of minimally invasive surgery, such as reduced pain and scarring, along with a quicker return to daily activity.

THE LAPAROSCOPIC ENVIRONMENT

Although this procedure mirrors the primary surgical goals while working as the minimally invasive counterpart to the open radical hysterectomy, performing the operation laparoscopically requires a keen understanding of the laparoscopic environment. Throughout the procedure, there is an incomplete view of the entire operative field. As a result, it is essential for the surgeon to have extensive anatomical knowledge and orientation to prevent getting lost in this truncated surgical environment. Keys to a safe and complete dissection include visually recognizing surgical landmarks; knowing and recognizing the upper, lower, and lateral limits of the dissection; and being able to recognize and isolate important structures such as the ureter and uterine artery. Surgeons also may experience disorientation from the lack of depth perception in the laparoscopic environment. Interpretation of the on-screen two-dimensional image and solid comprehension of surgical planes require training and experience. Despite these challenging aspects from the laparoscopic view, laparoscopy offers an unprecedented view of the deep pelvis while magnifying the operative field for precise dissection of fine structures.

Only overcome by dedicated practice, the use of laparoscopic instrumentation can present a number of challenges, including the hand-eye coordination required to adeptly manipulate instruments while referencing a video monitor, and the ability to use the optimal amount of force and pressure to perform operative as well as manipulative steps.

PREPARATION OF THE PATIENT

Cytological and histological exams are carried out, and if microinvasive tumors are detected by punch biopsy, a cone biopsy is performed to confirm the spread of the tumor. The course of investigations then examine for spread and extension of the tumor(s). The mobility of the cervix and the uterine body is established through digital exam (vaginal and rectal). Imaging techniques such as magnetic resonance imaging (MRI), computed tomography (CT), positron emission tomography (PET), and sonography are required to define the distribution of the tumor. Tumor markers such as SCC antigen and CEA are employed for squamous cell carcinoma, and CEA, CA125, and CA19-9 for adenocarcinoma. From this it is not only possible to establish the extent of the tumor spread, but also to detect recurrence at follow-up.

INSTRUMENTATION

Optical instruments:

- A high-definition video camera system along with 0°, 5 or 10 mm telescopes

Operative instruments:

- Three 5 mm and two 12 mm trocars
- An aspiration-irrigation unit equipped with a monopolar hook
- Various laparoscopic forceps including Maryland, bowel, and bipolar
- Laparoscopic scissors
- A needle driver
- A specimen retrieval tube (to be placed inside the 12 mm trocar) to prevent contamination of the port site
- An emergency hemostasis set consisting of vascular clamps, sponge, and a 10 mm aspiration nozzle

- A vessel sealing system (ENSEAL [Ethicon] and LigaSure Advance blunt tip [Covidien])
- Harmonic scalpel
- A vaginal pipe (Vagi-Pipe)

OPERATIVE PROCEDURE

POSITIONING OF THE PATIENT AND TROCAR PLACEMENT

The patient is placed in a mild Trendelenburg (10°) lithotomy position with legs extended slightly. A 5 or 12 mm umbilical trocar is placed along with two 3 or 5 mm trocars bilaterally at points 4 cm median to the iliac crest. Another trocar is set between these two. Finally, a fourth 12 mm trocar is placed in the left upper quadrant (Figure 30.1).

THE VAGINAL CUFF

Prior to beginning the abdominal procedure, a vaginal cuff is created. This preparatory step is to prevent the dissemination of tumor cells. Twelve 1.0 sutures are placed around the vagina at approximately 2–3 cm from the cervix. Pulling these sutures retracts the incision line of the vagina, a step that is useful when determining the incision line of the vagina later in the procedure. The vaginal mucosa is fully circumcised, and the vaginal cuff is closed with continuous running suture while the 12 initially placed sutures are removed (Figure 30.2).

PELVIC LYMPHADENECTOMY

The first step of the pelvic lymphadenectomy is the opening of the space between the round ligament and infundibulopelvic ligament to develop the paravesical space (Figure 30.3). After the paravesical space is developed, the entrance of the pararectal space is also developed (Figure 30.4). After development of the retroperitoneal

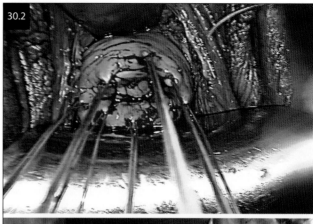

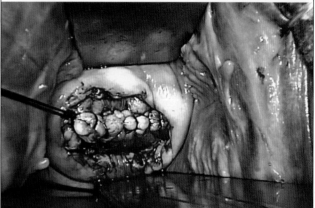

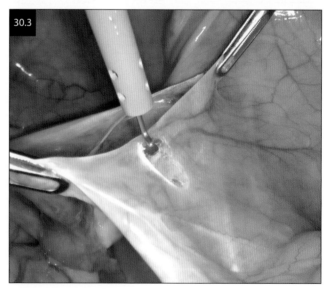

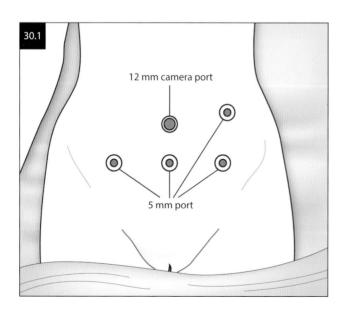

spaces, the laparoscopic procedure begins with the suspension of the umbilical ligaments, a method developed to assist in maintaining the operative field. A straight needle loaded with monofilament suture is pushed through the abdominal wall at the midline of the suprapubic area into the abdominal cavity. Under laparoscopic vision, the needle is passed under both umbilical ligaments and back through the abdominal wall where the sutures can pull the umbilical ligaments to the abdominal wall; as a result, this maintains a commendable operative field in the deep pelvis (Figure 30.5). Complete development of

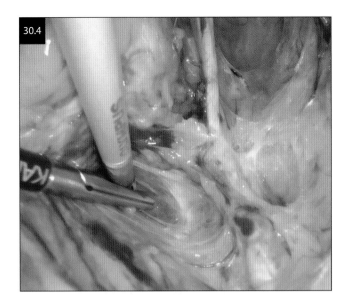

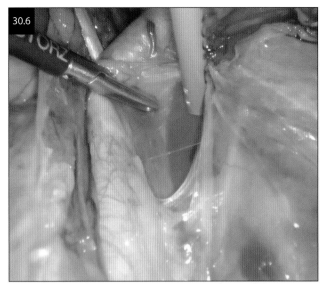

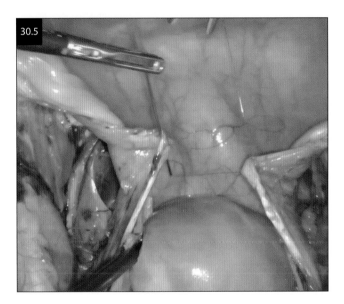

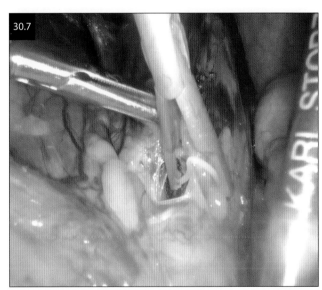

both retroperitoneal spaces elucidates the uterine artery and the cardinal ligament.

Separation of the connective tissue by blunt dissection continues until the obturator fascia is reached. The external iliac vessels are dissected off from the psoas muscle, and the obturator fossa is reached via this space between the external iliac vessels and the psoas muscle (Figure 30.6). The initial opening of this space makes it easier to extract the obturator lymph node from the obturator fossa through the interiliac space. The obturator lymph node is separated from the external iliac node. The upper limit of the external iliac node is clipped (Figure 30.7) and cut, and then the lymphatic chain is dissected from the external iliac vessels (Figure 30.8). The dissection continues until the circumflex iliac vein, the caudal landmark of this dissection, is reached. Although it is possible to dissect lymph nodes in a more caudal site, limiting the dissection here serves to reduce the incidence of lymphedema. The caudal and upper end of the external iliac node is sealed and transected using a vessel sealing system. The

obturator lymph node is dissected through the interiliac space. The obturator nodes are then detached from the obturator nerve and vessels (Figure 30.9), and the caudal end is sealed and cut. Thereafter, the deep lateral common iliac nodes are dissected (Figure 30.10), then the internal iliac nodes, and finally the cardinal nodes (Figure 30.11). These resected lymph nodes are retrieved via the retrieval pipe to prevent port site contamination.

RADICAL HYSTERECTOMY

In order to control the position of the uterine body and place appropriate tension on target structures in this step of the procedure, the uterine body is grasped from the upper left port with a forceps to move the uterine body into the correct location.

The ureter is dissected from the posterior layer of the broad ligament, and this dissection continues caudad until reaching the entrance of the ureteral tunnel (Figure 30.12).

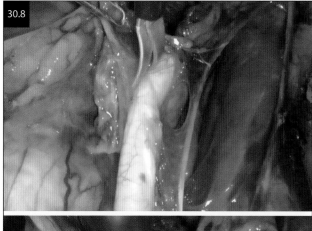

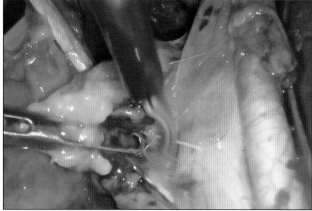

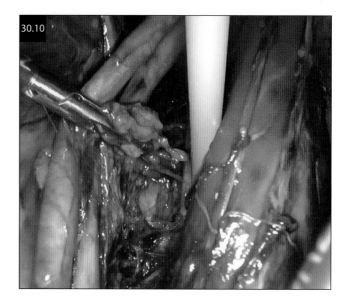

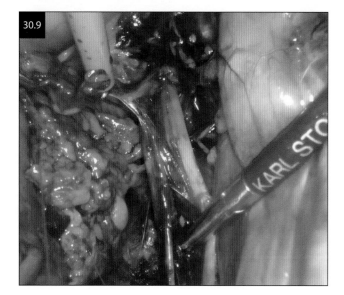

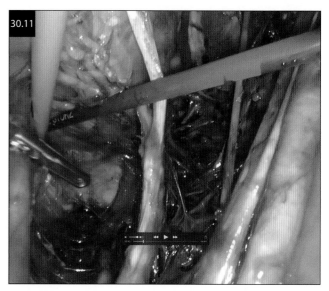

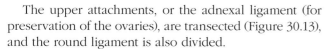

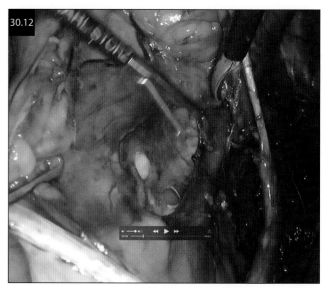

The upper attachments, or the adnexal ligament (for preservation of the ovaries), are transected (Figure 30.13), and the round ligament is also divided.

To dissect the bladder, the vesicouterine peritoneum is incised, and the bladder is dissected off from the cervix and vagina beginning at the midsection, and proceeding laterally, with a monopolar knife electrode (Figure 30.14).

The entrance of the ureteral tunnel is opened to expose the bladder pillar for dissection.

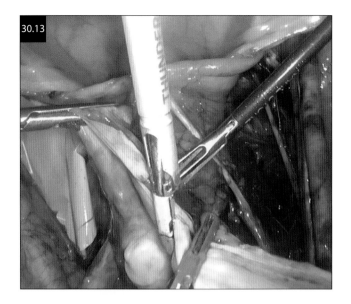

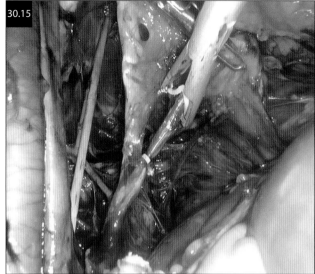

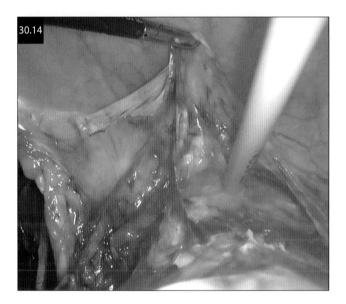

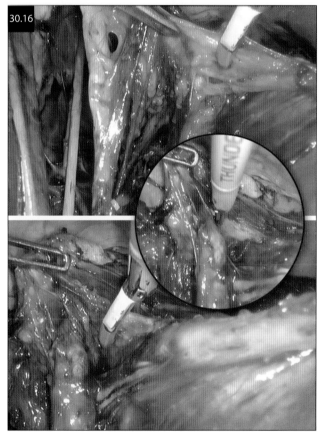

After pulling the umbilical ligament laterally, the uterine artery is separated from surrounding tissue, clipped at two sites, and then transected between these two clips with a vessel sealing system (Figure 30.15).

The assistant forceps are used to manipulate the cut end of the uterine artery anteriorly to create the ureteral tunnel. The ureter is unroofed by cutting the fibrous membrane median over the ureter, and the space between the ureter and the cervix is opened up. The superficial layer of the vesicouterine ligament is isolated step by step by blunt dissection and then transected using bipolar electrosurgery or with a vessel sealing system (VSS) (Figure 30.16). To prevent bleeding at this step, identification, isolation, and transection of the cervicovesical vessel are essential.

The uterine body is suspended by forceps or with a suture suspension to expose the Douglas peritoneum (Figure 30.17a) and to extend the parametria and the rectum by retracting with the assistant forceps. The Douglas peritoneum is incised with monopolar electrosurgery to dissect the rectum from the cervix (Figure 30.17b). The

expansion of the rectovaginal space eventually results in the exposure of the uterosacral ligament (Figure 30.18). This ligament is cut as close to the sacrum as possible using a vessel sealing system.

The fully developed paravesical and pararectal spaces expose the vascular part of the cardinal ligament. This vascular part (the deep uterine vein) is isolated, clipped in two places (Figure 30.19a), and then transected at the pelvic sidewall using a VSS (Figure 30.19b).

The course of the ureter is exposed by blunt dissection and by dissecting off the fibrous tissue around it. To

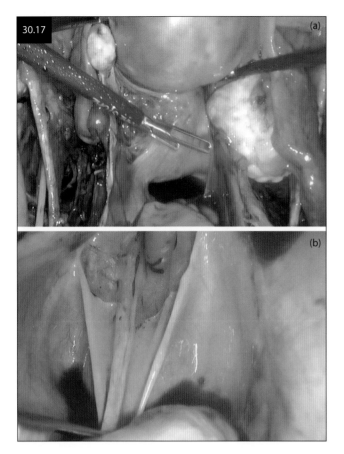

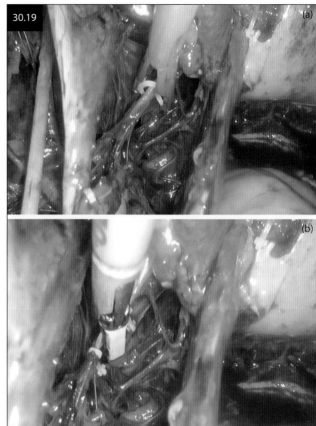

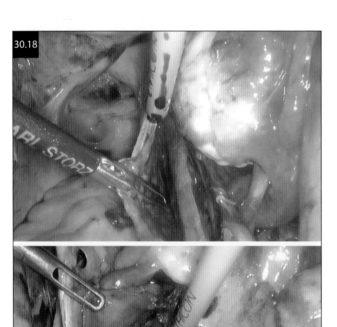

reach the posterior layer of the vesicouterine ligament, the triangular space between the ureter, bladder, and vagina is entered, and the stump of the cardinal ligament is pulled in a lateral direction to be transected with a VSS (Figure 30.20).

When transecting the paracolpium, initial suture ligation before transection with an energy device is preferable to prevent injury to surrounding tissue and to avert excessive bleeding (Figure 30.21).

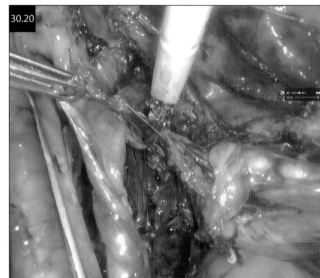

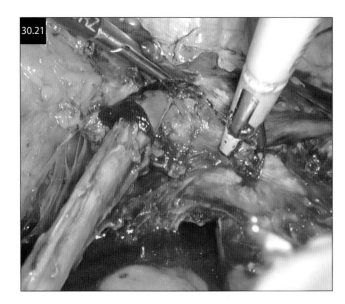

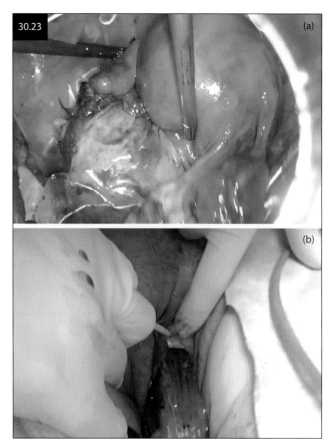

The final step before retrieving the specimen is the transection of the vagina. To achieve dissection of accurate length and to place tension on the vaginal wall, a vaginal pipe is inserted. The vagina is then transected using monopolar electrosurgery along with a vessel sealing system (Figure 30.22).

RETRIEVAL OF THE SPECIMEN AND HEMOSTASIS

For retrieval, the specimen is placed in a retrieval bag, which is made from a segment of a commercially available intestinal isolation bag sewn at the circumference with a purse-string suture (Figure 30.23a). After placing the specimen in the bag, the sutures are pulled to secure the bag, fed through the vaginal pipe, and then withdrawn to complete extraction (Figure 30.23b). The retrieval bag makes removal easy and ensures that the specimen is removed *en bloc* without dispersing tumor cells in the abdominal cavity or a port site. Once the

specimen has been retrieved, the abdominal cavity is irrigated, and the entire operative field is assiduously assessed for any signs of injury, bleeding, or leakage.

CLOSURE OF THE VAGINAL OPENING

Shortening of the vagina is a debilitating drawback of radical hysterectomy. To maintain some vaginal length, a new vaginal vault is created by using the pelvic peritoneum. The new dome of the vagina is made from the bladder and Douglas peritoneum to prevent shortening of the vagina. The edge of the Douglas peritoneum is sutured to the posterior cut edge of the vagina (Figure 30.24a), and then the edge of the bladder peritoneum is sutured to the rectum (Figure 30.24b). When closing the vagina, to prevent excessive bleeding from the paravaginal tissue, 1-0 synthetic absorbable sutures are placed at both edges of the vagina and then in between. To prevent prolapse or adhesion of the walls of this new vaginal vault, patients are required to have a prosthesis placed for approximately 3 months.

POSTDISSECTION

All of the dissection areas are carefully checked once again for bleeding, and the integrity of pelvic organs is confirmed (Figure 30.25). The quality of the dissection is also evaluated, and the specimen is checked to guarantee that the procedure has met the highest oncologic standards and requirements (Figure 30.26).

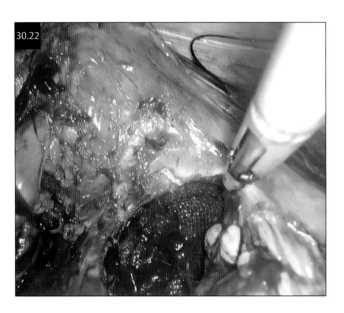

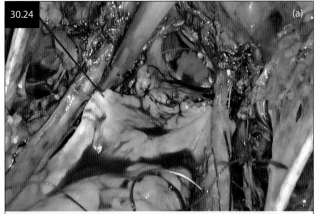

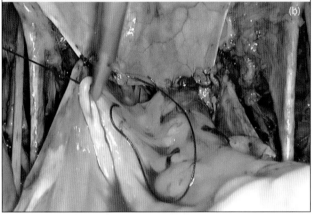

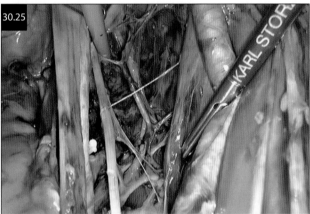

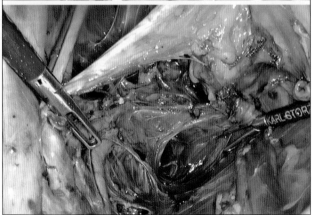

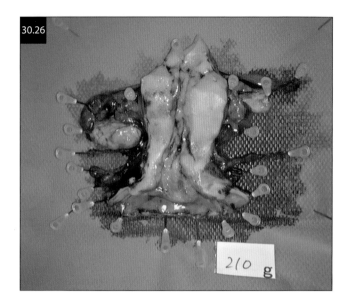

CLOSING OF ABDOMINAL PORT SITES

The final stage of the procedure is placing a drain and closing all abdominal port puncture sites. In the case of 12 mm port sites, the wounds are closed in two layers; first the fascia and then the skin incision are sutured. Smaller port sites—5 and 3 mm—are simply closed with staples.

DISCUSSION

The total laparoscopic approach offers a panoramic view of the operative field, while magnification helps define the pelvic anatomical structures including difficult to access zones deep in the pelvis. These advantages make it possible to perform complicated procedures that require attention to fine anatomical detail. This technique is characterized by the presurgical step of creating a vaginal cuff and the use of suspension techniques to maintain the operative field, tract organs toward or away from target zones, and place tension on target organs to help with accurate and expedient transection. Working to achieve the best comprehension of anatomy and a consistent approach to practicing new techniques that improve surgical skills will serve to advance this cornerstone of gynecologic surgery.

SUGGESTED READING

Andou M, Kanao H, Ota Y, Hada T. Laparoscopic radical hysterectomy. In: Abu-Rustum N, Barakat R, Levine D, eds. *Atlas of Procedures in Gynecologic Oncology.* 3rd ed. Boca Raton, FL: CRC Press; 2013:164–176.

Dargent D. A new future for Schauta's operation through presurgical retroperitoneal pelviscopy. *Eur J Gynaecol Oncol.* 1987;8:292–296.

Kato T, Murakami G, Yabuki Y. A new perspective on nerve-sparing radical hysterectomy: Nerve topography and over-preservation of the cardinal ligament. *Jpn J Clin Oncol.* 2003;33:589–591.

Nezhat CR, Burrell MO, Nezhat FR, et al. Laparoscopic radical hysterectomy with paraaortic and pelvic node dissection. *Am J Obstet Gynecol.* 1992;166:864–865.

Spirtos NM, Schlaerth J, Kimball R, et al. Laparoscopic radical hysterectomy (type III) with aortic and pelvic lymphadenectomy. *Am J Obstet Gynecol.* 1996;174:1763–1768.

Yabuki Y, Asamoto A, Hoshiba T, et al. Radical hysterectomy: An anatomic evaluation of parametrial dissection. *Gynecol Oncol.* 2000;77(1):155–163.

CHAPTER 31

LAPAROSCOPIC AND ROBOTIC-ASSISTED LAPAROSCOPIC LYMPHADENECTOMY IN GYNECOLOGIC ONCOLOGY

Farr Nezhat and Susan Khalil

In patients with gynecologic cancer, prognosis correlates with the extent of the disease according to the established International Federation of Gynecology and Obstetrics (FIGO) classification systems. Surgical staging is superior because it provides histologic verification of tumor extent. Lymph node status is one of the most important prognostic factors in gynecologic cancer, and surgical removal of pelvic and/or paraaortic lymph nodes for histologic assessment is part of staging gynecologic malignancies. Additionally, removal of bulky lymph nodes may have therapeutic benefit. Lymphadenectomy has generally been performed via laparotomy, leading to large incisions and significant intra- and perioperative morbidity.

Dargent and Salvat were the first to describe laparoscopic retroperitoneal lymphadenectomy for the management of gynecologic malignancies in 1989. In 1991, Querleu et al. reported transperitoneal pelvic lymphadenectomy in 39 patients with cervical cancer. The first laparoscopic intraperitoneal pelvic and paraaortic lymphadenectomy was reported by Nezhat et al. in 1991–1993 in a series of patients with cervical cancer undergoing laparoscopic radical hysterectomy and pelvic and paraaortic lymphadenectomy. Since that time, a number of other reports have described the safety and accuracy of laparoscopic lymphadenectomy for cervical, endometrial, and ovarian cancers. Numerous reports describe better magnification, fewer complications, and superior visualization of the anatomy provided by the video laparoscope in comparison with laparotomy.

Lymphadenectomy can be performed with conventional laparoscopy, or with robotic-assisted laparoscopy. However, the latter requires specific considerations for placement of the trocar sites to ensure optimal mobility of the robot arms, and in order to reach the operative field required to accomplish pelvic and paraaortic lymphadenectomy. The method for laparoscopic pelvic and paraaortic lymphadenectomy will be described, with a section following that describes trocar placement to accomplish lymphadenectomy with the same technique used in conventional laparoscopy. The trocar placement for laparoscopic pelvic and paraaortic lymphadenectomy is presented in Figure 31.1.

PELVIC LYMPHADENECTOMY

Pelvic and paraaortic lymphadenectomy is accomplished before or after hysterectomy and bilateral oophorectomy. The initial approach to pelvic lymphadenectomy is to expose the anterior and posterior leaves of the broad ligament by incising the round ligament and cutting the broad ligament in a cephalad fashion lateral and parallel to the infundibulopelvic ligament (Figure 31.2). An incision is made in the broad ligament lateral or parallel to the infundibulopelvic ligament to develop the paravesical space. Using the suction-irrigation probe, grasper, and scissors, the paravesical space is created. It is bordered medially by the obliterated hypogastric artery, bladder, and vagina and laterally by the pelvic sidewall. Creating the avascular paravesical space helps identify the obturator nerve and vessels, and pelvic vessels. The obliterated hypogastric artery and external iliac vein are landmarks to get to the paravesical space (Figure 31.3). The spaces lateral to this vessel and medial to the external iliac vein and obturator internus muscle are created with blunt and sharp dissection. Electrocoagulation should not be necessary as this space is generally avascular. Once this space is created, the bony lateral sidewall, the levator plate laterally, and the obturator nerve and vessels anteriorly should be visible (Figure 31.4). The pelvic lymph nodes can now be safely removed. Starting laterally over the psoas muscle and proceeding medially provide a safe approach that avoids the genitofemoral nerve (Figure 31.5). The external iliac nodes along the external iliac artery and vein are excised caudally from common iliac vessels to the level of the deep circumflex iliac vein seen crossing over the distal portion of the external iliac artery (Figure 31.6). This can usually be accomplished with blunt dissection with the suction irrigator and a grasper. Occasionally, unipolar scissors can be used to control small bleeders, or the capillary bleeding can be controlled with sponge gauze introduced through 10 mm trocar. It is important to remember that external iliac artery and vein do not have any contributories, and by staying parallel to the vessels, the lymph nodes can be removed *en bloc*.

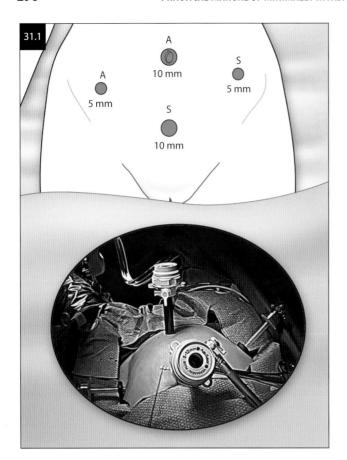

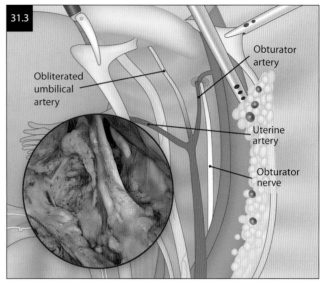

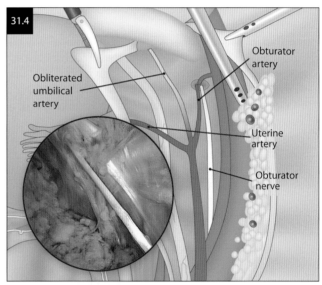

The obturator nerve is identified by blunt dissection below and between the obliterated umbilical artery and the external iliac vein (see Figure 31.4). Of note is that although the obturator vessels are usually posterior to the nerve, sometimes an aberrant obturator vein may enter the midpoint of the external iliac vein and is anterior to the nerve. The nodal tissue anterior and lateral to the nerve and medial and inferior to the external iliac vein is removed by blunt and sharp dissection. Venous anastomosis between the obturator and the external iliac veins are saved from injury. The obturator fossa lymph

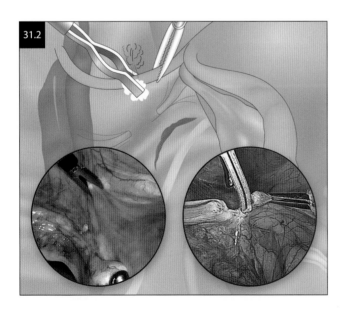

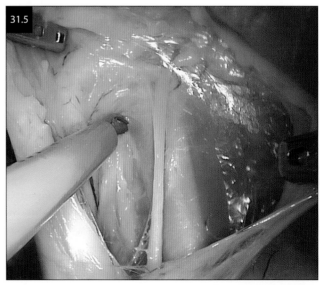

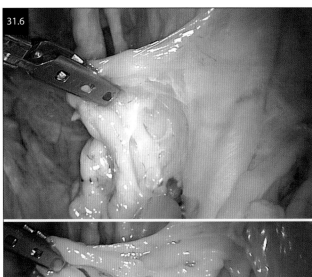

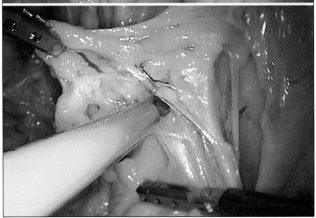

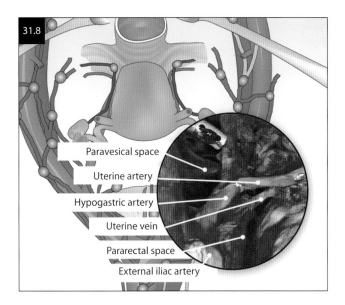

nodes are excised caudally to the pelvic sidewall where the obturator nerve exits the pelvis through the obturator canal and cephalad up to the bifurcation of the common iliac artery (Figure 31.7). Before the removal of each nodal bundle, each pedicle is ligated by electrocoagulation, endoscopic hemoclips, or harmonic sheers to prevent lymphocyst formation. The lymph node packets are removed in a bag through the largest trocar to avoid any contact between potentially malignant lymph node tissue and the abdominal wall. Using sharp and blunt

dissection, the nodes between the external iliac vessels and the obliterated hypogastric artery are removed. Hemoclips can be used as needed. The nodes along the hypogastric vessels are excised up to the bifurcation of the common iliac vessels as shown on the patient's right side (Figure 31.8). Caution is necessary to avoid injury to the obturator nerve and hypogastric vein.

To excise the lymph nodes around the common iliac artery, a plane is created between the posterior peritoneum and the adventitia overlying the common iliac artery. Another option is to extend the dissection over the common iliac vessels when removing the proximal portion of the external iliac nodes. Before the nodes are detached, the orientation of the ureter and ovarian vessels crossing the common iliac artery is identified (Figure 31.9). When one is performing a left pelvic lymph node dissection, it may be necessary to take down the rectosigmoid colon from the left pelvic sidewall to allow visualization of the pelvic vessels.

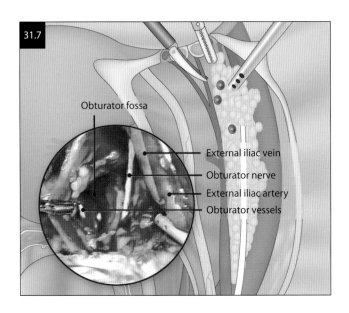

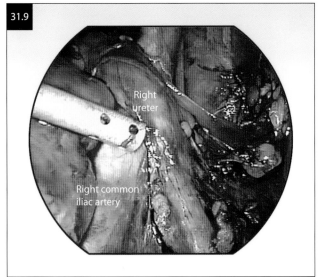

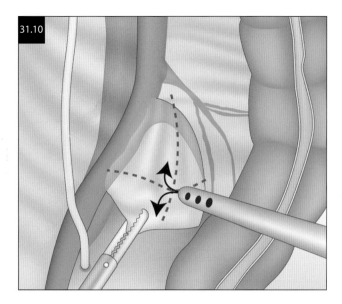

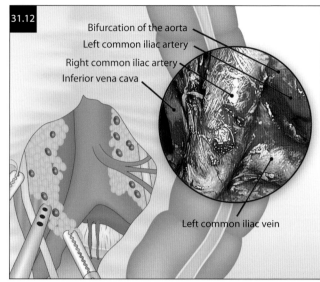

PARAAORTIC LYMPHADENECTOMY

There are several ways to begin the dissection: incising the peritoneum overlying the aorta, opening the peritoneum over sacral promontory, and extending the incision overlying the common iliac artery toward the aorta. The peritoneum over the sacral promontory or lower aorta is incised. The peritoneum can be lifted with the grasper and cut with the scissors. The underlying retroperitoneum is developed by blunt and sharp dissection or by hydrodissection (Figure 31.10). Next, the retroperitoneal space is created by using sharp and blunt dissection, to develop the space lateral to the aorta. Before cutting, it is essential to identify the right ureter, separate it from underlying tissue, and retract it laterally. The nodal tissue overlying the aorta, right common iliac artery, and sacral promontory is removed laterally toward the psoas muscle. Fatty and nodal tissue overlying the sacral promontory are removed. This tissue may contain hypogastric nerves. The left common iliac vein must be observed during this dissection (Figure 31.11). The dissection is continued cephalad to the level of the gonadal vein entering the vena cava, removing all lymphatic tissue anterior to and between the aorta and inferior vena cava (Figure 31.12). Again, it is essential to identify the right ureter along the inferior border of the dissection and the transverse duodenum along the superior margin of the dissection. Perforating vessels from the vena cava are electrocoagulated or ligated with hemoclips.

The removal of the left paraaortic nodes may be more difficult because of the location of the sigmoid colon. Attention is necessary to avoid injury to the left common iliac vein inferior mesenteric artery and the ureter. The left common iliac vein lies at the bifurcation of the aorta and under the left common iliac artery. The dissection proceeds from the left common iliac artery medially and the psoas muscle laterally toward the inferior mesenteric artery, excising the lymph nodes from below and above the inferior mesenteric artery (Figure 31.13). Attention should be paid to avoid injury to the left ureter and sigmoid colon laterally and lumbar vessels. Injuries

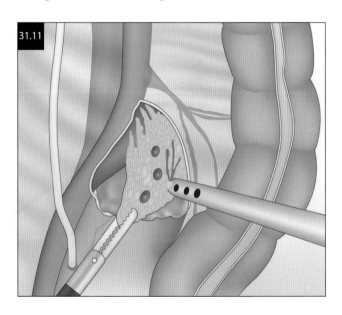

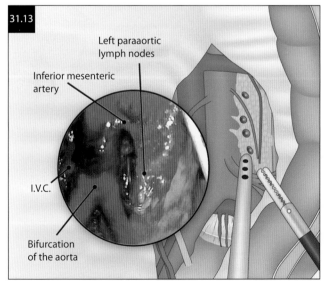

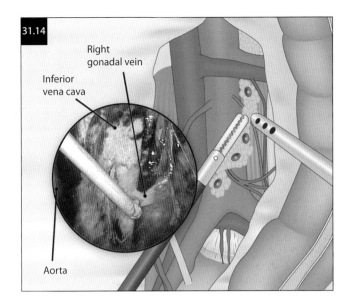

31.14

Right gonadal vein

Inferior vena cava

Aorta

to these vessels can be controlled by applying pressure and coagulation using bipolar forceps.

When paraaortic lymphadenectomy above the mesenteric artery is being performed, the peritoneal incision is extended to the level of the left renal vein and left ovarian vein (Figure 31.14). The ovarian vessels and the mesenteric artery are ligated, if necessary, to have better exposure to the lymph nodes and to prevent bleeding. After the lymphadenectomy is completed, the area is evaluated under decreased pneumoperitoneal pressure to ensure hemostasis.

As with pelvic lymphadenectomy, the peritoneum is not closed, and drains are not placed. An absorbable adhesion barrier can be applied to decrease postoperative adhesions (Figure 31.15). Our experience and published data in the literature suggest that the mean number of pelvic and paraaortic lymph nodes retrieved laparoscopically is similar to that of lymph nodes retrieved by laparotomy. One report addressed the fact that 25% of the pelvic lymph nodes were still present at laparotomy after laparoscopic lymphadenectomy; however, no patient with negative nodes at laparoscopy had positive nodes at laparotomy. The objective to remember is that the lymph node ratio (of significant nodes), and not retrieval of a high quantity of nodes, is important.

The rarity of pelvic sidewall recurrences in node-negative patients managed without a complete lymphadenectomy indicates that laparoscopy may enable us to remove the significant nodes even when the total number of nodes removed is low. If the requirement of clearly identifying the dorsal part of the obturator nerve and lumbosacral nerve is fulfilled, the risk of missing a positive pelvic lymph node is very low.

ROBOTIC-ASSISTED LYMPHADENECTOMY

Accurate port placement is essential in a robotic-assisted procedure. If the robotic ports are placed incorrectly, either operative arm collision will occur or the wristed instruments will not achieve their full dexterity. The robotic endoscope enters the abdominal cavity through a 10 or 12 mm cannula placed at or above the umbilicus. Robotic instruments enter through 5 or 8 mm steel cannulas. The placement of the accessory ports varies with the type of procedure planned.

Procedures involving structures in the pelvic cavity, such as pelvic lymphadenectomy, have similar port placements. A 12 mm port is first placed through the umbilicus for the robotic endoscope. Two 5 or 8 mm steel trocars are then placed 5 cm above and 1 cm medial to the anterior superior iliac crest. If the fourth robotic arm, which is available on the da Vinci S and Si systems, is used, the steel trocar can be placed in either the right or left lower or upper quadrant, inferior and lateral to the other robotic instrument port, at least 10 cm apart (Figure 31.16). Such placement enables optimal movement of the robotic arms, minimizes the risk of collisions, and enables access to the pelvic floor. Robotic monopolar scissors, hook, or spatula, and bipolar forceps may be

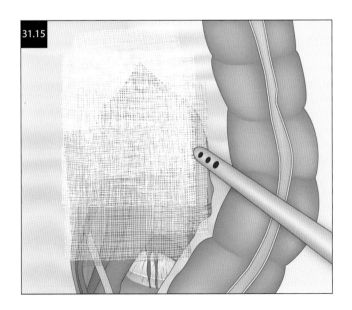

31.15

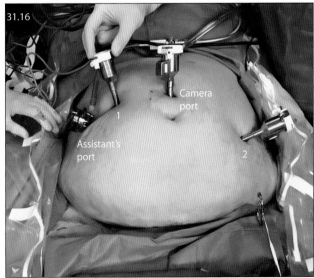

31.16

Camera port

1

Assistant's port

2

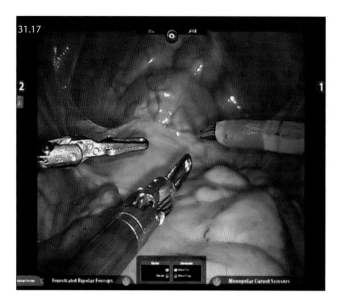

placed through the bilateral lower quadrant trocars. The electrosurgical scissors allow for dissection and resection, while the bipolar forceps are used for traction and electrodessication (Figure 31.17). A nonenergized instrument such as a forceps or retractor may be placed through the upper quadrant port. A 5–12 mm assistant port is also placed 1–2 cm above the camera port, between the camera port and one of the 8 mm trocars. Through this port, the assistant can introduce suture, instrumentation used for retraction, a suction-irrigator, vessel-sealing device, surgical clip applicator, or laparoscopic specimen bag.

For procedures extending above the pelvic brim, such as paraaortic lymphadenectomy, trocar placement must be modified, with the camera port placed approximately 5–8 cm above the umbilicus and the other trocars adjusted accordingly, based on the different camera port placement (Figure 31.18). Instruments introduced through the fourth robotic trocar or accessory port may be useful for retraction of omentum and the small bowel during paraaortic lymphadenectomy.

The docking of the da Vinci patient cart is often the most cumbersome and precise part of the procedure. The side-docking method has been incorporated into gynecologic surgery to aid in vaginal surgery, uterine manipulation, cystoscopy, or accessing the rectum. The parallel side-docking method has been used, where the base of the patient-side cart is directly adjacent to the base of the operating table. The column of the patient-side cart is advanced to the level of the midthigh if the camera port is inserted through the umbilicus. It may be adjusted accordingly if the camera port is moved superiorly to accommodate upper abdominal procedures. The camera arm is then aligned to the midline of the patient, and the remaining arms are attached systematically.

After docking the robot, the pelvic and paraaortic lymphadenectomy can then be performed in the manner described with conventional laparoscopy.

SENTINEL LYMPH NODE MAPPING

Sentinel lymph node (SLN) mapping has been proposed for use in endometrial and cervical cancer to assess the extent of lymph node metastasis without complete lymphadenectomy, which is based on the observation that tumor cells migrating from a primary tumor metastasize to one or a few lymph nodes before involving others. SLN mapping has been suggested as an intermediary in endometrial cancer between performing complete pelvic and paraaortic lymphadenectomy, versus its omission, thus aiding in planning adjuvant therapy. Its use has been previously established with breast cancer, and has been further applied to vulvar and cervical cancers.

Dye is injected into the cervix prior to the surgical procedure, and then identification of lymph nodes is made by visualizing a blue lymph node or lymphatics, or detection of radioactivity with a gamma-probe, or fluorescence with use of indocyanine green (ICG) dye and an endoscopic near-infrared imaging with robotic assistance (Figure 31.19). The learning curve suggested is at

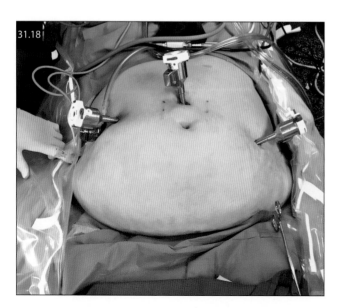

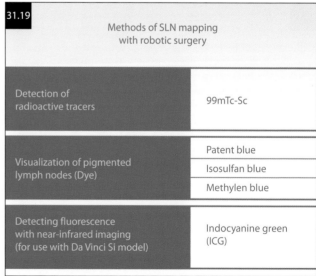

Methods of SLN mapping with robotic surgery	
Detection of radioactive tracers	99mTc-Sc
Visualization of pigmented lymph nodes (Dye)	Patent blue
	Isosulfan blue
	Methylen blue
Detecting fluorescence with near-infrared imaging (for use with Da Vinci Si model)	Indocyanine green (ICG)

TABLE 31.1

COMPARISON OF STUDIES USING ROBOTIC-ASSISTED LAPAROSCOPIC SURGERY WITH SLN MAPPING

	N	DYE	DETECTION RATE	SENSITIVITY	SPECIFICITY
HOWE ET AL.	100	PATENT BLUE, 99mTc-Sc	92%	89%	100%
ROSSI ET AL. (2012)	20	ICG(NIR)	88%	NOT DETERMINED	NOT DETERMINED
HOLLOWAY ET AL. (2012)	35	ISOSULFAN BLUE, ICG	100%	90%	100%

approximately 30 cases per surgeon before achieving a high detection rate (90%).

The application of SLN mapping to robotic-assisted laparoscopic staging was described in three studies, which are described in Table 31.1.

Laparoscopic lymphadenectomy is an evolving technique that plays an important role in the management of gynecologic malignancies, and its further evolution with robotic-assisted surgery. Pelvic and paraaortic laparoscopic lymphadenectomy appears to be a safe, adequate, and feasible procedure, with a low complication rate. Despite the degree of caution used, complications do occur during laparoscopic lymphadenectomy. In a series by Passover et al. (1998), 10 major vessel injuries were identified among 150 procedures. These included four vena cava, two right renal vein, two external iliac vein, one internal iliac artery, and one internal iliac vein injuries. A conversion to laparotomy was necessary in four cases. The mean hospital stay for patients undergoing laparoscopic lymphadenectomy was 3.2 days. Nezhat et al. (2005) reported in their series of patients managed with ultrasonically activated shears, who underwent pelvic and/or paraaortic lymphadenectomy for gynecologic malignancies, a 13% overall complication rate. This included three intraoperative complications, and the remainders were postoperative complications (Table 31.2). Other studies have also reported reduced length of hospital stay, and recovery times for patients managed laparoscopically. A study by Cardenas-Goicoechea et al. analyzed complications encountered with endometrial cancer staging and integration of robotic surgery in a minimally invasive program. Their findings were that the overall intraoperative complication rate was similar in both arms, three cases in the robotic arm ($n = 187$) versus seven cases out of the 245 cases in the laparoscopic arm (1.6% versus 2.9%, $p = 0.525$).

Both laparoscopic and robotic-assisted laparoscopic (or computer-enhanced telesurgery) lymphadenectomy provide additional modalities in extirpative procedures for gynecologic malignancies. Cho and Nezhat et al. performed a review of the literature on the role of robotic surgery in gynecologic malignancies, and their findings included that both conventional laparoscopic and robotic-assisted laparoscopic lymphadenectomy have been shown

to have decreased blood loss (96.5 versus 416.8 mL, robotic group versus laparotomy) and length of stay (1 versus 3.2 days, robotic versus laparotomy groups), compared to laparotomy. Additionally, the lymph node retrieval yield is greater with these approaches (17.5 versus 20.3 versus 13.1, median number of lymph nodes retrieved, robotic versus laparoscopic versus laparotomy groups).

The risks encountered include those traditionally attributed to laparoscopy, as well as those inherent to lymphadenectomy performed via laparotomy. In properly selected patients, when laparoscopic and robotic-assisted lymphadenectomy is performed by an experienced gynecologic oncologist, it provides adequate lymph node retrieval quantities, with an acceptable complication rate. The quicker recovery time associated with minimally invasive surgical procedures is of particular benefit for patients who require chemotherapy or radiation, thus decreasing the time from surgery to their initiation. Simple preventive measures allow patients to benefit from this technique while diminishing the likelihood of complications. With

TABLE 31.2

SUMMARY OF COMPLICATIONS

COMPLICATION	NUMBER
MAJOR	
VASCULAR INJURY	2
BOWEL OBSTRUCTION	1
TROCAR-SITE HERNIA	1
CYSTOTOMY	1
THROMBOEMBOLIC	1
PORT-SITE METASTASES	1
MINOR	
FEVER	4
SUBCUTANEOUS EMPHYSEMA	1
ABDOMINAL WALL ECCHYMOSIS	1
TOTAL	13

SOURCE: NEZHAT F ET AL. GYNECOL ONCOL. 2005;97(3): 813–819.

further development of the role of SLN detection methods, and their integration with minimally invasive surgical procedures, there is promise of enhancing lymph node yield while further decreasing risk of morbidity.

SUGGESTED READING

Cardenas-Goicoechea J, Soto E, Chuang L, Gretz H, Randall TC. Integration of robotics into two established programs of minimally invasive surgery for endometrial cancer appears to decrease surgical complications. *J Gynecol Oncol.* 24(1):21–28.

Cho JE, Nezhat FR. Robotics and gynecologic oncology: Review of the literature. *J Minim Invasive Gynecol.* 2009;16(6):669–681.

Dargent DF. Laparoscopic techniques for gynecologic cancer: Description and indications. *Hematol Oncol Clin North Am.* 1999;13:1–19.

Holloway RW, Bravo RA, Rakowski JA et al. Detection of sentinel lymph nodes in patients with endometrial cancer undergoing robotic-assisted staging: A comparison of colorimetric and fluorescence imaging. *Gynecol Oncol.* 2012;126(1):25–29.

How J, Lau S, Press J, Ferenczy A, Pelmus M, Stern J, Probst S, Brin S, Drummond N, Gotlieb W. Accuracy of sentinel lymph node detection following intra-operative cervical injection for endometrial cancer: A prospective study. *Gynecol Oncol.* 2012 Nov;127(2):332–337. doi: 10.1016/j.ygyno.2012.08.018. Epub 2012 Aug 19.

Melendez TD, Childers JM. Laparoscopic lymphadenectomy. *Curr Opin Obstet Gynecol.* 1995;7:307–310.

Nezhat CR, Burrell MO, Nezhat FR, Benigno BB, Welander CE. Laparoscopic radical hysterectomy with paraaortic and pelvic node dissection. *Am J Obstet Gynecol.* 1992;166:864–865.

Nezhat F, Yadav J, Rahaman J, Gretz H 3rd, Gardner GJ, Cohen CJ. Laparoscopic lymphadenectomy for gynecologic malignancies using ultrasonically activated shears: Analysis of first 100 cases. *Gynecol Oncol.* 2005;97(3):813–819.

Possover M, Krause N, Plaul K, Kuhne-Heid R, Schneider A. Laparoscopic para-aortic and pelvic lymphadenectomy: Experience with 150 patients and review of the literature. *Gynecol Oncol.* 1998;1:19–28.

Rossi EC, Ivanova A, Boggess JF. Robotically assisted fluorescence-guided lymph node mapping with ICG for gynecologic malignancies: A feasibility study. *Gynecol Oncol.* 2012;124(1):78–82.

CHAPTER 32

ROBOTICS: THE CLINICAL NUTS AND BOLTS TO APPLICATIONS IN MINIMALLY INVASIVE GYNECOLOGIC SURGERY

Kirsten Sasaki and Charles E. Miller

INTRODUCTION

Robotic-assisted laparoscopic surgery using the da Vinci Surgical System (Intuitive Surgical, Sunnyvale, California) has been approved by the U.S. Food and Drug Administration (FDA) for use in gynecology since April 2005. It provides an additional tool for performing minimally invasive gynecologic procedures, and has been widely adapted by new and established surgeons.

Whereas this is not the first robotic system used for gynecologic surgery, it is currently the only active platform. The da Vinci Surgical System offers technology that has never been used in robotic-assisted surgery. This includes three-dimensional, high-definition visualization, 10–15 times magnification, and 7° of freedom with wristed movements. Additional technologies include the ability to view radiologic images at the console, TilePro, da Vinci Firefly Fluorescence Imaging, and Single-Site robotic-assisted gynecologic surgery. This chapter reviews the clinical basics of employing robotic-assisted surgery in gynecologic surgery.

SURGEON CREDENTIALING

Each hospital has its own credentialing requirements, and Intuitive Surgical has developed a training pathway to assist with the initial educational process. This includes product training through an online curriculum, and modules with subsequent clinical training along with experienced robotic surgeons. After initial privileging, most hospitals have additional requirements to maintain these privileges.

When starting a new robotics program, it is essential that the operating room staff, nurses, and anesthesiologists are significantly involved. Initially challenging, it is a large but rewarding undertaking that requires investment and continuous commitment by all members of the robotic team.

PATIENT SELECTION

Robotic-assisted laparoscopic surgery has been adapted by all disciplines of gynecologic surgery, including benign gynecology, urogynecology, reproductive endocrinology and infertility, and oncology. Whereas it is a unique tool that can aptly assist minimally invasive surgery, it may not be the optimal approach for all patients. Since the patient is placed in a fixed and steep Trendelenburg position for the majority of the surgery, women with significant respiratory, cardiac, or neurologic disease may preclude this approach (Figure 32.1). Moreover, robotic-assisted laparoscopic surgery has yet to be approved for use in pregnant patients.

PATIENT SETUP

POSITIONING

As with conventional gynecologic laparoscopy, patients are placed in a modified dorsal lithotomy position. It is imperative to place the patient with her sacrum as close to the edge of the operating table as possible in order to ensure adequate space for uterine manipulation; recognizing that Trendelenburg often results in cephalad movement of the patient. While the use of positioning equipment and devices to prevent sliding cephalad will vary hospital to hospital, beanbags and nonskid foam are commonly employed. Since most robotic surgeons prefer that the arms are tucked and adducted to the patient's sides, proper arm placement and cushioning are necessary to help prevent nerve compression and subsequent injury.

UTERINE MANIPULATION

Depending on the procedure, a uterine manipulator is not only useful but essential for successful execution and completion of the surgery. Since the surgeon sits some distance from the bedside and is unable to control uterine manipulation without leaving the console, it is essential to have an experienced professional at this position. The choice of manipulator is dependent on surgeon preference and availability; for example, when performing a total robotic hysterectomy, it is useful to have a manipulator that has a vaginal ring, such as that on the V-Care (ConMed Endosurgery, Utica, New York), Fornisee (LSI Solutions, Victor, New York), or RUMI (Cooper Surgical,

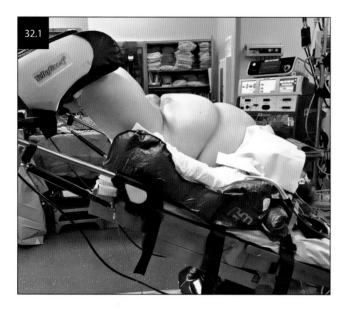

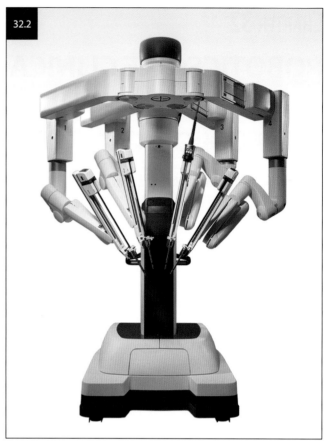

Shelton, Connecticut) with KOH Cup (Cooper Surgical, Shelton, Connecticut) to also push the uterus and cervix cephalad and away from the ureters on colpotomy.

ROBOTIC COMPONENTS

The da Vinci system is composed of three components that work together: the patient cart, the da Vinci vision tower, and the surgeon console.

PATIENT CART

The patient cart has three or four arms that dock onto the camera and robotic trocars placed at the bedside (Figure 32.2). The robotic instruments are placed through these trocars and are manipulated by the surgeon seated at the console. Compared to conventional laparoscopy, these instruments have 7° of freedom versus 4°, scaled down motion, and tremor filtration. Robotic-assisted surgery also eliminates the fulcrum effect of laparoscopy, in which the instrument moves in the opposite direction of the hand movement, thus providing the surgeon the ability to operate as if performing open surgery in a minimally invasive manner. Docked to the patient cart is the camera trocar, through which the da Vinci vision system is placed.

DA VINCI VISION TOWER

The Vision Tower represents the brain of the robot (Figure 32.3). This system is composed of two cameras, each with a separate light source, that provide three-dimensional, high-definition images to the surgeon console. On the Si system, there are two cameras available in different sizes, 8.5 and 12 mm. There is a 0° lens and a 30° lens for each size, which can be placed up or down depending on the location of the surgical anatomy. For the newer Xi system, there is only a 8 mm camera option.

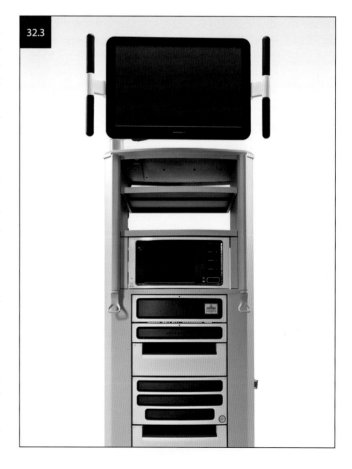

SURGEON CONSOLE

The surgeon console is placed away and in direct line of site from the patient cart and operating bed. The console houses the binocular viewer, and camera and instrument controls that are manipulated through the use of pedals and hand controls (Figure 32.4). Through these controls the surgeon is able to manipulate all of the instruments and camera to magnify the view up to 15-fold. The ability to sit while operating provides multiple ergonomic advantages, both physical and cognitive, compared to conventional laparoscopy.

Available for the da Vinci Si and Xi systems is the option for a dual console. This enables two surgeons to operate at the console together, and is useful when training residents and new robotic surgeons (Figure 32.5).

TROCAR PLACEMENT

CAMERA TROCAR

As with traditional laparoscopy, the camera trocar is the first to be placed. Depending on the platform acquired by the hospital, there may be one or two camera sizes available. For the Si system, there are two sizes of cameras available, 8.5 and 12 mm. With the new Xi platform, only an 8 mm camera is available. For a hysterectomy or myomectomy, this trocar is generally placed 8–10 cm from the fundus of the uterus. For smaller uteri, this trocar can often be placed at the umbilicus, but for larger uteri,

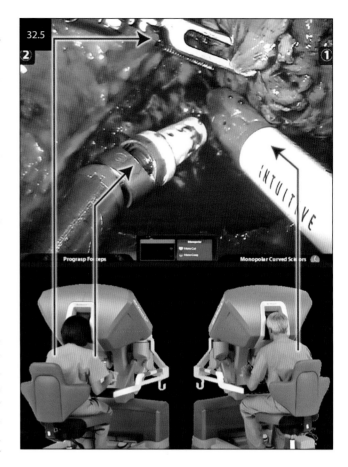

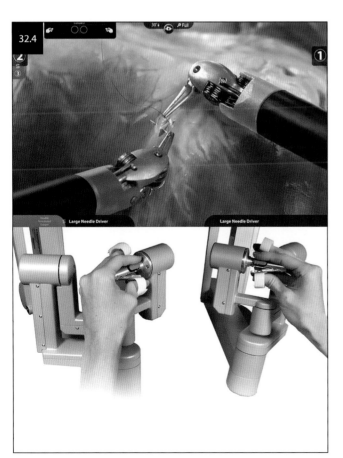

it may require placement supraumbilically (Figure 32.6). After the camera is inserted and the abdomen and pelvis are surveyed, the location of the additional trocars can be determined. It is important to measure and determine the location of the robotic trocars after the abdomen is insufflated, as this location changes with insufflation.

For the Si system, the choice between the 8.5 and 12 mm camera depends on the surgeon's preference, procedure, and hospital availability. Some surgeons prefer to use an 8.5 mm camera when no transabdominal

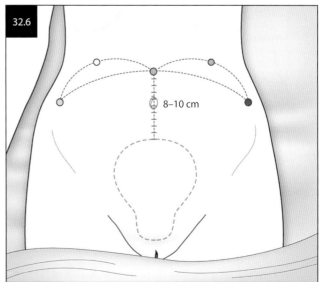

morcellation is necessary (i.e., total hysterectomies or supracervical hysterectomies with transcervical morcellation), and reserve the 12 mm camera for myomectomies or hysterectomies that require transabdominal morcellation, as this requires at least a 12 mm incision.

Additionally, with the new da Vinci Xi platform, the instrument and camera trocars are all 8 mm and interchangeable. Therefore, depending on the anatomy, one can change the orientation of instruments as well as the focus of visualization.

ROBOTIC TROCARS

The decision to use three or four arms depends on multiple factors including surgeon preference and experience, surgical procedure, and abdominal and pelvic anatomy (Figure 32.7). Regardless of how many arms are used, it is essential to position them approximately 8 cm apart in order to avoid collisions of the robotic arms. The lateral trocars can often be placed at or below the level of the camera trocar. If four arms are used, the fourth arm should be placed opposite of the assistant trocar and slightly cephalad to the camera trocar (Figure 32.8).

There are two robotic trocar sizes, 5 and 8 mm. Most robotic-assisted gynecologic procedures are performed with the 8 mm robotic instruments, but some pediatric surgeons use the 5 mm instruments. Not all instruments are available in the 5 mm size, and in order to utilize the 7° of freedom, these instruments must protrude into the robotic trocar more than the 8 mm instruments, thus limiting surgical workspace.

ASSISTANT TROCAR

As with trocar number, the decision to use an assistant trocar depends on multiple factors. Some surgeons prefer to use an assistant trocar for traction, needle introduction and removal, and suction/irrigation, but with the introduction of the robotic suction/irrigation device for the da

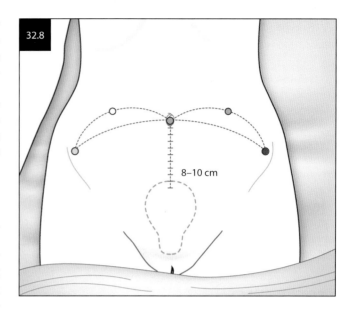

Vinci Si system, this trocar is not always necessary. If it is placed, it can often be placed at the same level on the opposite side of the fourth arm (Figure 32.8).

INSUFFLATION AND SMOKE EVACUATION

Depending on the number of trocars and use of an assistant trocar, the location of the insufflation and smoke evacuator can differ. If using a three-port technique without an assistant trocar, the insufflation is often attached to a port on the robotic trocar with the smoke evacuator attached to the camera trocar. If an assistant trocar is placed, the insufflation is attached to this trocar.

DOCKING

Prior to docking the robot, the bed should be lowered and the patient should be placed in enough Trendelenburg so that the surgeon can complete the procedure. Patients are often placed in at least 20° of Trendelenburg, but it is essential to communicate with the anesthesiologist at this point to ensure that the patient can tolerate this position for the duration of the procedure. The stirrups should be lowered so the legs are not hyperflexed at the hips.

The patient cart can be brought in straight or at an angle to the bed, also known as side-docking (Figure 32.9). When "straight" docking is preferred, the robotic cart center column and camera port should be aligned (Figure 32.10). The patient cart should be brought in until the camera arm is nearly touching the camera port, and the camera arm should be in the blue "sweet spot."

When side-docking, the operating bed can be rotated, or if the room configuration allows, the cart can be angled so that it is brought in at a 30°–45° angle to the bed. This often means that the legs of the base straddle one corner of the operating bed. Side-docking provides more room for the person performing the uterine manipulation. When side-docking, it is not necessary to keep the robotic arms within the "sweet spot" bands.

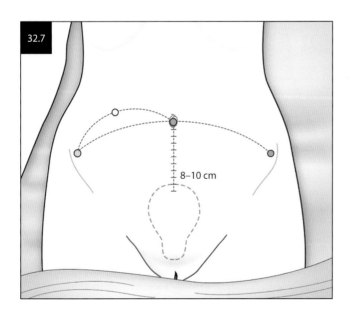

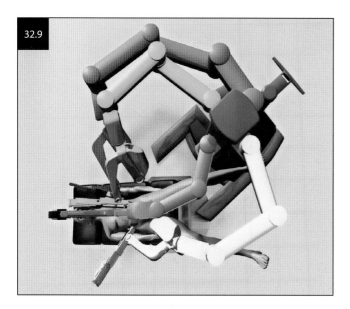

32.9

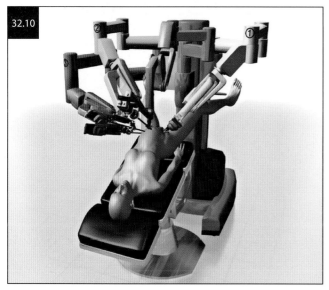

32.10

Once docked, the operating bed cannot be moved, as this can affect the placement and depth of the trocars, causing possible abdominal or pelvic injury.

For some gynecologic oncology procedures, including paraaortic lymph node dissections and excision of upper abdominal metastasis, redocking of the robot may be required over the patient's head in order to access the upper abdomen. With the newer Xi system, redocking is not necessary as the technology enables multi-quadrant surgery without redocking.

INSTRUMENTATION

There are currently multiple instrument combinations available for a robotic-assisted hysterectomy. Some popular bipolar electrosurgical instruments include the Maryland forceps, PK dissecting forceps (Olympus, Southboro, Massachusetts), and fenestrated forceps. Common monopolar electrosurgical instruments are the curved scissors, also known as Hot Shears, hook, and

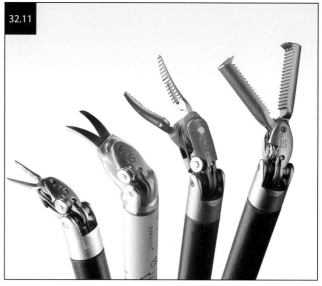

32.11

spatula (Figure 32.11). Additional instruments include the Harmonic Ace (Ethicon, Cincinnati, Ohio) and for the Si system the EndoWrist One Vessel Sealer, which provides bipolar cautery and the ability to cut in one instrument. If using the Si system, they both currently lack the 7° of movement that the other instruments provide, but the EndoWrist Vessel Sealer is available with wristed motion for the Xi system. One way to overcome this limitation is to switch the instrument to the opposite robotic arm throughout the procedure. Similar to the approach for a traditional laparoscopic hysterectomy, these instruments are used to divide the round ligament, create a bladder flap, and skeletonize and desiccate the uterine vessels. For the vaginal cuff closure, two needle drivers are available, the mega and the large needle driver (Figure 32.12). They both come with the option to have a suture cutting ability, but careful suture manipulation is necessary as one can inadvertently cut the suture prematurely. Some surgeons prefer to use two needle drivers, while others may use a grasping instrument, such as the ProGrasp,

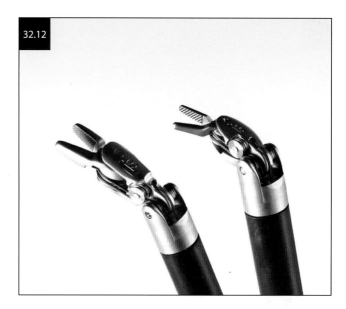

32.12

Cadiere, or long-tip forceps, in the nondominant hand. Suturing technique will vary by surgeon, but interrupted sutures of Vicryl are often placed, as knot tying becomes less of an obstacle with robotics than traditional laparoscopy. As the image is magnified up to 15 times, it is essential to take adequate bites of tissue beyond the desiccated margin in order to minimize vaginal cuff dehiscence.

Especially for larger uteri, lateral visualization can sometimes be difficult if no assistant port is placed for traction. This can be overcome with traction from a robotic arm, using one of the EndoWrist graspers, such as the cobra grasper or single-tooth tenaculum, and with use of a 30° lens.

For procedures that require complex and delicate tissue dissection, the Black Diamond Micro Forceps and Fine Tissue Forceps are available. In addition, when cautery is not optimal, but vessel sealing is needed, the robot now offers small, medium, and large clip appliers.

ADDITIONAL TECHNOLOGY

DA VINCI SURGICAL SKILLS SIMULATOR

Simulators have been created to improve robotic training while avoiding the risk of harm to patients and cost to the health-care system. Intuitive Surgical has a simulator that attaches to the da Vinci Si, Si-e, and Xi consoles and enables surgeons to perform over 25 exercises and procedures that focus on different skill sets specific to the robot. This simulator uses three-dimensional software by MIMIC Technologies (Seattle, Washington) and the face, content, and predictive validity have been demonstrated (Figures 32.13 and 32.14).

TILEPRO

Available for the S, Si, and Xi systems, TilePro allows surgeons to view radiologic images at the surgeon console. This can be useful for mapping intramural fibroids

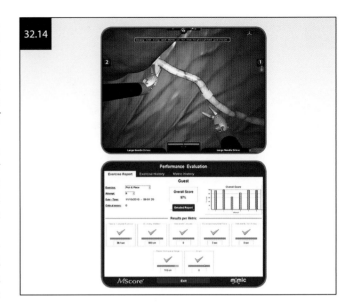

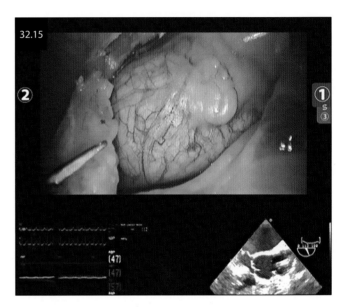

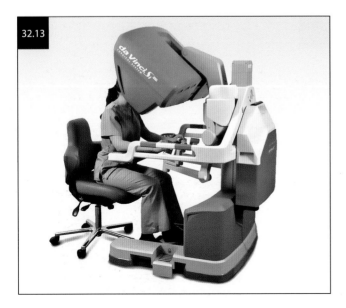

and has been used in urologic surgery to identify tumor margin (Figure 32.15).

DA VINCI FIREFLY FLUORESCENCE IMAGING

The Firefly fluorescence technology can be used to assist in identifying blood vessels during surgical dissection. Indocyanine green dye is injected intravenously through a peripheral line and binds to albumin. Using an excitatory light source, the artery and, subsequently, vein are easily identified (Figures 32.16 and 32.17). This can facilitate gonadal vein transections, can facilitate dissection of the presacral space, and has been used to identify tumor margin for resection. It is currently available for the Si and Xi systems.

SINGLE-SITE

The most recent addition to gynecologic robotic surgery is the ability to perform single-site robotic-assisted surgery

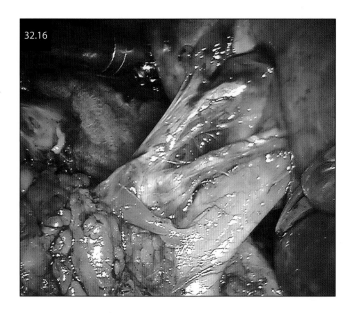

32.16

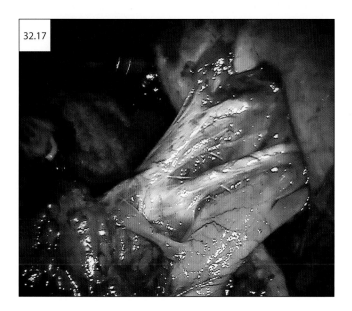

32.17

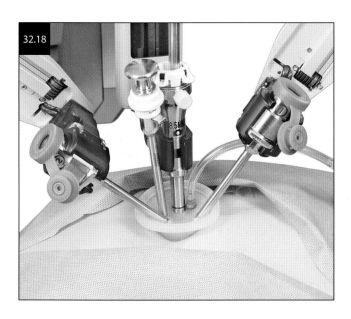

32.18

on the da Vinci Si system and now Xi system (Figure 32.18). It is currently being used to perform benign hysterectomies and adnexal surgery. Through a concealed 2–2.5 cm umbilical incision, a single gel port is placed, allowing the camera, robotic, and assistant trocars to be placed. Although the only currently available wristed Single-Site instrument is the wristed needle driver, which offers up to 45° of motion in all directions, a large obstacle of Single-Site is overcome with the elimination of cross-body confusion. It also maintains the three-dimensional visualization and magnification of the traditional robotic platform.

ACKNOWLEDGMENTS

We would like to thank Dr. Aarathi Cholkeri-Singh for her assistance with editing this manuscript.

SUGGESTED READING

Autorino R, Kouk J, Stolzenburg J et al. Current status and future directions of robotic single-site surgery: A systematic review. *Eur Urol.* 2012;63:266–280.

Bedaiwy M, Volsky J, Sandadi S et al. The expanding spectrum of robotic gynecologic surgery: A review. *Middle East Fertil Soc J.* 2012;17:70–78.

Chen CC, Falcone T. Robotic gynecologic surgery: Past, present and future. *Clin Obstet Gynecol.* 2009;52:335–343.

Escobar P, Fader A, Paraiso M et al. Robotic-assisted laparoendoscopic single site surgery in gynecology: Initial report and technique. *J Min Inv Gyn.* 2009;16:589–591.

Fanning J, Fenton B, Purohit M. Robotic radical hysterectomy. *Am J Obstet Gynecol.* 2008;198:649.e1–649.e4.

Finan MA, Rocconi RP. Overcoming technical challenges with robotic surgery in gynecologic oncology. *Surg Endosc.* 2010;24:1256–1260.

Lee G, Lee M, Clanton T et al. Comparative assessment of physical and cognitive ergonomics associated with robotic and traditional laparoscopic surgeries. *Surg Endosc.* 2014;28:456–465.

Leon Woods D, Hou JY, Riembers L et al. Side-docking in robotic-assisted gynaecologic cancer surgery. *Int J Med Robot.* 2011;6:57–60.

Palep J. Robotic assisted minimally invasive surgery. *J Minim Access Surg.* 2009;5:1–7.

Quemener J, Boulanger L, Rubod C et al. The place of robotics in gynecologic surgery. *J Visc Surg.* 2012;149:e289–e301.

Silverman S, Orbuch L, Orbuch I. Parallel side-docking technique for gynecologic procedures utilizing the da Vinci robo. *J Robotic Surg.* 2012;6:247–249.

Tinelli A, Malvasi A, Gustapane S et al. Robotic assisted surgery in gynecology: Current insights and future perspectives. *Recent Pat Biotechnol.* 2011;5:12–24.

Tusheva OL, Cohen SL, Wang KC. Robotic approach to management of fibroids. In: Istre O, ed. *Minimally Invasive Gynecological Surgery.* London: Springer-Verlag; 2015:111–123.

Visco AG, Advincula AP. Robotic gynecologic surgery. *Obstet Gynecol.* 2008;1112:1369–1384.

Yim GW, Kim YT. Robotic surgery in gynecologic cancer. *Curr Opin Obstet Gynecol.* 2012;24:14–23.

CHAPTER 33

ROBOTIC HYSTERECTOMY

Fatih Şendağ and Ali Akdemir

INTRODUCTION

Given its proven association with reduced morbidity, faster recovery, shorter hospitalization, less infection, and better cosmesis, laparoscopic surgery has played a key role in gynecology for more than two decades. In many centers, laparoscopy is now the preferred surgical approach for both basic and advanced operations including the full gamut of hysterectomy, myomectomy, pelvic floor repair, resection of endometriosis, and even oncological surgeries. But, laparoscopy also presents some well-known technical challenges for the surgeon, including the need to switch from three-dimensional (3D) to two-dimensional (2D) views, the loss of depth perception, the amplification of tremor or movement by long and rigid instruments, diminished tactile feedback, and the fulcrum effect from trocar position. Compared to laparotomic instrumentation, laparoscopic instruments are typically restricted to only 5 degrees of freedom (DOF), including pitch, jaw, rotation, extraction/instruction, and instrument actuation. To overcome these technical challenges, comparatively unique and novel psychomotor skills are required. In fact, psychomotor fatigue from the technical challenges of surgery can contribute to poor decision making and ergonomically generated injuries including disc prolapse and joint arthropathies. All of these factors can retard adoption by making the learning curve of laparoscopic surgery significantly longer. In part generated by these potential obstacles, robotic surgical systems have been successfully introduced into surgical practice. Since U.S. Food and Drug Administration (FDA) approval for clinical use in 2000 and then for hysterectomy in 2005, the da Vinci Robotic Surgical System (Intuitive Surgical, Sunnyvale, California) has been successfully integrated into the gynecologic armamentarium for assisting the full spectrum of laparoscopic procedures. The underlying reasons for the rapid adaptation originate from the advantages of a robotic surgical system, including improved surgeon dexterity, surgical precision, and ergonomics. Enhanced visualization with a 3D view eliminates the loss of depth perception related to conventional laparoscopy. Moreover, motion scaling and adjustable tremor filtration properties of the system provide significant surgical instrument stabilization and minimize the fulcrum and leverage effect. Furthermore, instruments for the robotic surgical system are considerably different from those used in conventional laparoscopy.

The wrist function at the tip of the instrument provides an additional 2 DOF (extension/flexion and tilt function), which mimics the movements of the surgeon's hand in full range of motion (Figure 33.1). Since surgery is performed while sitting at a dedicated console during the procedure, the typical ergonomic challenges of traditional laparoscopy are essentially eliminated by these advantages. Collectively, these technical advantages can rapidly empower a gynecologic surgeon with limited experience using conventional laparoscopic surgery to perform more advanced procedures. Nevertheless, these advantages must be weighed against the demonstrated disadvantages of robotic surgery, including the high costs associated with purchasing the robotic system along with disposable instruments and drapes, and annual maintenance fees.

The da Vinci Surgical System consists of a console, a laparoscopic tower, and a patient side cart with robotic arms. The bulky structure of the system, high cost, and lack of haptic feedback are the leading drawbacks of the robotic surgical system. Among these, the lack of tactile feedback or haptics creates the most significant challenge for the robotic surgeon. Whereas this is widely accepted as a handicap, especially for the novice robotic surgeon, it has been demonstrated that surgeons performing robotic surgery can quickly adjust and adapt to this limitation by developing a "visual haptic" created by integrating the magnified and 3D vision system along with the benefits of advanced instrumentation. This chapter addresses the use of the da Vinci Robotic Surgical System, models S, Si, and Xi, to perform minimally invasive types of hysterectomy.

ROBOTIC HYSTERECTOMY

Hysterectomy is the most frequently performed major gynecologic surgery. Vaginal, laparoscopic, and abdominal methodologies are currently being used to perform hysterectomy. Whereas it is widely recommended to perform vaginal hysterectomy whenever possible, the comparatively higher morbidity associated with laparotomy relegates abdominal hysterectomy as the least desirable approach. Since this morbidity results from an abdominal incision, the use of a laparoscopic approach is preferred whenever the vaginal approach is precluded by technical issues or lack of surgical experience. With

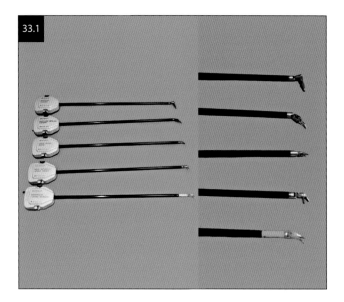

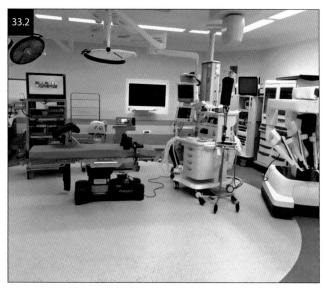

the introduction of the robotic surgical system, rates for laparoscopic hysterectomies have continued to increase over the last decade. It has been reported that among the approximately 500,000 hysterectomies performed annually in the United States, the use of robotically assisted hysterectomy increased from 0.5% in 2007 to 9.5% for all hysterectomies in 2010. These trends undoubtedly continue to evolve. It was reported that only 3 years after the first robotic procedure was introduced at hospitals where robotically assisted hysterectomy was subsequently performed, 22.4% of all hysterectomies were robotically assisted procedures. The rapid adoption of this technique is undoubtedly related to how effectively it decreases the gap between expert and novice surgeon in the field of minimal invasive surgery. Regardless, when compared to the use of conventional laparoscopy to perform benign hysterectomy, the robotic surgical system has not been shown to result in improved clinical outcomes.

TECHNIQUE FOR ROBOTIC HYSTERECTOMY

OPERATING ROOM PREPARATION

As with any surgical procedure, the preparation of the operating room (OR) and patient are of utmost importance. Since the da Vinci Surgical System has a bulky structure and consists of three units, it is of paramount importance to prepare in one dedicated OR. The OR should have enough space to include adequate setup for the robotic surgical system (console, patient cart, and tower), the assistant console if a dual console is used—all without compromising the patient safety and function of the OR staff. Additionally, a conventional laparoscopic setup including towers and screens should be included in the OR for the surgical team (Figure 33.2). Moreover, the system connection cables should be covered and secured to provide complete functionality without any chance for interruption.

PATIENT PREPARATION

After general anesthesia with endotracheal intubation is administered, the patient is placed in a dorsal lithotomy position with the buttocks slightly extending beyond the operating table to improve the effectiveness of the uterine manipulator. The arms are padded and tucked at the sides along the body (Figure 33.3). Further precautions include shoulder braces, chest straps, an underbody foam mattress, or any combination of these, to secure and prevent sliding head-ward during deep Trendelenburg position. A Foley catheter is placed into the bladder. An orogastric tube may be inserted to deflate the stomach in order to minimize the risk for injury related to the primary peritoneal access.

UTERINE MANIPULATOR

The primary purpose of the uterine manipulator is to improve surgical exposure by using traction and

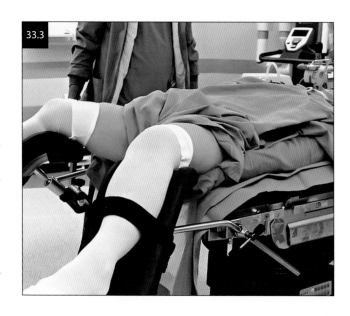

countertraction. Moreover, the cup of the manipulator helps delineate the vaginal fornices, which facilitates circumferential colpotomy, while displacing the ureters laterally. To place the manipulator, the cervix is first objectively evaluated to select the appropriate colpotomy ring. The cervix is then secured with a single-tooth tenaculum, and the uterine cavity is sounded to choose the appropriate tip size. After assembly, the uterine manipulator is sequentially placed transvaginally and then into the uterine cavity (Figure 33.4). Vaginal examination should then be performed to ensure that the colpotomy ring is appropriately positioned.

PLACEMENT OF TROCARS AND DOCKING

Port positions are usually dependent upon the size of the uterus. The numbers of trocars as well as robotic instruments are decided by the custom and practice of the surgeon. Some may prefer to use three robotic arms in order to reduce cost. Four robotic arms can be employed during more complex or advanced surgeries based on the surgeon's preference. In most cases, the primary trocar is placed transumbilically and used for a camera. Second and third robotic instrument 8.5 mm ports are then placed approximately 10 cm lateral and 2–3 cm below the camera port on both sides. An assistant trocar is then inserted between the camera port and either the left or the right ports depending on the location of the bedside assistant. This trocar is usually 10–12 mm to facilitate unimpeded passage of suture needles, tissue extraction, and as a port for suction and irrigation (Figure 33.5). In the case of a larger uterus, all trocars are placed more cephalad in order to provide sufficient working space between the robotic instruments and the target tissue. When using the da Vinci Surgical System S and Si, the size of the primary trocar is 12 mm. However, with the da Vinci Surgical System Xi, the size of the primary trocar is 8.5 mm, similar to other robotic instrument ports. This is one of the main differences between the Xi and S–Si

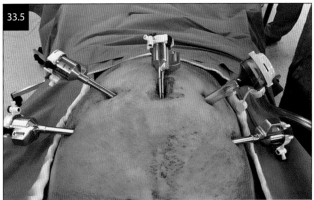

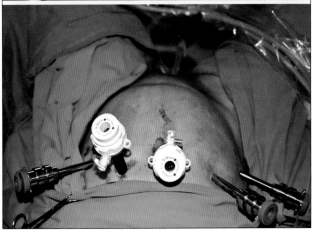

systems. As a result, in the Xi system, the endoscope can be attached to any arm, providing flexibility for visualizing the surgical site. If needed, a fourth robotic trocar is usually inserted 8–10 mm lateral and 2–3 cm inferior to the lateral robotic trocars. Since robotic trocars must be inserted with the thick black band on the neck of the cannula at the level of the abdominal fascia to maintain the pivot point for the trocar, all robotic port placements must be performed under direct vision (Figure 33.6). After the ports are inserted, the abdominopelvic cavity is

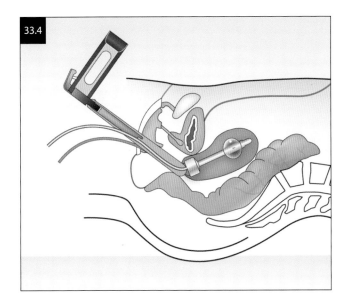

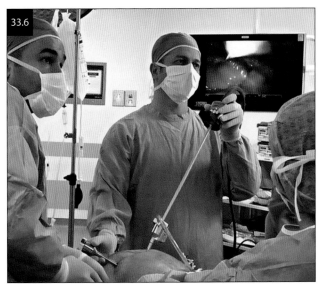

visualized for additional pathologies, such as adhesions. Adhesions may be separated before docking using conventional laparoscopic instruments if they are judged to go beyond the movement range of the robotic surgical system. The patient is then placed in deep Trendelenburg position. This is required to retract the intestines and bowel cranially to improve pelvic exposure. Docking and attaching each robotic trocar to the respectively assigned robotic arm are then completed (Figure 33.7). The robotic endoscope is attached to the umbilical trocar, while the right and left operating robotic arms are attached directly to the right and left lateral robotic ports. A patient side-cart is either brought between the patient's legs (central docking) or to the patient's side (side-docking). Side-docking may be more appropriate whenever an assistant has to hold the uterine manipulator. We recommend the use of a 30° robotic endoscope in the up position during docking. This facilitates proper placement of the robotic trocars and setting of the robotic instruments (Figure 33.8). The robotic EndoWrist instruments are then loaded into the robotic arms and inserted into the surgical field. At this point, the primary surgeon leaves the sterile field and sits at the console. A monopolar scissors on the right and a bipolar instrument (Maryland or fenestrated) on the left are the most commonly used configurations for hysterectomy. Moreover, an EndoWrist needle holder will be required for cuff closure as the final step of the procedure. If a fourth arm is needed, a single-tooth tenaculum and ProGrasp forceps are also commonly employed

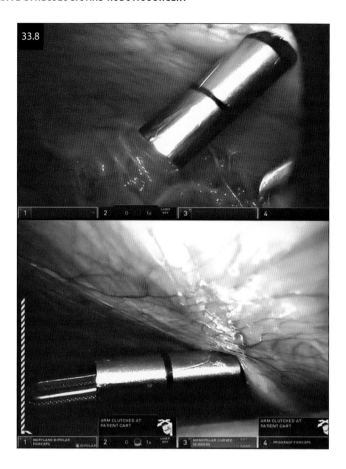

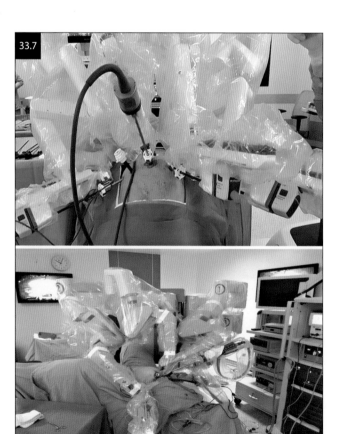

(Figure 33.9). When the setup and all initial steps are complete, the robotic endoscope is then switched to a 0° optic, and the hysterectomy procedure is initiated.

OPERATING TECHNIQUE

Pelvic visualization is performed to confirm the correct placement of the uterine manipulator. Lysis of adhesions to restore normal anatomical relationships should be performed at the outset of the hysterectomy. Mobilization of the left pericolic reflection between

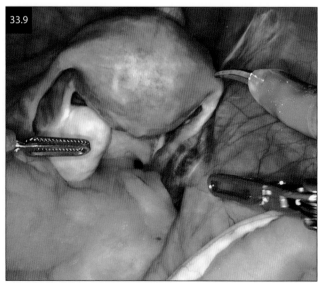

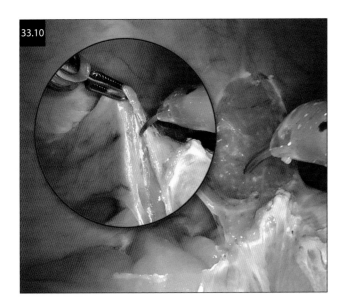

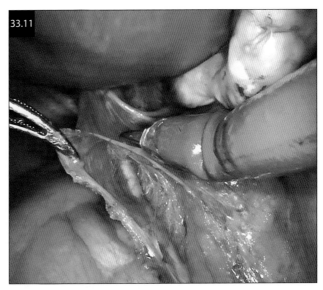

the left pelvic sidewall and the rectosigmoid colon can facilitate surgical exposure of the left infundibulopelvic (IFP) and round ligament (RL) (Figure 33.10). The ureteral course is then bilaterally identified. Although there is no evidence-based precedent, retroperitoneal dissection can be used to identify the ureters. This dissection is carried out starting at the level of the pelvic brim just medial to the IFP ligament. At this point, the assistant pushes the uterus cranially and to the contralateral side, as the ovary is lifted up. In the case of using a fourth robotic arm, this instrument grasps the ovary and lifts it up to improve the exposure. In either case, the peritoneum covering each ureter is opened and dissected downward toward the uterosacral ligament. Appearing as small retroperitoneal bubbles, this dissection is facilitated by the gas of the pneumoperitoneum. Using this type of retroperitoneal dissection, the ureter subsequently falls downward, and it is distanced from the IFP ligament as well as uterine vascular structures (Figure 33.11). If retroperitoneal ureterolysis is not performed, these structures should be visually identified and their pathways charted from the pelvic brim toward the bladder.

If the ovaries are preserved, each fallopian tube is first lifted to expose the mesosalpinx, which is sequentially cut using monopolar electrosurgery down to the level of the round ligament. Bipolar electrosurgery can be employed to control any bleeders (Figure 33.12).

If ovaries are removed, after identifying the course of the ureter, the IFP ligament is then coagulated with the bipolar robotic instrument just lateral to the ovary. After adequate coagulation, the IFP ligament is then cut using the monopolar robotic scissors. Effective coagulation and cutting of the main vascular supplies are quite important, since conventional bipolar energy is commonly utilized without the benefit of true vessel sealing now provided by more advanced bipolar electrosurgical instrumentation. Ideally, the surgeon should perform coagulation in small steps in order to prevent bleeding

(Figure 33.13). Laparoscopic clips for small vessel ligation can be used through the assistant port. The round ligament is then grasped and coagulated with bipolar robotic instrument 2–3 cm medial to the pelvic sidewall and then cut with monopolar scissors (Figure 33.14). The anterior leaf of the broad ligament is then identified and incised from the round ligament up to the vesicouterine peritoneal fold. Proper uterine manipulation is maintained using the fourth robotic instrument or by the assistant surgeon. Since the posterior leaf of the broad ligament was already cut during the retroperitoneal dissection for ureteral identification, the next step is to mobilize the bladder off of the lower uterine segment. For this purpose, the uterus is pushed cranially and slightly posterior to improve the exposure of the base of the vesicouterine space and vesicouterine peritoneal fold. The bladder and the peritoneum are then secured with a grasping instrument (the assistant or the fourth robotic instrument) in the midline, and lifted to the anterior abdominal wall. The peritoneum

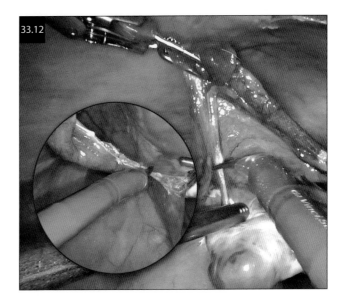

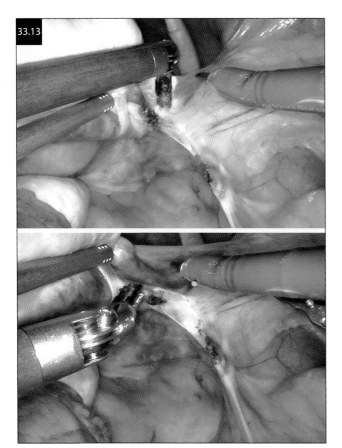

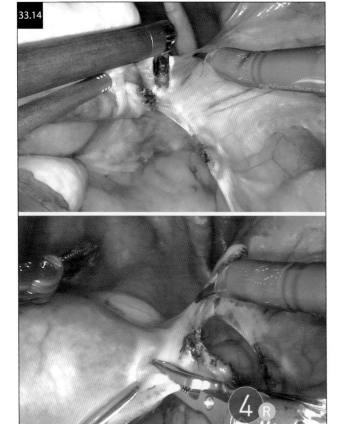

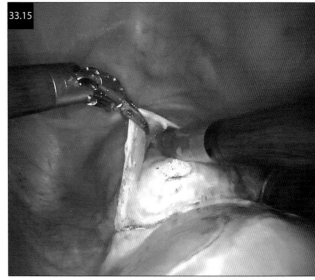

is then coagulated and cut to access the vesicovaginal plane. The vesicovaginal plane is then dissected, and vesicouterine ligaments are bilaterally coagulated and then cut. The dissection of this plane is started medially and finished laterally (Figure 33.15). The uterine vessels are then isolated and secured. To do this, the uterus is first moved to the contralateral side by the assistant. The uterus is then grasped at the cornu and moved to the contralateral side to improve exposure of the ipsilateral uterine vessels. The posterior peritoneum is cut above the uterosacral ligament to help identify and ultimately skeletonize the uterine vessels (Figure 33.16). The ascending branch of the uterine artery is skeletonized as much as possible to provide access for adequate coagulation using the bipolar robotic instrument. Before coagulating the uterine artery, the colpotomy cup should be carefully identified to previsualize the line for colpotomy. The uterine vessels should then be grasped, coagulated, and cut high and medial to the colpotomy cup (Figure 33.17). If necessary, additional

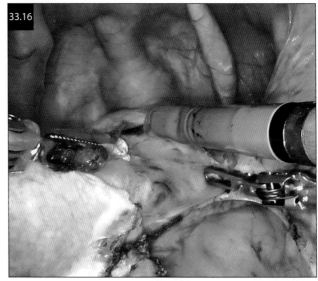

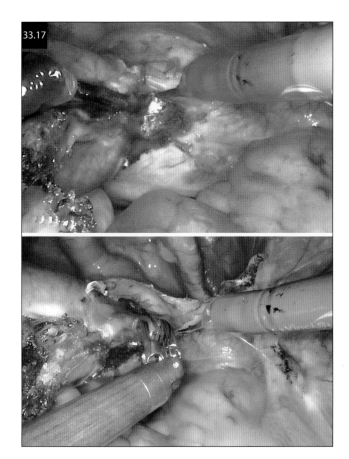

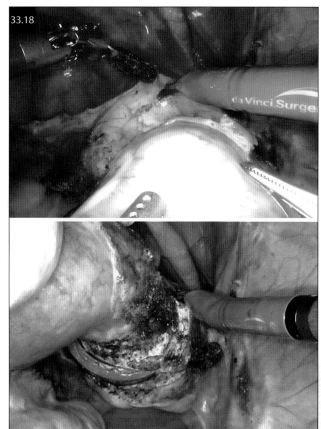

tissue purchases should be taken medial to the uterine pedicle. This reduces the risk for ureteral injury. At this step, the uterus is moved to the contralateral side, and the operating steps are repeated on the contralateral side of the uterus. The uterus is then pushed cranially and posteriorly to facilitate an anterior colpotomy by using the colpotomy cup as a guidepost. The assistant should manipulate the uterus to clearly identify the colpotomy line over the cup. The colpotomy is then advanced laterally and posteriorly (Figure 33.18). During the posterior colpotomy, either the first assistant or the fourth robotic arm grasps the uterus and provides tension to improve the exposure on the posterior side of the uterus. In case of a large uterus, starting with the posterior colpotomy may be preferable. Since monopolar instrumentation is primarily used in robotic hysterectomy, one of the main obstacles is the smoke produced during colpotomy. Aspirating smoke through an assistant port can improve vision at the surgical field. The uterus is then removed through the vagina. Before closing the vaginal cuff, maintaining the pneumoperitoneum is crucial. For this purpose, the uterus may be left in the vagina as a natural tissue occlusion, or a surgical glove filled with surgical gauze can be inserted into the vagina. The vaginal cuff is then closed after the monopolar robotic scissors is switched with the robotic EndoWrist needle holder. Since the robotic surgical system significantly improves a surgeon's dexterity, the vaginal cuff can be efficiently closed with intracorporeal suturing using the robotic surgical system. The suture material and

needle can be introduced and removed from the abdomen through the assistant port. The vaginal cuff is typically closed using interrupted figure-of-8 stiches with a delayed absorbable suture material. Alternatively, it can be closed with a running suturing technique using a barbed suture material. The anterior vaginal wall should be held by the assistant surgeon or the fourth robotic arm to improve exposure during vaginal cuff closure. It should be kept in mind that since the robotic endoscope provides a magnified view, it can lead to underpurchasing of tissue during suturing, potentially contributing to

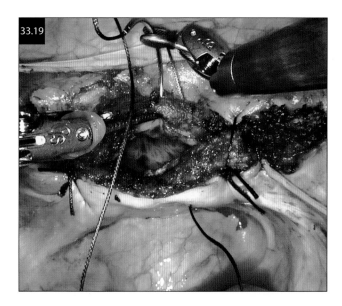

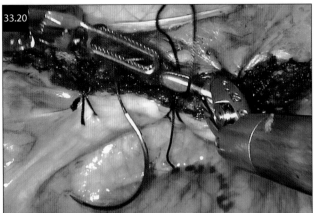

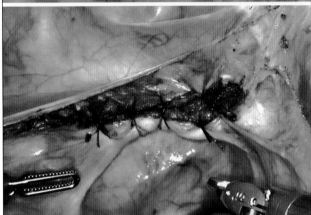

The trocars are then removed, and facial defects at the larger trocar incisions are closed to decrease the risk of port site hernia.

SUGGESTED READING

Cohen SL, Vitonis AF, Einarsson JI. Updated hysterectomy surveillance and factors associated with minimally invasive hysterectomy. *JSLS*. 2014;18(3).

Gala RB, Margulies R, Steinberg A et al. Society of Gynecologic Surgeons Systematic Review Group. Systematic review of robotic surgery in gynecology: Robotic techniques compared with laparoscopy and laparotomy. *J Minim Invasive Gynecol*. 2014;21(3):353–361.

Investor FAQ. Intuitive Surgical. "da Vinci Products FAQ." Intuitive Surgical. Accessed 11/10/2015.

Jonsdottir GM, Jorgensen S, Cohen SL et al. Increasing minimally invasive hysterectomy: Effect on cost and complications. *Obstet Gynecol*. 2011;117:1142–1149.

Kenngott HG, Fischer L, Nickel F, Rom J, Rassweiler J, Müller-Stich BP. Status of robotic assistance—A less traumatic and more accurate minimally invasive surgery? *Langenbecks Arch Surg*. 2012;397(3):333–341.

Sendag F, Akdemir A. Robotic suturing in laparoscopic surgery. In: Jain N, ed. *State-of-the-Art Atlas and Textbook of Laparoscopic Suturing in Gynecology*, 2nd ed. JAYPEE; 2014:232–248.

Sendag F, Zeybek B, Akdemir A, Ozgurel B, Oztekin K. Analysis of the learning curve for robotic hysterectomy for benign gynaecological disease. *Int J Med Robot*. 2014;10(3):275–279.

Wright JD, Ananth CV, Lewin SN et al. Robotically assisted vs laparoscopic hysterectomy among women with benign gynecologic disease. *JAMA*. 2013;309:689–698.

Wright JD, Burke WM, Wilde ET et al. Comparative effectiveness of robotic versus laparoscopic hysterectomy for endometrial cancer. *J Clin Oncol*. 2012;30(8):783–791.

postoperative cuff dehiscence. Ideally, tissue purchase during suturing should be at least 5 mm lateral to the suture line (Figures 33.19 and 33.20). After closing of the vaginal cuff, the pelvic cavity is assessed for adequate hemostasis. The robotic instruments are then removed under direct vision, and the patient cart is undocked.

CHAPTER 34

ROBOTIC MYOMECTOMY

Kirsten Sasaki and Charles E. Miller

INTRODUCTION

Uterine fibroids, or leiomyoma, can affect up to 80% of women and cause symptoms including but not limited to menorrhagia, metrorrhagia, anemia, pelvic pain and pressure, urinary frequency, and infertility. For women who wish to preserve their fertility, myomectomy is the most common surgical treatment option. Depending on the location of the fibroid(s) and the experience and skill of the physician, the surgical approach can include hysteroscopy, laparotomy, minilaparotomy, laparoscopy, or robotic-assisted laparoscopy. This chapter discusses the important preoperative, intraoperative, and postoperative components of a robotic-assisted myomectomy.

PATIENT EVALUATION

Prior to taking a patient to the operating room for a robotic myomectomy, a thorough evaluation of her uterus and fibroids is necessary. After a complete history and physical exam, all patients should undergo some form of pelvic imaging to help "map" out fibroid(s) location and size. It can help the surgeon create a plan for the procedure and provide the patient with more information regarding the possible length and complexity of the surgery. Transvaginal ultrasound (TVUS), magnetic resonance imaging (MRI), and three-dimensional saline-infused sonohysterogram are the most useful imaging techniques. Three-dimensional saline-infused sonohysterogram is especially useful to determine penetration of a fibroid into the myometrium, and whether a submucosal fibroid is best managed by hysteroscopy or laparoscopy (Figure 34.1). With increasing fibroid burden, MRI can provide more information regarding the precise location and number of fibroids. Although both MRI and ultrasound can help in distinguishing fibroid and adenomyosis, MRI appears to be more helpful in the diagnosis of a uterine sarcoma. If there is concern for extrauterine fibroids, MRI is also a better modality for characterizing these locations, as they can be in the broad ligament, attached to the abdominal wall or gastrointestinal tract. However, with MRI, additional cost must be considered, and thus should be used only when information through ultrasound and saline infused sonohysterogram (SIS) evaluation is not forthcoming.

Patients with anemia may be treated with a GnRH agonist, such as leuprolide acetate, preoperatively in order to build up their blood stores for improved perioperative outcomes. Although not approved by the U.S. Food and Drug Administration (FDA) for this indication, some practitioners will also use a GnRH agonist to decrease fibroid volume prior to surgery. However, leuprolide acetate is generally avoided in patients undergoing myomectomies as this can distort the tissue planes, potentially making the procedure more difficult with increased operative time and blood loss. Other patients may be prescribed oral or intravenous iron or epoetin to increase preoperative hemoglobin levels. An additional option is preoperative storage of blood in patients who are anticipated to need intraoperative or postoperative transfusions secondary to multiple and/or large fibroids and chronic anemia.

PATIENT SETUP

After the patient is intubated and a nasogastric or orogastric tube is placed, each patient is placed in the dorsal, supine lithotomy position. After the abdomen and vagina are prepped, a Foley catheter is placed into the bladder and secured into place. A bimanual exam is performed to evaluate the version and flexion of the uterus relative to the vagina and cervix. A speculum is used to visualize the cervix, and a single-tooth tenaculum is placed on the anterior lip. The uterus is gently sounded to measure cavity length, and hysteroscopy is performed to diagnose and treat pathology within the endometrial canal. A uterine manipulator is subsequently placed. The uterine manipulator selected should allow instillation of dye to evaluate the patency of the fallopian tubes if fertility is desired. Moreover, the manipulator must be long enough to enter the uterine cavity to enable uterine manipulation. The final step is to place the patient in a proper position that enables uterine manipulation.

Depending on the direction the surgeon prefers to dock the robot, the operating room bed may be rotated approximately 30°–45° away from the robotic arms.

SUBMUCOSAL FIBROIDS

If the patient is noted on preoperative evaluation to have any submucosal fibroids, a hysteroscopy with possible myomectomy is performed after the tenaculum is placed and the cervix is gently dilated to or just greater than the

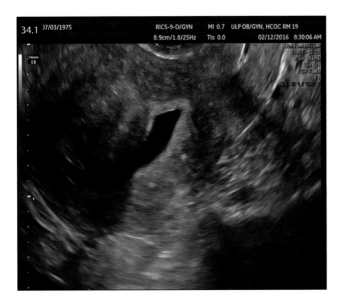

size of the operative hysteroscope. Type 0 or I submucosal myomas will most likely be removed hysteroscopically, while the approach to type II submucosal myomas depends on the size, location, and surgeon preference. Hysteroscopic myomectomy can be performed via the resectoscope (monopolar or bipolar) or hysteroscopic morcellation. After the hysteroscopic portion is complete, a uterine manipulator will be placed as outlined in the previous section.

PORT PLACEMENT

Standard placement

The umbilicus is everted with towel clamps and a Veress needle is placed mid-umbilically to obtain pneumoperitoneum, to a pressure of 25 mm Hg. The Veress needle is then removed and a trocar is inserted at the umbilicus. This trocar is placed at a 90° angle to the abdominal wall, to avoid a lesser angle bringing the camera too close to the uterus. Depending on surgeon preference, obtaining pneumoperitoneum and initial trocar

placement can be done without a Veress needle through an open procedure. After the laparoscope is inserted and the abdomen and pelvis have been surveyed, the uterus is pushed cephalad with the manipulator to ensure there is enough working room between the robotic camera and the fibroids. In general, one should have approximately 6–8 inches between the camera and uterine fundus. If the camera appears too close to the specimen, then the robotic camera trocar should be placed slightly left of the midline superiorly. After this is confirmed, one 8 mm robotic trocar is placed generally at the level of the camera trocar on each side of the abdomen. These trocars are generally placed 10–12 cm lateral from the camera trocar under direct visualization (Figure 34.2). It is important that these trocars are placed above and lateral to the pathology. As a myomectomy relies on dissecting along the right tissue plane between the uterus and the fibroid pseudocapsule, traction and countertraction are essential to the procedure. Therefore, some surgeons may place a 5 or 12 mm assistant trocar in the upper quadrant between the camera and left robotic port, or a third robotic arm in the right or left lower quadrant (Figure 34.3).

Special cases

High risk of abdominal wall adhesions

In patients with vertical laparotomy incisions, multiple surgeries that put them at high risk for abdominal wall adhesions, including ruptured appendices and tubo-ovarian abscesses, or umbilical hernias with or without repair, a left upper quadrant entry is often used. If the patient has a history of splenomegaly or surgery in the left upper quadrant of the abdomen, initial port placement may be required in the right upper quadrant. If proceeding in the left upper quadrant, a Veress needle is placed inferior to the last rib along the midclavicular line or at Palmer point to obtain pneumoperitoneum. A 5 mm trocar is then placed with an optical view trocar. Although important for most laparoscopic procedures,

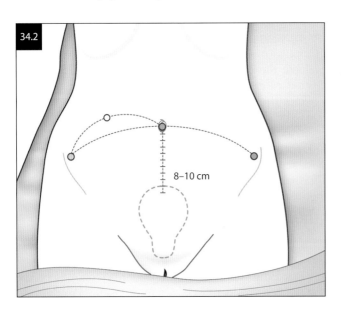

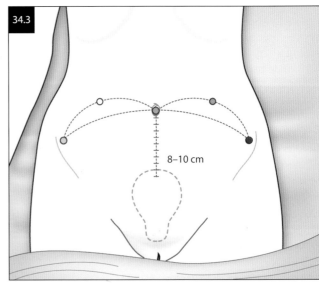

it is especially important to confirm with the anesthesiologist that the patient has an orogastric or nasogastric tube in place prior to placing this trocar. The same 12 and 8 mm robotic trocars are then placed, and adhesions are taken down as necessary prior to docking the robot. Alternatively, three 8 mm trocars are placed across the upper abdomen, and a 12 mm trocar is placed at the umbilicus, and used later to perform morcellation (see Figure 34.3).

Large uteri

In patients with a uterus that measures 18–20 weeks' gestation or larger, the camera trocar should be placed superior to the umbilicus. Many surgeons prefer to obtain pneumoperitoneum at the umbilicus with the Veress, and a 5 mm trocar can be placed at this site in order to assess the size and mobility of the uterus. The 8.5 or 12 mm camera trocar can be inserted under direct visualization approximately 6–8 cm superior to the uterus. If one is confident about the size of the uterus, one may forgo the 5 mm umbilical trocar and place the 12 mm camera trocar at the appropriate location, but this can be difficult without direct visualization of the uterus and fibroids beforehand. The 8 mm robotic trocars should be placed with enough room to operate for the most cephalad and caudad fibroids. This often places the trocars midway between the umbilicus and the camera trocar. Ultimately, given current tissue removal techniques, at least a 12 mm trocar must be placed for morcellation. Cosmetically, and secondary to risk of subsequent hernia formation, consider a 12 mm trocar at the umbilicus.

DOCKING

Prior to docking the robot, the patient's bed should be lowered toward the floor as much as possible and then placed in the Trendelenburg position. Depending on the type of operating room bed, the patient may require the maximum Trendelenburg offered by the bed in order to confirm adequate visualization of the pelvis, but sometimes less may be sufficient. Depending on the preference of the surgeon and the accommodations of the operating room, the robot can be brought into dock along the midline or to the side of the patient. As constant uterine manipulation is required throughout the procedure, many surgeons prefer to dock from the side, thus providing the person performing the uterine manipulation adequate room for comfort and maneuverability (Figure 34.4).

DISSECTING OUT FIBROIDS

Now that the robot is docked, an operative plan is made in terms of the order of the fibroids to be removed and how the hysterotomy will be made. This is imperative in order to minimize the number of incisions, thus limiting blood loss and operative time, and maintaining uterine integrity. Ideally, depending on the location, multiple

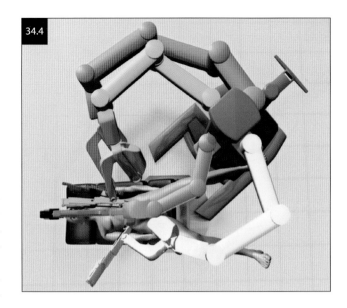
34.4

fibroids should be removed through a single incision. After the operative plan is created and communicated to the bedside assistants, dilute vasopressin, a potent vasoconstrictor, is often injected to minimize blood loss, although an off-label use. There are numerous dilutions that can be used, including 1 mL (20 units) in 100–200 cc of sterile saline. A small stab incision is made on the skin, and an 18-gauge spinal needle is introduced under direct visualization. The needle is manipulated using a grasper in the robotic arm and placed between the uterine serosa and fibroid pseudocapsule (Figure 34.5). After aspirating to confirm the needle is not intravascular, the dilute vasopressin is injected until blanching is noted throughout and around the fibroid. It is important to alert the anesthesiologist that dilute vasopressin is being injected, as it can cause transient tachycardia, hypertension, arrhythmias, and bronchospasm. If injected intravascularly, there is further risk of potential pulmonary edema, acute coronary spasm, and myocardial ischemia. Vasopressin injection may also be completed prior to

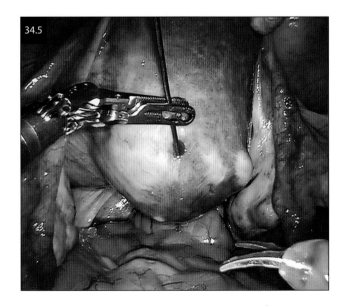
34.5

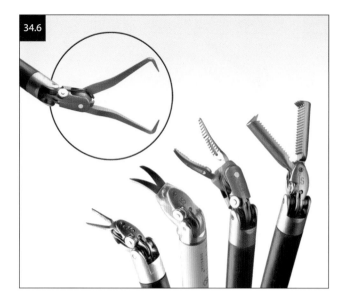

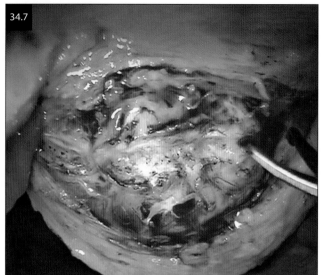

docking the robot, as at times the robotic arms can prevent one from obtaining the optimal angle for insertion of the needle.

Multiple robotic instruments can be used for a robotic myomectomy, but many surgeons find the best dissection results with a single-tooth tenaculum in their nondominant hand and a Hot Shears (Intuitive Surgical, Sunnyvale, California), or Harmonic Ace (Ethicon, Cincinnati, Ohio) in their dominant hand. If a third robotic arm is used, a ProGrasp or other grasping forceps, such as the long-tip forceps, can be useful to provide retraction and countertraction (Figure 34.6). The monopolar energy can be set up to 38 W on cut and 38 W on coagulate, which is the highest setting supported by Intuitive Surgical (Sunnyvale, California). Generally, the cutting current is utilized.

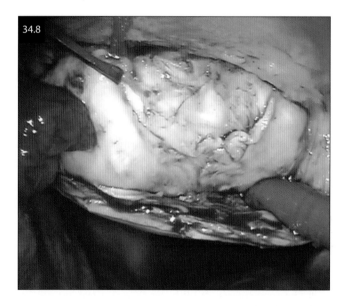

Intramural fibroids

For fibroids that are predominantly intramural, the direction of the incision can vary depending on the location within the uterus and the relative location of other fibroids. When two fibroids are adjacent to one another, one can often make a single incision to enucleate both fibroids. The incision is made using the cut function of the monopolar scissors and is generally as long as the fibroid (Figure 34.7). Once the pseudocapsule of the fibroid is entered, the tenaculum should be placed on the fibroid as close to the visible edge of the fibroid as possible (Figure 34.8). With traction applied to essentially "roll" the fibroid out of the capsule, the monopolar scissors or harmonic scalpel are used to separate any tissue fibers holding the fibroid in place (Figure 34.9). If the fibroid is not easy to enucleate from the pseudocapsule, one may not be deep enough, and additional dissection may be required.

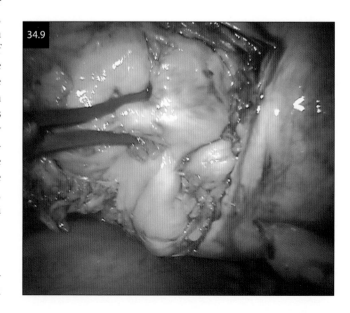

Subserosal fibroids

After injecting the uterine serosa with dilute vasopressin near, but not into, the stalk or base of the fibroid, a circumferential incision can be made approximately 2 cm above the base of the fibroid into the uterine serosa. This is to ensure that enough uterine serosa remains so that the incision can be reapproximated without excessive tension. One should not inject vasopressin directly into the base of the subserosal fibroid, as invariably the area is very vascular.

Extrauterine fibroids
Round ligament fibroids

These fibroids can often be treated similarly to intrauterine fibroids; care must be taken to identify the course of the ureter prior to creating the incision and the uterine vessels during the course of dissection. It is often best to make a horizontal incision, as the fibroid is often either incorporated with the uterus or directly adjacent to it. The decision to make the incision anteriorly or posteriorly on the broad ligament is based on which surface is distorted the most by the fibroid (Figure 34.10).

Parasitic fibroids

These fibroids are often iatrogenic in nature, as many arise after a prior laparoscopic or robotic myomectomy or hysterectomy with morcellation, but can sometimes occur *de novo*. They often implant in the pelvis, along the anterior abdominal wall, bowel, and bladder, but can also implant in the upper abdomen along the paracolic gutters and even under the diaphragm. If they are implanted on a thin stalk, this can be coagulated at the base, and the fibroid can be easily removed, but depending on the complexity of the implantation and location, consultation with colorectal surgery, urology, and possibly cardiothoracic surgery is warranted.

ENUCLEATION OF THE FIBROIDS

Enucleating the fibroids can sometimes be a formidable task and may require constant tension on the fibroid and simultaneous pulling by the robotic arm

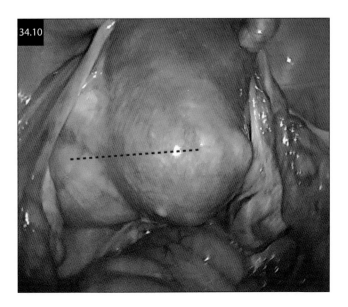

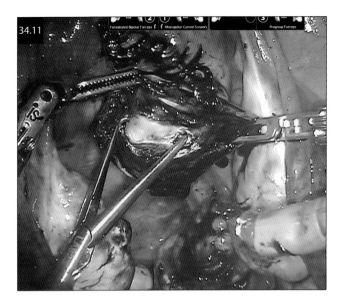

and coagulation/cutting using the unipolar scissors or harmonic scalpel. The upward tension on the fibroid can be achieved by placing the myoma screw or single-tooth tenaculum into the fibroid through the ancillary port and having the assistant provide the tension on the fibroid, or by applying the tension by the third robotic arm. The second robotic arm is used for countertension on the myometrium, while the right hand is used to cut the fibroid attachments using the harmonic scalpel or the unipolar electrode (Figure 34.11).

ADDITIONAL TECHNOLOGY

As mentioned above, fibroids can distort the orientation of the uterus making it difficult to determine the best approach to a myomectomy. One additional technology that the da Vinci Xi and Si systems offer is the ability to simultaneously view radiographic images with the three-dimensional endoscopic view, using Tile-Pro. This has been used extensively for radical and partial robotic-assisted nephrectomies, and has assisted in guiding surgeon dissection and location of tumor margin without having to leave the console to view radiographic images (Figure 34.12).

KEEPING TRACK OF FIBROIDS

Smaller fibroids can sometimes be removed immediately after dissection through a robotic or assistant trocar; very large fibroids can often be placed in the cul-de-sac or upper quadrants after dissection, as they are very unlikely to be lost. The majority of fibroids will require removal, at the completion of the procedure. In order to keep track of all removed fibroids, the circulator or scrub nurse must document throughout the procedure the total number of fibroids dissected out, those removed at the time of dissection, and those fibroids that remain *in situ*. If fibroids are too large to be removed, they can be loosely sutured to the abdominal wall. A 0 silk suture on

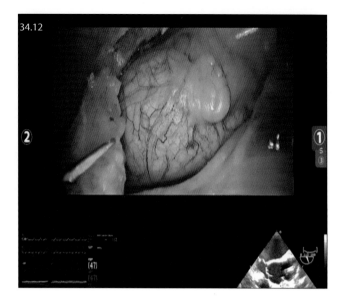

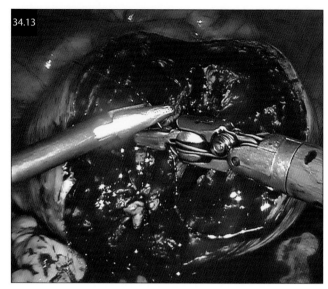

a Keith needle can be introduced through the abdominal wall, and the fibroids can be strung on this suture as they are excised. The needle is then secured into the anterior abdominal peritoneum until all fibroids are removed. The suture is often placed through the left lower quadrant in order to avoid interfering with visualization and further dissection.

SUTURING UTERUS

There are numerous combinations of instruments that can be used for suturing, but a popular combination for suturing the myometrium and sometimes endometrium is the mega needle driver in the dominant hand and ProGrasp in the nondominant hand. Some surgeons prefer to use two needle drivers or a needle driver and a long tip forceps, so trial and error is sometimes required in order to determine the best combination for each surgeon.

If an assistant trocar is placed, needles can be introduced and retrieved through this site. If only two robotic trocars are used, CT-1 and CT-2 needles can be introduced through these trocars, or through the camera trocar, but using the camera trocar can be more time consuming and potentially dangerous, as they are not introduced under direct visualization. If no assistant trocar is used, the needles are "parked" to the anterior abdominal wall and retrieved at the end of the case through the 12 mm trocar laparoscopically, after the robot is undocked.

Endometrial closure

Prior to choosing the suture, it should be determined whether the endometrial cavity has been entered. Sometimes it is rather obvious, as the uterine manipulator can be visualized, but at times it is more subtle. Methylene blue or indigo carmine can be injected through the uterine manipulator to determine exactly where the cavity was entered. If this is confirmed, the endometrium is reapproximated with an absorbable suture that causes minimal tissue reaction. Many surgeons prefer 3-0

Polydiaxanone Suture (PDS) (Ethicon, Cincinnati, Ohio) or any other delayed absorbable suture for this closure in an interrupted or mattress fashion placed into the myometrium, just above the endometrium (Figure 34.13). This suture does not need to be airtight, but should reapproximate the tissue.

Myometrial closure

After the endometrium is reapproximated, or if it does not require reapproximation, the myometrium should be closed in multiple layers. A variety of sutures can be used, but many surgeons prefer to use barbed suture. There are two types of barbed suture currently available, the V-Loc (Covidien, Mansfield, Massachusetts) and STRATAFIX (Ethicon, Cincinnati, Ohio). These sutures provide continuous, uniform tension across the suture line, and although much easier with the assistance of the robot, do not require any knot tying. For deeper fibroids, two or more layers may be required to reapproximate the myometrium (Figure 34.14). Although it may seem easier to use a longer suture when a large or deep defect requires closure, it is sometimes easier to use multiple 6 or 9 inch sutures, as suture management can be difficult. Alternatively, one can use a monofilament suture such as PDS, which slides through tissue easier than a braided suture. Depending on surgeon preference, "0" to 3-0 suture is utilized.

Serosal closure

After the myometrium is reapproximated, the serosa is closed in a baseball stitch fashion with either a 3-0 or 4-0 suture (Figure 34.15). This stitch minimizes the amount of suture at the surface, thus reducing adhesions. Again, a barbed suture can be used for this purpose, as the monofilament suture causes minimal inflammation and tissue abrasion. It is important to pull this suture through the tissue delicately yet firmly so excess suture and thus barbs are not left exposed, as it can increase the risk of postoperative adhesion formation.

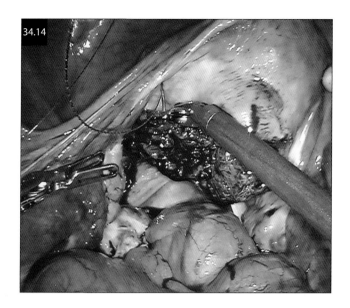

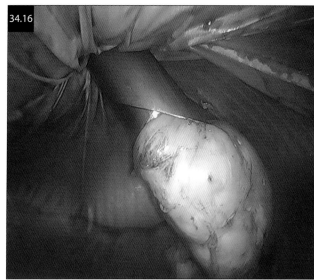

REMOVING FIBROIDS

After uterine reconstruction is complete, the 12 mm trocar is removed and the fascia dilated with uterine dilators to accommodate the morcellator. The robot can be undocked and the morcellation can be achieved with the laparoscopic camera. Recently, the U.S. Food and Drug Administration issued warnings regarding the use of laparoscopic power morcellation, due to the potential for undiagnosed malignancies to be disseminated in the abdomen and pelvis. Due to this announcement, some hospital systems and manufacturers have prohibited power morcellation and removed morcellators from the market. Conversely, some surgeons have collaborated with one another and manufacturers to determine ways to safely morcellate in a contained manner. Regardless of the method used to remove fibroids, it is essential that each patient is well informed of the risks, benefits, and alternatives that are available.

Several devices exist, and surgeon preference and device availability will often dictate what is used. Once

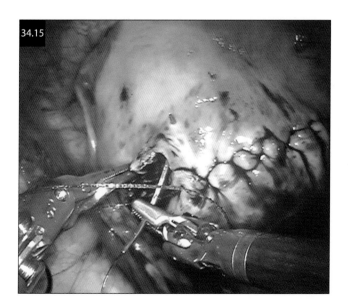

the morcellator is introduced, some have found it easier to navigate if the person operating the morcellator and the camera holder stand on the same side of the patient. This prevents the morcellator operator from having to pick up objects with a "backward" view of the camera. One technique of contained power morcellation involves placing a specimen bag in the abdomen, placing all of the fibroids in the bag, and then bringing the open end of the bag out of the abdomen. Either through a larger incision at the umbilicus that accommodates the morcellator and an angled scope, or by placing an accessory port into the bag, the specimen can be morcellated in a contained fashion while under constant, direct visualization (Figure 34.16).

PREVENTING ADHESIONS

Many surgeons prefer to place adhesion barriers, such as oxidized methylcellulose, Interceed (Ethicon Gynecare, Somerville, New Jersey) over the suture lines, although this is not currently an approved use by the FDA. It is important to remember that if Interceed is used, it should be placed on top of the hemostatic surface, and contact with blood should be avoided (Figures 34.17 and 34.18). Others will create a solution of saline and Seprafilm (Genzyme, Cambridge, Massachusetts) and spray it over the surgical site, but it should be noted that this is an off-label use.

PORT CLOSURE

Ports that are greater than 10 mm are at increased risk for hernia formation, and many recommend reapproximation of the fascia at these ports. There are several fascial device closures on the market that can assist with this process, including the Carter Thomason CloseSure system (Cooper Surgical Inc., Trumbull, Connecticut), or they can be closed with sutures from above.

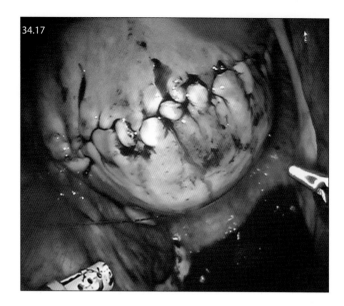

34.17

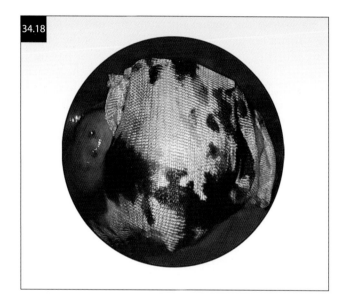

34.18

POSTOPERATIVE CONSIDERATIONS

As many patients who undergo myomectomies are interested in fertility, they should all be extensively counseled regarding the recovery period prior to attempting pregnancy. This period is often 3 months but is also surgeon and provider dependent. Many surgeons will obtain an ultrasound at this point to assess for uterine healing. Early data indicate that the uterine rupture rate after robotic-assisted myomectomies is similar to that after laparoscopic and open myomectomies. Once a successful pregnancy is achieved, if the myometrium was compromised during the myomectomy, the patient cannot labor and requires a cesarean section for delivery.

ACKNOWLEDGMENTS

Thank you to Dr. Aarathi Cholkeri-Singh for assisting in the editing of this chapter.

SUGGESTED READING

Catenacci M, Flyckt R, Falcone T. Robotics in reproductive surgery: Strengths and Limitations. *Placenta.* 2011;32:S232–S237.

Cohen LS, Valle RF. Role of vaginal sonography and hysterosonography in the endoscopic treatment of uterine myomas. *Fertil Steril.* 2000;73: 197–204.

Cohen S, Einarsson J, Wang K, et al. Contained power morcellation within an insufflated isolation bag. *Obstet Gynecol.* 2014;124:491–497.

Dueholm M, Lundorf E, Hansen ES et al. Accuracy of magnetic resonance imaging and transvaginal ultrasonography in the diagnosis, mapping and measurement of uterine myomas. *Am J Obstet Gynecol.* 2002;186:409–415.

Falcone T, Parker W. Surgical management of leiomyomas for fertility or uterine preservation. *Obstet Gynecol.* 2013;121:856–868.

Food and Drug Administration. FDA discourages use of laparoscopic power morcellation for removal of uterus or uterine fibroids. *FDA News Release.* April 17, 2014.

Greenberg J. The use of barbed sutures in obstetrics and gynecology. *Rev Obstet Gynecol.* 2010;3:82–91.

Hobo R, Netsu S, Koyasu Y, et al. Bradycardia and cardiac arrest caused by intramyometrial injection of vasopressin during a laparoscopically assisted myomectomy. *Obstet Gynecol.* 2009;113:484–486.

Kho K, Nezhat C. Parasitic myomas. *Obstet and Gynecol.* 2009;114:611–615.

Levens E, Wesley R, Premkumar A, et al. Magnetic resonance imaging and transvaginal ultrasound for determining fibroid burden: Implications for research and clinical care. *Am J Obstet Gynecol.* 2009;200:537.e1–e7.

Lonnerfors C, Persson J. Robot-assisted laparoscopic myomectomy; a feasible technique for removal of unfavorably localized myomas. *Acta Obstet Gynecol.* 2009;88:994–999.

Nezhat F, Admon D, Nezhat C, et al. Life-threatening hypotension after vasopressin injection during operative laparoscopy, followed by uneventful repeat laparoscopy. *J Am Assoc Gynec Lap.* 1994;2:83–86.

O'Donovan P, Miller CE. *Modern Management of Abnormal Uterine Bleeding.* London: CRC Press; 2008.

Ostrzenski A. Uterine leiomyoma particle growing in an abdominal-wall incision after laparoscopic retrieval. *Obstet Gynecol.* 1997;89:853–854.

Parker W. The utility of MRI for the surgical treatment of women with uterine fibroid tumors. *Am J Obstet Gynecol.* 2012;206:31–36.

Paul P, Koshy A. Multiple peritoneal parasitic myomas after laparoscopic myomectomy and morcellation. *Fertil and Steril.* 2006;85:492–493.

Quaas A, Einarsson J, Srouki S, et al. Robotic myomectomy: A review of indications and techniques. *Rev Obstet Gynecol.* 2010;3:185–191.

Rogers C, Laungani R, Bhandari A, et al. Maximizing console surgeon independence during robot-assisted renal surgery by using the fourth arm and TilePro. *J Endouro.* 2009;23:115–121.

Senapati S, Advincula A. Surgical techniques: Robot-assisted laparoscopic myomectomy with the da Vinci Surgical System. *J Robotic Surg.* 2007;1:69–74.

Sinha R, Hegde A, Mahajan C. Parasitic myoma under the diaphragm. *J Min Inv Gynecol.* 2007;14:1.

Sroga J, Patel S. Robotic applications in reproductive endocrinology and infertility. *J Robotic Surg.* 2008;2:3–10.

CHAPTER 35

ROBOTIC SACROCOLPOPEXY

Dobie Giles

HISTORY

Pelvic organ prolapse (POP) is a common condition with over 28 million women in the United States noted to have some aspect of this pelvic floor disorder. With an aging population, the U.S. Census population projections predict an increase in the pelvic floor disorders to over 43 million women by 2050. Today, approximately 160,000 surgeries are performed annually for POP. Unfortunately, about one in three women who have undergone surgery for prolapse or incontinence will undergo a repeat operation within 4 years.

Apical support has traditionally been treated with either a sacrocolpopexy or uterosacral suspension. This chapter focuses on sacrocolpopexy. In 1957, Arthure was the first to describe attaching the vagina and uterine complex to the anterior longitudinal ligament of the sacrum. In 1962, Lane suggested the use of an intervening graft between the vagina and the anterior longitudinal ligament to reduce excessive tension. The ideal fixation site at the sacrum has been debated. In 1973, Birnbaum recommended attachment to the S3-S4 region. However, by 1981 Sutton suggested the S1-S2 region because this location allowed for better visualization of the middle sacral artery without significantly changing the vagina axis.

As minimally invasive technology has advanced to allow for performance of complex surgical procedures, Nezhat published the first series of 15 patients to undergo laparoscopic sacrocolpopexy with 100% success rate at 3–40 months follow-up in 1994. Robotic surgery was later approved by the U.S. Food and Drug Administration for gynecologic surgery in 2005, and Elliott was the first to publish on a series of 30 patients undergoing robotic sacrocolpopexy in 2006.

PATIENT SELECTION

Traditionally, recurrent apical prolapse has been the indication for sacrocolpopexy. Recently, however, several authors suggest this procedure as a primary treatment of uterovaginal prolapse with or without retention of the uterus. If the concomitant hysterectomy is performed with sacrocolpopexy, total laparoscopic hysterectomy (with colpotomy and removal of the cervix) appears to increase the risk of mesh erosion. Therefore, most authors recommend a supracervical hysterectomy with attachment of the cervix and vagina to the sacral promontory.

PATIENT POSITIONING

The patient should be positioned on the operating table in the dorsal lithotomy position using boot-type stirrups. The arms are tucked to allow easy access to the patient. The use of foam or gel material is beneficial to prevent slippage while in Trendelenburg. The amount of Trendelenburg varies, but it should be enough to allow for visualization of the pelvis. A three-way catheter is placed and may be retrograde filled to aid in identifying the plane of dissection between the bladder and vagina. A probe is placed into the vagina to aid in dissection, and occasionally a rectal probe is utilized to help develop the rectovaginal space.

PORT PLACEMENT

The 12 mm camera port is typically placed at the umbilicus but may be placed more cephalad if a large uterus is encountered. Two 8 mm robotic ports are placed approximately 8–10 cm lateral and inferior to the camera port (one on each side).

The third robotic port is placed lateral and superior to the first robotic port on the ipsilateral side of the body relative to the patient cart, and a 10–12 mm assistant port is placed lateral and superior to the camera port on the opposite side of the body relative to the patient cart (Figure 35.1).

BOWEL MANIPULATION

After all ports are placed, the sigmoid should be retracted to the left to aid in development of the presacral space. The fourth arm can be used to provide this retraction by grasping an epiploic appendage. An alternative to this retraction technique is to place a straight needle with suture through the anterior abdominal wall, through an epiploic appendage, and back out through the abdominal wall.

SACRAL DISSECTION

After the bowel has been retracted to the left, the relevant anatomic structures should be identified, including the right ureter and the iliac (Figure 35.2). The sacral promontory should be palpated, typically by the bedside assistant due to the lack of haptic feedback for the

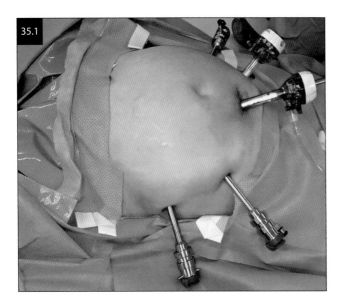

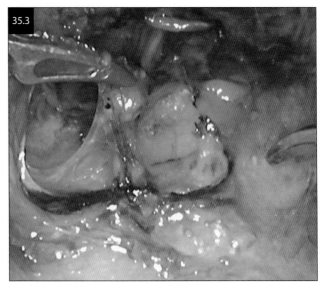

console surgeon. The peritoneum is elevated away from the underlying structures (Figure 35.3) and incised caudally. (This is more difficult in obese patients due to the amount of adipose tissue.) Extending the peritoneal incision caudally allows the CO_2 gas to aid in dissection of the presacral space. Be aware of the left iliac vein, which is inferior and medial to the left iliac artery. Continue to open the peritoneum and presacral adipose tissue until the anterior longitudinal ligament is identified (Figure 35.4). The middle sacral artery courses through this area of suture placement, and it can be cauterized prior to suture placement if necessary. Open the remainder of the peritoneum from the sacral promontory to the vaginal cuff, remaining cognizant of the path of the right ureter (Figure 35.5).

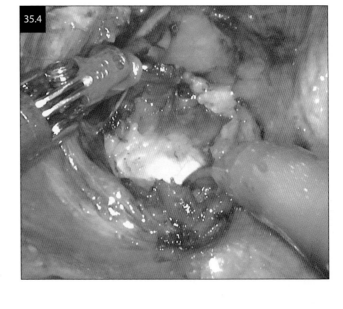

ANTERIOR DISSECTION

With a probe in the vagina, incise the peritoneum over the apex and dissect caudally. The goal is to continue

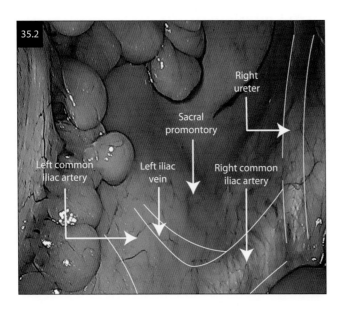

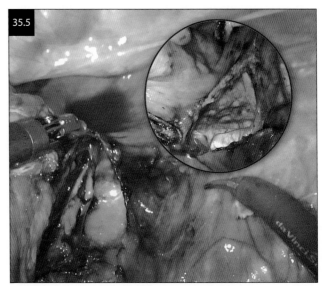

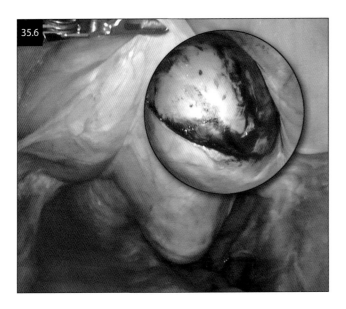

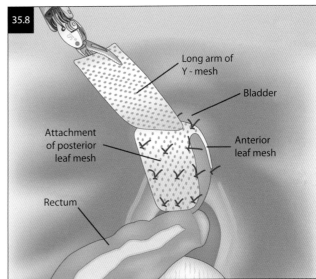

this dissection to the trigone. The fourth arm may be used to provide countertraction of the bladder anteriorly (Figure 35.6). The catheter bulb can be utilized to assist in identifying the area of the trigone. As the trigone is approached, lateral dissection is limited because of the risk of ureteral damage. At times, backfilling the bladder through the three-way Foley catheter aids in identifying dissection planes.

POSTERIOR DISSECTION

A rectal probe may assist in dissection (Figure 35.7). Dissect the rectovaginal space as caudally as possible depending on the length of the vagina. Some authors advocate dissection to the perineal body.

CHOICE OF SUTURE

Attachment of the mesh to the anterior and posterior vagina (Figure 35.8) can be achieved with numerous types

of sutures. Some advocate delayed absorbable, while others prefer permanent. Barbed sutures have been utilized as well. The mesh is typically attached to the vagina with four to eight sutures per side (Figure 35.9). A 30° scope angled up can improve visualization of the posterior dissection (Figure 35.10). Typically four to six sutures are placed posteriorly. Attachment to the sacrum is accomplished with two permanent sutures through the anterior longitudinal ligament (Figure 35.11). Sacral tacking is also acceptable. However, care should be taken to avoid deep penetration of the disc spaces as serious complications such as discitis have been reported. The mesh should be adjusted to provide support without tension to the vagina, as this has been associated with increased risk of stress urinary incontinence. Care must be taken not to put too much tension on the mesh since the mesh will shrink over time. The surgeon should perform a vaginal exam to verify correct tension. The peritoneum is then closed with an absorbable suture in a running fashion (Figure 35.12). This closure retroperitonealizes the mesh

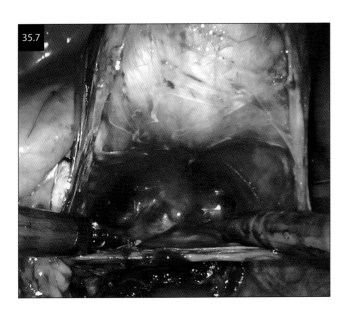

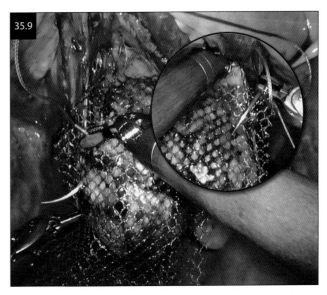

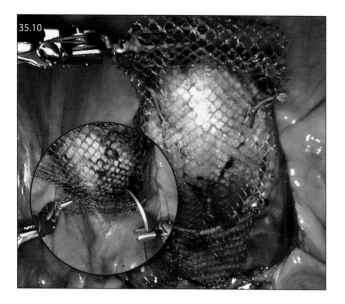

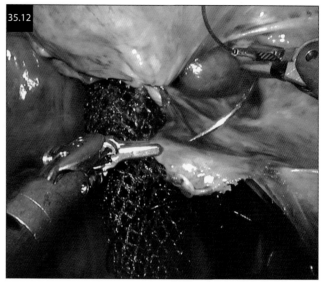

along the right pelvic sidewall and is advocated to avoid bowel complications (Figure 35.13).

CYSTOSCOPY

Cystoscopy should be performed at the completion of the procedure to ensure no damage or kinking occurred to the ureters or bladder. Intravenous indigo carmine (3–5 mg) is given, and then utilizing a 70° cystoscope, the bladder and trigone are carefully inspected. Vigorous, equal, bilateral efflux of indigo carmine should be noted as well as confirming that no inadvertent damage to the bladder has occurred.

COMPLICATIONS

The most serious complication of sacrocolpopexy is vascular injury. This complication can occur with dissection of the presacral space or suture placement and typically results from injury to the iliac vessels or

injury to the middle sacral artery or vein. The first step in management is to control bleeding using direct pressure. The addition of a hemostatic matrix may also be beneficial. If the bleeding originates from the middle sacral artery or vein, one can use electrical energy or place a sacral tack.

The rectum is also susceptible to injury when dissecting the rectovaginal space. If a rectal injury occurs, most would recommend closing the injury and proceeding with a uterosacral suspension instead of placing a foreign material. If the bladder is injured, a two-layer closure with absorbable suture is usually sufficient. If accidental entry into the vagina occurs, then the defect can be closed with interrupted sutures. Do not affix the mesh to the vaginotomy so as to decrease risk of mesh erosion.

SACROHYSTEROPEXY

Patients may choose to retain their uterus for a number of reasons. Costantini reported on the largest series of

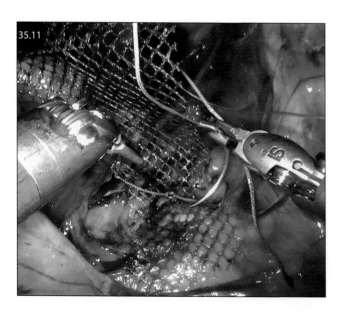

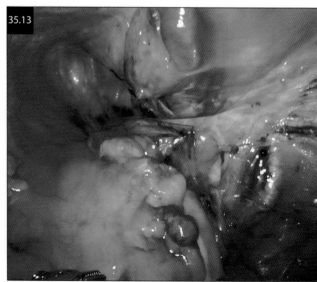

55 patients with a 60-month follow-up. Successful pregnancies have been reported, but the data are limited.

OUTCOMES

Abdominal sacrocolpopexy is considered the gold standard for prolapse repair and has a reported success rate between 78% and 100%. The Cochrane review analyzed 40 randomized controlled trials involving 3773 women and demonstrated that abdominal sacrocolpopexy had a better success rate than vaginal repairs with less recurrent vault prolapse and less dyspareunia. There are no Cochrane review data available on the success rate of minimally invasive sacrocolpopexy. Several studies have shown the short-term success of minimally invasive sacrocolpopexy to be comparable to abdominal sacrocolpopexy. One disadvantage to robotic sacrocolpopexy has been associated with increased cost when compared to laparoscopic sacrocolpopexy. Paraiso et al. reported on the only blinded RCT of 78 patients, which showed a longer operating room time associated with robotic sacrocolpopexy with no difference in success rates.

CONCLUSION

Robotic sacrocolpopexy is a safe procedure for apical vaginal prolapse. This procedure has been performed since 2006 with good short-term results, but long-term data are needed.

SUGGESTED READING

Collins SA. Complex sacral abscess 8 years after abdominal sacral colpopexy. *Obstet Gynecol.* 2011;118:451–454.

Diwadkar GB, Chen Chi Chiung Grace, Paraiso Marie Fidela R et al. An update on the laparoscopic approach to urogynecology and pelvic reconstructive procedures. *Curr Opin Obstet Gynecol.* 2008;20:496–500.

Flynn MK, Mark ER, Allen AW et al. Abdominal surgery for pelvic organ prolapse. *J Pelvic Med Surg.* 2007;13(4):157–170.

Frick AC, Paraiso Marie Fidela R et al. Laparoscopic management of incontinence and pelvic organ prolapse. *Clin Obstet Gynecol.* 2009;52(3):390–400.

Klauschie JL, Cornella JC. Surgical treatment of vaginal vault prolapse: A historic summary and review of outcomes. *Female Pelvic Med Reconstr Surg.* 2012;18(1):8–15.

Maher C, Feiner B, Baessler K, Adams EJ, Hagen S, Glazener CM. Surgical management of pelvic organ prolapse in women. *Cochrane Database Syst Rev.* 2010:(4):CD004014.

Novara G, Artibani W. Surgery for pelvic organ prolapse: Current status and future perspectives. *Curr Opin Urol.* 2005;15:256–262.

Paraiso MF, Jelovesek JE, Frick A, Chen CCG, Barber MD. Laparoscopic compared with robotic sacrocolpopexy for vaginal prolapse. A randomized controlled trial. *Obstet Gynecol.* 2011;118:1005–1013.

Tan-Kim J, Menefee Shawn A, Luber Karl M et al. Robotic-assisted and laparoscopic sacrocolpopexy: Comparing operative times, costs and outcomes. *Female Pelvic Med Reconstr Surg.* 2011;17(1):44–49.

Chapter 36

ROBOTICALLY ASSISTED RADICAL HYSTERECTOMY

Antonio Gil-Moreno, Javier F. Magrina, Paul Magtibay III, Paul M. Magtibay, and Melchor Carbonell-Socias

TECHNIQUES

The terminology of the autonomic pelvic nerves, for purposes of the nerve-sparing technique and according to the Anatomic Terminology of 1978, consists of the superior hypogastric plexus (sympathetic), pelvic splanchnic nerves (parasympathetic), and inferior hypogastric plexus (sympathetic and parasympathetic). Figure 36.1a represents the superior and inferior hypogastric plexus and splanchnic nerves that originate from S2, S3, and S4, viewed from the right side of the pelvis. The inferior hypogastric plexus (IHP) has been mobilized laterally from the right uterosacral ligament. In Figure 36.1b, the pelvic splanchnic nerves are seen joining the IHP in a perpendicular fashion (a, superior vesical artery; b, inferior hypogastric plexus; c, pelvic splanchnic nerve; d, ureter; e, hypogastric nerve; f, uterine artery; g, pararectal space).

In the nerve-sparing technique (C1) the inferior hypogastric plexus, the pelvic splanchnic nerves and the inferior hypogastric efferent nerves to the bladder and vagina are preserved, as opposed by the conventional C2 technique. In the B or modified radical hysterectomy technique, identification of the autonomic nerves is not required. Whenever possible, the nerve-sparing technique is preferable since postoperative bladder function, rectal function, and vaginal lubrication remained unchanged without compromising recurrence or survival. This technique is more commonly used in Japan, where it originated (Tokyo method), and in some European centers in Italy, Belgium, Germany, and Spain. It is becoming more commonly used in the United States due to the spread of robotic technology among gynecologic oncologists.

INDICATIONS

The extent of paracervical resection described with the robotic technique here is designated as radical hysterectomy type C1 of the revised classification of radical hysterectomy. The nerve-sparing technique was first introduced in this standard classification.

The B or modified radical hysterectomy technique is indicated for patients with cervical cancer ≤2 cm, and the type C1, which is detailed in this chapter, is indicated for cases >2 cm diameter, up to 4 cm. The extent of vaginal resection is dependent on the location of the tumor margins. The location of the ectocervical margin of the tumor will dictate whether a small or a longer segment of vaginal cuff is needed for adequate margins. In patients with a margin near or involving the vaginal fornix, a longer segment of vagina will be necessary.

PATIENT PREPARATION

A preoperative medical examination is routinely performed 1 or 2 days before the surgery day to identify any subclinical conditions that may represent a risk or the need for a change in anesthesia. The day before surgery, the patient has normal oral intake until midnight. She is allowed clear oral liquids until 2 hours before surgery, which is the time when she is admitted to the hospital. Cefotetan 1 g or Cefazolin 2 g IV is given 1 hour before surgery in the preoperative area and repeated 3 hours into the operation.

PATIENT POSITIONING

The patient is placed in the semilithotomy position using Allen stirrups. Arms are tucked in bilaterally. Arms and legs are foam padded to protect injury. To prevent sliding during the much needed Trendelenburg position during the procedure, an egg crate mattress is fastened with wide tape to the operating room table, and the patient's bare back lays directly on it. An antiskid foam material (Tyco/Kendall Prod #3-472, Mansfield, Massachusetts) has been evaluated for this purpose and found to be satisfactory. This also avoids the risk of cervical plexus injury associated with the use of inappropriately placed shoulder straps. A Foley catheter is inserted into the bladder. The patient is placed in Trendelenburg prior to prepping and draping to determine if there is any degree of sliding. She is then returned to a flat position and prepped and draped as customary.

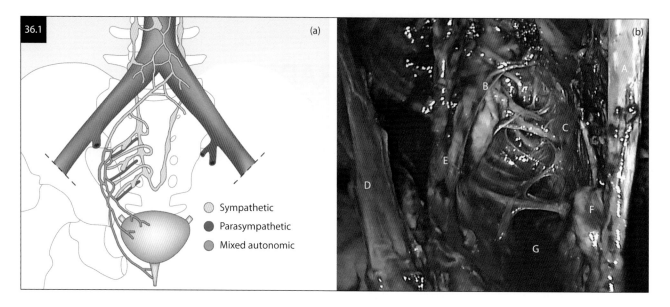

ENTRY

A transumbilical open technique with a 12 mm trocar (8 mm with the da Vinci Xi) is used for all patients. The incision is made at the deepest part of the umbilicus, where one finds the shortest distance between the skin and the abdominal wall fascia. The upper abdomen is explored in the supine position. The patient is then placed in the Trendelenburg position, enough to displace the sigmoid and small bowel out of the pelvis and allow a safe pelvic operation.

ROBOTIC COLUMN POSITION

The da Vinci Si or da Vinci Xi robotic systems (Intuitive Surgical, Sunnyvale, California) are adequate for the operation. The da Vinci robotic column is side-docked to the patient's right knee. This allows direct access to the vagina for the identification of the vaginal fornices with a vaginal probe (Apple Medical Rectal Probe, Marlborough, Massachusetts) and removal of the uterus by the assistant. Our preference is the use of a vaginal probe and not a uterine manipulator, since it provides similar information with minimal time to insert.

TROCAR PLACEMENT

Two robotic trocars (8 mm each) are introduced 8 cm to the right and left of the umbilical optical trocar and at the same level of the umbilicus. An assistant trocar (10 mm) is placed midway and 2 cm cranial to the umbilical and left trocar in all patients. Another robotic trocar (8 mm), designated as the right or fourth robotic arm, is introduced 7–8 cm lateral and 3 cm cranial to the umbilical trocar. The configuration of the trocars for radical hysterectomy and pelvic lymphadenectomy is like a crescent with upper convexity, and it is presented in Figure 36.2. The Xi system has an easier docking mechanism as compared to the Si system.

INSTRUMENTS

The robotic instruments as well as the surgeon console are the same for the Si and Xi systems. An EndoWrist PK grasper (Intuitive Inc., Sunnyvale, California) is used on the left robotic arm, and an EndoWrist monopolar scissors or spatula (Intuitive Inc., Sunnyvale, California) is used in the right robotic arm. The EndoWrist Prograsper (Intuitive Inc., Sunnyvale, California) is used in the right lateral robotic arm to assist with retraction. An EndoWrist needle holder (Intuitive Inc, Sunnyvale, California) is used to replace the monopolar scissors/spatula to suture the vaginal cuff.

The assistant sits to the left of the patient and performs the functions of sealing and division of vascular pedicles with a vessel sealer device, suction and irrigation, removal of small specimens, additional tissue retraction, and insertion and removal of sutures for closure of the vaginal cuff. A second assistant, sitting between the legs of the patient, manipulates a vaginal probe (Apple

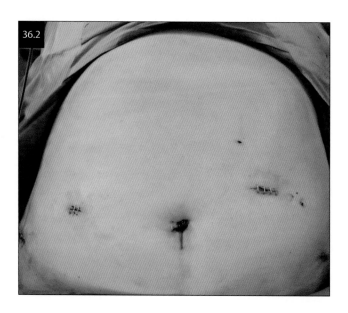

Medical, Marlborough, Massachusetts) for bladder dissection and during colpotomy and removes the uterus and lymph nodes vaginally (with Endobags). The nurse sitting to the right of the patient cleans the lens of the laparoscope, switches the monopolar scissors or spatula for a needle holder, and maintains pneumoperitoneum during vaginal transection. A colpo-occluder balloon (RUMI Colpo-occluder, Cooper Medical, Trumbull, Connecticut) is placed in the vagina to maintain pneumoperitoneum after removal of the specimen. No uterine manipulator is used.

OPENING THE LATERAL PELVIC SPACES

After inspection of the abdominal cavity to exclude carcinomatosis, an incision is made with the monopolar scissors or spatula over the peritoneum, lateral and parallel to the infundibulopelvic ligament, starting at a level cranial to the pelvic brim and continuing in a caudal direction lateral to the external iliac vessels toward the outer third of the round ligament. The round ligament is then transected and the incision continued over the anterior leaf of the broad ligament in the direction of the vesico-uterine fold (Figure 36.3).

The bifurcation of the common iliac artery is identified at the pelvic brim. The dissection is continued immediately over the hypogastric (internal iliac) artery in a caudal direction until the anterior bifurcation is found by simply separating the loose connective tissue with the PK grasper. The superior vesical artery (a branch of the umbilical artery) is followed to the upper lateral aspect of the bladder. The ureter is identified attached to the pelvic peritoneum, and the main blood vessels are also identified (Figure 36.4).

DEVELOPMENT OF PARAVESICAL SPACE

Anterolateral to the superior vesical artery and medial to the external iliac vein, we find a safe point of entry to the

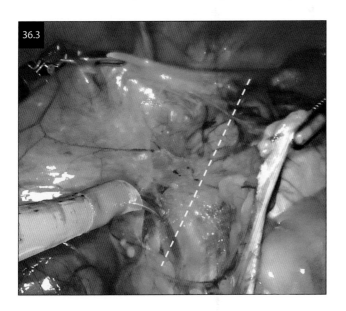

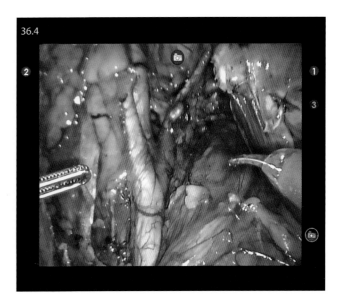

paravesical space. The space is created by dissecting in a dorsal and caudal direction the loose connective tissue, by traction and countertraction medially and laterally, respectively, in successive steps, until the pelvic floor (levator ani muscle) is reached. The external iliac vessels and obturator nodes constitute the lateral wall, the paracervical tissue or parametrium the posterior aspect, the bladder the medial wall, and the pubic bone the anterior boundary. Dissection of the left side is shown in Figure 36.5a (A, paravesical space; B, pararectal space; C, superior vesical artery; D, uterine artery; E, uterine vein; F, internal iliac artery; G, external iliac vein; H, external iliac artery). The dissection of the uterine vessels (left side) is shown in Figure 36.5b (A, paravesical space; B, deep uterine vein; C, uterine artery).

DEVELOPMENT OF PARARECTAL SPACE

The ureter is found attached to the lateral pelvic peritoneum and is traced until crossing the uterine artery. Immediately posteromedial to the superior vesical artery, medial to the hypogastric artery, and lateral to the ureter, we find the safe point of entry to the pararectal space. Separating the loose connective tissue in a caudal and dorsal direction by medial and lateral traction and countertraction, respectively, in successive steps, the space is developed. The right and left pararectal spaces are shown in Figure 36.6a and b. The hypogastric artery and vein lay on the lateral wall, the rectum medially, the sacrum posteriorly, and the parametrium anteriorly.

As part of the nerve-sparing technique, the pelvic splanchnic nerves (parasympathetic) are identified in the dorsal and lowermost aspect of the pararectal space. They originate from S2, S3, and S4 anterior roots of the sacral plexus and can be seen coursing toward the medial and lower aspect of the parametrium. The left pelvic splanchnic nerves can be appreciated at the lowermost and dorsal aspect of the pararectal space

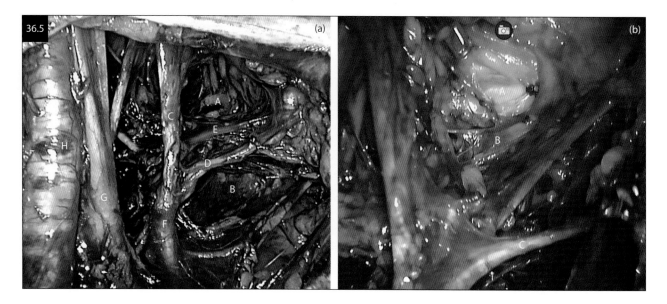

(Figure 36.7a: A, deep uterine vein; B, left hypogastric vein; C, left pararectal space; D, splanchnic nerves; Figure 36.7b: A, left pararectal space; B, deep uterine vein; C, splanchnic nerves). There they join the inferior hypogastric nerve, which contains sympathetic nerves coming from the superior hypogastric plexus. The right pelvic splanchnic nerves can be appreciated at the lowermost and dorsal aspect of the pararectal space coursing to the dorsal and medial aspect of the parametrium, where they fuse with the hypogastric nerve, forming the pelvic plexus. Figure 36.7c shows the anatomical view of pelvic autonomic nerves, right side (radical hysterectomy type C1): A, superior vesical artery; B, intern obturator muscle; C, obturator fossa; D, transected uterine artery; E, inferior hypogastric plexus; F, obturator vein; G, obturator nerve; H, ureter; I, pelvic splanchnic nerve; J, external iliac vein; K, hypogastric nerve; and L, pararectal space.

The ventral branches of the inferior hypogastric plexus provide innervation to the uterus (uterine branches), and its caudal (efferent) branches supply the bladder (vesical branches) and vagina (vaginal branches).

MANAGEMENT OF THE ADNEXA

In case of adnexal removal, a peritoneal window is made between the ureter and the infundibulopelvic ligament, which is then divided with a vessel sealer at the level of the pelvic brim. This window prevents ureteral injury at this level. If the adnexa are preserved, the tuboovarian pedicles are divided, as well as their peritoneal attachments, and placed above the pelvic brim. If there are other risk factors, an ovariopexy may be carried out in order to remove the ovary of a possible field of pelvic radiation.

PELVIC AND AORTIC LYMPHADENECTOMY

A systematic bilateral pelvic lymphadenectomy from the common iliac artery to the inferior boundary of the

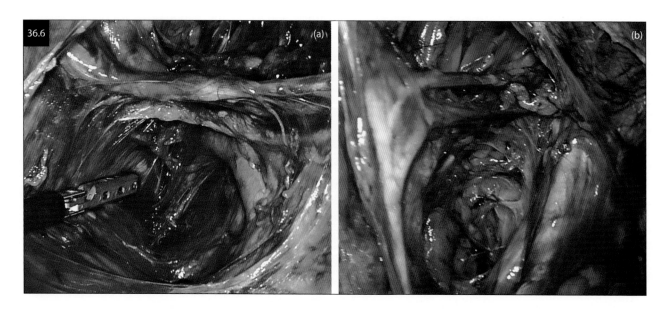

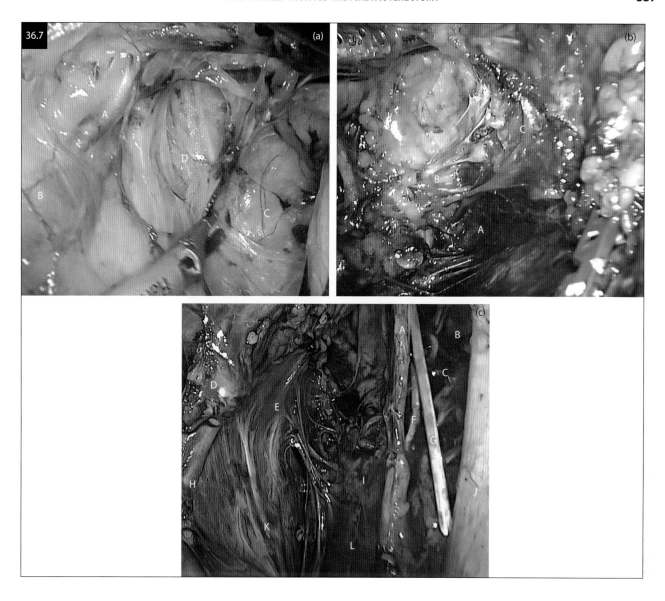

circumflex iliac vein is performed after the sentinel node procedure. If the sentinel node is positive, the patient will receive radiotherapy, and radical hysterectomy should be avoided due to the increased morbidity of using both treatment modalities. In these cases, systematic pelvic and paraaortic lymphadenectomy is done to limit the irradiation field.

Pelvic lymphadenectomy is usually performed first, because it facilitates the identification of retroperitoneal anatomical structures, especially the autonomic pelvic nerves. The external iliac nodes, from the bifurcation of the common iliac vessels to the inguinal ligament, the obturator nodes above and below the obturator nerve, the ventral and lateral nodes of the hypogastric artery, and the ventral and lateral common iliac nodes from the middle of the common iliac vessels, are removed bilaterally using the PK grasper and monopolar scissors/spatula. We have the capability to obtain a frozen section of the removed nodes, which facilitates whether additional pelvic nodes and the aortic nodes need removal.

In the presence of positive sentinel node or positive pelvic nodes, a bilateral aortic lymphadenectomy is carried out up to the renal vessels. Using the same trocar placement and instruments, the inframesenteric nodes can be safely removed. For the infrarenal nodes, the robotic system arms are undocked and the operating table rotated 180°, resulting in the robotic column being now located at the patient's head or lateral to the right shoulder. You can also change the location of the robot (lateral to the right shoulder) without having to rotate the operating table. Two to three trocars are placed suprapubically, one or two for the assistant and one for the endoscopic camera (12 mm, but 8 mm with da Vinci Xi). The robotic arms are redocked, and using the same robotic instruments, the aortic lymphadenectomy is extended to the infrarenal nodes, up to the level of the renal vessels. The benefit of removing positive aortic nodes has been addressed in recent literature. Our technique and experience with infrarenal aortic lymphadenectomy and rotation of the operating table have also been described.

The new da Vinci Xi system allows rotation of the robotic arms after undocking them from the pelvic position without the need to rotate the operating table or modify the location of the robot column. Once the arms are rotated 180° they are docked again. However, it still requires the placement of additional trocars suprapubically for the optical trocar and assistant.

IDENTIFICATION AND DIVISION OF THE PARAMETRIUM

The parametrium is the dorsal continuation of paracervical tissue, inserting into the upper third of the vagina and lower cervix and reaching in a posterolateral direction the pelvic wall. It inserts in the pelvic wall in a triangular fashion, its apex resting at the level of the anterior division of the hypogastric artery and the base, on the lateral pelvic wall. The parametrium separates the paravesical from the pararectal space, and once divided there will be a single pelvic lateral space. In the division of the right parametrium, the divided ends of the uterine artery

are noted. The vascular portion of the parametrium has been divided with the sealer vessels to the level of the deep uterine vein. The transection is then carried out in a medial and dorsal direction to preserve the pelvic plexus. The hypogastric nerve is retracted medially by the grabber, exposing the pararectal space (Figure 36.8a). The left parametrium is shown in Figure 36.8b (A, paravaginal space; B, pararectal space).

The nervous part or nerve-containing portion of the parametrium is located at its dorsal aspect, where dense connective tissue is present. By preserving this lower dense part, the splanchnic nerves are spared.

In the nerve-sparing technique, the uterine artery is divided selectively by the assistant with the use of a vessel sealing device and continues with the division of the parametrium dorsally with successive applications (Figure 36.8c). The vascular or ventral portion of the parametrium is divided only up to the level of the deep uterine vein, which is transected at its origin from the internal iliac vein. Below that level, thicker, dense connective tissue is identified at the beginning of the nerve-containing

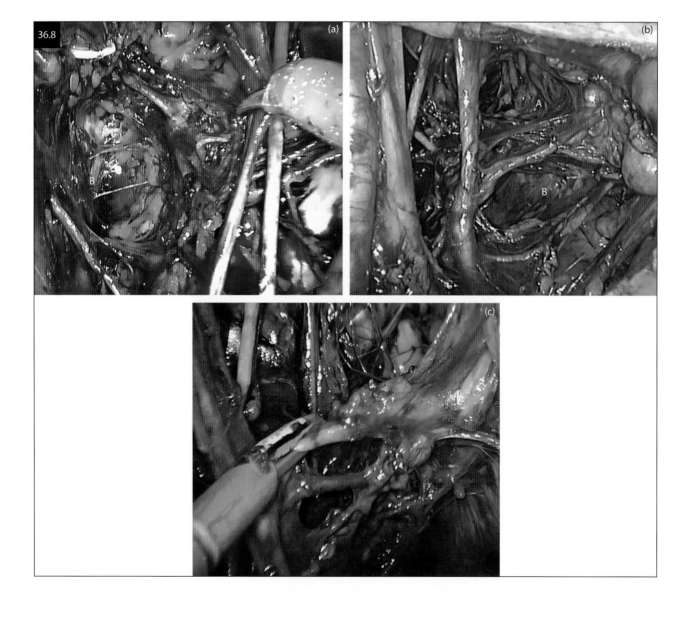

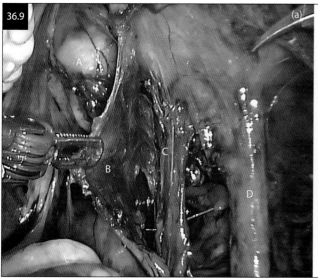
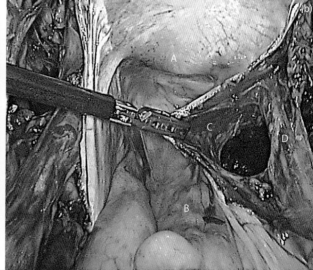

section of the parametrium (parasympathetic splanchnic pelvic nerves).

MOBILIZATION OF THE URETER FROM THE MEDIAL ASPECT OF THE PELVIC PERITONEUM

The ureter is mobilized from the pelvic peritoneum by coagulating with the monopolar scissors or spatula at its peritoneal attachments, about 5 mm ventral and parallel to its course, and developing a dissecting plane between the ureter and the pelvic peritoneum. The dissected anatomical view on the right side is shown in Figure 36.9a (A, Douglas space; B, peritoneal leaf; C, inferior hypogastric nerve; D, ureter). Figure 36.9b represents the anatomical view from the right side: A, posterior view of the uterus; B, sigma; C, peritoneal leaf; D, ureter. This dissection is carried caudally until the uterine artery is identified. A ureter that appears "naked" (markedly white) has been dissected in the wrong plane, and because its adventitia has been removed, it carries the risk of ischemia with subsequent development of stricture or fistula if the "naked" area includes a long segment.

The pelvic peritoneum is divided at the level of the planned division of the uterosacral ligaments, and the division is carried until it reaches the upper border of the uterosacral ligament.

DEVELOPMENT OF THE RECTOVAGINAL SPACE AND DIVISION OF THE UTEROSACRAL LIGAMENTS

By downward traction on the peritoneum at the most caudal portion of the posterior cul-de-sac, and upward traction on the uterus with the robotic grasper, a transverse incision is made with the monopolar scissors or spatula across the most dependent portion of the cul-de-sac and anterior to the rectum. The transected edges of the peritoneum will separate due to the traction on the tissues.

The loose connective tissue of the rectovaginal space is separated by traction and countertraction in a ventral and dorsal direction, respectively. When dissecting in this space, the surgeon must be aware that the fat belongs to the rectum. In the rare case where the anterior rectal wall cannot be clearly identified, a rectal probe (Apple Medical Rectal Probe, Marlborough, Massachusetts) inserted in the rectum and advanced to that level will facilitate its identification. The rectum is displaced dorsally at its lateral borders where it is in contact with the uterosacral ligaments, and the uterosacral ligaments become apparent. The inferior hypogastric nerves are identified on the lateral aspect of the uterosacral ligament (Figure 36.10). Figure 36.11 represents the posterior view of the uterus, left side (A, Douglas space; B, uterosacral ligament; C, inferior hypogastric nerve; D, ureter).

The PK grasper is used to create a space between the inferior hypogastric nerves and the lateral aspect of the

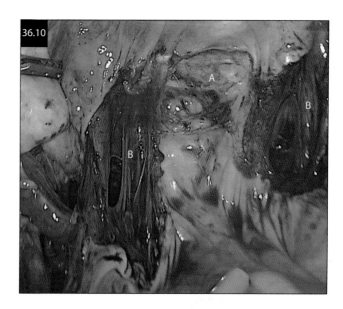

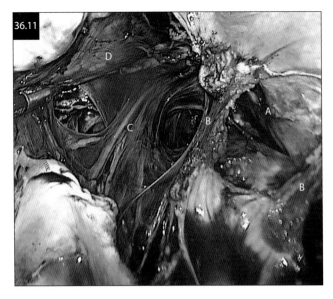

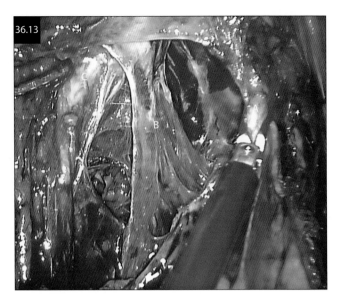

uterosacral ligament by blunt dissection. These nerves are isolated and separated from the uterosacral ligaments and must be preserved (Figure 36.12). Figure 36.12 represents the dissection and identification of the left inferior hypogastric nerve. A space has been developed between the soft lateral aspect of the uterosacral ligament containing the hypogastric nerve and the left uterosacral ligament. The uterosacral can then be divided, preserving the inferior hypogastric nerve (A, Douglas space; B, uterosacral ligament; C, inferior hypogastric nerve; D, ureter; E, obturator nerve; F, vein obturator).

The uterosacral ligaments are selectively divided (without including the inferior hypogastric nerves) at the level of the anterior rectal wall and to their attachment to the posterior vaginal wall with the vascular sealer (Figure 36.13).

DEVELOPMENT OF THE VESICOVAGINAL SPACE

With ventral traction on the bladder using the Prograsp, and dorsal and cranial traction on the uterus by the

assistant, the monopolar scissors are used to transect the peritoneum transversally at the level of the vesicouterine fold (Figure 36.14). The edges of the transected peritoneum will separate due to the traction on the tissue. With the monopolar scissors/spatula, the loose connective tissue between the bladder and vagina is dissected by traction and countertraction in a ventral and dorsal direction, respectively. Short touches of the monopolar scissors or spatula are applied when necessary. To assist in the dissection, a vaginal probe (Apple Medical Rectal Probe, Marlborough, Massachusetts; Koh inflatable ring; Cooper Surgical Colpopneumo occluder, Trumbull, Connecticut) is introduced into the vagina by the assistant and advanced toward the anterior vaginal wall. This facilitates the identification of the anterior vaginal wall and its separation from the bladder wall.

The dissection is carried until the full upper third of the vagina is exposed. It is important to remain in the midline of the vesicovaginal space until the lower limit of the dissection is reached, since there are no blood vessels in that area. The vesicouterine ligaments

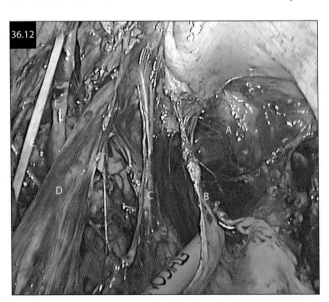

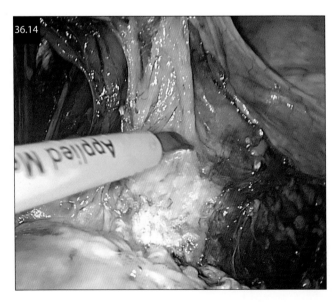

containing blood vessels are the lateral limits of the vesicovaginal space.

DISSECTION OF THE PARAMETRIAL URETER (URETERAL TUNNEL)

The ureter is followed until its entrance into the parametrial tunnel. A space is created with the monopolar scissors or spatula, and the PK grasper is immediately placed above the ureter at the 12 o'clock position until the instrument appears on the vesicovaginal space (Figure 36.15). The space is widened until the posterior blade of the vessel sealer can be introduced in the created space above the ureter.

The ventral part of the vesicouterine ligament is then transected. These steps are repeated until the ventral vesicouterine ligament is transected completely and the ureter is unroofed (Figure 36.16). It is then mobilized laterally by dividing with the monopolar device its loose attachments to the dorsal aspect of the vesicouterine ligament, until the latter is exposed and identified. While the assistant is holding the ureter ventrally, the avascular space located immediately below the entrance of the ureter into the bladder is identified and widened with the monopolar spatula/scissors, clearly delineating the dorsal vesicouterine ligament (Figure 36.17), which is transected by the assistant using a vessel sealer.

The dorsal and lateral portions of the posterior vesicouterine ligament contain the vesical branches of the inferior hypogastric plexus, which provide innervation to the bladder and vagina. There they can be identified and separated by blunt dissection from the vascular portion of that ligament. By selectively dividing the vascular part of the ligament, the vesical and vaginal autonomic nerves can be spared. This results in complete mobilization of the ureter from the vesicouterine ligament and parametrium with preservation of the vesical branches of the inferior hypogastric plexus. Additionally, the blood supply to the distal portion of the ureter is preserved,

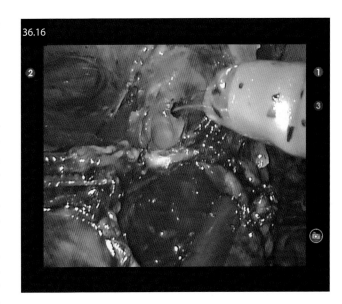

reducing the risk of ischemia and the potential for subsequent stricture or fistula formation. The entire right anterior vesicouterine ligament has been divided with successive applications of the Enseal. The parametrial portion of the right ureter is exposed to its insertion into the bladder. The parametrial ureter has been retracted medially, exposing the posterior vesicouterine ligament. At the junction of the ureter into the bladder and the lateral edge of the vagina, an avascular space is identified. It is the entry point for the division of the posterior vesicouterine ligament (Figure 36.18).

The right posterior vesicouterine ligament has been divided, and the ureter is now totally free from its attachments and can be further elevated ventrally (Figure 36.19).

DIVISION OF PARAVAGINAL TISSUE

With the transected parametrium retracted ventrally and the ureter laterally, the paravaginal tissue is exposed. The vesical branches of the inferior hypogastric plexus

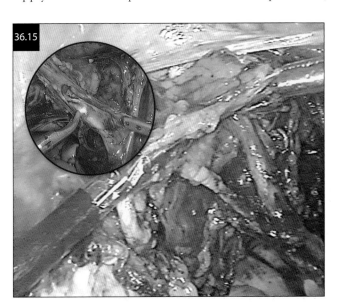

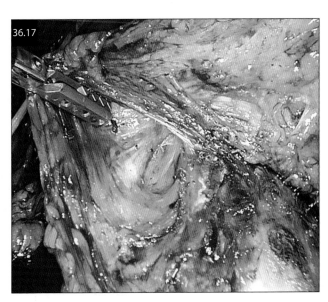

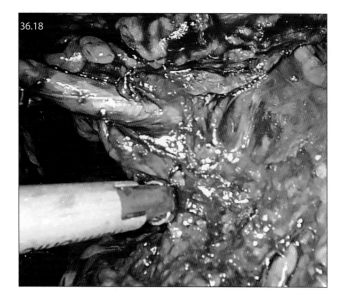

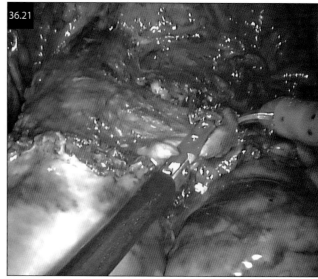

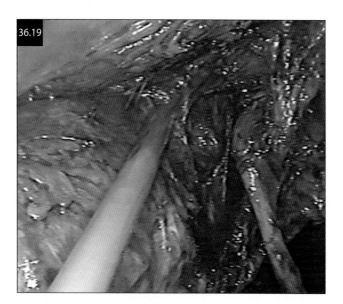

run along the lateral edge of the vagina where they are identified and gently mobilized dorsally, below the lower portion of the transected parametrium and below the planned level of transection of the vagina. Figure 36.20 represents the view of the right side of the pelvis. The distal fibers of the inferior hypogastric plexus run toward the vagina and bladder along the dorsal vesicouterine ligament and the lateral wall of the vagina (A, bladder; B, inferior and middle vesical veins; C, distal fibers of the inferior hypogastric plexus to the bladder and vagina— vesical plexus or bladder branch; D, vaginal cuff; E, ureter; F, hypogastric nerve). The paravaginal tissue is then divided with one or two applications, until the lateral aspect of the vagina is reached (Figure 36.21).

TRANSECTION AND CLOSURE OF THE VAGINA

The level of transection of the vagina is determined by the proximity of the tumor margin to the vaginal fornices (Figure 36.22). To assist in identifying the level of the

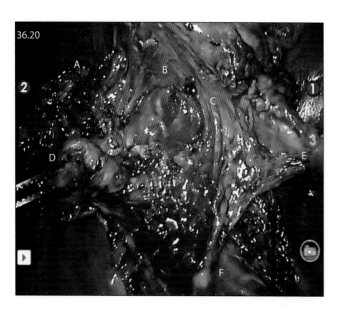

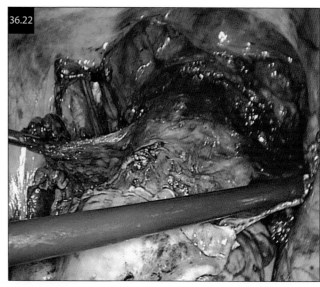

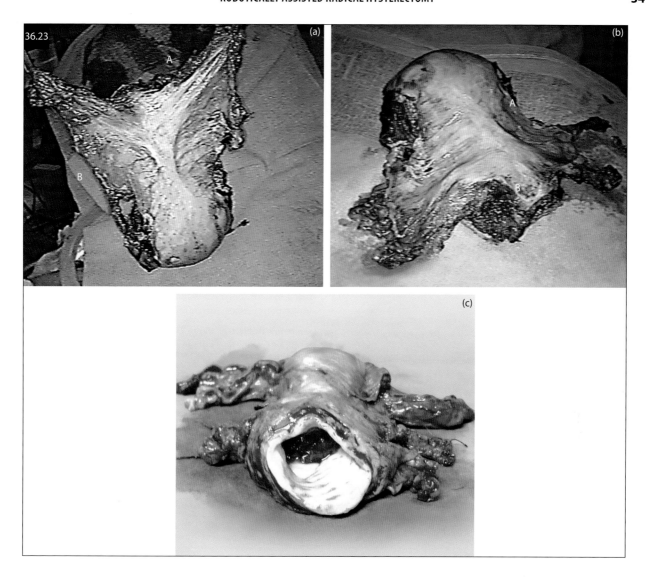

cervicovaginal junction, the vaginal probe is advanced by the assistant toward the anterior vaginal fornix. It is important to consider that margins obtained with a stretched vagina will be shorter once the tension is removed. The monopolar scissors/spatula is used to transect the vagina circumferentially, starting at the 12 o'clock position. Excessive coagulation of the transected vaginal edge is to be avoided, since this may result in extensive thermal damage, subsequent necrosis, formation of granulation tissue, and possible vaginal cuff dehiscence or evisceration.

The assistant removes the uterus with the help of a Schroeder tenaculum (Aesculap, Germany) introduced vaginally. It is also possible to remove the lymph nodes with bags. A surgical specimen of a radical hysterectomy is shown in Figure 36.23a and b, and the specimen using the traditional technique with nerve sparing is shown in Figure 36.23c.

VAGINAL CUFF CLOSURE

The vaginal cuff is closed laparoscopically with a continuous running suture using 2-0 V-loc (Medtronic, Boulder, Colorado) or Stratafix (Ethicon, Sommerville, New Jersey), starting at the right angle and incorporating a minimum of 5 mm of vagina with each bite and 5 mm of separation in between sutures, in order to avoid vaginal failure. Once the left angle is reached, three more passes of the suture are taken to the right side to prevent the closure becoming loose.

The pelvis is inspected for hemostasis by irrigating with saline solution. By lowering the CO_2 pressure, any bleeding site will become clearly visible. No drains are used, and the lateral pelvic peritoneum is left open (Figure 36.24).

In the nerve-sparing technique, the pelvic autonomic nerves can be seen extending from the lateral wall of the rectum to the bladder, passing along the lateral aspect of the vaginal cuff. Figure 36.25 shows the view of the right side of the pelvis. The inferior hypogastric plexus (IHP) has been mobilized laterally from the right uterosacral ligament. The pelvic splanchnic nerves are seen joining the IHP in a perpendicular fashion (A, superior vesical artery; B, inferior hypogastric plexus; C, pelvic splanchnic nerve; D, ureter; E, hypogastric nerve; F, uterine artery; G, pararectal space).

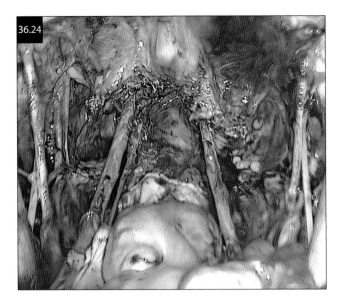

TROCAR SITES CLOSURE

The fascia at the umbilical incision (12 mm) is closed with a running suture using 0 Vicryl UR 6 needle (Ethicon, Sommerville, New Jersey). The skin is closed with a subcuticular continuous suture of 4-0 Vicryl (Ethicon, Sommerville, New Jersey).

POSTOPERATIVE COURSE

Clear liquids are started upon awakening from anesthesia if the patient is not nauseated. A regular diet is started the next morning for breakfast. Deambulation is started as soon as possible. The Foley catheter is removed at the beginning of deambulation, and residual urine measurements obtained on two separate occasions should be less than 100 mL before discharge. A postoperative visit is performed at 1 and 2 weeks after discharge to check the residual urine (must be less than 100 mL), and at 6 weeks from surgery to inspect the vaginal vault.

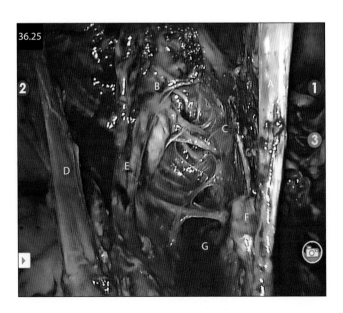

ACKNOWLEDGMENTS

Our deepest gratitude to Regina Montero, RN, and Karen Mills, RN, who so efficiently prepared and organized the laboratory to allow us to demonstrate this technique in a fresh cadaver using the same instrumentation and same setting as would be used if performed in an operating room.

SUGGESTED READING

Díaz-Feijoo B, Correa-Paris A, Pérez-Benavente A, et al. Prospective randomized trial comparing transperitoneal versus extraperitoneal laparoscopic aortic lymphadenectomy for surgical staging of endometrial and ovarian cancer: The STELLA Trial. *Ann Surg Oncol.* 2016;23(9):2966–2974.

Ercoli A, Delmas V, Gadonneix P, et al. Classical and nerve-sparing radical hysterectomy: An evaluation of the risk of injury to the autonomous pelvic nerves. *Surg Radiol Anat.* 2003;25:200–206.

Gil-Ibañez B, Díaz-Feijoo B, Perez Benavente A, et al. Nerve sparing technique in robotic-assisted radical hysterectomy: Results. *Int J Med Robot.* 2013;9(3):339–344.

Gil-Moreno A, Magrina JF, Pérez-Benavente A, et al. Location of aortic node metastases in locally advanced cervical cancer. *Gynecol Oncol.* 2012;125(2):312–314.

Gold MA, Tian C, Whitney CW, Rose PG, Lanciano R. Surgical versus radiographic determination of para-aortic lymph node metastases before chemoradiation for locally advanced cervical carcinoma. A Gynecologic Oncology Group study. *Cancer.* 2008;112:1954–1963.

Havenga K, Maas CP, DeRuiter MC, Welvaart K, Trimbos JB. Avoiding long-term disturbance to bladder and sexual dysfunction in pelvic surgery, particularly with rectal cancer. *Semin Surg Onc.* 2000;18:235–243.

Hockel M, Horn L-C, Hentschel B, Hockel S, Naumann G. Total mesometrial resection: High resolution nerve-sparing radical hysterectomy based on developmentally defined surgical anatomy. *Int J Gynecol Cancer.* 2003;13:791–803.

Hockel M, Konerding MA, Heubel CP. Liposuction-assisted nerve-sparing extended radical hysterectomy: Oncologic rationale, surgical anatomy, and feasibility study. *Am J Obstet Gynecol.* 1988;178:971–976.

Klauschie J, Wechter ME, Jacob K, et al. Use of anti-skid material and patient-positioning to prevent patient shifting during robotic-assisted gynecologic procedures. *J Minim Invasive Gynecol.* 2010;17(4):504–507.

Landoni F, Maneo A, Cormio G, et al. Class II versus Class III Radical hysterectomy in stage IB-IIA cervical cancer: A prospective randomized study. *Gynecol Oncol.* 2001;80:3–12.

Leblanc E, Narducci F, Frumovitz M, et al. Therapeutic value of pretherapeutic extraperitoneal laparoscopic staging of locally advanced cervical carcinoma. *Gynecol Oncol.* 2007;105:304–311.

Magrina JF, Goodrich MA, Lidner TK, Weaver AL, Cornella JL, Podratz KC. Modified radical hysterectomy in the treatment of early squamous cervical cancer. *Gynecol Oncol.* 1999;72:183–186.

Magrina JF, Long JB, Kho RM, Giles DL, Montero RP, Magtibay PM. Robotic transperitoneal infrarenal aortic lymphadenectomy: Technique and results. *Int J Gynecol Cancer.* 2010;20(1):184–187.

Michalas S, Rodolakis A, Voulgaris Z, Vlachos G, Giannakoulis N, Diakomonalis E. Management of early-stage cervical carcinoma by modified (Type II) radical hysterectomy. *Gynecol Oncol.* 2002;85:415–422.

Querleu D, Morrow CP. Classification of radical hysterectomy. *Lancet Oncol.* 2008;9:297–303.

Raspagliesi F, Ditto A, Fontanelli R, et al. Nerve-sparing radical hysterectomy: A surgical technique for preserving the autonomic hypogastric nerve. *Gynecol Oncol.* 2004;93:307–314.

Sakakamoto S, Takizawa K. An improved radical hysterectomy with fewer urological complications and with no loss of therapeutic results for invasive cervical cancer. *Ballieres Clin Obstet Gynecol.* 1988;2:953–962.

Sakuragi N, Todo Y, Kudo M, Yamamoto R, Sato T. A systematic nerve-sparing radical hysterectomy technique in invasive cervical cancer for preserving postsurgical bladder function. *Int J Gynecol Cancer.* 2005;15:389–397.

Trimbos JB, Mass CP, DeRuiter MC, Peters AAW, Kenter GG. A nerve-sparing radical hysterectomy; Guidelines and feasibility in Western patients. *Int J Gynecol Cancer.* 2001;11:180–186.

Yang Y-C, Chang C-L. Modified radical hysterectomy for early Ib cervical cancer. *Gynecol Oncol.* 1999;74:241–244.

Chapter 37

HEMOSTATIC AGENTS IN LAPAROSCOPIC SURGERY

Pattaya Hengrasmee, Traci Ito, and Alan Lam

BACKGROUND

"*Haemostasis*," derived from the Greek terms "*haima*" meaning blood and "*stasis*" meaning standstill, means the stoppage of bleeding. As hemorrhage is an inherent risk of all forms of surgery, the need to achieve rapid and reliable hemostasis is paramount for patient's safety. This is particularly the case in laparoscopic surgery, as minimal access restricts the rapid use of hemostatic mechanisms by compression, clamping, and suturing.

MECHANISMS OF HEMOSTASIS

During surgery, hemorrhage can result from either failure to control significant arterial and venous sources or failure of normal clotting mechanism. The natural physiological mechanism of hemostasis generally involves three crucial steps: vasoconstriction, platelet plug formation, and blood coagulation.

Vascular spasm is the first response of blood vessels to injury, which helps reduce the amount of blood flow to the damaged area (Figure 37.1). The second hemostatic mechanism involves *platelet plug formation*, whereby platelets in the circulation adhere to the damaged endothelium and form a temporary seal or plug to cover the defect in the vessel wall (Figure 37.2). The third and most enduring mechanism involves the *coagulation* cascade (Figure 37.3) in which fibrinogen is converted to fibrin to form a molecular glue that reinforces the platelet plug.

HEMOSTATIC AGENTS FOR USE IN SURGERY

When normal physiology fails to provide adequate hemostasis during surgery, additional measures are required to achieve effective and rapid hemostasis. The currently available techniques and agents to help achieve hemostasis can be broadly categorized into mechanical instruments, topical hemostatic agents, and systemic hemostatic agents (Table 37.1).

MECHANICAL TOOLS

Mechanical tools are hemostatic techniques of choice for controlling significant arterial and venous bleeding. They comprise direct pressure, suturing, ligature, hemoclips, staplers, electrosurgery (monopolar and bipolar), ultrasonic energy, and various electrosurgical vessel-sealing devices. With sutures, surgeons can confidently ligate blood vessels of any size. Similarly, properly applied vascular clips or staples can ligate vessels up to 8 mm. Recent advances in energy-dependent devices such as advanced bipolar technology (Ligasure, Enseal, Gyrus PK) and adaptive tissue technology with ultrasonic shears (Harmonic ACE) can now seal vessels up to 7 mm. Potentially, the most important factors in determining the choice of each device are efficacy, reproducibility, ergonomic comfort, extent of unintended collateral damage, and cost effectiveness. The vessel sealing devices are covered in Chapter 7.

TOPICAL HEMOSTATIC AGENTS

In circumstances when conventional surgical techniques are not feasible, such as bleeding near vital structures, bleeding at needle-holes, bleeding from raw surface areas, bleeding in friable tissue, or bleeding in patients with abnormal coagulation, topical hemostatic agents serve as adjunctive treatments. Knowledge of the available agents for laparoscopic surgery is strongly recommended.

Topical hemostatic agents have been defined by the U.S. Food and Drug Administration (FDA) as "devices intended to produce hemostasis by accelerating the clotting process of blood." These were classified by the FDA in October 2006 as class II devices, which means "higher risk devices requiring greater regulatory controls to provide reasonable assurance of the device's safety and effectiveness."

The most important characteristics of an ideal hemostatic agent include high efficacy, nonantigenicity or biocompatibility, complete absorbability, quick preparation, easy application, and cost effectiveness. Currently, no single hemostatic agent satisfies all these criteria. The available products in the market vary in composition, mechanism of action, method of use, efficacy, preparation, specific advantages, and adverse reactions. They can be broadly divided into three categories: physical, biologic, and synthetic agents.

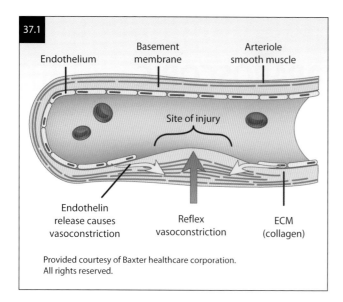

37.1

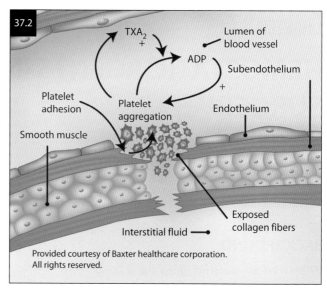

37.2

Direct tamponade

It is well-established that applying pressure alone to a bleeding area may provide adequate hemostasis. This technique is widely used in open surgery by applying surgical sponges or gauzes to the area of bleeding. This same technique may be adapted in laparoscopic surgery by placing a dry gauze through a 10 mm or larger trocar into the peritoneal cavity and then pressing it directly against the area of bleeding. The sponge can be removed after the bleeding is under control by grasping the end of it and withdrawing through the same trocar (Figure 37.4).

Physical and absorbable agents

Absorbable agents act by initiating the coagulation cascade through a contact activation (intrinsic) pathway and/or promoting platelet aggregation on a physical matrix. Available products currently on the market are discussed in the next paragraph.

Gelatin (Gelfoam, Gelfilm; Pfizer, Belgium, NV) and Surgifoam (Ethicon Inc., San Lorenzo, Puerto Rico) (Figure 37.5) have the advantages of being nonantigenic and having neutral pH, which allows congruent use with other biologic agents. Of note, given the neutral pH, the gelatin matrices do not directly activate the clotting cascade. In

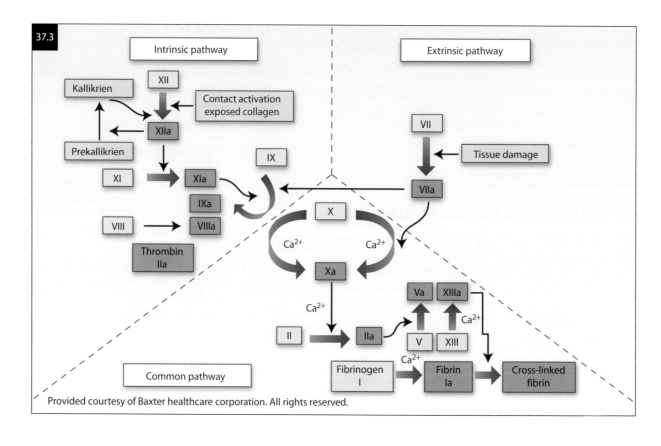

37.3

TABLE 37.1

HEMOSTATIC AGENTS

I.   MECHANICAL INSTRUMENTS

    DIRECT TAMPONADE

    SURGICAL CLIPS

    ELECTROSURGICAL INSTRUMENTS

II. TOPICAL HEMOSTATIC AGENTS

    1. BIOLOGICAL ABSORBABLE AGENTS

    GELATIN

        GELFOAM

        SURGIFOAM

    OXIDIZED REGENERATED CELLULOSE (ORC)

        SURGICEL

        FIBRILLAR, SURGICEL, NU-KNIT

        SURGICEL SNoW

    MICROFIBRILLAR COLLAGEN

        AVITENE

        HELITENE

    MICROPOROUS POLYSACCHARIDE (MPH)

        ARISTA

    GELATIN-THROMBIN MATRIX

        FLOSEAL

        VITAGEL

    RECOMBINANT HUMAN THROMBIN

        RECOTHROM

    FIBRIN DRESSINGS

        TACHOSIL

    FIBRIN SEALANT

        TISSEEL

    2. SYNTHETIC HEMOSTATIC AGENTS

    POLYETHYLENE GLYCOL HYDROGEL

        COSEAL

    CYANOACRYLATES

        DERMABOND

    GLUTARALDEHYDE CROSS-LINKED ALBUMIN

        BIOGLUE

III. SYSTEMIC HEMOSTATIC AGENTS

    ANTIFIBRINOLYTICS

        TRANEXAMIC ACID

    PROCOAGULANTS

        VASOPRESSIN

        RECOMBINANT FACTOR VIIA

          CONCENTRATE

        rFVIIA

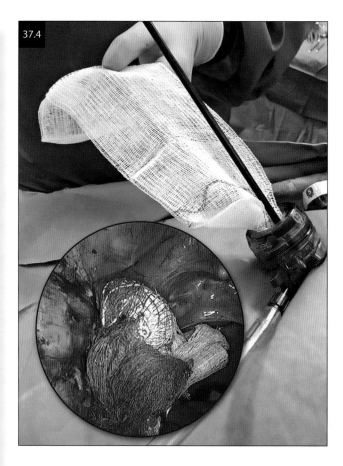

comparison to collagen and cellulose-based agents, this material has a propensity to double in volume and can potentially cause complications secondary to compression in confined areas and near nerves. Correct application involves applying pressure for several minutes to optimize hemostasis. Laparoscopic use of gelatin is simple given its malleable properties when moistened. This allows passage through the trocars. Careful mention of gelatin use should be made in operative documentation as it takes 4 to 6 weeks to be fully absorbed.

Oxidized regenerated cellulose (ORC) (SNoW Ethicon, Inc., San Lorenzo, Puerto Rico) (Figure 37.6) acts as a platform on which platelets can aggregate to form a clot. ORCs are uniquely acidic and activate the clotting cascade, thereby providing additional hemostasis by

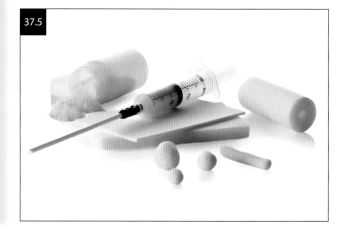

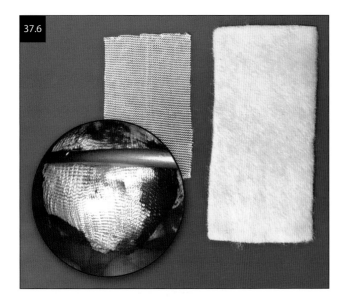

inducing vasoconstriction. The lower pH also denatures blood proteins and allows the agent to have bactericidal properties. Placement through trocars is easy as the material is yielding to the surrounding tissue. The disadvantage of the acidic pH is inactivation of other biologic agents such as thrombin, increased tissue inflammation, and delayed wound healing. Absorption time ranges from 2 to 6 weeks and is dependent on the volume used during surgery. These types of Surgicel are slightly different. NuKnit is stronger than the original and achieves hemostasis 30% faster. Fibrillar is a cotton-like material, which can be peeled off layer by layer. SNoW achieves hemostasis 43% faster than the Surgicel Original, making it an attractive option for sites of heavier bleeding.

Microfibrillar collagen (Avitene; Bard Davol, Warwick, Rhode Island) and Helitene (Integra Lifesciences, Plainsboro, New Jersey) (Figure 37.7) stimulates platelet adherence and activation, leading to platelet aggregation and thrombus formation. As a result, this can be used to successfully control diffuse areas of parenchymal oozing and is even effective in the context of profound heparinization.

Arista AH Absorbable Hemostat (BARD, Davol Inc., Warwick, Rhode Island) (Figure 37.8) is a polysaccharide produced from potato starch. This functions as a molecular filter and isolates platelets, erythrocytes, and other proteins. As a result, when Arista AH is applied, the absorption of water causes the agent to concentrate blood solids, which then form a gel matrix to promote clot formation. Due to this mechanism of action, Arista can expand up to 15 times its dry volume. Absorption of the Arista starts immediately and usually lasts about a day. Arista is used as an adjunctive hemostatic device to assist in control of capillary venous and arterial bleeding when other bleeding control modalities are ineffective or impractical. Arista should not be injected into blood vessels or be used in surgical situations where it may enter the blood vessel, as it could form a clot.

Biologic hemostatic agents

The mechanism of action is dependent on the composition of each agent. Thrombin is an enzyme that is produced from prothrombin and is responsible for the conversion of fibrinogen to fibrin. Examples of these agents that take advantage of thrombin's ability to form a fibrin clot are topical thrombin and fibrin sealants. Additionally, when thrombin is combined with either gelatin or collagen, the agent directly stimulates

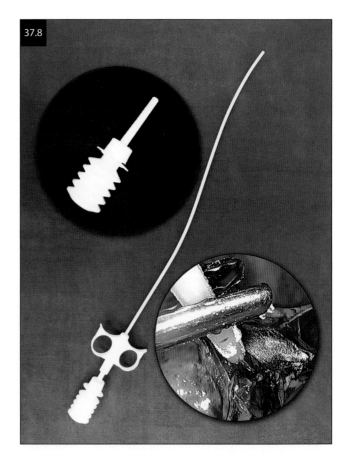

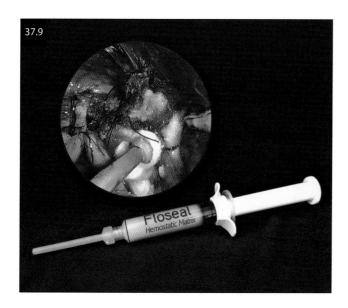

37.9

the coagulation cascade and provides a physical matrix for clotting initiation. Examples of these agents include Floseal (Baxter, Hayward, California), a gelatin-thrombin matrix (Figure 37.9), and Vitagel (Stryker, Malvern, Pennsylvania), a collagen-thrombin gel (Figure 37.10).

The first generation of topical thrombin was derived from bovine plasma, which has been shown to induce immunologic response leading to coagulopathy and thrombosis. This agent's use is most studied in the realm of vascular surgery. Even the human plasma-derived thrombin poses the risk of infectious disease transmission. Due to these concerns, researchers have recently developed the latest generation of recombinant thrombin known as Recothrom (Bristol Myers Squibb, Princeton, New Jersey), which is a recombinant human thrombin, to overcome the two disadvantages.

Fibrin sealants are composed of thrombin and plasma-derived fibrinogen. They have been found to be effective in heparinized patients and in controlling venous oozing from raw surfaces, such as retroperitoneal space, vaginal cuff, myomectomy bed, and after hematoma evacuation. The ingredients are supplied in separate vials with a dual-syringe delivery system that admixes the two components immediately before use.

The combination of thrombin and gelatin offers better control of moderate arterial bleeding than fibrin sealants due to the ability to swell and expand. This property is a benefit of the gelatin particles that provide an additional tamponading effect.

Collagen-thrombin gel or platelet sealants are a combination of microfibrillar collagen, thrombin, and the patient's plasma-derived fibrinogen and platelets. Platelets from patients can help strengthen clots. However, the need for blood centrifugation and pre-use processing makes the product less attractive.

TISSEEL (Baxter Healthcare, Westlake Village, California) (Figure 37.11) is an example of a two-component fibrin sealant. The first component is a sealer protein solution that contains a synthetic Aprotinin, factor XIII, and fibrinogen. The second component is the thrombin solution, which has human thrombin and calcium chloride. The solutions are frozen and therefore must be defrosted prior to use. The two components work symbiotically at the time of application.

TISSEEL is effective because thrombin transforms the fibrinogen in the sealer protein solution into fibrin monomers that cross-link to form a fibrin clot. In addition, the synthetic aprotinin is a protease inhibitor that delays degradation of fibrin. These unique properties make TISSEEL an attractive option in patients on anticoagulation and those with coagulopathy.

Contraindications for application include patients with a known hypersensitivity to synthetic aprotinin or brisk arterial or venous bleeding. TISSEEL is denatured when exposed to alcohol, iodine, or heavy metals. It also cannot function in the presence of oxidized regenerated cellulose-containing agents.

Other biologic hemostatic agents are available in a dressing form. This category includes fibrin dressings

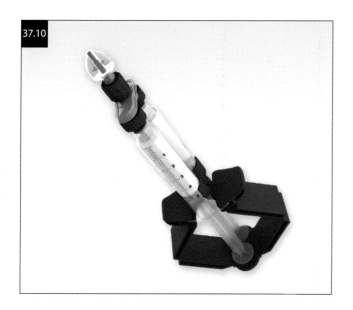

37.10

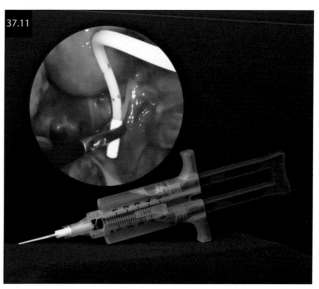

37.11

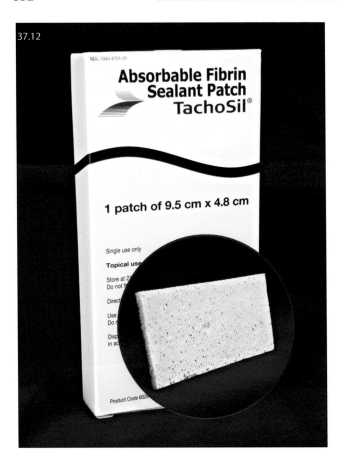

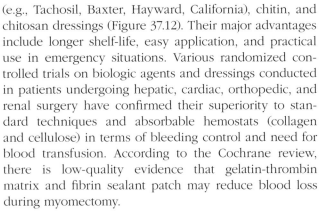

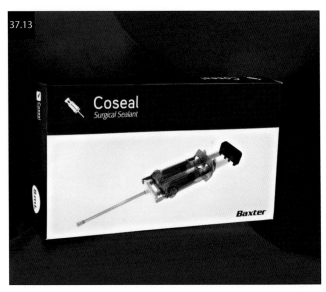

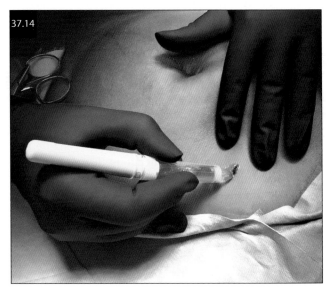

(e.g., Tachosil, Baxter, Hayward, California), chitin, and chitosan dressings (Figure 37.12). Their major advantages include longer shelf-life, easy application, and practical use in emergency situations. Various randomized controlled trials on biologic agents and dressings conducted in patients undergoing hepatic, cardiac, orthopedic, and renal surgery have confirmed their superiority to standard techniques and absorbable hemostats (collagen and cellulose) in terms of bleeding control and need for blood transfusion. According to the Cochrane review, there is low-quality evidence that gelatin-thrombin matrix and fibrin sealant patch may reduce blood loss during myomectomy.

Synthetic hemostatic agents

Currently available synthetic hemostatic agents vary considerably in compounds, properties, and features. Among these, polyethylene glycol hydrogel (Coseal, Baxter Hayward, California) (Figure 37.13) is one of the most commonly used agents. It provides hemostasis by formation of synthetic tissue sealant, as well as provides a barrier to cell ingrowth and adhesion formation. Although Coseal's anastomotic sealing performance is equivalent to that of Gelfoam/thrombin, its main advantages are speed in achieving hemostasis, nonexothermic process, and no inflammatory reaction. Nevertheless, due to its unique characteristic of four times swelling, the product should not be applied in a confined space to avoid compressive complication to nerves and

vulnerable structures. Other synthetic products include cyanoacrylates (Dermabond, Ethicon) (Figure 37.14), glutaraldehyde cross-linked albumin (BioGlue, Cryolife Kennesaw, Georgia), and mineral zeolite (QuikClot, Z-Medica, Wallingford, Connecticut).

Systemic hemostatic agents, "pharmacotherapy," aim to produce hemostasis by preventing or reversing defects associated with coagulopathy. Most prospective studies have focused on the efficacy of individual drugs given prophylactically or preoperatively in patients with known coagulation defect. Pharmacologic interventions for decreasing blood loss can be broadly divided into antifibrinolytics and procoagulants.

Antifibrinolytics

The most commonly prescribed medication in gynecological practice is *tranexamic acid*, which is a synthetic lysine analogue. Its mechanism of action is to competitively bind to lysine-binding sites of plasminogen and plasmin, inhibiting activation of the plasminogen to the active fibrinolytic enzyme plasmin. It also helps improve hemostasis by preventing plasmin-induced platelet activation. Most clinical research on tranexamic acid has been carried out in patients undergoing cardiac and orthopedic surgeries. Fewer data have confirmed its effectiveness in gynecologic surgery and postpartum hemorrhage. Regarding the most recent Cochrane database, there is low-quality evidence that tranexamic acid (Lysteda, Ferring) may reduce blood loss during myomectomy.

Procoagulants

Vasopressin is a nanopeptide, synthesized as a prohormone in the posterior hypothalamus, and is transported along the supraoptic hypophyseal tract to the posterior pituitary. Vasopressin acts on V1, V2, V3, and oxytocin-type receptors (OTR) with a half-life of 10 to 35 minutes before being metabolized by vasopressinases in the liver and kidney. Its mechanism for hemostasis involves stimulation of V2 and OTR. V2 receptors located on endothelial cells are essential for the release of factor VIII and von Willebrand factor, which further enhance platelet aggregation. Activation of OTRs which are predominantly found on myometrium and vascular smooth muscle such as capillaries, small arterioles, and venules can raise intracellular calcium, resulting in vasoconstriction. However, these receptors are also located on endothelial cells in which their activation can cause increased production of nitric oxide, which is a potent vasodilator. The off-label use of vasopressin during myomectomy procedure has shown favorable outcomes in terms of significantly less blood loss when compared to placebo and a comparable result when compared to uterine artery tourniquet technique. Additionally, there is moderate-quality evidence from the Cochrane database that vasopressin may reduce blood loss during myomectomy. Care should be taken when injecting this agent into any vascular tissue, as intravascular injection can lead to bradycardia from increased afterload and rarely cardiovascular collapse. Injection of vasopressin should always be preceded by aspiration to prevent intravascular injection. There is no established maximum safe dose for vasopressin. The typical solution is prepared by adding one 20 unit (1 mL) ampule of vasopressin to 100 cc of normal saline. The half-life of intramuscular vasopressin is 10 to 20 minutes, and the duration of action is 2–8 hours.

Recombinant factor VIIa concentrate (rFVIIa) has been approved by the FDA for the treatment of bleeding related to hemophilia with factor inhibitors. Its mechanism of action is to enhance the coagulation cascade through the formation of tissue factor–factor VIIa complex at the site of endothelial damage, resulting in a substantial rise in thrombin production at the surface of platelets. The off-label use of rFVIIa may be effective in certain cases, such as intracranial hemorrhage and rescue therapy for excessive bleeding. Its application should be restricted to situations in which the risk for continuing bleeding unresponsive to transfusion therapy clearly outweighs the risk for serious thrombotic complications.

SUMMARY

Hemorrhage is an intrinsic risk of all forms of surgery. The minimal access nature of laparoscopic surgery presents unique challenges in which meticulous surgical techniques are required to control hemorrhage. Besides physical techniques, both topical and systemic hemostatic agents are useful adjunctive agents. Knowledge of the available agents, their mechanisms of action, and their risks and benefits are crucial for optimal and appropriate utilization when required.

SUGGESTED READING

Abbott WM, Austen WG. The effectiveness and mechanism of collagen-induced topical hemostasis. *Surgery.* 1975;78:723–729.

Achneck HE, Sileshi B, Jamiolkowski RM, Albala DM, Shapiro ML, Lawson JH. A comprehensive review of topical hemostatic agents: Efficacy and recommendations for use. *Ann Surg.* 2010;251(2):217–228.

Celebi N, Celebioglu B, Selcuk M, Canbay O, Karagoz AH, Aypar U. The role of antifibrinolytic agents in gynecologic cancer surgery. *Saudi Med J.* 2006;27(5):637–641.

Fletcher H, Frederick J, Hardie M, Simeon D. A randomized comparison of vasopressin and tourniquet as hemostatic agents during myomectomy. *Obstet Gynecol.* 1996;87(6):1014–1018.

Glickman M, Gheissari A, Money S, Martin J, Ballard JL. A polymeric sealant inhibits anastomotic suture hole bleeding more rapidly than gelfoam/thrombin: Results of a randomized controlled trial. *Arch Surg.* 2002;137(3):326–331.

Hedner U, Erhardtsen E. Potential role for rFVIIa in transfusion medicine. *Transfusion.* 2002;42(1):114–124.

Kanake P, Eaton MP. Systemic strategies for reducing blood loss in surgery. *Anes News.* 2013;39(1):1–7.

Kim HJ, Fraser MR, Kahn B, Lyman S, Figgie MP. The efficacy of a thrombin-based hemostatic agent in unilateral total knee arthroplasty. *J Bone Joint Surg Am.* 2012;94(13):1160–1165.

Kongnyuy EJ, Wiysonge CS. Interventions to reduce haemorrhage during myomectomy for fibroids. *Cochrane Database Syst Rev.* 2014;(8):CD005355.

Kordestani SS, Noohi F, Azarnik H, et al. A randomized controlled trial on the hemostasis of femoral artery using topical hemostatic agent. *Clin Appl Thromb Hemost.* 2012;18(5):501–505.

Lamberton GR, Hsi RS, Jin DH, Lindler TU, Jellison FC, Baldwin DD. Prospective comparison of four laparoscopic vessel ligation devices. *J Endourol.* 2008;22(10):2307–2312.

Lawson JH, Spotnitz WD, Albala D, et al. Regulation of absorbable hemostatic agents: Guidance for encouraging innovation without compromising patient safety. Unpublished communication from Dr. Lawson 2007.

Mayer SA, Brun NC, Begtrup K, et al. Efficacy and safety of recombinant activated factor VII for acute intracerebral hemorrhage. *N Engl J Med*. 2008;358(20):2127–2137.

Nasso G, Piancone F, Bonifazi R, et al. Prospective, randomized clinical trial of the FloSeal matrix sealant in cardiac surgery. *Ann Thorac Surg*. 2009;88(5):1520–1526.

Parker WH, Sharp HT, Falk SJ. Techniques to reduce blood loss during abdominal or laparoscopic myomectomy. http://www.uptodate.com/contents/techniques-to-reduce-blood-loss-during-abdominal-or-laparoscopic-myomectomy.

Porter RS, ed. Hemostasis. In: *The Merck Manuals Online Medical Library*. http://www.merck.com/mmpe/sec11/ch134/ch134a.html.

Sarfati MR, Dilorenzo DJ, Kraiss LW, et al. Severe coagulopathy following intraoperative use of topical thrombin. *Ann Vasc Surg*. 2004;18:349–351.

Sharma JB, Malhotra M. Topical oxidized cellulose for tubal hemorrhage hemostasis during laparoscopic sterilization. *Int J Gynaecol Obstet*. 2003;82:221–222.

Sharma JB, Malhotra M, Pundir P. Laparoscopic oxidized cellulose (Surgicel) application for small uterine perforations. *Int J Gynecol Obstet*. 2003;83:271–275.

Sharman A, Low J. Vasopressin and its role in critical care. *Contin Ed Anaesth Crit Care Pain*. 2008;8(4):134–137.

Tomizawa Y. Clinical benefits and risk analysis of topical hemostats: A review. *J Artif Organs*. 2005;8:137–142.

Wagner WR, Pachence JM, Ristich J, et al. Comparative in vitro analysis of topical hemostatic agents. *J Surg Res*. 1996;66:100–108.

Xu J, Gao W, Ju Y. Tranexamic acid for the prevention of postpartum hemorrhage after cesarean section: A double-blind randomization trial. *Arch Gynecol Obstet*. 2013;287(3):463–468.

Chapter 38

COMPLICATIONS OF LAPAROSCOPIC SURGERY

Erica C. Dun and Ceana H. Nezhat

INTRODUCTION

Complications are possible with any surgical procedure, whether the procedure is performed by laparotomy or laparoscopy. Patients and even some physicians believe that laparoscopic surgery carries a lower risk of adverse events than "open" surgery, but this is a false assumption. Minimally invasive surgery does not necessarily equate to minimal risk. Catastrophic complications can occur with laparoscopic surgery, and often signs and symptoms become apparent after the patient is discharged from the hospital. Knowledge of anatomy, proper instrumentation, preoperative planning, and surgical expertise are the best tools to prevent complications and achieve optimal surgical outcomes.

The literature addressing laparoscopic surgery complications is extensive. Therefore, this chapter provides a brief overview of the most common laparoscopic complications, prevention, and how to recognize complications if they occur (Table 38.1).

PREVENTION OF COMPLICATIONS

While some complications are unavoidable and stem from circumstances beyond the surgeon's control, the majority are preventable. One important step toward the prevention of these complications is having a system in place that actively checks and double checks steps that may lead to problems. This system should begin with preoperative planning, continues with intraoperative management, and finally culminates in postoperative follow-up.

PREOPERATIVE PREVENTION OF COMPLICATIONS

HISTORY AND PHYSICAL

Taking a thorough patient history is critical for preoperative surgical risk assessment. Any history of previous abdominal or pelvic surgeries, as well as factors such as pelvic inflammatory disease (PID), peritonitis, and endometriosis may increase the complexity of any case. Medical comorbidities, especially cardiovascular and pulmonary disease, should be thoroughly investigated and the patient's risk stratified for the procedure. Previous problems with anesthesia should be carefully evaluated

in consultation with an anesthesiologist who will be participating in the case. Patients with high body mass index (BMI), especially those over 350 pounds, require focused preoperative planning and may benefit from a bariatric operating table and bariatric bed.

COUNSELING AND CONSENT

The decision to undergo surgery should be reached by the patient and the physician. The procedure should be explained in detail, including the risks, benefits, and alternatives. A patient's initial understanding and expectations of the procedure, surgical outcomes, and postoperative recovery are all governed by the preoperative discussion. In addition to the surgical consent, a consent for possible blood transfusion should be included as part of the preoperative discussion. Consenting for possible transfusion serves as a reminder to clarify any possible preferences for transfusion, including autologous blood, and refusal of all or certain blood products due to religious beliefs (i.e., Jehovah's Witnesses) or health concerns.

PREOPERATIVE MECHANICAL BOWEL PREPARATION

Historically, preoperative mechanical bowel preparation using a hyperosmotic laxative was routinely used across surgical subspecialties and was thought to improve the surgical view and bowel handling, and lower the risk of complications. Recently, in the fields of colorectal surgery and urology, the mantra of preoperative mechanical bowel preparation has been directly challenged and found to have no demonstrable benefit for the surgical view, to facilitate open surgery, or to decrease the incidence of anastomotic leakage or wound infection after elective surgery. In fact, the most current guidelines reflect this research and recommend that mechanical bowel preparation should not be routinely used before open colorectal surgery. However, it is still recommended in laparoscopic colorectal surgery to facilitate manipulation of the bowel. In the field of laparoscopic gynecologic surgery, a single-blinded randomized controlled trial showed that there was no significant difference in surgical view and bowel handling between patients who underwent fasting versus low residual diet versus low residual diet plus mechanical bowel preparation. Similar to the colorectal and urology

TABLE 38.1

LAPAROSCOPIC COMPLICATIONS

- POSITIONAL
- EQUIPMENT
- ABDOMINAL ENTRY
- TROCAR PLACEMENT
- ELECTRICAL ENERGY
- VASCULAR COMPLICATIONS
- BOWEL COMPLICATIONS
- GENITOURINARY COMPLICATIONS

literature, the study reported a significant and higher incidence of postoperative patient discomfort such as headache, thirst, weakness, and fatigue among women who had a preoperative low residual diet plus mechanical bowel preparation.

SURGICAL INSTRUMENTATION AND OPERATING ROOM PREPARATION

Whereas the primary surgeon is ultimately in charge of the operative procedure, a team approach with communication and shared understanding of the surgical plan will not only serve to minimize complications, but will facilitate prompt and efficient action should a problem arise. Key technical equipment such as monitors and cameras should be customarily checked prior to the patient's arrival in the operating room. The operating table position should be configured for gynecologic surgery, preparing for dorsal lithotomy as the bottom of the table is then lowered or removed.

Most surgeons develop a preference list for surgical procedures with instruments and equipment they typically use for their procedures. Equipment may be unavailable, out for repair, or discontinued. Therefore, surgeons must be familiar with and knowledgeable of the surgical instrumentation available in the hospital and should be able to use alternative instrumentation if necessary.

PATIENT POSITIONING

Nerve injuries are not unique to laparoscopic surgery but are more common after prolonged cases (Table 38.2). Proper patient positioning is vital to prevent these complications. The presence of any preoperative neuropathic symptoms should be documented. Previous spine, arm, shoulder, hip, or knee surgery should be noted, and positioning the patient while awake should be considered. Judicious use of padding (cloth, towels, foam mats, egg crates, gel pads) can help decrease the risk of nerve injury. Use of shoulder braces to prevent patients from slipping down on the operating room table should be avoided because of the high incidence of brachial plexus compression injuries. These injuries occur if the shoulder brace is positioned medial close to the neck and may press on the brachial plexus when the patient is placed in Trendelenburg position. If the shoulder braces are used, they should be positioned on the acromion. Obese patients are more prone to slip when placed in Trendelenberg position. Placing the patient on a nonslip gel or foam mat on the operating room table helps prevent movement cephalad when the patient is placed in steeper Trendelenburg position. Moreover, tucking the arms bilaterally with the hands adducted reduces the risk of brachial plexus traction injury from lateral abduction.

Boot-type stirrups (Figure 38.1) that support the foot and calf are preferred, distributing pressure more evenly and allowing for controlled and limited abduction. This type of stirrup reduces the risk of stirrup slippage and accidental dropping of the leg during adjustment. Care should still be taken to properly position the patient's legs in these types of stirrups. The peroneal nerve at the lateral head of the fibula may be at risk when there is undue pressure between the outer knee and the boot stirrup. Femoral neuropathy may occur, particularly in very thin patients, when this large, relatively avascular nerve is stretched around the inguinal ligament during exaggerated positions in dorsal lithotomy. Sciatic nerve compression occurs when the nerve is stretched at the sciatic notch. Both injuries occur when the patient's hips

TABLE 38.2

SUMMARY OF NERVE COMPLICATIONS DUE TO MALPOSITIONING

COMPLICATION	POSTOPERATIVE CLINICAL PRESENTATION
BRACHIAL PLEXUS COMPRESSION	SENSORY DEFICITS ALONG THE MEDIAL ASPECT OF THE ARM, FOREARM, AND HAND; SERIOUS INJURIES RESULT IN MUSCULAR WEAKNESS OF THE ARM AND HAND
PERONEAL NERVE COMPRESSION	SENSORY DEFICIT IN THE LATERAL AND ANTERIOR ASPECT OF LOWER LEG; MORE SEVERE INJURY CAN RESULT IN INABILITY TO DORSIFLEX THE FOOT OR "FOOT DROP"
FEMORAL NERVE COMPRESSION	SENSORY DEFICITS OVER THE ANTERIOR THIGH AND MEDIAL ASPECTS OF THE LOWER LEG; SEVERE INJURY PRESENTS WITH MUSCULAR WEAKNESS OF THE QUADRICEPS MUSCLE AND DECREASED PATELLAR REFLEXES
SCIATIC NERVE COMPRESSION	SENSORY DEFICITS OVER THE CALF AND ON THE DORSUM, SOLE, AND LATERAL SIDE OF THE FOOT; SEVERE INJURY MAY RESULT IN INABILITY TO FLEX THE KNEE

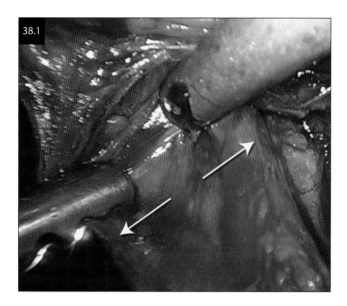

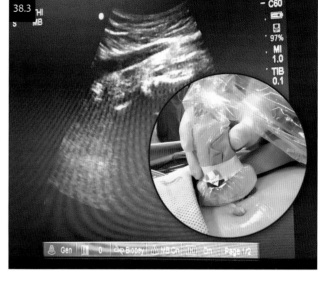

and knees are hyperflexed. Padding the sacrum and keeping the hips as flat as possible will decrease the risk of these neuropathies. Most compression injuries resolve spontaneously. Nevertheless, the injury should be documented and followed postoperatively until it resolves.

ABDOMINAL ENTRY

More than half of all complications related to laparoscopy are associated with the entry technique. Preventing complications associated with initial peritoneal entry

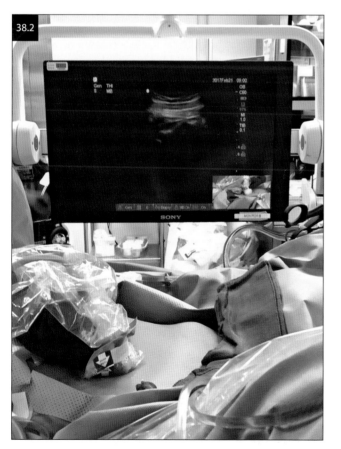

is a primary concern for laparoscopic surgeons. Every surgeon should have a customary technique but should also be familiar with alternative techniques. The most important factor with regard to safe entry during peritoneal access is the surgeon's familiarity and proficiency. The chosen technique is predicated on a combination of patient surgical history, body habitus, gynecologic pathology, and surgeon experience.

In patients with suspected adhesions, prior to placing the initial trocar, a preoperative periumbilical ultrasound-guided saline infusion (PUGSI) can be performed in the operating room as a tool to predict obliterating subumbilical adhesions for women at high risk, i.e., prior laparoscopy or laparotomy (Figures 38.2 and 38.3). The technique involves the injection of a small amount of sterile saline into the area of laparoscopic entry to determine whether obliterating (dense) subumbilical adhesions can be detected perioperatively based on either loculation or lack of dispersion of injected fluid as seen on ultrasound. A study of this technique revealed that the PUGSI test was able to detect most cases of subumbilical obliterating adhesion, demonstrating a sensitivity close to 100%.

There are many techniques for abdominal entry; however, no significant differences in rates of complications have been demonstrated between the various methods used (Table 38.3). The closed entry technique with a Veress needle consists of blindly inserting the Veress needle to insufflate the abdominal-pelvic cavity. Open laparoscopy, as described by Hasson, has been shown to minimize vascular injuries but does not necessarily reduce bowel injuries. Direct trocar entry is performed by elevating the anterior abdominal wall away from the viscera, and then using a see-through trocar with endoscope attached to enter the abdomen. This technique is becoming more popular. Advantages of the direct trocar entry technique are visualizing the layers of the abdominal wall as the trocar passes through and immediately detecting vascular or bowel injuries.

TABLE 38.3

COMPLICATION RATES BASED ON TECHNIQUE OF ABDOMINAL ENTRY

TECHNIQUE	COMPLICATION RATE PER 1000
VERESS NEEDLE	0.3–2.7
OPEN LAPAROSCOPY	0.6–12.0
DIRECT TROCAR	0.6–1.1
FIRST TROCAR	1.9–2.7
ACCESSORY TROCAR	0.8–6.0

SOURCE: FROM JACOBSON MT ET AL. *JSLS.* 2002;6(2):169–174. WITH PERMISSION.

Microlaparoscopy, using a 3 mm trocar to enter the abdomen, has been described as an alternative entry technique. The small 3 mm trocar is placed, and a 3 mm laparoscope inserted to confirm its location in the abdomen. Alternative entry sites such as the left upper quadrant (Palmer point), may be considered in cases involving a large uterus, pregnancy, challenging umbilical entry, or prior abdominal or pelvic surgeries that may cause adhesions around the umbilical area (Figure 38.4).

A detailed knowledge of both the superficial and deep abdominal wall vessels is essential for safe accessory trocar placement. Transillumination with a laparoscope can be used to delineate the superficial epigastric vessels, whereas direct observation is usually required to identify the course of the inferior epigastric vessels. In obese patients, landmarks on the interior of the abdominal wall, such as the medial umbilical ligaments, can help delineate the location of the inferior epigastric vessels.

There are certain principles that may help avoid injuries, if systematically practiced. Three-dimensional knowledge of anatomy of the abdomen and pelvis is important in order to avoid hazardous regions prior to inserting trocars. Inadvertent placement of the Veress needle into a vein during attempted peritoneal insufflation can result in fatal gas embolism. Veress needle injury to retroperitoneal vessels can result in minimal hemoperitoneum with a large retroperitoneal hematoma that is difficult to visualize at laparoscopy. Catastrophic bleeding occurs when the primary trocar injures a major artery or vein deep to the umbilicus. The location of the aortic bifurcation varies depending on the patient's body habitus. In the majority of patients, the aortic bifurcation is at the fourth lumbar vertebrae and does not correlate with BMI. However, the aortic bifurcation with respect to the umbilicus inversely correlates to the patient's BMI. In nonobese women, the mean location of the umbilicus has been measured to be 0.4 cm caudal to the aortic bifurcation. In overweight women, the mean umbilical location was 2.4 cm caudal to the bifurcation, and in obese patients it was 2.9 cm caudal to the bifurcation. The depth of the abdominal wall to the aortic bifurcation may be as much as 6 cm or more below the umbilicus in an obese patient, whereas it may be as close as 1.5 cm in a thin patient (Figure 38.5).

The following pearls can increase safety during peritoneal access:

1. Maintain the patient in a flat and centered position on the operating table during placement of the primary cannula. Avoid premature Trendelenburg position because the sacral promontory and retroperitoneal vessels are rotated closer in line with the axis of the overlying umbilicus (Figure 38.6).
2. If the anatomy is considered and the appropriate access site and angle (90° to the abdominal wall) are chosen, there should be no need to use longer needles or trocars.
3. Consider alternate sites for needle and trocar insertion in patients with potentially difficult peritoneal access, including very thin or obese patients, and for those having undergone abdominal surgery.

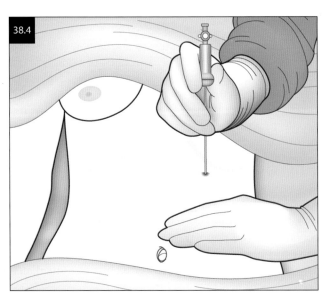

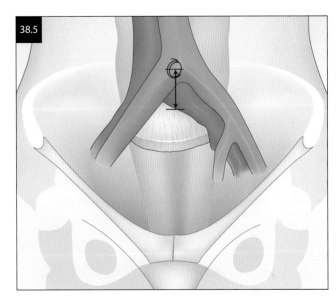

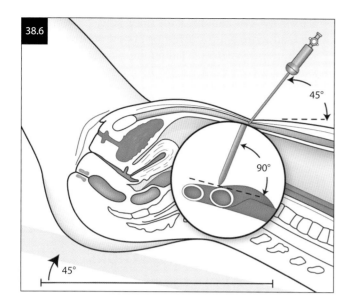

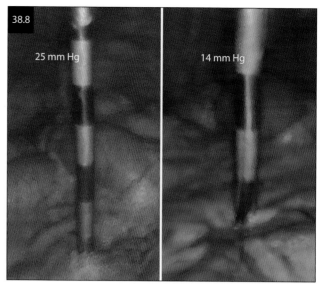

4. A spinal needle with a syringe filled with saline or local anesthetic can be used to explore the region underlying the intended insertion site. Inject and then aspirate, looking for either bowel contents or blood (Figure 38.7). A sufficient volume must be injected to permit aspiration of thick material such as fecal matter.

5. Insufflate the abdomen to a relatively high pressure (e.g., 25 mm Hg) for a short period of time to maximize peritoneal volume and to permit maximal counterpressure to increase proprioception while inserting the trocar (Figure 38.8).

6. Determine the estimated depth of the peritoneal cavity and note it on the trocar or Veress needle, and then use slow, steady pressure on the instrument to insert it just to that predetermined depth. Holding the index finger along the trocar shaft can help control the force and depth of insertion. For surgeons with smaller hands, holding the shaft with the nondominant hand can provide similar control to reduce risk for retroperitoneal injury (Figure 38.9). If resistance is felt during the trocar insertion or the trocar hits a hard surface after the

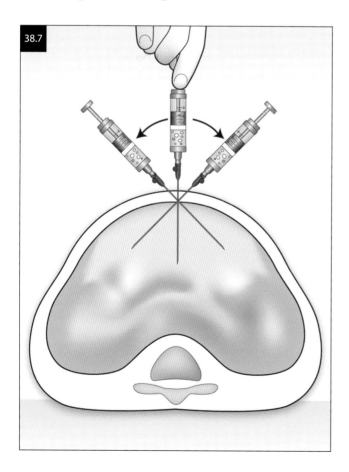

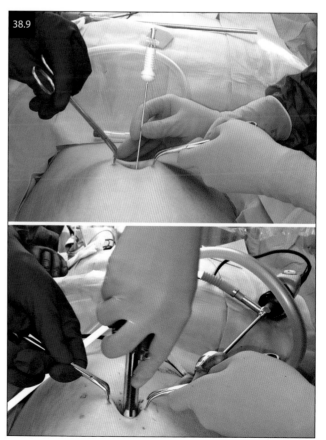

laparoscope is introduced, the patient should be expeditiously placed in steep Trendelenburg position and the bowel mobilized to directly inspect the retroperitoneal space directly below the pathway of the primary trocar.

7. Avoid multiple passes with the Veress needle or the trocar.

8. Albert Einstein said the "Definition of insanity is doing the same thing over and over again and expecting different results." This is reasonable advice for laparoscopic peritoneal entry. If abdominal access is difficult at one location, consider alternate sites or methods rather than risking injury by repeating attempts at insertion in the same place.

9. Inspect the region underneath the insertion site immediately upon placement of the laparoscope with the patient in the supine position. Look for discoloration, blood, debris, or bowel contents. Bleeding may be an ominous sign and mandates careful inspection of the retroperitoneum for hematoma formation. Similarly, damage to the bowel is most easily identified early in the procedure before the patient has been placed in steep Trendelenburg position and the bowel contents swept out of the visual field. This step allows early recognition and treatment.

10. Always place all secondary ports under direct vision (Figure 38.10).

11. Carefully consider the location in order to avoid the inferior and superficial epigastric vessels, pelvic sidewall, and bladder. A spinal needle with a syringe filled with saline can also be used to explore the areas of secondary trocar placement. After insertion of the secondary ports, the laparoscope can be inserted through the secondary port to inspect the initial port site for bleeding or inadvertent insertion through the bowel. This technique of "port hopping" should frequently be utilized for adhesiolysis to clear omental and bowel adhesions prior and during port placement. For patients with prior pelvic surgery, the bladder may be scarred or pulled up toward the lower uterine segment. Filling the bladder may help to identify its borders before insertion of a midline suprapubic trocar.

12. Finally, at the conclusion of the procedure, remove the laparoscope under direct vision, looking at each layer of the abdominal wall as the primary trocar sleeve is removed, and ensure that a through-and-through injury has not occurred or no loops of bowel have been pulled through the port site. For more detailed explanation of entry techniques, see Chapter 5.

INTRAOPERATIVE COMPLICATIONS

ADHESIOLYSIS AND RESTORATION OF ANATOMY

After reassurance of a nontraumatic abdominal entry, the abdomen and pelvis are surveyed for pathology. Endometriosis, PID, and prior surgeries all contribute to distortion of the normal anatomy of the pelvic organs, blood vessels, ureters, and bowel. Adhesiolysis and ureterolysis with meticulous restoration of anatomy should first be undertaken before beginning the procedure. Once normal anatomy has been restored, key anatomic landmarks should be identified and recognized, including anterior and posterior cul-de-sac, ureters, and major blood vessels. This process, though tedious, will aid in the correct identification of pelvic structures and decrease the risk of unintended injuries.

COMPLICATIONS OF ELECTRICAL ENERGY

Knowledge of electrosurgery and tissue effects is essential to properly apply monopolar, bipolar, ultrasonic, and laser energy. Unintended electrosurgical injuries can occur due to defects in insulation that cause sparking, direct coupling with another instrument (Figure 38.11),

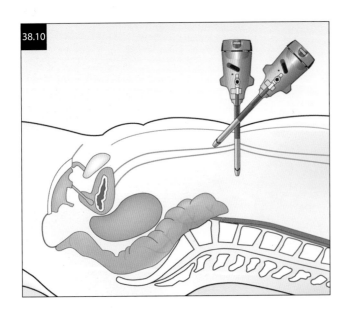

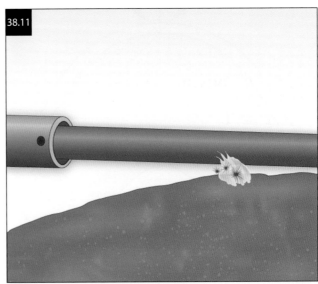

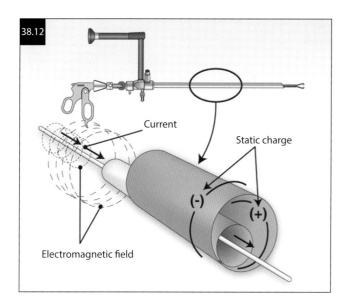

38.12

Current

Static charge

(-)   (+)

Electromagnetic field

indirect (capacitive) coupling (Figure 38.12), probe activation when at a distance from tissue (creating an "open circuit"), overheating of the active electrode tip (when covered with dried blood or debris), and the use of coagulation-type current to achieve the same effect as cutting current. There are two important principles to keep in mind when using any type of energy during laparoscopy. The first is always keep the tips of the instruments in the center of the screen when applying energy. The second is ideally avoid using two different energy sources in the abdomen at the same time. It is easy to get confused and activate the wrong energy source, causing unintended and disastrous effects on the wrong tissue. For more detailed explanation of electrosurgery, see Chapter 6.

VASCULAR COMPLICATIONS

Vascular injuries (Table 38.4) occur most commonly during laparoscopic entry while placing the Veress needle or primary trocar. In addition, major vessel injuries have been reported with a variety of instruments including scissors, electrosurgery, stapling devices, and lasers.

They occur in three major areas: pelvic sidewall, intraperitoneal parenchyma, and retroperitoneum. Veins have thinner walls compared to arteries, and the vena cava and its branches are at greater risk of laceration during dissection and resection. Pneumoperitoneum increases the intraabdominal pressure and can lead to tamponade bleeding. Injury to structures may not be evident until the postoperative period. Before closure, release of the pneumoperitoneum and inspection of the pelvis under low-pressure conditions or under fluid can help to identify these problems intraoperatively.

The most commonly injured vessels during trocar insertion are the right common iliac artery and the left common iliac vein. These vessels are in close proximity; the right common iliac artery crosses over the left common iliac vein in the midline beneath the umbilicus (Figure 38.5). Retroperitoneal vessel injury may be concealed and insidious, and require immediate action including laparotomy to control. Immediate fluid and blood resuscitation and manual pressure on the aorta underneath the renal arteries should be applied until a surgeon experienced in vascular surgery can assess the bleeding with the primary surgeon.

If vascular injury occurs, an experienced laparoscopic surgeon may attempt the laparoscopic vessel repair. The first step is to occlude the vessel with an atraumatic grasper to stop the active bleeding. After irrigation with fluids and aspiration of blood, bleeding vessels are identified and hemostasis is established either with laparoscopic suturing or vessel clips (Figure 38.13). The choice of suture for the vessel repair should be a permanent 6-0 suture. In case of small arterial or venous bleeders, bipolar current, Endoloop, or mechanical pressure can be utilized. If there is a small diffuse bleeding, a Ray-Tec gauze can be placed through the 10 mm trocar into the abdominal cavity, and the pressure can be held with the gauze until the bleeding stops (Figure 38.14). Hemostatic agents consisting of thrombin and gelatin matrix can be used for small vessel bleeding (see Chapter 37).

TABLE 38.4

COMMON LOCATIONS OF VASCULAR INJURY

- PELVIC SIDE WALL
  - EXTERNAL ILIAC ARTERY AND VEIN
- INTRAPERITONEAL VESSEL INJURY
  - MESENTERY
  - OVARIAN ARTERY
  - UTERINE ARTERY
- RETROPERITONEAL INJURY
  - COMMON ILIAC ARTERY AND VEIN
  - VENA CAVA
  - AORTA

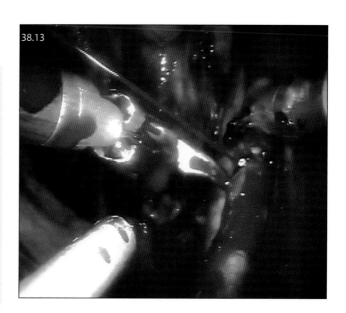

38.13

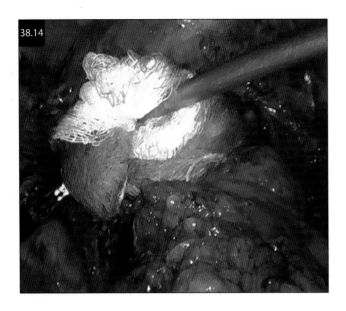

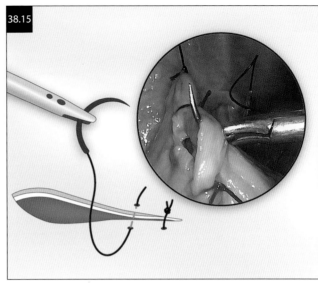

BOWEL COMPLICATIONS

The risk of bowel injury during minor laparoscopic procedures is 0.08%, and the risk for major operative laparoscopic procedures is 0.3%. Bowel perforations by scissors or tearing, if not recognized at the time of surgery, typically result in early and severe postoperative abdominal pain, and patients do not make a normal recovery. They may not develop severe illness immediately. Fever, absent bowel sounds, and acute abdomen should provoke suspicion in the early postoperative period. Delayed perforation may occur in patients where adhesiolysis or attempts at hemostasis were accompanied by the use of electrosurgery. Devascularization and coagulative necrosis may result in perforation days after the procedure. The average time from small bowel injury to diagnosis is 2–3 days for needle and cannula injuries and 10–12 days for electrosurgery injuries. Delayed diagnosis of a bowel injury can result in major sepsis and mortality rates up to 20%.

Small, nonleaking Veress needle injuries of less than 5 mm diameter in healthy large bowel tissue can be managed expectantly. Small or large bowel injuries, if recognized during the laparoscopic surgery, can be fixed laparoscopically (Figure 38.15). The choice of suture should be 3-0 Vicryl in two layers. Injured bowel may be pulled out through an expanded 10 mm incision and fixed by conventional suturing technique. Sutured bowel can be carefully pushed back inside the abdomen, avoiding a laparotomy incision. See Chapter 29 on bowel surgery.

GENITOURINARY COMPLICATIONS

Bladder injury most commonly occurs in the setting of suprapubic trocar placement or dissection of the bladder from the lower uterine segment in women with prior pelvic surgery or cesarean sections, which can cause the bladder to scar or be pulled superiorly. The bladder is

a forgiving organ; if the injury is detected intraoperatively, it can be repaired laparoscopically in two layers using absorbable sutures. The choice of suture should be absorbable suture (3-0 Vicryl or 3-0 Monocryl) running stitch (Figure 38.16). After the repair is completed, the integrity of the bladder can be tested by backfilling the bladder up to 200 cc with dilute methylene blue. Depending on the size of the cystotomy, a Foley catheter should be placed to decompress and drain the bladder for at least 10 days. Prior to removing the catheter, a retrograde cystogram should be performed to ensure that the bladder is well-healed and without defects.

Ureteral injury occurs in 0.5%–1.5% of open gynecological surgeries, and is slightly higher for laparoscopic surgeries. According to the most recent study by Adelman et al., the overall urinary tract injury rate for laparoscopic hysterectomy was 0.73%. The bladder injury rate ranged from 0.05% to 0.66% across procedure types, and the ureteral injury rate ranged from 0.02% to 0.4% across procedure types.

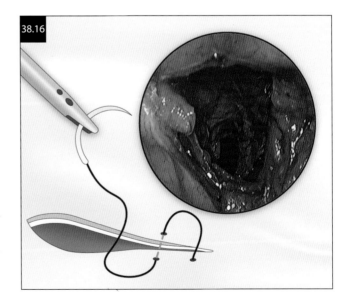

Though visualization is improved, laparoscopy has two drawbacks that contribute to injury: loss of depth perception from the two-dimensional video screen, and the inability of the surgeon to palpate various structures with his or her own finger. The ureter is particularly vulnerable to injury at three locations: (1) at the pelvic brim as the infundibulopelvic ligament is divided; (2) at the ovarian fossa, during resection of ovaries or ovarian remnants that are bound by adhesions to the pelvic side wall; and (3) lateral to the cervix during division or coagulation of the uterine artery, the uterosacral ligament, or the cardinal ligament. The best way to prevent ureteral injury is to identify the ureters at the beginning of the procedure and be certain of their location at all times during the procedure. Aside from knowing the location of the ureters, there are several techniques to prevent ureteral injury. In difficult cases where there is fibrosis and scarring, routine dissection of the pelvic ureters can be performed so that their location is clear throughout the entire surgical procedure (Figure 38.17).

If there is any concern about possible ureteral injury, an intraoperative cystoscopy is recommended. Indigo carmine is administered intravenously, and after 5–10 minutes blue-colored urine should be visualized jetting out of the ureteral orifices. Ureteral efflux can be retarded by excessive bladder volume or peritoneal insufflation. After 15 minutes if no urine is visualized from the ureteral orifice, a ureteral stent could be passed in a retrograde fashion to evaluate for obstruction. If there is injury, the site of injury may be laparoscopically identified by the blue-colored urine leaking from the transected ureter or presence of hydroureter. If resistance is met or if the location of the catheter is uncertain, a retrograde pyelogram should be performed by injecting contrast dye through the catheter. Thermal injury to the ureter may be difficult to diagnose intraoperatively. Signs and symptoms of thermal injury usually do not appear until 10–14 days after surgery. Injuries recognized and repaired intraoperatively have the best

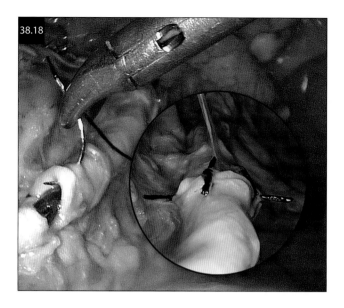

prognosis. A delay in diagnosis can lead to progressive deterioration of renal function. As many as 25% of unrecognized ureteral injuries result in eventual loss of the affected kidney. Depending on the location and the extent of the injury, the ureter can be repaired after passing a stent or implanted in the bladder. In case of partial ureteral injury, the ureteral stent should be passed and the injury can be repaired laparoscopically with 6-0 Vicryl suture. If the ureter is completely resected, it should be dissected and freed from any tension, and then the ureteral stent should be passed under laparoscopic guidance. The 3-0 suture should be passed through the adventitia and muscularis layer in order to reapproximate the cut ends of the ureter and to hold the cut parts together while the final repair is performed. Four 6-0 or 5-0 absorbable sutures should be placed consecutively at 6, 9, 3, and 12 o'clock through the full thickness of the wall to reconnect the ureter (Figure 38.18). The ureteral stent can then be removed 14 days after the repair.

CHECKING OF UNRECOGNIZED INJURIES

While an unintended injury is an unfortunate occurrence, an unrecognized injury carries more serious as well as long-term problems. As Benjamin Franklin said, "An ounce of prevention is worth a pound of cure." As a result, surgeons should take precautions to ensure that unrecognized injuries have not occurred. For example, if there is doubt regarding the location of the bladder edges, backfilling the bladder through a Foley catheter would help to identify the margins. Lowering the abdominal pressure to 8 mm Hg or less may reveal bleeding from a peritoneal edge or vessel that was tamponaded by the pneumoperitoneum. If extensive dissection of the pelvic sidewall was performed or electrosurgery was used close to the ureter, cystoscopy with direct visualization of ureteral patency can assist in diagnosing ureteral injury. Directly visualizing ancillary trocar removal

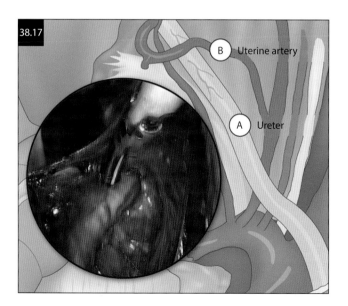

B Uterine artery

A Ureter

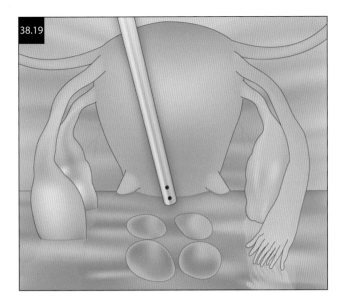

would reduce the possibility of unrecognized abdominal wall vessel injury. Dissection of endometriosis or adhesions from the posterior cul-de-sac may expose the bowel to injury. Sigmoidoscopy is a helpful test to detect defects in the rectum and sigmoid colon through visually inspecting the interior at the site of dissection. Another check is performed by filling the pelvis with saline irrigation while simultaneously occluding the distal portion of the sigmoid and placing air in the rectum through the sigmoidoscope or a Foley catheter. If there is a hole in the bowel, air bubbles will escape from the hole (Figure 38.19).

POSTOPERATIVE PREVENTION OF COMPLICATIONS

Unrecognized injury may occur outside the field of view during laparoscopy. Therefore, vigilant attention to unexpected postoperative signs or symptoms and early recognition of complications are absolute necessities for the gynecologic laparoscopist. The surgeon should be aware of the timeline of occurrence for some of the most common complications.

Vascular or vessel injuries are the most urgent and life-threatening injuries. They present immediately and are recognized either in the postanesthesia care unit or within the first 24 hours postoperatively with abnormal or unstable vital signs or a significant drop in blood count.

Bladder injury also presents in the immediate postoperative period with decreased urine output, abdominal distension, and constant leakage through the vaginal cuff after hysterectomy. Ureteral injury usually occurs within the first 48–72 hours postoperatively, but may present later. Fever, flank pain, peritonitis, and abdominal distention should be recognized as concerning signs. These injuries may also present with leukocytosis and hematuria. If these injuries were not recognized intraoperatively, intravenous pyelogram (IVP) can assist with diagnosis.

Bowel complications may occur days to weeks after the initial surgery, leading to delayed and insidious complications. The patient may present with obvious symptoms such as fever, abdominal tenderness, and an elevated white count, but may also present with mild complaints of malaise or nausea. Worsening and/or persistent pain after laparoscopic surgery necessitates immediate and thorough examination to exclude bowel trauma.

CONCLUSION

While laparoscopic surgery has provided dramatic advances in the field of gynecology, it is not without risks or complications. Using a systematic approach to each procedure by commencing with detailed preoperative evaluation and patient counseling and ending with assiduous attention to surgical detail, complications can be better anticipated and steps taken to minimize and recognize them in a timely fashion.

SUGGESTED READING

Adelman MR, Bardsley TR, Sharp HT. Urinary tract injuries in laparoscopic hysterectomy: A systematic review. *JMIG.* 2014;21(4):558–566.

Ahmad G, Oflynn H, Duffy JM, Phillips K, Watson A. Laparoscopic entry techniques. *Cochrane Database Syst Rev.* 2012;15:2.

Bhoyrul S, Vierra MA, Nezhat CR, Krummel TM, Way LW. Trocar injuries in laparoscopic surgery. *J Am Coll Surg.* 2001;192(6):677–683.

Brill AI. Electrosurgery: Principles and practice to reduce risk and maximize efficacy. *Obstet Gynecol Clin North Am.* 2011;38(4):687–702.

Brill AI, Nezhat F, Nezhat CH, Nezhat C. The incidence of adhesions after prior laparotomy: A laparoscopic appraisal. *Obstet Gynecol.* 1995;85(2):269–272.

Brosens I, Gordon A, Campo R, Gordts S. Bowel injury in gynecologic laparoscopy. *J Am Assoc Gynecol Laparosc.* 2003;10(1):9–13.

Camran C, Nezhat F, Nezhat C, eds. *Nezhat's Video-Assisted and Robotic-Assisted Laparoscopy and Hysteroscopy.* 4th ed. New York, NY: Cambridge University Press; 2013.

Harkki-Siren P, Kurki T. A nationwide analysis of laparoscopic complications. *Obstet Gynecol.* 1997;89:108–112.

Hasson HM. A modified instrument and method for laparoscopy. *Am J Obstet Gynecol.* 1971;110:886–887.

Hurd WW, Bude RO, DeLancey JO, Pearl ML. The relationship of the umbilicus to the aortic bifurcation: Implications for laparoscopic technique. *Obstet Gynecol.* 1992;80(1):48–51.

Jacobson MT, Osias J, Bizhang R et al. The direct trocar technique: An alternative approach to abdominal entry for laparoscopy. *JSLS.* 2002;6(2):169–174.

Nezhat CH. Direct microlaparoscopy is an alternative to open laparoscopy. *American Association of Gynecologic Laparoscopists 27th Annual Meeting*, Atlanta, GA, November 14, 1998.

Nezhat CH, Bastidas JA, Pennington E, Nezhat FR, Raga F, Nezhat CR. Laparoscopic treatment of type IV rectovaginal fistula. *J Am Assoc Gynecol Laparosc.* 1998;5(3):297–299.

Nezhat CH, Cho J, Morozov V, Yeung P. Preoperative periumbilical ultrasound-guided saline infusion (PUGSI) as a tool in predicting obliterating subumbilical adhesions in laparoscopy. *Fert Steril.* 2009;91(6):2714–2719.

Nezhat CH, Dun EC, Katz A, Wieser FA. Office visceral slide test compared with two perioperative tests for predicting periumbilical adhesions. *Obstet Gynecol.* 2014;123(5):1049–1056.

Nezhat CH, Nezhat F, Nezhat C, Rottenberg H. Laparoscopic repair of a vesicovaginal fistula. *Obstet Gynecol.* 1994;83(5 Pt 2):899–901.

Nezhat F, Brill AI, Nezhat CH, Nezhat A, Seidman DS, Nezhat C. Laparoscopic appraisal of the anatomic relationship of the umbilicus to the aortic bifurcation. *J Am Assoc Gynecol Laparosc.* 1998;5(2):135–140.

Sandadi S, Johannigman JA, Wong VL, Biebea J, Altose MD, Hurd WW. Recognition and management of major vessel injury during laparoscopy. *J Minim Invasive Gynecol.* 2010;17(6):692–702.

Swank HA, Mulder IM, la Chapelle CF, Reitsma JB, Lange JF, Bemelman WA. Systematic review of trocar-site hernia. *Br J Surg.* 2012;99(3):315–323.

Won H, Maley P, Salim S, Rao A, Campbell NT, Abbott JA. Surgical and patient outcomes using mechanical bowel preparation before laparoscopic gynecologic surgery. *Obstet Gynecol.* 2013;121(3):538–546.

INDEX